Textbook of

Radiological Safety

Textbook of
Radiological Safety

Second Edition

Kuppusamy Thayalan MSc DipRP MPhil PhD
Founder and President, Radiologic Physics Foundation
Former Professor, Madras Medical College
Chennai, Tamil Nadu, India
kthayalan@gmail.com

Foreword

Paul Ravindran

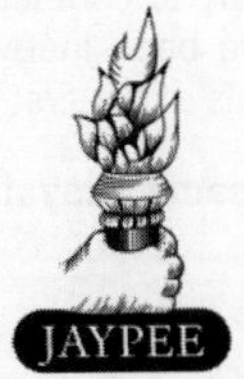

JAYPEE BROTHERS MEDICAL PUBLISHERS
The Health Sciences Publisher
New Delhi | London

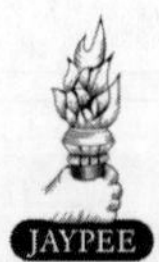

Jaypee Brothers Medical Publishers (P) Ltd

Headquarters
EMCA House
23/23-B, Ansari Road, Daryaganj
New Delhi 110 002, India
Landline: +91-11-23272143, +91-11-23272703
+91-11-23282021, +91-11-23245672
E-mail: jaypee@jaypeebrothers.com

Corporate Office
Jaypee Brothers Medical Publishers (P) Ltd.
4838/24, Ansari Road, Daryaganj
New Delhi 110 002, India
Phone: +91-11-43574357
Fax: +91-11-43574314
E-mail: jaypee@jaypeebrothers.com

Overseas Office
JP Medical Ltd.
83, Victoria Street, London
SW1H 0HW (UK)
Phone: +44-20 3170 8910
E-mail: info@jpmedpub.com

EU GPSR Authorised Representative
Logos Europe, 9 rue Nicolas Poussin
17000, La Rochelle, France
Phone: +33 (0) 6 67 93 73 78
E-mail: Contact@logoseurope.eu

Website: www.jaypeebrothers.com
Website: www.jaypeedigital.com

© 2024, Jaypee Brothers Medical Publishers

The views and opinions expressed in this book are solely those of the original contributor(s)/author(s) and do not necessarily represent those of editor(s) or publisher of the book.

All rights reserved by the author. No part of this publication may be reproduced, stored or transmitted in any form or by any means, electronic, mechanical, photocopying, recording or otherwise, without the prior permission in writing of the publishers.

All brand names and product names used in this book are trade names, service marks, trademarks or registered trademarks of their respective owners. The publisher is not associated with any product or vendor mentioned in this book.

Medical knowledge and practice change constantly. This book is designed to provide accurate, authoritative information about the subject matter in question. However, readers are advised to check the most current information available on procedures included and check information from the manufacturer of each product to be administered, to verify the recommended dose, formula, method and duration of administration, adverse effects and contraindications. It is the responsibility of the practitioner to take all appropriate safety precautions. Neither the publisher nor the author(s)/editor(s) assume any liability for any injury and/or damage to persons or property arising from or related to use of material in this book.

This book is sold on the understanding that the publisher is not engaged in providing professional medical services. If such advice or services are required, the services of a competent medical professional should be sought.

Every effort has been made where necessary to contact holders of copyright to obtain permission to reproduce copyright material. If any have been inadvertently overlooked, the publisher will be pleased to make the necessary arrangements at the first opportunity.

***Textbook of Radiological Safety* / Kuppusamy Thayalan**

First Edition: 2010

Second Edition: **2024**

Reprint: 2025, 2026

ISBN: 978-93-5465-855-6

Printed at K.K. Printers, Kundli, Haryana-131 028.

Dedicated to

My late mother

Mrs K Arukkani

My late father

Mr K Kuppusamy

and

Demised brother

Pulavar K Krishnasamy

Foreword

I am really honored to write the Foreword for the Second edition of the very useful "*Textbook of Radiological Safety*" by Professor Kuppusamy Thayalan. I have known him since 1986 when I took up the field of Medical Physics. He is an excellent teacher admired by students of radiation oncology, medical physics, and radiation technology. His passion for teaching and his interest to share his knowledge with the younger generation, has led him to write several books related to radiological physics. His books are very popular with the students and have been prescribed by Universities in India as textbooks and reference books.

Radiation safety is an important subject in three main fields of medicine, radiation oncology, diagnostic radiology and in nuclear medicine and for three levels of professionals, viz., postgraduate medical students and technologists in these fields, and medical physicists. It is interesting to note that this book not only addresses the radiation physics related to these three fields of medicine in detail but is also well-designed so that it will be useful for all the professionals in the field. Quality assurance of medical radiation equipment is essential and this book deals with these aspects in depth.

It is heartening to see that this book provides in detail the radiation protection procedures and rules in radiology, radiation therapy, and nuclear medicine. In addition, topics such as regulation of medical radiation facilities and facility design have been included which will be very useful for the management of the hospital. I am also impressed by the way Dr Kuppusamy Thayalan has brought out the important points in each of the chapters and the order in which the chapters are organized. I am convinced that this book will be very helpful for the students in these fields.

I am pleased to recommend this book for the medical and health professional and for all those interested in radiological safety.

Paul Ravindran PhD Dip RP FCCPM
Chief Medical Physicist and Principal—Allied Health Sciences
Christian Institute of Health Sciences and Research
Dimapur, Nagaland, India
Formerly Professor of Radiation Physics, Christian Medical College
Vellore
Consultant Radiotherapy Medical Physicist, DMRP
International Atomic Energy Agency
Vienna, Austria

Preface to the Second Edition

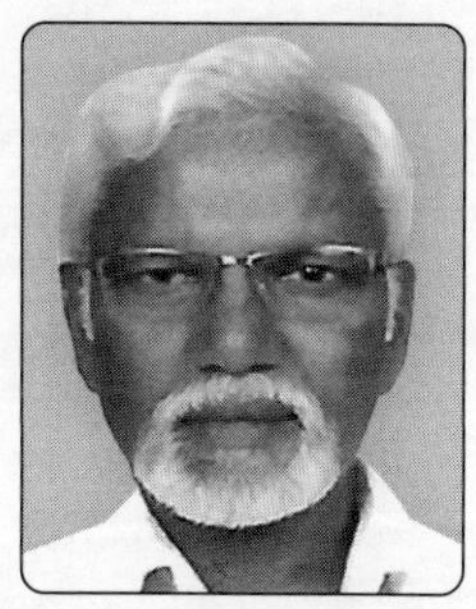

After the discovery of X-rays, radioactivity, and radium, radiation has been used in medicine both in diagnostic and therapeutic application. Since radiation has both risk and benefit, there is a need to use radiation judiciously to the patients. Many early users of radiation were affected by radiation-induced stochastic and deterministic effects. International recommendations and National regulation demand certain standards in medical use of ionizing radiation. Hence, there is a need to understand the concepts of radiation, and its optimal use to protect not only the hospital workers but also the patients and public at large.

Therefore, an attempt is made to bring together all essential topics of radiation protection and safety under one title. This is a second edition of my previous book published in 2010. Since then, a lot of developments have taken place in medicine which warranted this revision. Attempts have been made to incorporate the recent developments in the above areas.

The book consists of 19 chapters and number of figures and tables for easy understanding. The book addresses fundamental concepts, radiation biology, radiation protection standards, radiation hazards and evaluation, disposal of radioactive waste, transport of radioactive material, radiation regulation, radiation emergencies and medical management and emergency response plans and preparedness. Planning a radiation facility, quality assurance, shielding calculation and model layout plans are also given in much detail. For easy understanding, the above information is given under separate headings: Diagnostic radiology, nuclear medicine, and radiation therapy.

This book is targeted to postgraduates (MD/DNB) of radiology, nuclear medicine, radiation oncology, and medical physics (MSc) students of Indian Universities and abroad. It will be useful to prepare RSO examinations for medical physicists and nuclear medicine technologists. Worked examples are given wherever it is needed.

I hope this book may be of much useful to improve the ethics, regulation, and standards, especially optimal use of radiation, protection of personnel, patient, and the public without losing the quality of patient care.

I am looking forward to healthy comments and suggestions from the readers.

Kuppusamy Thayalan
(January, 2023)

Preface to the First Edition

It gives me immense pleasure to come out with a Textbook on Radiological Safety, a unique textbook. It is my long-felt dream to have a complete book, on radiological safety, covering the entire fields of radiology, i.e., diagnostic radiology, nuclear medicine and radiotherapy.

Radiation is analogous to fire which has both beneficial and harmful effects. The inherent philosophy is to minimize the hazards and maximize the benefits in order to bring down radiation doses within the regulatory control limits by which we can ensure the safety of the occupational workers as well as the patient and public. Hence, it is important that every one should be aware of the safety concepts, dose limits, regulation, waste disposal, etc., to establish a safe work culture while handling radiation sources in the hospital. As such, no single document is available for the above purposes, and the information is collected from safety codes and guides of international and national agencies like IAEA, NCRP, and AERB.

An attempt has been made to bring all the relevant information including safety terminology, biological effects, exposure control, monitoring, planning of the installation, quality assurance, regulation, personnel safety, transport, waste disposal and radiation emergency, etc., in the form of a book. The whole objective is to remove misconception about radiation and prepare the minds of younger generation to face the future challenge confidently. This book is intended for postgraduates of medical physics, diagnostic radiology, nuclear medicine and radiotherapy. This book may also find a place for the preparation of RSO examinations for medical physicists.

Moreover, an attempt has been made to bring quantitative data from international reports and recommendations, wherever necessary, with practical examples and illustrations. This may enable the new entrants to plan a radiation facility, carry out quality assurance and radiation survey without much cumbersome and perform the day-to-day medical physicist's job with ease and involvement. Large numbers of tables and figures are incorporated wherever necessary for better understanding of the reader.

I am very much thankful to my family members for their support and cooperation. I also acknowledge the assistance offered by the Dr Kamakshi Memorial Hospital staff, especially the medical physics colleagues, in the preparation of the text. I also thank Mrs G Shakunthala for neatly typing the manuscript.

I also acknowledge my teachers, by whom I got inspiration and passion toward teaching. I invite the readers to offer constructive comments for the future improvement of the book.

Kuppusamy Thayalan

Acknowledgment

I am thankful to my wife Tamilselvi, son Parthiban, and daughter Kayal Vizhi for their love, support, and cooperation. I am also thankful to my brothers, K Ramaiyan and K Annadurai for the moral support and guidance.

I also thankful to Dr RK Jeevanram, Scientific Officer (retired), Indira Gandhi Centre for Atomic Research, Kalpakkam for having corrected the script and offered suggestions. I acknowledge Dr Kamakshi Memorial Hospital Pvt Ltd and the Managing Director, Dr TG Govindarajan, and my medical physics colleagues, Ms X Sidonia Valas, Ms T Ruthra and K Palanisamy and interns Mr M Mozhi Alagan and Ms A Keerthana for their assistance and support during the book writing process.

I am much thankful to Dr Paul Ravindran, Senior Medical Physicist who has written foreword to the second edition of this book.

I am also thankful to Shri Jitendar P Vij (Group Chairman), Mr Ankit Vij (Managing Director), Ms Chetna Malhotra (Senior Director—Professional Publishing, Marketing, and Business Development), Ms Pooja Bhandari (Production Head), and of M/s Jaypee Brothers Medical Publishers (P) Ltd, New Delhi, India, for publishing this book as usual, neat and elegant manner.

Contents

PLATE 1

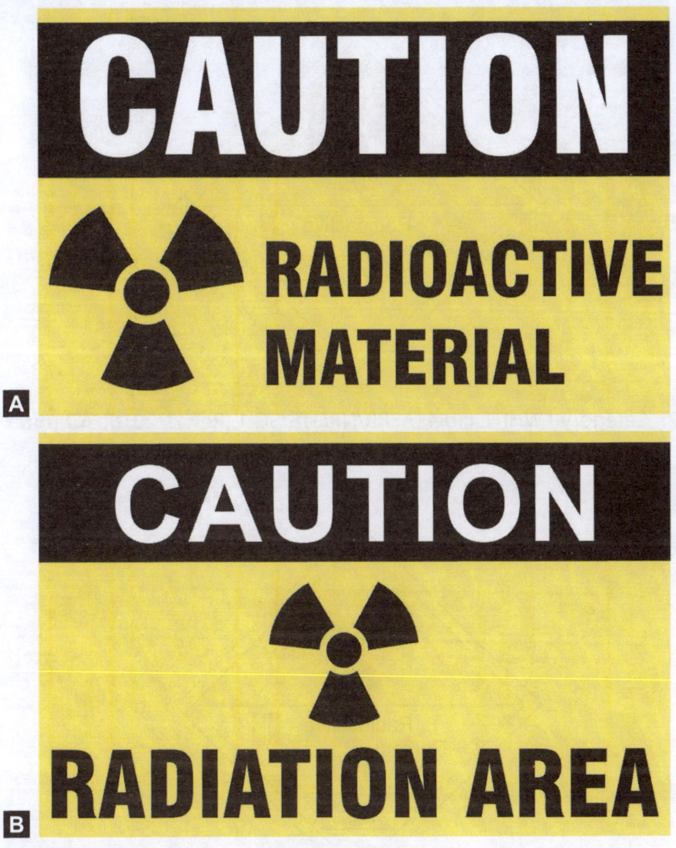

FIGS. 8.2A AND B: (A) Placard for storage and transport containers, (B) Placard for radiation areas/rooms with trefoil symbol. ***(Chapter 8)***

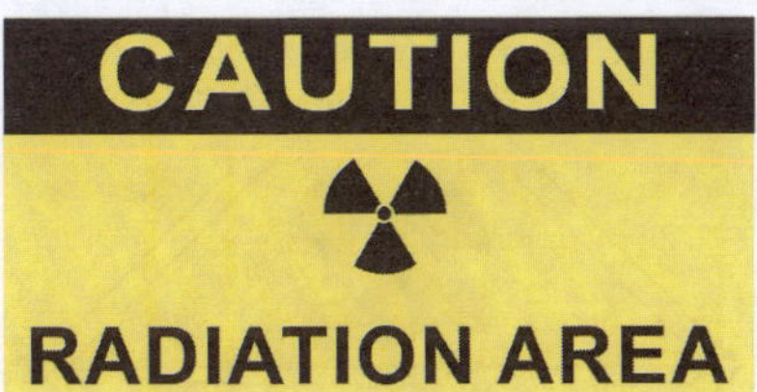

FIG. 11.3: Radiation warning placard. ***(Chapter 11)***

PLATE 2

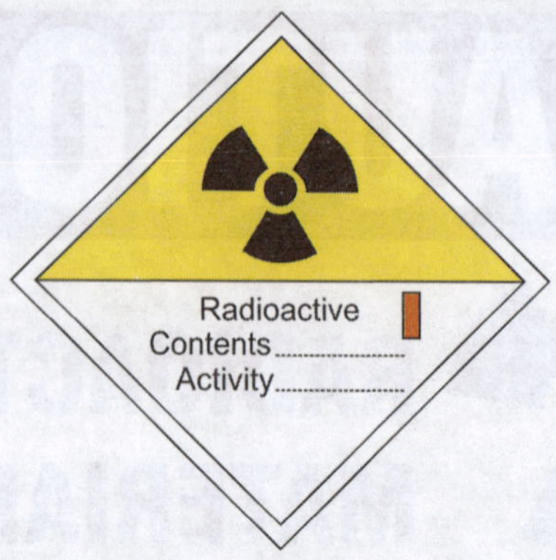

FIG. 16.2: Category-I WHITE label [AERB/NRF-TS/SC-1 (Rev.1), 2016]. ***(Chapter 16)***

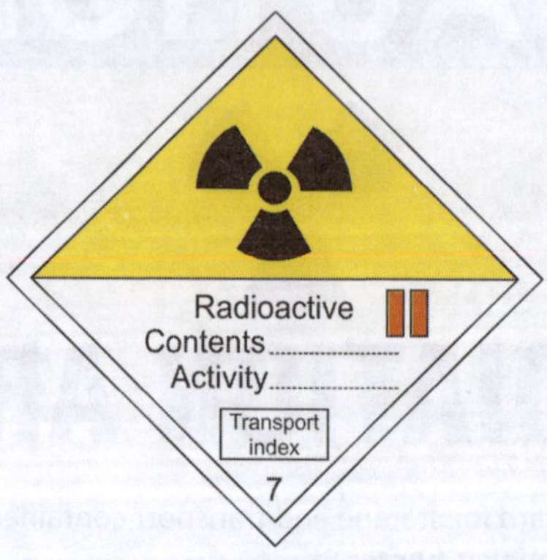

FIG. 16.3: Category-II YELLOW label [AERB/NRF-TS/SC-1 (Rev.1), 2016]. ***(Chapter 16)***

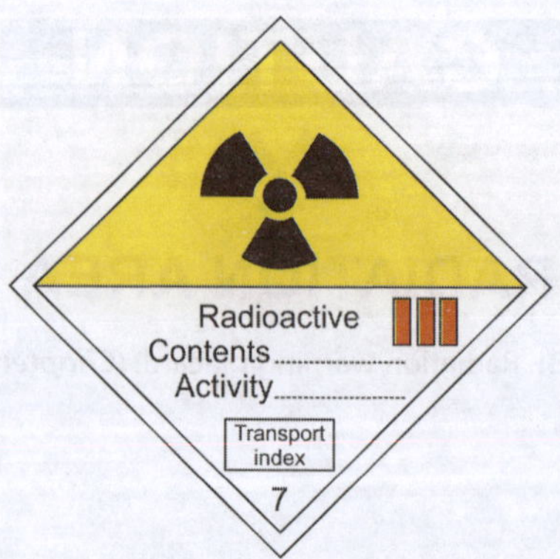

FIG. 16.4: Category-III YELLOW label [AERB/NRF-TS/SC-1 (Rev.1), 2016]. ***(Chapter 16)***

PLATE 3

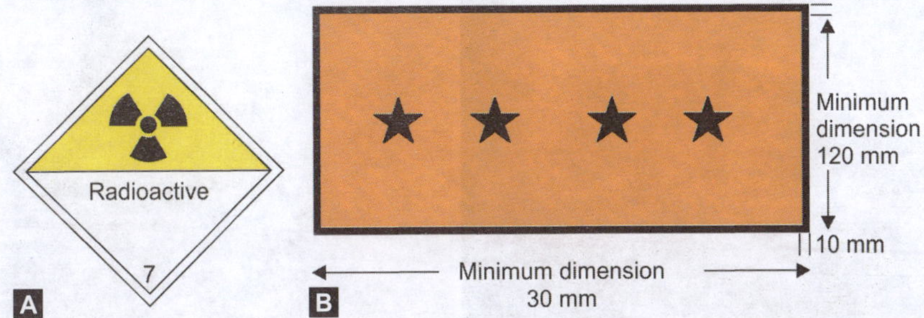

FIGS. 16.6A AND B: (A) Placard, and (B) Placrad for separate display of UN number [AERB/NRF-TS/SC-1 (Rev.1), 2016]. ***(Chapter 16)***

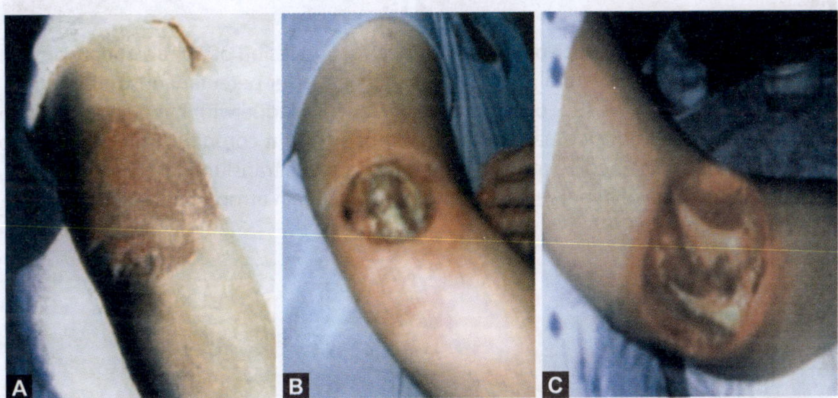

FIGS. 18.1A TO C: 49-year-old woman with 8-year history of refractory supraventricular tachycardia; Photographs show: (A) sharply demarcated erythema above right elbow at 3 weeks after radiofrequency cardiac catheter ablation; (B) tissue necrosis 5 months after procedure; and (C) deep ulceration with exposure of the humerus at 6.5 months. ***(Chapter 18)***

Courtesy: AJR:177, July 2001.

PLATE 4

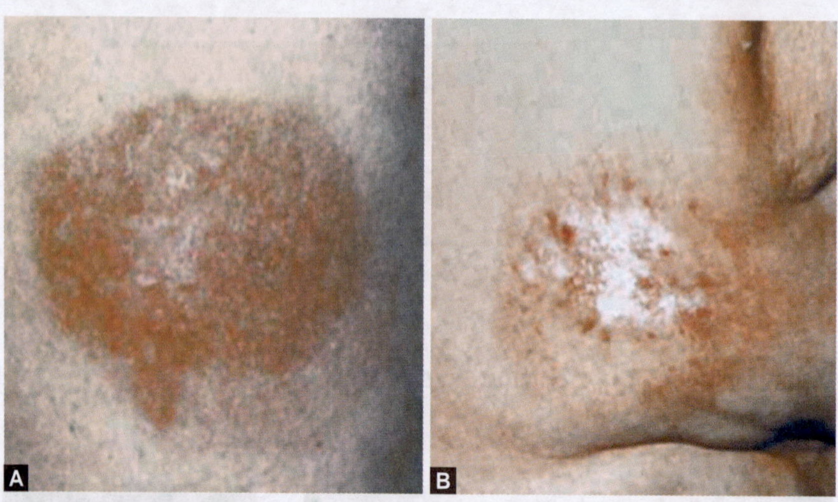

FIGS. 18.2A AND B: (A) 56-year-old man with obstructing lesion of right coronary artery. Photograph of right posterolateral chest wall at 10 weeks after percutaneous transluminal coronary angioplasty shows 12 × 6.5 cm hyperpigmented plaque with hyperkeratosis below right axilla; (B) A 75-year-old woman with 90% stenosis of right coronary artery. Photograph of right lateral chest obtained 10 months after percutaneous transluminal coronary angioplasty shows area of hyper- and hypopigmentation, skin atrophy, and telangiectasia (poikiloderma). ***(Chapter 18)***

Courtesy: AJR:177, July 2001.

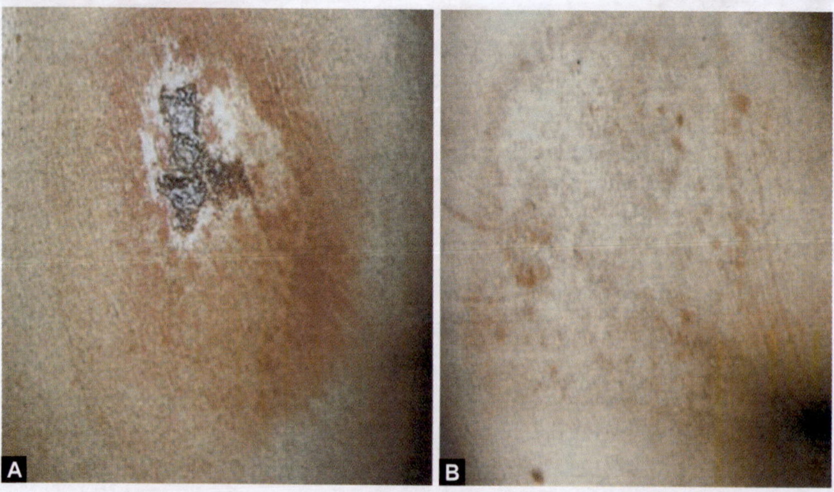

FIGS. 18.3A AND B: (A) Skin necrosis (erythema and hyperpigmentation), 3 years after angioplasty examination; (B) A17-year-old girl with history of cardiac arrhythmia underwent two cardiac ablation procedures in 13 months. Photograph taken 2 years after last intervention shows atrophic indurated plaque with skin telangiectasia at right lateral chest wall involving posterolateral aspect of breast. Induration resulted in limited movement of right arm. Risk of breast cancer is increased. ***(Chapter 18)***

Courtesy: AJR:177, July 2001.

PLATE 5

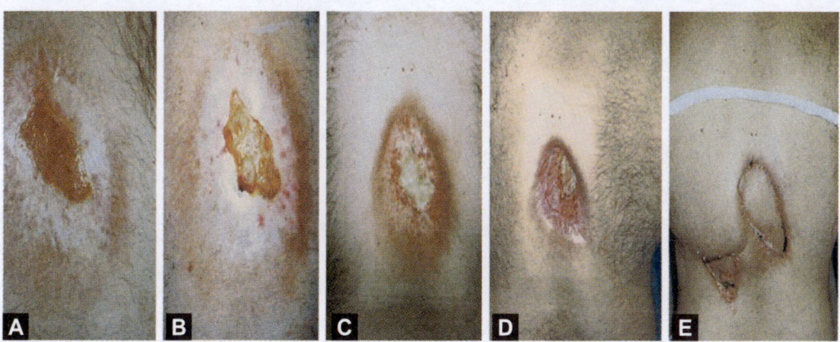

FIGS. 18.4A TO E: A 49-year-old man with history of liver cirrhosis and intractable upper gastrointestinal bleeding who underwent two transjugular intrahepatic portosystemic shunt (TIPS) placements and one attempted TIPS placement within a week. Photographs show progression of ulceration. (A) Secondary ulceration with surrounding rings of depigmentation and hyperpigmentation 6 months later; (B) Small blisters developed at 7.5 months after procedure. Wound is very painful; (C) Wound has progressed in size and depth at 10 months; (D) Nonhealing ulcer with exposure of deep tissues, including spinous process of vertebra, at 22 months; (E) At 23 months, musculocutaneous skin grafting was performed. Disfigurement is permanent. ***(Chapter 18)***

Courtesy: AJR:177, July 2001.

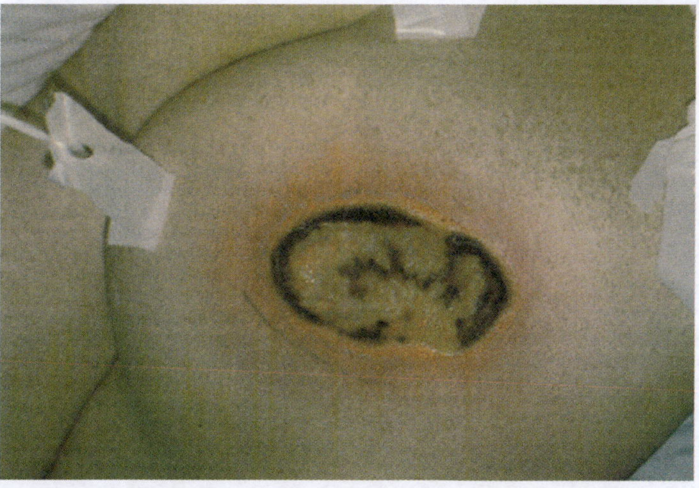

FIG. 19.1: Iridium source kept in the back pocket caused radiation burn in the buttock of a worker. ***(Chapter 19)***

Courtesy: IAEA-TECDOC-1205, IAEA, 2001.

CHAPTER 1

Radiation Quantities and Units

INTRODUCTION

Radiation was used in medicine soon after the discovery of X-rays by *WC Roentgen* on November 15, 1895. The use of X-rays in India began in 1900 at the Government General hospital, presently the *Barnard institute of Radiology and Oncology*, Chennai.

Radiation hazards were realized in the beginning of 20th century. The X-rays were used indiscriminately in the early years and have caused visible damage to several physicians and X-ray enthusiasts. Within 6 months of their use, several cases of erythema, dermatitis, and alopecia were reported among X-ray operators and their patients. In 1902, the first X-ray-induced skin cancer was reported. In 1921, *W. Ironside Bruce*, a first-generation radiologist in London (Charing Cross Hospital), died of aplastic anemia at the age of 45. Within 5 years, about 170 cases of radiation injuries were reported and by 1922, about 100 radiologists had died from radiation over exposures. *Thomas Alva Edison's* assistant *Clarence Madison Dally* died at his age of 39 with mediastinal cancer caused by X-ray exposure (1904). *Marie Curie* and her daughter *Irene* died out of leukemia caused by excessive radiation. Similarly, several lives were lost due to excessive use of radium and X-rays.

Above experiences, outcome of radiobiological experiments and improved knowledge of health effects of radiation demanded radiation protection. In 1915, the *British Roentgen Society* made the first radiation protection recommendations. To regulate the safe use of radiation, the *British X-ray and Radium Protection Committee* was formed (1921) and first recommendation report came in 1931. It was renamed as International X-ray and Radiation Protection Committee (IXRPC) in 1928, and later transformed as *International Commission on Radiological Protection (ICRP)* in 1950.

RADIATION FLUENCE AND FLUX

There are two types of radiation, namely: (i) photons and (ii) particles. Photons such as X- and gamma (γ)-rays travel as waves and transfer energy from one point to another point. Particles such as electron (e), proton (p), and alpha (α) interact with matter directly and produce ionization. Radiation is a double-edged weapon, analogous to fire which possess both benefits and risks.

When radiation travels in a medium, it has both fluence and flux. The fluence (Φ) is the number of photons or particles passing per unit area and its unit is m^{-2}:

$$\Phi = \frac{\text{Photons}}{\text{Area}} \tag{1.1}$$

It is a measure of photon intensity in m^2 area perpendicular to its path. The photon flux (φ) is the fluence rate that is number of photons passing in unit area per unit time:

$$\varphi = \frac{\text{Photons}}{\text{Area} \times \text{Time}} \tag{1.2}$$

It is expressed in $m^{-2}s^{-1}$.

Energy Fluence and Flux

The amount of energy (E) passing per unit area is called energy fluence (Ψ):

$$\left(\frac{\text{Photons}}{\text{Area}} \times \frac{\text{Energy}}{\text{Photons}} \right) \tag{1.3}$$

It is measured in Joules or MeV per m^2. The energy fluence of a monoenergy radiation beam is simply the product of fluence and photon energy. In the case of polyenergetic beam, number of photons of each energy is multiplied by its energy and their sum gives energy fluence. The energy fluence per unit time is called energy flux or energy fluence rate.

INVERSE SQUARE LAW

Radiation intensity (exposure rate) from a point source decreases with distance due to divergence of the beam. It is governed by the *inverse square law,* which states that the exposure rate from a point source of radiation is inversely proportional to the square of the distance. If the exposure rate is X_1 at distance d_1, then the exposure rate X_2 at another distance d_2 is given by:

$$X_1 \propto \frac{1}{d_1^2}, X_2 \propto \frac{1}{d_2^2}$$

$$\frac{X_2}{X_1} = \frac{d_1^2}{d_2^2}$$

$$X_2 = X_1 \left(\frac{d_1}{d_2} \right)^2 \tag{1.4}$$

Let 100 mR/h is the radiation exposure at 1 m for a point source **(Fig. 1.1)**. The radiation exposure at 2 m is found to be 25 mR/h by inverse square law. Hence, if distance is doubled, the radiation is reduced by a factor of 4.

This relationship is valid for point sources only, whose dimensions are very small compared to distance under consideration. Thus, the relationship is not valid near (<1 m) a patient injected with radioisotopes since the exposure rate decreases less rapidly than inverse square law.

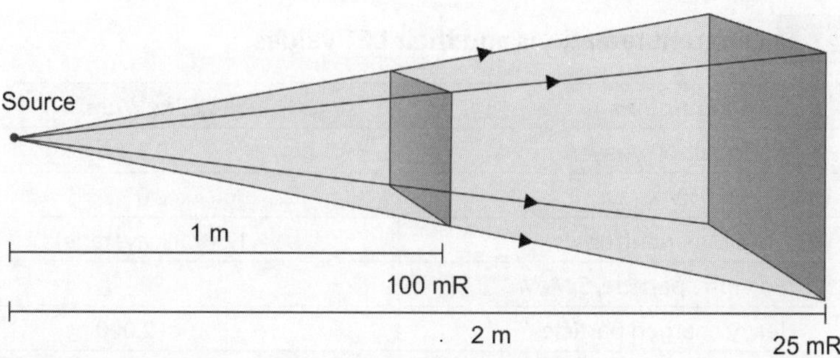

FIG. 1.1: Inverse square law: Exposure rate from a point source decreases with distance due to divergence of the beam.

Worked Example 1.1

The exposure rate from a telecobalt radiation source is 100 cGy/min at 100 cm. What would be the exposure rates at—(i) 90 cm and (ii) 110 cm, respectively?

(i) $X_1 = 100$ cGy/min, $d_1 = 100$ cm, $d_2 = 90$ cm, $X_2 = ?$

$$X_2 = X_1\left(\frac{d_1}{d_2}\right)^2$$

$$X_2 = 100\left(\frac{100}{90}\right)^2$$

$$= 123.5 \text{ cGy/min}$$

(ii) $X_1 = 100$ cGy/min, $d_1 = 100$ cm, $d_2 = 110$ cm, $X_2 = ?$

$$X_2 = X_1\left(\frac{d_1}{d_2}\right)^2$$

$$= 100\left(\frac{100}{110}\right)^2 = 82.6 \text{ cGy/min}$$

Answer: The radiation exposure rates at 90 cm and 110 cm are 123.5 cGy/m and 82.6 cGy/m, respectively.

LINEAR ENERGY TRANSFER

When radiation (photon/particle) passes through a medium, it loses energy. It depends on the distance it travels and the density of the ionization on the track. The linear energy transfer (LET) refers to local energy loss along the track. The track is divided into equal length and energy deposited in each length gives the LET value. Different radiations interact differently with medium **(Table 1.1)**. X- and γ-rays give raise to electrons, which are sparingly ionizing. Neutrons are 2,000 times heavier than electrons, interact with protons, and produce recoil protons, which do further ionization. Alpha particles are highly charged, heavy, and slow-moving particle, which produces dense ionizations in their path. It is four times heavier than neutron and 8,000 times that of electron. More densely ionizing radiation deposits greater amount of energy along the track. X- and γ-rays are called low LET radiations, neutron as intermediate LET, and alpha as high LET radiations.

TABLE 1.1 Different radiations and their LET values.

Radiation	*LET keV/μm*
Cobalt-60 γ-rays	0.3
250 kV X-rays	2.0
14 MeV neutrons	12 (track average)
^{210}Po alpha particle, 5 MeV	90
Heavy charged particle	100–2,000

(LET: linear energy transfer)

Courtesy: Eric J Hall, 2006.

Specific Ionization

Specific ionization (SI) refers to total number of ion pairs produced per unit path length by both primary and secondary ionization events along a charged particle track. The energy expended per ionization event (W) is the ratio of LET and SI:

$$W = \frac{LET}{SI} \tag{1.5}$$

It is independent of type of energy of the incident particle. Its value is 33.7 eV per ion-pair for air. It is different from the ionization potential (I) which is the average energy required to cause ionization in a metal. Its range is 10–15 eV for gases.

ATTENUATION

Attenuation is the reduction of radiation intensity while radiation travels in a medium. There are two types of attenuation coefficients namely linear and mass attenuation coefficients when photon interacts with matter. Linear attenuation coefficient provides a measure of the fractional attenuation per unit length of material traversed. Mass attenuation coefficient provides a measure of the fractional attenuation per unit mass of material encountered.

Linear Attenuation Coefficient

When photon travels in medium, only a fraction is transmitted through the medium whereas some fraction is absorbed, and some fraction is scattered in the medium. Thus, the intensity of the transmitted beam is lesser than the incident beam. Such reduction of photons intensity is called attenuation, which is an exponential function and is given by the equation **(Figs. 1.2A and B)**. The attenuation is the product of absorption and scattering:

$$I = I_0 \, e^{-\mu x} \tag{1.6}$$

In which I_0 and I are the initial and final intensity after a thickness x and μ is the linear attenuation coefficient. *Linear attenuation coefficient* (μ) is defined as the reduction in radiation intensity per unit path length, expressed in cm^{-1}. It depends on the radiation quality and density of the medium. The linear attenuation coefficient is found to increase linearly with density (ρ).

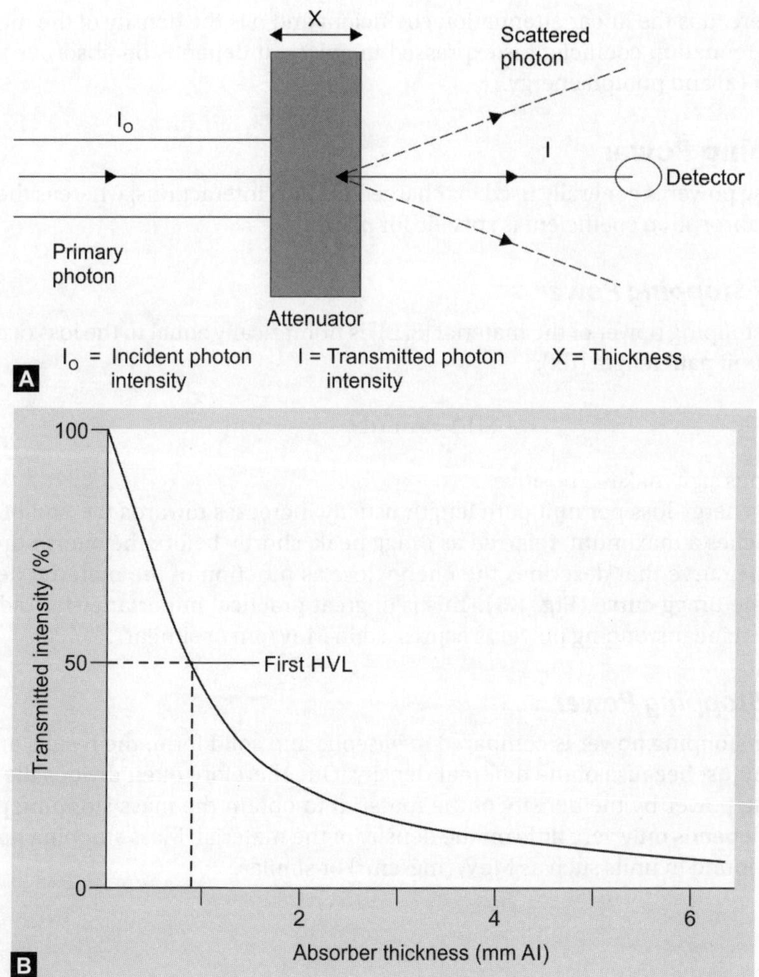

FIGS. 1.2A AND B: Attenuation of radiation in a medium, (A) Absorption and scattering of radiation while traveling in a medium of thickness X, (B) Percent transmitted intensity decreases exponentially as a function of absorber thickness.

Complete absorption of photons in a medium requires infinite thickness since attenuation of photon in a medium is exponential. That means that photon beams cannot be stopped fully in a medium. However, it is possible to reduce the photons to a desired level by providing a suitable thickness of the absorber.

Mass Attenuation Coefficient

When photons travel in any medium, the intensity of the photons decreases as it traverses through the medium. If thickness of the medium is expressed in mass/area, it is referred as mass attenuation coefficient (μ_m):

$$\mu_m = \frac{\mu}{\rho} \tag{1.7}$$

Where, μ is the linear attenuation coefficient and ρ is the density of the material. Mass attenuation coefficient is expressed in cm^2/g. It depends on absorber atomic number (z) and photon energy.

Stopping Power

Stopping power is generally used for charged particle interactions, whereas the mass energy absorption coefficient is specific for photons.

Linear Stopping Power

Linear stopping power of the material [S(E)] is numerically equal to the loss of energy dE per unit path length (dx):

$$S(E) = -dE/dx \tag{1.8}$$

The minus sign makes S positive.

The energy loss per unit path length usually increases towards the end of range and reaches a maximum, referred as Bragg peak, shortly before the energy drops to zero. The curve that describes the energy loss as function of the material depth is called the Bragg curve **(Fig. 1.3)**. This is of great practical importance for radiation therapy. Linear stopping power is expressed in MeV/cm or similar.

Mass Stopping Power

If linear stopping power is compared in gaseous and solid form, the results are very different just because of the different density. One therefore often divides the linear stopping power by the density of the material to obtain the mass stopping power, which depends only very little on the density of the material. Mass stopping power is usually found in units such as $MeV/(mg/cm^2)$ or similar.

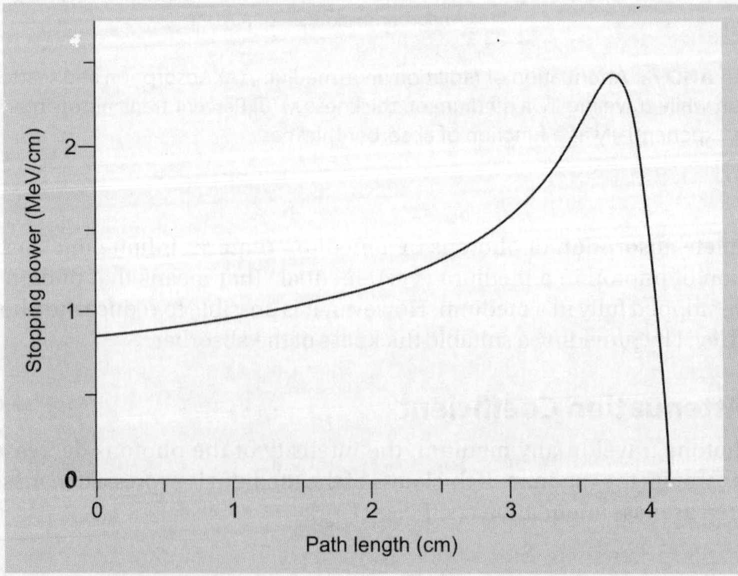

FIG. 1.3: Bragg curve and peak for alpha particle of 5.49 MeV in air, showing energy loss as function of depth in a medium.

Stopping Power and Linear Energy Transfer

Stopping power refers to the rate of energy loss per unit path length by the particle beam traversing the surrounding media, LET refers to the linear restricted stopping power that is the energy absorbed by the media per unit of distance travelled by the ionizing radiation.

Stopping power includes both collisional and radiation losses along the track. Collisional loss decreases with energy, whereas the radiation loss increases with energy. Stopping power is density dependent and usually called as mass collision stopping power and mass radiative stopping power:

$$\left(\frac{S}{\rho}\right)_{tot} = \left(\frac{S}{\rho}\right)_{col} + \left(\frac{S}{\rho}\right)_{rad} \tag{1.9}$$

$$S_{col} = S_{col} < \Delta + S_{col} > \Delta$$

The restricted collisional stopping power (LET) is given by: LET = $S_{col} < \Delta$ in which Δ is generally set at 100 keV.

Half-value Thickness

The thickness of material that attenuates radiation beam intensity by 50% of the original intensity is referred as *half-value layer or half-value thickness (HVT)*. HVT of a given medium is different for different photon energy. X-ray beam is heterogeneous; hence, HVT is quoted in terms of effective photon energy. Effective energy of a heterogeneous photon beam is that energy of a homogeneous photon beam at which μ of the homogeneous beam matches with that of the heterogeneous beam. The linear attenuation coefficient for effective photon energy is related to HVT as follows:

$$\mu_{eff} = \frac{0.693}{HVT} \tag{1.10}$$

The reduction factor offered by one HVT is 2 and by 2 HVT is 2×2 or 2^2. Hence, reduction factor for n HVT of shielding material is 2^n. For diagnostic X-ray beam energies, the HVL for soft tissue ranges from 2.5 to 3.0 cm. **Table 1.2** indicates the decrease of radiation intensity with increasing HVTs (for heavily filtered X-ray beam).

For a given photon beam energy, the HVT is different for different medium. It depends on the atomic number (Z) and density of the medium. More thickness of low Z material is required to equal the photon reduction offered by a high Z material. HVT increases with increase of photon energy. Hence, for a given thickness, low-energy photons undergo more attenuation than that of high-energy photons.

Beam Hardening

When heterogeneous X-ray beam passes through a medium, attenuation of soft energy takes place in the initial layers of the medium. As a result, the effective energy of the beam or HVT increases as it traverses through the medium. This effect, which happens only in the heterogeneous X-ray beam, is called *beam-hardening effect*. As the beam is filtered more and more, the emerging beam becomes more homogeneous, and HVT remains constant.

Soft-energy photons in the X-ray beam do not have sufficient energy to penetrate the patient body but contribute skin entrance dose to the patient. Since they are not useful for imaging, removal of soft-energy photons is required for patient safety point of view. It is achieved by providing additional filters in the beam path.

TABLE 1.2 Relation between half value layer and % of transmission.

Number of HVTs	*Transmission (%)*
0	100.0
1	50.0
2	25.0
3	12.50
4	6.25
5	3.12
6	1.56
7	0.78
8	0.39
9	0.19
10	0.09
(HVT: half-value thickness)	

TABLE 1.3 HVT and TVT values of concrete, steel, and lead for ^{192}Ir, ^{137}Cs and ^{60}Co.

Source	*Concrete (mm)*		*Steel (mm)*		*Lead (mm)*	
	HVT	*TVT*	*HVT*	*TVT*	*HVT*	*TVT*
^{192}Ir	43	152	13	43	6	16
^{137}Cs	48	175	16	53	6.5	22
^{60}Co	62	218	21	71	12	41
(HVT: half-value thickness; TVT: tenth value thickness)						
Courtesy: IAEA Safety series 47.						

Tenth Value Layer

There is another term called *tenth value layer or thickness (TVL or TVT)*, which reduces the photon intensity to one-tenth of its original intensity value. In other words, it gives the thickness of material that attenuates radiation beam by 90%. The reduction factor offered by one TVT is 10, and by 2 TVT is 10×10 or 10^2 and 10^n for n TVT and so on. The TVL and HVT can be related by using the equation:

$$\mathrm{TVT} = \frac{2.303}{\mu} \tag{1.11}$$

$$\mathrm{TVT} = \frac{2.303}{0.693/\mathrm{HVT}} = 3.32\,\mathrm{HVT}$$

This relation is applicable only for a homogeneous X-ray and gamma beam with exponential attenuation. For a given material, both HVT and TVT depend upon the energy of incident radiation and nature of medium **(Table 1.3)**. These parameters are useful in calculating thickness of shielding material or barrier while designing installations.

INTERACTION OF PHOTON WITH MATTER

Photons mainly interact with matter by photoelectric absorption, Compton scattering, and pair production, which are much important in medical applications. However, other interactions such as coherent scattering and photonuclear disintegration are there but less important.

Photoelectric Absorption

In the photoelectric effect (PE), a photon of energy E collides with an atom and ejects one of the bound electrons from the K or L shells **(Fig. 1.4)**. The ejected electron is called photoelectron and it has kinetic energy equal to E-orbital binding energy. In this process, all the incident photon energy is transferred to the electron. The incident photon must have energy equal or greater than the orbital binding energy of the electron, to perform PE.

After the PE, the atom is said to be ionized and there is vacancy in the orbit. This vacancy is filled by an electron of lower binding energy from higher orbit. This will create a cascade of electron transition event from outer orbit to inner orbit. The difference in binding energy is released as *characteristic X-rays or Auger electrons.* PE involves tightly bound electrons, which are mostly available in K shell; hence, most photoelectric interactions occur at the K shell.

The probability of photoelectric cross-section per unit mass is proportional to Z^3/E^3, where Z is the atomic number and E is the incident photon energy. As the X-ray photon energy increases, PE decreases, resulting decreased subject contrast. As atomic number increases, the photoelectric absorption increases, resulting higher subject contrast. That is why barium (Z = 56) and iodine (Z = 53) are used as contrast agents, which maximize the PE.

Even though PE decreases with increase of energy, there are few exceptions. The relation between probabilities of photoelectric absorption with photon energy is plotted, as exponential curve **(Fig. 1.5)**. It refers that as the photon energy increases, the attenuation decreases exponentially. However, if the photon energy is equal or greater the K-shell binding energy, the absorption increases steeply, and the curve appears with discontinuities. The above sharp discontinuity in the attenuation plot is called as *K-edge absorption.* Elements exhibit K-absorption edges, e.g., binding

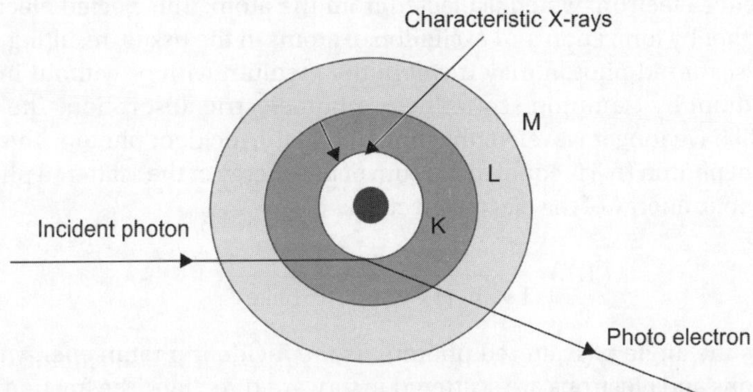

FIG. 1.4: Photoelectric absorption: Photon supply full energy and ejects electron from the K shell of the atom.

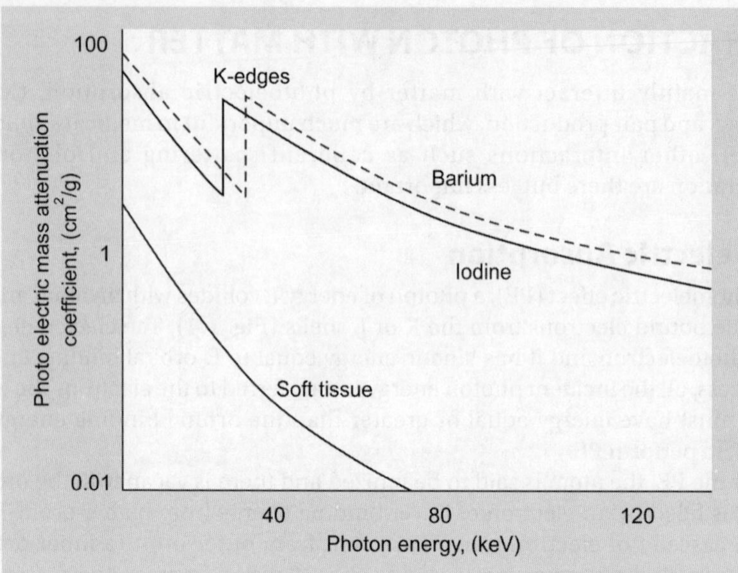

FIG. 1.5: Photoelectric absorption as a function of photon energy in soft tissue, iodine and barium, appearance of K-edges for iodine and barium.

energy of the K-shell in iodine is 33.2 keV, which will have six times higher absorption at the K-edge.

The photon energy corresponding to an absorption edge increases with atomic number. The absorption edges of elements H, C, N, and O present in the soft tissue are well below <1 keV. The iodine, barium, and lead absorption edges are 33.2, 37.4, and 88 keV, respectively. The PE is very important in soft tissue imaging for photon energy <50 keV. It will differentiate attenuation between two tissues with slightly varying atomic number.

Compton Scattering

In Compton scattering, photon interacts with a free electron (valence) of an atom and gets scattered with partial energy **(Fig. 1.6)**. The other part of energy is given to the valence electron, which is ejected from the atom. The ejected electron loses energy further by ionization and excitation of atoms in the tissue, resulting to patient dose. The scattered photon may travel in the medium with or without interaction in the medium by Compton scattering or photoelectric absorption. The scattered photon will have longer wavelength compared to the incident photon. The energy of the incident photon (E_0) is equal to the sum of the energy of the scattered photon (E_{sc}) and the kinetic energy of the ejected electron:

$$E_{SC} = \frac{E_0}{1 + \left[E_0 (1 - \cos\theta) \div 511\,\text{keV} \right]} \tag{1.12}$$

where, θ is the angle of scattered photon. As the incident photon energy increases, both photons and electrons are scattered in forward direction. The fraction of energy transferred to the scattered photon decreases with increase of incident photon energy, for a given angle of scatter.

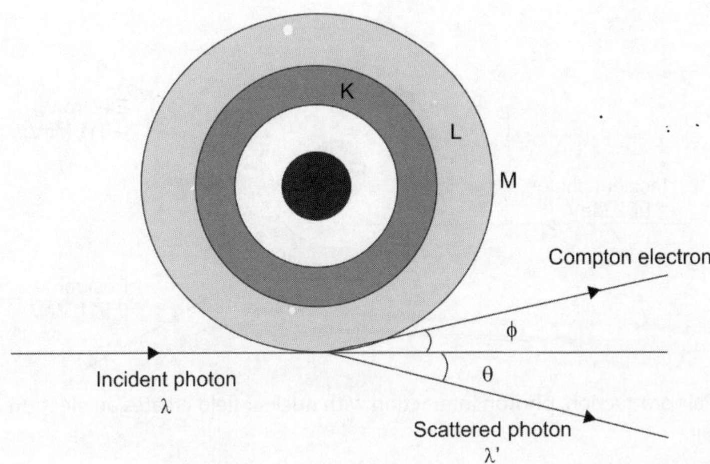

FIG. 1.6: Compton scattering: Photon interacts with a free electron (outer orbit), share partial energy and gives compton electron.

If the photon makes a direct hit on the electron, the electron will travel straight forward ($\phi = 0$) and the scattered photon will be scattered back with $\theta = 180°$. In this collision, the electron will get its maximum energy, while the scattered photon goes with minimum energy. If the photon makes a grazing hit with the electron, the electron will be emitted at right angles ($\phi = 90°$) and the scattered photon will go in the forward direction ($\theta = 0$). In this collision, the electron receives minimal energy, and the scattered photon goes with maximum energy.

The Compton scattering involves an interaction between a photon and a free electron, resulting ionization of atom. The incident photon energy is shared between the scattered photon and ejected electron. The probability of Compton scattering depends upon the electron density (*number of electrons per gram × density*) in the medium. Except hydrogen, the electron density is constant for tissue; hence, it is independent of atomic number (Z). Probability of Compton interaction decreases with increase of X-ray energy, and it is $\propto 1/E$. The probability per unit volume is proportional to the density of the material. Hydrogenous material has higher probability for Compton scattering.

Compton scattering occurs in all energies in tissue, and it is important in X-ray imaging. It is a predominant interaction in the diagnostic energy range with soft tissue (100 keV to 10 MeV). Scattered X-rays provide no useful information, only reduce image contrast, and create radiation hazards in radiography and fluoroscopy. In fluoroscopy, large amount of radiation is scattered from the patient and contributes to occupational radiation exposure.

Pair Production

A photon having an energy >1.02 MeV, which passes near the nucleus of an atom, is subjected to strong nuclear field **(Fig. 1.7)**. The photon may suddenly disappear and create a positron and electron pair, which is called pair production. For each particle, 0.511 MeV energy is required and the excess energy >1.02 MeV would be shared between the positron and electron as kinetic energy. The interaction is between a photon and the nuclear field. This process is an example for the conversion of energy into mass as predicted by *Albert Einstein*. The threshold energy for the

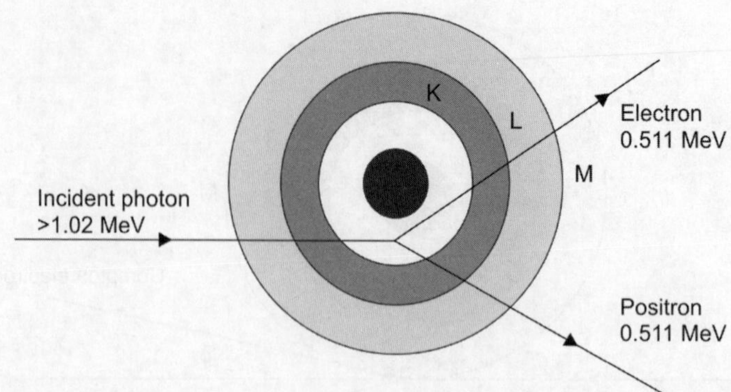

FIG. 1.7: Pair production, photon interaction with nuclear field creates an electron and positron pair.

pair production process is 1.02 MeV. The probability of pair production increases with energy for a given material and increases with atomic number (Z^2). It is very important for photons having energy >5 MeV.

The electron loses energy in the medium by further excitation and ionization and filling vacancy in the orbital shells. The positron travels in the medium and loses its energy by ionization, excitation, and bremsstrahlung process. Finally, the positron combines with a free electron and produces two photons of energy of 0.511 MeV, which are ejected in opposite directions. The above process is called the *positron annihilation*. This is an example of conversion of mass into energy and is the basis for *positron emission tomography (PET)*.

Interaction of Alpha and Beta Particles with Matter

Charged particles interact with matter by electrical forces and lose kinetic energy via excitation and ionization. Ionization is the removal of an electron from a neutral gaseous atom. Alpha particles ionize by attracting an electron from an atom. Beta particles ionize by repelling an electron from an atom. Excitation is the movement of an electron from a lower energy level to a higher energy level by absorbing energy. It makes an atom move from a ground state to an excited state. Beta particles interact with radiative losses in addition to excitation and ionization.

Radiative loss is the collision between two charged particles in which part of the kinetic energy of the particles is converted into electromagnetic radiation. That is the electromagnetic radiation is produced by the deceleration of a charged particle when deflected by another charged particle, typically an electron by an atomic nucleus. This is known as Bremsstrahlung meaning "braking radiation" or "deceleration radiation". The moving particle loses kinetic energy, which is converted into radiation (i.e., a photon), thus satisfying the law of conservation of energy.

Bremsstrahlung has a continuous spectrum, which becomes more intense and whose peak intensity shifts towards higher frequencies as the change of the energy of the decelerated particles.

Interaction of Neutron with Matter

Neutrons have no net electric charge; they are neither attracted nor repelled by atomic nuclei. They interact with target matter via nuclear forces, some neutrons are captured, and target nuclei may be converted into radioactive product. The above type of event is called neutron activation. Nuclear forces are very short range of few fermis (1 fermi = 10^{-15} m) and the sizes of nuclei are typically 100,000 times smaller than the distances between them. Neutrons can, therefore, travel long distances in a medium without being scattered or absorbed, i.e., they are highly penetrating (to depths of 0.1–0.01 m). For example, attenuation of low-energy neutrons by Al is ≈1%/mm compared to >99%/mm for X-ray.

Interaction of neutrons with matter can cause reactions, which gives rise to other forms of radiation such as protons. Common neutron reactions are (n,γ), and (n,p) reactions. In the (n,γ) reaction, product nuclei become different isotope of the same chemical element with prompt emission of gamma rays. In (n,p), target, nuclei captures neutron, emit protons, and product nuclei do not represent same chemical element. The amount of activity induced by bombarding depends on the—(i) intensity of the particle beam, (ii) number of target nucleus in the sample, and (iii) probability of particle interaction with target nuclei.

Activation Cross-section

Probability of neutron interaction is determined by activation cross-section (σ). It refers to probability of a given type of nuclear reaction while a particle is bombarding a target nucleus to induce radioactivity. Activation cross-section is the effective area of the target nucleus to a bombarding particle. To characterize the probability that a certain nuclear reaction will take place, it is customary to define an effective area of the target nucleus in terms of cross-section. Nuclear cross-section can be quantified physically in terms of characteristic area where a larger area means a larger probability of interaction:

$$\sigma = \frac{R}{I} \tag{1.13}$$

where R is the number of reactions per unit time per nucleus, and I is the number of incident particles per unit time per unit area.

There are two types of interaction cross-section, namely—(i) macroscopic cross-section (Σ) and (ii) microscopic cross-section (*σ*). Macroscopic cross-section is the probability of interaction per unit length in a material and its unit is cm^{-2}. Microscopic cross-section is the probability of interaction per nucleus of material and its unit is barn (b) and 1 b = 10^{-28} m^2 or 1 millibarn = 10^{-31} m^2. It is appreciable at low energy and in low Z materials.

The activation cross-section for a given particle depends on—(i) type of bombarding particle, (ii) type of reaction involved, and (iii) energy of the bombarding particle. However, cross-section is a strong function of bombarding particle energy.

RADIATION QUANTITIES AND UNITS

Quantities are used to measure a physical entity by estimating a measurable physical effect of the physical entity, e.g., mass and heat. In such cases, the amount of physical entity and its effect should have a linear relationship. Quantities of radioactivity and radiation of interest are—(i) amount of nuclear disintegration takes place per unit time, (ii) ionizing photons present in the field, (iii) energy transferred from radiation to the tissue, (iv) energy absorbed in the tissue, and (v) biological effectiveness of energy absorption. These quantities are activity, exposure, kerma, terma, absorbed dose, equivalent dose, and effective dose.

Activity

Activity refers to number of unstable nuclei that regain stability through radio disintegration per unit time. The quantity of radiation released from the radioactive source is directly proportional to the activity. The unit of activity is curie (Ci) and it is defined as the number of disintegration per second from 1 gram of radium-226 and it is found to be 3.7×10^{10} (*Marie Curie*). The SI unit of activity of Becquerel (Bq) = 1 disintegration per second (dps). In practice, mega Becquerel (MBq) and giga Becquerel (GBq) are used as units; 1 μCi = 37 kBq, 1 mCi = 37 MBq, and 1 Ci = 37 GBq.

Exposure

The term exposure (X) refers to amounts of ionizing photons present in air. Exposure is quantified from the ionization events produced by charged particle, which are liberated by ionizing photons in air. Average energy required to produce ionization in air is 35 eV. The unit of exposure is roentgen (R).

One roentgen shall be the quantity of X or gamma radiation such that the associated corpuscular emission per 0.001293 grams of air (1 cc of dry air at NTP = 273 K and 760 mm Hg), produces in air, ions carrying 1 electrostatic unit (esu) of quantity of electricity of either sign. In the case of vented ion chamber, the temperature and pressure variation can alter the amount of air molecules present in the chamber. Hence, temperature and pressure corrections are required.

The unit may also be defined in terms of SI unit as 1 roentgen is equal to amount of photons that produce 1 Coulomb of charge in 1 kilogram of air:

$$1\ \text{R} = 2.58 \times 10^{-4}\ \frac{\text{c}}{\text{kg}}\ \text{of air} \tag{1.14}$$

Here, the volume is replaced by mass of air, which is not affected by temperature and pressure variations. Exposure and exposure rate meters are calibrated in terms of roentgen. However, in practice milliroentgen (mR) is often used as unit = 1/1,000 roentgen. Exposure rate is the exposure measured in roentgen per minute (R/m) or mR/h. It is used as readings in survey meters during equipment calibration and radiation survey.

Limitations of roentgen unit includes; it is not a unit of dose, which is a measure of absorbed energy. It is defined only for X and gamma radiations in air not in tissue. Charge measurement is not possible above 3 MV due to loss of electronic equilibrium, hence, it can be used only up to photon energy of 3 MeV.

Kerma

Uncharged particles such as photon and neutron transfer kinetic energy to electrons or protons while travelling in a medium. Transferred energy appears as kinetic energy of the electrons. This kinetic energy causes ionization events in the medium. During this process, some electrons lose energy as bremsstrahlung X-rays. Thus, the energy transferred to the medium is not fully absorbed in the medium. The energy absorbed by matter (absorbed dose) is different from total energy transferred by the radiation to the matter, referred as kerma.

Kerma (K) is the *K*inetic *E*nergy *R*eleased in unit *Ma*ss in a medium. It describes the initial interaction of photon with an atom that takes place at a point in medium. It

TABLE 1.4 Air-kerma rate constant of few radionuclides used in nuclear medicine.

Radionuclides	*Air-kerma rate constant (mGy.m²/GBq-h)*
^{18}F	0.1351
^{60}Co	0.3090
^{68}Ga	0.1290
$^{99}Mo/^{99m}Tc$	0.0336
^{131}I	0.0522
^{137}Cs	0.0821
^{125}I	0.0377

Courtesy: Simon R Cherry, 2012.

is a measure of kinetic energy transferred to the charged particles. The unit of kerma is gray and 1 Gy = J/kg.

If kerma is measured in air, it is called air kerma, which describes the radiation intensity in air, and one air kerma = 114 R. If the medium is tissue, it becomes tissue-kerma. The measurement kerma per minute or hour (Gy/m or Gy/h) is called kerma rate. If it is measured in air, it is referred as air kerma rate. X-ray output, dose area product (DAP) meter, and free air ionization chamber readings are read in air kerma rate.

Air-kerma Rate Constant

Air kerma rate constant (Γ) is defined as the air kerma measured at a distance 1 m from an unshielded 1 GBq point source of a radionuclide in mGy per hour. It is expressed in mGy.m²/GBq-h **(Table 1.4)**. The air kerma rate (KR) at a distance d, from an activity (A) of a radionuclide having an air kerma rate constant (Γ), is given by:

$$KR = \frac{A\Gamma}{d^2} \tag{1.15}$$

Air-kerma Strength

Air-kerma strength (S_k) is the product of air-kerma rate in free space and square of the distance (d) between a source and calibration point (AAPM, TG-32). It is measured in air along the transverse axis of an encapsulated source. This distance is usually taken as 1 m and unit is μGym^2h^{-1} or cGy cm^2h^{-1}, expressed by the symbol U (1 U= μGym^2h^{-1} = one unit of air-kerma strength).

Terma

It is the total energy released per unit mass (Terma), which includes the energy retained by the scattered photons. In other words, it is the energy removed from the primary beam:

$$T_n(d) = \Psi_n(d)\left(\frac{\mu}{\rho}\right)_n \tag{1.16}$$

where, Ψ_n is the energy fluence at depth d and n is the component of energy fluence. Terma is larger than kerma by a factor of μ/μ_{tr}. It includes coherent scattering, since it is negligible at MV beams, KERMA=TERMA, it is used as modulating the energy deposition kernel in convolution for dose calculation.

Absorbed Dose

When radiation passes through a medium, energy is transferred to the medium referred as kerma. The transferred energy is not fully absorbed the medium because of bremsstrahlung X-ray production. Dose difference between kerma and bremsstrahlung loss is referred as absorbed dose (D). It refers to amount of energy absorbed per unit mass of a medium. It is defined as ratio of mean energy ($d\bar{\varepsilon}$) imparted by the ionizing radiation in a volume element and the mass (dm) of matter in that volume:

$$D = \frac{d\bar{\varepsilon}}{dm} \tag{1.17}$$

The unit of absorbed dose is J/kg with a special name gray (Gy). The old unit of absorbed dose is rad (*r*adiation *a*bsorbed *d*ose) and 1 rad (r) = 100 ergs/g. The unit rad is related to gray as follows:

$$1\,\text{Gy} = 1\,\text{J/kg} = \frac{10^7\,\text{erg}}{10^3\,\text{g}} = 10^4\,\frac{\text{erg}}{\text{g}} = 100\,\text{rads}$$

In practice, milligray (mGy) and microgray (μGy) are used. Thus, 1 Gy = 100 rad and 1 mGy = 100 mrad.

Absorbed dose is obtained from the mean value of the stochastic quantity of the imparted energy and does not reflect the fluctuations of the interaction events in tissue. It can be measured by primary standards. Radiological protection involves low doses and measured absorbed dose can be correlated with radiation detriment for stochastic effects in the tissue with required accuracy. It is independent of type of radiation and medium.

Roentgen-rad Conversion Factor

The absorbed dose (D) is related to the exposure (X) as follows:

$$D = f \times X \tag{1.18}$$

i.e., absorbed dose = f × exposure

where, f is the roentgen-to-rad conversion factor. In diagnostic X-ray energies, the f-factor for air, muscle, and other soft tissue is close to 1. Hence, the exposure is equal to the absorbed dose for diagnostic energy. However, the factor is 4.4 for bone

TABLE 1.5 **f-factor for a range of photon energies and absorbed media.**

Photon energy (keV)	*Fat (Z = 5.9)*	*Muscle (Z = 7.5)*	*Bone (Z = 13.8)*
30	0.53	0.92	4.4
50	0.66	0.94	3.6
100	0.91	0.96	1.5
150	0.96	0.96	1.1

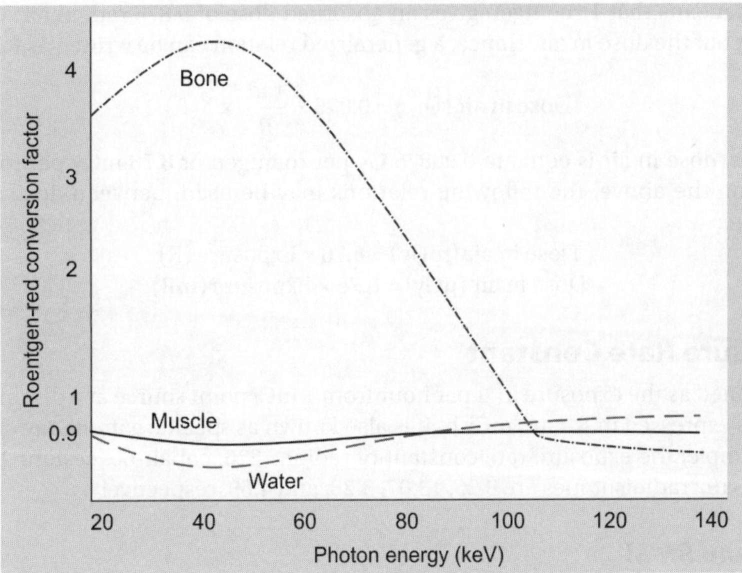

FIG. 1.8: Roentgen-rad conversion factor as a function of photon energy in water, muscle and bone.

at 30 keV, because of higher photoelectric absorption **(Table 1.5)**. The variation of roentgen-rad conversion factor with photon energy is given in **Figure 1.8**.

Absorbed Dose from Exposure

The absorbed dose in air is the product of charge produced per unit mass and energy required to produce a unit charge:

$$D_{air} = X\left(\frac{W}{e}\right)_{air} \tag{1.19}$$

where, W/e = 33.97 J/c is the energy deposited in air per Coulomb charge produced. D_{air} is equal to collision kerma under charged particle equilibrium (CPE). To convert it into dose in medium, the D_{air} is multiplied by the ratio of mass collision stopping powers:

$$D_{med} = D_{air}\left(\frac{L}{\rho}\right)_{air}^{med} \tag{1.20}$$

where, $\frac{L}{\rho}$ is the restricted mass collision stopping power.

Worked Example 1.2

Calculate the dose in air from exposure?

Let D_{air} be the dose in air, in Gy, and X is the exposure, R, then—

The charge in 1 roentgen exposure (R) is = 2.58×10^{-4} C kg^{-1}

The average energy (W/e) deposited in air per ion pair is = 33.97 JC^{-1}

The total energy associated with 1 roentgen exposure is given by:

$$1\ roentgen = (W/e) \times R = 33.97\ JC^{-1} \times 2.58 \times 10^{-4}\ C\ kg^{-1}$$
$$= 0.00876\ Jkg^{-1} = 0.00876\ Gy - 0.876\ rad$$

This means that 1 roentgen gives an absorbed dose of 0.876 rad, in air, which is nothing but the dose in air. Hence, a generalized relation can be written as follows:

$$\text{Dose in air } (D_{air}) = 0.876 \times \frac{\text{rad}}{\text{R}} \times X(\text{R})$$

Thus, dose in air is equal to 0.00876 Gy per roentgen or 8.76 mGy per roentgen. Based on the above, the following relations may be used, between dose and the exposure:

$$\text{Dose in air (mGy)} = 8.76 \times \text{Exposure (R)}$$
$$\text{Dose in air } (\mu\text{Gy}) = 8.76 \times \text{Exposure (mR)}$$

Exposure Rate Constant

It is defined as the exposure in R per hour from 1 mCi point source at a distance 1 cm and it is expressed in R-cm^2/mCi-h. It is also known as specific gamma ray constant. For example, the exposure rate constant of radium-226, cobalt-60, cesium-137, and iridium-192 radioisotopes are 8.25, 13.07, 3.26, and 4.69, respectively.

RHM and RMM

If the exposure rate constant is defined for 1 Ci source at 1 m, then it is called RHM (roentgen–hour–meter). It is defined as the exposure (R) per hour from 1 Ci point source at a distance 1 m and it is expressed in R-m^2/Ci-h. In practice, RHM of a given radioisotope can be obtained by dividing the exposure rate constant by a factor 10. Hence, the RHM of radium-226, cobalt-60, cesium-137, and iridium-192 radioisotopes are 0.825, 1.307, 0.326, and 0.469, respectively. Mostly, RHM is employed for calibration purposes in brachytherapy and industrial radiography.

Instead of hour, one can also express it for 1 minute, then it is called RMM (roentgen–minute–meter). It is defined as the exposure per minute from 1 Ci point source at a distance 1 m and it is expressed in R-m^2/Ci-min. For example, if the RHM of the Cobalt radioisotope is 1.307, the corresponding RMM value is 1.307/60 = 0.0217. RMM is the most preferred and useful terminology in telecobalt source calibration.

RMM and Curie

In the case of Cobalt, 0.0217 RMM corresponds to 1 Ci; hence, 1 RMM = (1/0.0217) = 46.08 Ci. Similarly, it can be applied to different radioisotopes **(Table 1.6)**.

TABLE 1.6 RHM and RMM of different radioisotopes.

Radioisotope	*Exposure rate constant R-cm^2/mCi-h*	*RHM*	*RMM*	*Activity (Ci) equivalent to 1 RMM*
Radium-226	8.25	0.825	0.0137	72.99
Cobalt-60	13.07	1.307	0.0217	46.08
Cesium-137	3.26	0.326	0.0054	185.18
Iridium-192	4.69	0.469	0.0078	128.20
Fluorine-18	5.66	0.566	0.0094	106.38

(RHM: roentgen–hour–meter; RMM: roentgen–minute–meter)

Worked Example 1.3

If a cobalt teletherapy source is purchased with 200 RMM capacity, what is the corresponding activity of the source in Ci?

1 RMM = 46.08 Ci

200 RMM = 46.08 × 200 = 9,216 Ci

Worked Example 1.4

If a cobalt teletherapy source is purchased with 12,000 Ci capacity, what is the corresponding RMM value?

46.08 Ci = 1 RMM

12,000 Ci = (1/46.08) × 12,000 = 260.4 RMM

CHARGED PARTICLE EQUILIBRIUM

The energy deposited in a volume is equal to the difference between energy entering the volume and the energy leaving the volume. Under charged particle equilibrium (CPE), the energy entering in and out is equal. Then the energy deposited in the volume is equal to the energy transferred (ε_{tr}) to the charged particle. Considering that there is no bremsstrahlung production then the dose (D) is equal to collision kerma (K_c) which is equal to kerma (K):

$$D = K = K_c \tag{1.21}$$

If bremsstrahlung production is considered, the dose is equal to collision kerma, but it is smaller than kerma:

$$D = K_c, \text{ but } D < K_c \tag{1.22}$$

The assumption in the above equation is that no charged particle enters or leaves the volume. If charged particle enters the volume and secondary charged particle exits the volume, the dose is not equal to collision kerma:

$$D \neq K_c \tag{1.23}$$

The primary photon fluence decreases with depth so that number of charged particles entering successive layers decrease as depth increases due to attenuation. The equivalence of dose to collision kerma takes place slightly upstream. This is said to be transient CPE. Here, the dose is proportional to kerma.

DOSIMETRIC QUANTITIES

Equivalent Dose

Specific ionizations produced per path length or energy transfer rate is different for different radiations. Alpha-like heavy ionizing particle transfers more energy per unit path length in the medium. Particle offering higher SI will produce more tissue damage in their proximity. Hence, biological effectiveness of alpha particle is more compared to sparingly ionizing radiation such as X and gamma rays. Absorbed dose does not convey the above biological effectiveness of the radiation. To account the biological effectiveness of different radiation based on SI and LET properties, the term equivalent dose was proposed.

TABLE 1.7 **Radiation-weighting factors (W_R).**

Radiation type	W_R
Photons	1
Electrons and muons	1
Protons and charged pions	2
Alpha particles, fission fragments, heavy ions	20
Neutrons	A continuous function of neutron energy

Courtesy: ICRP-103, 2007.

Thus, the biological effectiveness of radiation depends not only on absorbed dose but also on the type of radiation energy. Hence, ICRP-60 (1991) introduced radiation-weighting factors for different radiation **(Table 1.7)**. It will modify the dose to reflect the relative effectiveness of the type of radiation causing biological damage. Earlier, it was related to the radiation quality factor (Q) as a function of LET. The equivalent dose (H_T) is the product of absorbed dose and radiation-weighting factor:

$$H_T = \Sigma_R D_{T,R} \times W_R \tag{1.24}$$

where, $D_{T,R}$ is the average absorbed dose delivered by a radiation type R in the volume of tissue or organ T, and W_R is the weighting factor for the radiation type.

The unit of equivalent dose if J/kg and the special name Sievert (Sv) after *Rolf Sievert*, the Swedish Scientist: 1 Sievert (Sv) = 1 J/kg. In practice, milli-Sievert (mSv) unit is used, and 1 mSv = 100 mrem, where rem (*r*oentgen *e*quivalent *m*en) is the special unit of equivalent dose used earlier.

The conversion of absorbed dose into equivalent dose is valid only for low dose and low-dose rate that too limited to radiation protection purposes. The given radiation-weighting factors are not valid for high dose and high-dose rate range. In medical X-rays, 1 roentgen exposure provides an energy absorption of about 97.8 erg in 1 g of tissue. It is almost equal to 1 rad = 97.8 ≈100 ergs. If it is multiplied by the radiation-weighting factor of X-rays which is = 1, then the equivalent dose is 1 rem. Hence, for radiation protection purpose: 1 roentgen = 1 rad = 1 rem. Therefore, roentgen and rad units are interchangeably used in diagnostic X-rays.

Effective Dose

Radiation exposure can be either whole body or partial body in nature. Whole body exposure is uniform whereas partial body is nonuniform. Radiosensitivity of different tissues in the human body is different and radiation-induced effects vary with sensitivity of the organ. Hence, radiation exposure of individual tissues contributes differently to the total detriment of heath of the individual. It depends upon the seriousness of the damage in individual tissues and its curability. The equivalent dose for various tissues may differ markedly.

Radiation can cause both deterministic and stochastic effects. Aim of radiation safety is to prevent deterministic effect and minimize stochastic effect. To reduce the probability of stochastic effect, equivalent dose limit is recommended. Human body consists of multiple tissues or organs. The total stochastic effect risk of all individual organs should not exceed the risk of an exposed person to a whole-body exposure that amounts to recommended equivalent dose limit.

TABLE 1.8 **Tissue-weighting factors (W_T).**

Tissue	W_T	ΣW_T
Bone-marrow, colon, lung, stomach, breast, remainder tissues*	0.12	0.72
Gonad	0.08	0.08
Bladder, esophagus, liver, thyroid	0.04	0.16
Bone surface, brain, salivary glands, skin, kidneys, brain	0.01	0.04
Total		1.0

*Mean doses to adrenals, extrathoracic (ET) region, gallbladder, heart, kidneys, lymphatic nodes, muscle, oral mucosa, pancreas, prostate, small intestine, spleen, thymus, and uterus/cervix.

Courtesy: ICRP-103, 2007.

To account this nonuniform nature of irradiation and organ sensitivity variation, ICRP-60 (1991) introduced the tissue-weighting factors (W_T) as given in **Table 1.8**. Effective dose (E) is given by:

$$E = \Sigma_T W_T \times H_T \tag{1.25}$$

where, W_T is the weighting factor for tissue T and $\Sigma W_T = 1$, H_T is mean equivalent dose received by the tissue, and E is summed overall organs and tissues of the human body for which specific detriment value can be calculated. W_T represents the contributions of individual organs and tissues to overall radiation detriment from stochastic effects, averaged over all ages and sexes. The unit of effective dose is J/kg with a special name Sievert (Sv) as stated earlier.

Worked Example 1.5

In a CT scan study, the tissues breast, lung, bone marrow, and thyroid receive dose of 21, 23.5, 5.17, and 2.30 mSv, respectively. Calculate the effective dose with tissue-weighting factors.

$$E = \Sigma W_T \times H_T$$

$$= (21 \times 0.12) + (23.5 \times 0.12) + (5.17 \times 0.12) + (2.3 \times 0.04) = 6.05 \text{ mSv}$$

The effective dose is 6.05 mSV.

Annual Limit on Intake

Nuclear Regulatory Commission (NRC) has introduced annual limit on intake (ALI). ALI is that quantity of radionuclides, which is taken into the body by inhalation, ingestion, or through the skin over 1 year, and would result in a committed dose equal to relevant dose limit. It will limit the radioactive activity so that no workers will exceed the limits. ALI is expressed in μCi and data is provided for wide variety of radionuclides for inhalation and ingestion pathways.

Derived Air Concentration

To regulate the airborne activity, derived air concentration (DAC) is used. It is the concentration of a given radionuclide in air, which, if breathed by a reference man for 2,000 hours under conditions of light work, results in an intake of one ALI. It is calculated by dividing ALI by the volume of air inhaled by a reference man in a working year and its unit is Bq/m^3 or μCi/mL. For example, ALI and DAC values of I-131 for occupational workers, via ingestion, are 30 μCi, and 2×10^{-8} μCi/mL, respectively (NRC data).

Personnel Dose Equivalent

Personnel dose equivalent (PDE) is a dose equivalent in soft tissue, at an appropriate depth—d, below a specified point on the body and its unit is Sievert (Sv). It is denoted by the symbol $H_P(d)$, was defined by ICRP for individual monitoring. Two operational quantities are defined, namely—(i) $H_P(0.07)$, and (ii) $H_P(10)$. The H_P (0.07) dose equivalent is an operational quantity for individual monitoring for the assessment of dose to skin and hands and foot. H_P (10) dose equivalent is an operational quantity for individual monitoring for the assessment of effective dose.

Personnel dose equivalent can be assessed indirectly with a thin tissue equivalent detector, which is worn at the surface of the body. It is covered with suitable tissue equivalent material. The depth is usually where the radiation dosimeter is worn. In the case of superficial organs, depths of 0.07 mm for skin and 3 mm for eye lens are used. It is referred as shallow depth dose equivalent.

In the case of assessment of deep organs, a depth of 10 mm is used which is referred as deep dose equivalent. If the personnel dosimeter is worn on a position of the body, the value of H_P (10) provides an effective dose value, which is precise enough for radiological protection. In the above, it is assumed that the dose is low with uniform whole-body exposure.

Operational quantities are measurable and instruments for radiation monitoring are calibrated in terms of these quantities. Neutron and gamma radiations contribute both shallow and deep doses, whereas beta is completely absorbed at skin level.

Total Effective Dose Equivalent

Total effective dose equivalent (TEDE) is the quantity defined by *Nuclear Regulatory Commission (NRC, US)*. It is used to monitor and control human exposures to ionizing radiations. It is the sum of the effective dose equivalent from external exposure and committed effective dose equivalent (CEDE) from internal exposure. Thus, it addresses all known radiation exposures both from external and internal. It is useful to monitor occupational exposures especially in nuclear medicine and interventional radiology.

Committed Absorbed Dose

If an individual is subjected to a radiation burden over a period, then committed absorbed dose is used. It is the absorbed dose the individual receives because of the intake of radioactive material. The individual will continue to receive a dose of radiation if the traces of radioactivity remain within the body:

$$D(\tau)=\int_{t_0}^{t_0+\tau} D(t)dt \tag{1.26}$$

where t_0 is the time of intake, is the absorbed dose at time t, and τ is the time elapsed after an intake of radioactive substance. If is not specified, it is generally taken as 50 years and 70 years for adult and children, respectively. Committed dose is a measure of stochastic risk due to intake of radioactive material into the human body.

Similarly, committed dose equivalent (CDE) and CEDE can be defined. The CDE is specified to know the effect of single organ or tissue exposure over a period. It is obtained by multiplying the equivalent dose by elapsed time ($H_T \times \tau$). For example, if the dose to the lung is 2 mSv due to radon inhalation, then the committed equivalent dose after 60 years is 2 × 60 = 120 mSv.

The CEDE (E_τ) is the product of committed organ or tissue dose and tissue-weighting factor, i.e., $E_{(\tau)} = H_T \times W_T$. For example, a lung exposed to 2 mSv will have its committed effective dose 2 × 0.12 = 0.24 mSv, since lung-weighting factor is 0.12.

Collective Dose

To assess the overall effect of radiation dose on a large group of persons exposed to radiation, ICRP, 1991 recommended collective dose. It accounts the group of persons exposed to radiation and period of exposure. It also represents sum of all individual doses from the source over a specified period. If N is the number of individuals in a population receiving mean organ equivalent dose H_T, over a period τ, then the collective equivalent dose (S_T) is given by:

$$S_T = \Sigma H_{T(\tau)} \times N \tag{1.27}$$

It describes both internal and external dose measurements and its unit is person-Sievert. If 10,000 people receive a mean effective dose of 0.01 Sv, then the collective effective dose is 10,000 × 0.01 = 100 man-Sievert, and old unit is man-rem.

The collective effective dose (S) due to individual effective dose values between E_1 and E_2 is given by:

$$S(E_1, E_2, \Delta T) = \int_{E_1}^{E_2} E \frac{dN}{dE} dE \tag{1.28}$$

where $\frac{dN}{dE}$ refers to number of individuals who are exposed to an effective dose between E and E+ΔE over a period ΔT.

Collective effective dose is intended for use in optimization, especially in radiological protection. It is useful in planning complex work involving varying number of workers and to determine the optimum balance between relatively large exposures to a few workers and lower exposures to a larger number of workers. In public exposures, it is used part of optimization for planned, existing, or emergency exposure situations. Collective effective dose is also useful to compare studies to find radiological impact of different sources of exposure. It is not intended for epidemiological analysis and prediction of health effects in populations.

Worked Example 1.6

If the committed equivalent dose to the lung is 2 mSv from radon inhalation, what is the collective equivalent dose for India like population of 1,200 million?

Committed equivalent dose = 2 mSv = 2×10^{-3} Sv

Population = 1,200 million = $1{,}200 \times 10^6$

Collective equivalent dose (S) = $E_{(\tau)} \times N$

$= 2 \times 10^{-3}$ Sv $\times 1{,}200 \times 10^6$

= 2,400,000 man-Sievert

If we consider the estimate of cancer induction is 80 per person-Sv, then the expected radiation-induced cancer due to radon exposure in India would be about 2,400,000/80 = 30,000. Thus, CEDE can be used as a method to assess the impact of human health from population radiation exposures.

In uranium miners, CEDE is small due to relatively small size of the workforce involved in the occupation. Total annual CEDE for all occupationally exposed workers is about 2,000 person-Sv, for all occupations, whereas the annual CEDE attributable to natural background radiation for the same population is about 3,200 person-Sv. It means that the occupational workers getting an additional 62.5% (2,000/3,200) over the natural background. In general, CEDE is decreasing in medicine due to small size of the exposed population and improved health physics practices.

Genetically Significant Dose

Genetic significant dose, or genetically significant dose (GSD), was initially defined by United Nations Scientific Committee on the Effects of Atomic Radiation (UNSCEAR) in 1958. It represents an estimate of the genetic significance of gonad radiation doses. Annual GSD is calculated by weighting the individual gonad doses received during radiation imaging by the number of individuals examined, and accounting for the number of offspring in every individual.

The GSD is defined as that equivalent dose that, if received by every member of the population, would be expected to produce the same genetic injury to the population as do the actual doses received by the irradiated individuals. It is expressed in Sievert (Sv). It is used to assess the genetic risk or detriment to the whole population from radiation exposure, especially in medicine. It assumes a linear dose-effect relationship. For example, the patients who undergo X-ray examinations may receive a dose of about 10.0 mGy. If the same dose was received by every member of the population, it would be expected to produce the same total genetic effect on the population. The GSD accounts the childbearing potential of the patient population.

In GSD, the equivalent dose to the gonads of each exposed individual is weighted for the number of progenies expected for a person of that sex and age. Annual GSD from all radiation sources is about 1.3 mSv that includes 1.02 mSv (78%) from natural background and 0.28 mSv (22%) from technological sources (NCRP Report 93, 1987). Among the technological sources, the major contributor is diagnostic X-rays, 0.20 mSv (15%). Among the 15%, one-third is attributable to male and two-thirds to females. The higher proportion of female component is due to the location of the ovaries within the pelvis, which places them in the primary beam during most abdominal-pelvic examinations.

Detriment and Nominal Risk Coefficient

Detriment is the term used to quantify the harmful effects (stochastic effect) of radiation at low doses. It considers the severity of disease in terms of—(i) lethality, (ii) quality of life, and (iii) years of life lost. Risk of genetic disorders and harm arising from them up to second generation is also considered in arriving the detriment. ICRP-103 provided calculation of detriment adjusted nominal risk coefficients, which are averaged across populations, all ages and both sexes. They are not intended to use in estimating risk of individuals.

As per ICRP-103, detriment adjusted nominal risk coefficient per Sv for cancer is 5.5% and 4.1% for whole population and adults respectively, whereas it is 0.2% and 0.1% per Sv for heritable effects. Total detriment risk coefficient for whole population and adults is 5.7% and 4.2% per Sv, respectively. The risk coefficient values are lower than that of ICRP-60. The values are based on improved epidemiological analysis and use of incidence rather than mortality data. Lower values of heritable effects are based on available experimental data. To conclude heritable effect, risk is small at low doses compared to the natural frequency of genetic diseases.

As Low as Reasonably Achievable

The term, as low as reasonably achievable (ALARA), was introduced by ICRP-26. It states that doses to patients and staff should be kept as low as reasonably achievable. It is known that the dose limits for workers and public are regarded to be upper limits rather than acceptable doses. In fact, majority of occupational exposures in medicine result in lower doses well below the limits. All users of radiation should carry out good health physics practices and safety program so that the radiation exposures to workers and public are kept by ALARA principle. Every reasonable effort must be made to reduce radiation levels below the stated dose limits within economic and social limits.

As low as reasonably achievable principle should be the focus while making policies, procedures, and practices for radiation facilities. The employee and employer should make commitment to minimize radiation exposures to staffs and the public. ALARA concept is equivalent to that of ICRP's optimization of protection. ICRP not only emphasizes ALARA to the staff and public, but also to the patients, especially in diagnostic and interventional procedures.

Dose and Dose Rate Reduction Effectiveness Factor

Risk factors obtained for cancer induction from Japanese data is related to high dose rate conditions. There is difficulty in using this data for low LET radiations with low dose rate. Radiobiological studies suggest that dose and dose rate effectiveness factor (DDREF) is required to estimate cancer risk at low dose rate. It reduces effectiveness of low LET radiation for cancer induction. ICRP recommends DDREF of 2 for low LET radiations. It is applicable for all absorbed doses <0.2 Gy and for all exposures of dose rates <0.1 Gy/h. There is no DDREF factor for high LET radiation.

PROBLEMS

1. What would be the radiation level at 1 meter from a 15 Ci ^{192}Ir source? (RHM of ^{192}Ir = 0.49R/Ci at 1 m)

   Answer: 7.5 R/h

2. What would be the radiation level (R/h) at a distance of 10 meters from a 10 Ci ^{192}Ir source? (RHM of ^{192}Ir = 0.49R/Ci at 1 m)

   Answer: 50 mR/h

3. What is the distance in meter required to reduce the radiation level from a 5 Ci ^{60}Co source to 2.5 mR/h? (RHM of ^{60}Co = 1.3R/Ci at 1 m).

   Answer: 51 meters

4. While handling a ^{137}Cs source with 2-feet manipulator rod, the radiation level at the operator's position is 100 mR/h. What would be the radiation level at the operator's position if he uses 8-feet manipulator rod instead of the 2-feet rod?

   Answer: 6.25 mR/h

5. While handling a 5 Ci ^{192}Ir with a 0.5-m manipulator rod, within how much time the operator will receive the weekly maximum permissible dose? (RHM of ^{192}Ir = 0.49 R/h-Ci at 1 m, weekly permissible dose 100 mR)

   Answer: 36 seconds

6. While handling a 5 Ci ^{192}Ir with 0.5-m manipulator rod, the operator takes 15 seconds for a single exposure operation, and the weekly permissible dose will be received even with two such exposures. If a 2-m manipulator rod is used instead of 50-cm rod, how much is the allowed time?

   Answer: 8 minutes

7. If the radiation exposure from a source at 1 meter is 100 mR, how much is the exposure at 25 cm?

   Answer: 6.25 mR

8. A source has an exposure rate of 40,000 R/h at some distance. How much shielding material in TVT and HVT is required to reduce the exposure rate to 100 R/h?

   Answer: 2 TVT + 2 HVT

9. What is the thickness lead required in TVT to reduce the dose rate from 5 Ci ^{192}Ir source to 2.5 mR/h at a distance of 1 m from the source? (RHM of ^{192}Ir = 0.49 R/Ci at 1 m).

   Answer: 3 TVT of lead

10. What is the thickness of concrete shielding required to reduce the dose rate from 10 Ci ^{60}Co source to 0.25 mR/h at a distance of 5 m from the source? (RHM for ^{60}Co = 1.3 R/Ci at 1 meter).

    Answer: 3 TVT + 2 HVT concrete thickness

11. What would be radiation level at a distance of 2 meter from a 15 Ci ^{137}Cs source provided with a 3-inch steel shielding? (RHM of ^{137}Cs = 0.32 R/Ci at 1 meter, reduction factor for steel = 15.5).

    Answer: 80 mR/h

12. Calculate the amount of shielding thickness in terms of steel which will reduce the dose rate from a 5 Ci ^{60}Co source to 2 mR/h at 1 m (RHM of ^{60}Co = 1.3 R/Ci at 1 meter, TVT of steel for ^{60}Co = 6.6 cm, HVT of lead for ^{60}Co = 2 cm).

    Answer: 23.8 cm

13. The radiation level at a particular distance from a lead source container having a ^{192}Ir source is 100 mR/h (TVT of lead for ^{192}Ir = 1.6 cm, HVT of lead for ^{192}Ir = 0.5 cm)
    (i) What is the amount additional thickness of lead to be provided to the container to reduce the radiation level to 0.5 mR/h at the same distance?
    (ii) Instead, if 2 inch of the lead shielding is removed from the container, what would be the radiation level at the same distance?

    Answer:
    (i) 3.7 cm
    (ii) 200 R/h

14. Calculate the shielding requirement in terms of HVT and TVT to reduce an X-ray exposure level of 500 mR/h to 2.5 mR/h (assume it is a 150 kV X-ray beam, further filtration do not change the HVT).

    Answer: 2 TVT + 1 HVT

15. The measured output of a telecobalt machine is 200 RMM. What will be the exposure rate at 1 meter if lead sheets of thickness 6 cm are interposed between the unit and the detector?

Answer: 6.25 R/m

16. The exposure rate of ^{137}Cs source at a point is 120 mR/h. How much lead should be interposed between the source and the point so that exposure level could be brought down to 0.25 mR/h at that point (HVT of lead –0.6 cm).

Answer: 5.4 cm

17. The exposure rate from a telecobalt machine is 200 RMM. What are the exposures rates at—(i) 1 cm, (ii) 2 meter, (iii) 3 meter, and (iv) 4 meter?

Answer: (i) 2,000,000 R/m, (ii) 50 R/m, (iii) 22.2 R/m, and (iv) 12.5 R/m

18. The exposure rate at 2 meter from the source is 120 mR/h. For how long the engineer can work at distance of—(i) 3 meter and (ii) 5 meter, without exceeding the dose equivalent limits? (Dose equivalent limit 20 mSv/year)

Answer: (i) 46 min/week, (ii) 122 min/week

19. The exposure rate from a source at a point where the engineers are doing servicing is 120 mR/h. On an average for how much time can the engineer work at this point without exceeding the dose equivalent limits?

Answer: 4 min/day

BIBLIOGRAPHY

1. Bushberg JT, Seibert JA, Leidholdt EM, Boone JM. The essential physics of medical imaging, 3rd edition. Philadelphia: Wolters Kluwer/Lippincott Williams & Wilkins; 2012.
2. Dowsett DJ, Kenny PA, Johnston RE. The physics of diagnostic imaging, 2nd edition. UK: Hodder Arnold; 2006.
3. ICRP. (2018). The use of effective dose as a radiological protection quantity. ICRP publication 120, Annals of ICRP-Draft recommendations, 2018. [online] Available from https://www.icrp.org/page.asp?id=382. [Last accessed September, 2022].
4. ICRP. International Commission on radiological Protection ICRP-103 annals of ICRP. Oxford, United Kingdom: Pergamon Press; 2007.
5. IRCP. International Commission on radiological Protection ICRP-26 annals of ICRP. Oxford, United Kingdom: Pergamon Press; 1977.
6. IRCP. International Commission on radiological Protection ICRP-60 annals of ICRP. Oxford, United Kingdom: Pergamon Press; 1991.
7. Sherer MAS, Visconti P, Ritenour ER, Haynes KW. Radiation protection in medical radiography, 7th edition. Maryland Heights: Elsevier; 2014.
8. Thayalan K. Basic radiological physics, 2nd edition. New Delhi: Jaypee Brother's Medical Publishers; 2017.
9. US Nuclear Regulatory Commission. (2011). Safety culture policy statement, NUREG/BR-0500. [online] Available from https://www.nrc.gov/reading-rm/doc-collections/nuregs/brochures/br0500/index.html. [Last accessed September, 2022].
10. Cherry SR, Sorenson JA and Phelps ME. Physics of Nuclear Medicine, 4th Edition, Elsevier Saunders, 2012.

CHAPTER 2

Radiation Biology

INTRODUCTION

Radiation biology deals with the study of the nature of damage caused by ionizing radiation on body tissues. The degree of response of body tissue against radiation exposure depends on various factors such as type of radiation, amount of dose, dose rate, fractionation, nature of exposure (whole body/partial body), cell cycle, presence of radioprotectors or sensitizers, and age of the exposed individual, etc. This chapter gives an overview of radiobiology related to medical exposures of ionizing radiation.

CELL

Cells are divided into two types, namely prokaryotic, e.g., bacteria, and eukaryotic, e.g., animal cell. Human body is a multicellular organism, and the size of each cell is around 10^{-15} μm. Adult human body contains about 10^{14} cells. Cell is a structural and functional unit of every living organism (*Robert Hooke*, 1665). Cells of similar nature constitute a tissue and different tissues form an organ. Many organs constitute a system, namely integumentary, skeletal, muscular, nervous, endocrine, circulatory, lymphatic, respiratory, digestive, urinary and reproductive systems.

Body cells are classified into somatic cells and germ cells. All cells of the body are considered as somatic cells except the cells, which participate in the reproductive process. The cells which are involved in the reproductive process are called germ cells. They are sperm in males and ovum in females. Human body contains 23 pairs of chromosomes. Among these, 22 pairs are called autosomes and one pair is called sex chromosomes. Male has 22 pairs of autosomes and one pair of sex chromosomes, namely X and Y chromosomes. Female has 22 pairs of autosomes and one pair of X chromosomes as sex chromosomes.

Mammalian cell consists of a nucleus, cytoplasm, internal membrane, and outer plasma membrane (**Fig. 2.1**). Cytoplasm is a viscous liquid occupies about 70% of cell volume and consists various organelles such as mitochondria, rough and smooth endoplasmic reticulum, Golgi complex, lysosome, and ribosome. Each organelle has a specific function of its own. For example, ribosome plays a role in protein synthesis, Golgi complex modifies proteins before use, mitochondria provides the necessary energy for cell function, and lysosomes are the digestive organelle of the cell.

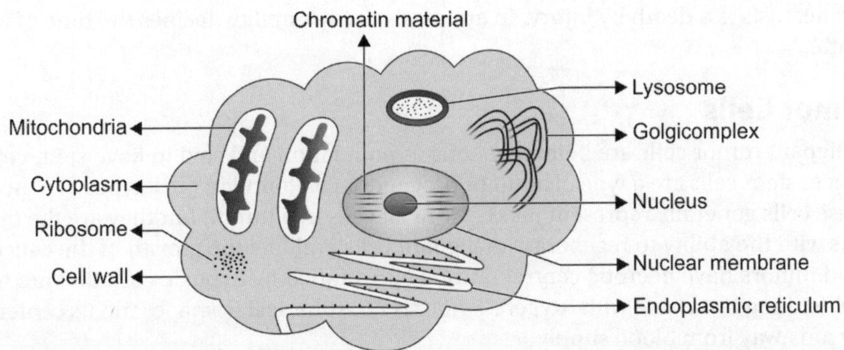

FIG. 2.1: Mammalian cell structure containing, nucleus, cytoplasm, internal membrane, and outer plasma membrane.

Nucleus and Deoxyribonucleic Acid

The nucleus is a control center of the cell, contains deoxyribonucleic acid (DNA), and nucleolus. It has machinery for DNA replication and ribonucleic acid (RNA) transcription and processing. It is enveloped in a double membrane and the outer membrane is fused with endoplasmic reticulum.

Deoxyribonucleic acid is double-stranded form, having helical structure with series of repeating nucleotides arranged in certain sequence. Nucleotide contains a nucleobase [adenine (A), guanine (G), cytosine (C), or thymine (T)], a pentose sugar, and phosphorous. Nucleotide present on one strand is connected to the nucleotide present on the opposite strand by hydrogen bond. Sections of DNA contain information for specific functions called genes. The double-stranded DNA is in the form of helical structure with a width of about 2 nm and is wound around histones, which undergo condensation to form chromatin. It appear as beads-on-a-string with dimension of 11 nm. It is closely packed as series of looped domains wound in a tight helix. Extended form of chromosome has the dimension of 300 nm, whereas the final condensed metaphase chromosome is 1,400 nm. Any damage to DNA molecule such as single-strand break (SSB) is recognized by repair enzymes and repairs perfectly. However, if the damage is severe like double-strand break (DSB), the repair may be a right repair or wrong repair. The wrong repair may lead to cell death or mutation.

Cell Cycle and Death

Cell undergoes cell division to produce two daughter cells. During this process, the cell undergoes various phases such as G1 (gap 1), S (synthesis), G2 (gap 2), and M (mitosis). The G1, S, and G2 are said to be interface of the cycle. During the S phase, the DNA molecule is replicated into two molecules. Cell cycle is regulated by *cyclin-dependent kinase (Cdk)*. The length of each phase varies with the type of cells, mitosis is the shortest phase (hour), and S phase lasts for 6–8 hours. Cell cycle variation is generally due to the differences in the length of G1 phase.

Mitosis is further divided into four phases, namely *prophase, metaphase, anaphase, and telophase. Mitotic index* is the ratio of cells in mitosis to the total number of cells in the sample. Cell division process of germ cell is referred as meiosis, and it has two stages, namely meiosis I, and meiosis II.

Cell death may be in three ways, namely—(i) autophagy, (ii) necrosis, and (iii) apoptosis or programmed cell death. Autophagy is the process of self-degradation, and necrosis is a death by injury. In apoptosis, body's ability decides the time of cell death.

Tumor Cells

Malignant tumor cells are heterogeneous in population and said to have stem cells. Cancer stem cells are a type of adult or progenitor cell found in most types of cancer. These cells generally represent just 1–3% of all cells in a tumor, but they are the only cells with the ability to regenerate malignant cells and fuel the growth of the cancer. Solid tumors have necrotic central portion surrounded by hypoxic cells that are not proliferating but viable with oxygen. Tumor is not spherical in shape, and its center is 200 μm away from blood supply.

Tumor staging is the estimation of extent of the tumor spread. There are four stages, namely stage 1, stage 2, stage 3, and stage 4. *Union for International Cancer Control* (*UICC*) has suggested TNM staging based on primary tumor (T), nodal spread (N), and distant metastasis (M) status. In addition, American Joint Committee on Cancer (AJCC) staging, and Fédération Internationale de Gynécologie et d'Obstétrique (FIGO) staging for gynecological cancer are available. Detailed discussion of tumor staging is beyond the scope of this text.

INTERACTION OF RADIATION WITH CELLS

Radiation deposits energy in tissues randomly via excitation, ionization, and thermal heating. Time interval between the radiation exposure and manifestation of effects is divided into four stages, namely (i) physical stage, (ii) physiochemical stage, (iii) chemical stage, and (iv) biological stage. In physical stage, biomolecules, which absorb energy, result in excited and ionized molecules (10^{-13} s). Physiochemical stage involves formation of free radicals and primary lesions in target molecules (10^{-10} s). In chemical stage, primary lesions result in molecular alterations (10^{-6} s). In biological stage, the molecular alteration causes biological effects (seconds-years). Biological effects include lethality, mitotic inhibition, division delay, chromosome aberration, and mutation.

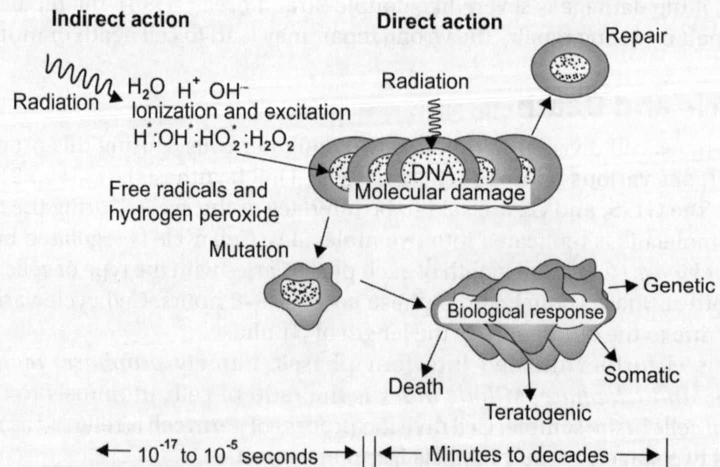

FIG. 2.2: Interaction of radiation in cell: Physical, chemical, and biological response of ionizing radiation by both direct and indirection action.

Direct and Indirect Action

Radiation causes biologic effects by interacting with the target molecules either directly or indirectly **(Fig. 2.2)**. Direct action is dominant in high-linear energy transfer (LET) radiations. For example, an alpha particle breaks the chemical bonds directly in a DNA molecule. In indirect action, radiation interacts with water molecules in the cell and produces free radicals, a process known as *radiolysis of water*. Free radicals are atoms or molecules or ions with an unpaired electron in the outermost shell. They are highly reactive, interact with biomolecules, and cause damage. Indirect action is a dominant process in low LET radiations. The damaging effect of free radical is enhanced in the presence of oxygen.

Radiolysis of Water

Human body cell is composed of about 80% water. The absorption of radiation by water molecule results in ion pairs (H_2O^+, H_2O^-), which are unstable and form free radicals such as H* (hydrogen), OH* (hydroxyl), and hydrated electron (e^-_{aq}).

$$H_2O + \text{X-ray} \rightarrow H_2O^+ + H_2O^-$$

$$H_2O^+ \rightarrow H^+ + OH^*$$

$$H_2O^- \rightarrow H^* + OH^- \qquad (2.1)$$

CELL SURVIVAL CURVES

If cells are irradiated with ionizing radiation it will result in partial cell death and partial survival of cells. Cells that lose reproductive capacity and fail to divide further are called dead cells. Cells that retain reproductive capacity and able to divide indefinitely are called surviving cells. There is direct relation between number of cells killed and the radiation exposure. Radiation dose and the surviving fraction (SF) of cells can be plotted in a semi-log paper, which is referred as *survival curve*. This curve is useful to understand the radiosensitivity, repair, and recovery ability of the cell. SF is a fraction of cells that survive after radiation exposure:

$$SF = \frac{\text{Number of colonies counted}}{\text{Number of celles seeded} \times \text{Plating efficiency}} \qquad (2.2)$$

where, plating efficiency (PE) is the percentage of seeded cells that survive to form colonies under control conditions, which is obtained by in vitro study. To express this in mathematical terms, *(i) point heat theory, (ii) target theory, and (iii) linear quadratic (LQ) theory* were proposed. As per point heat theory, absorption of radiation enhances temperature, which is responsible for the inactivation of cells, which was not successful.

Target Theory

Target theory (*Crowther and Lea*) assumes critical targets in cell, which needs to be hit to kill the cells. This theory includes single-target, multitarget, and multihit models. Single target model does not account for dose rate, fractionation, and irradiation environment. Multitarget model assumes more than one target and the survival curve appears with shoulder. Cell inactivation needs at least one hit to each target in cell. It fails to explain the experimental results of survival fraction of cells. Multihit theory assumes single target, which needs more than one hit. In general, survival curve exhibits initial linear part, shoulder, and final linear part. D_0 is the dose required to reduce the survival from 1 to 0.37, often referred as D_{37}. The number of targets (n) in the cell is a measure of width of the shoulder. However, there is no shoulder for radiations of high LET. The initial slope of the survival curve is not explained by the above models.

Linear Quadratic Model

Linear quadratic model accounts both single-hit and two-hit events in cell death. Single hit refers to initial part of the survival curve where cell killing is linear. At higher doses, two-hit events are involved, which are quadratic in nature. It believes that cell killing is caused by DSBs, which have both linear and quadratic part in the survival curve **(Fig. 2.3)**. The linear part is due to single ionizing event, quantified by αD, where α is the probability for such events per unit dose. The quadratic part is due to two separate ionizing events quantified by βD^2, where β is the probability of such events per unit dose. The α damage is irreparable, whereas β damage is reparable. The surviving fraction (S) of cells is given by:

$$S = e^{-(\alpha D + \beta D^2)}$$

Or,

$$-\ln S = (\alpha D + \beta D^2) \tag{2.3}$$

The LQ model explains the cell killing in a better way in the low-dose region (0–3 Gy) and clinically much useful. The dose D at which cell killing due to linear and quadratic component is equal is given by:

$$\alpha D = \beta D^2 \text{ or } D = \frac{\alpha}{\beta} \text{ ratio} \tag{2.4}$$

This ratio varies with the type of cells. For early reacting normal tissues and tumor cells, $\frac{\alpha}{\beta}$ ratio is high and for late reacting normal tissue, $\frac{\alpha}{\beta}$ ratio is low. Studying the $\frac{\alpha}{\beta}$ ratio is useful to compare the radiosensitivity of different cell lines as the shape of the survival curve is determined by this ratio. As per this model, the shape of the curve is continuously bending which is not observed experimentally. It is also against the belief that cell killing is an exponential function of dose represented by a straight line in a semi-log plot. Although this model has certain drawbacks mentioned above, it is sufficient to explain the cell killing for doses used in fractionation applied in clinical radiotherapy.

DNA DAMAGE AND ITS REPAIR

Deoxyribonucleic acid (DNA) is the most important target molecule, which undergoes variety of changes such as intramolecular cross-linking, intrastrand cross-linking, degradation, etc., due to radiation. Intramolecular cross-linking refers to the cross-linking that occurs between bases on the same strand of a DNA. Intermolecular cross-linking includes DNA–DNA, and DNA–protein cross-link. In intrastrand cross-linking, two adjacent thymine bases on the same strand of DNA get linked to each

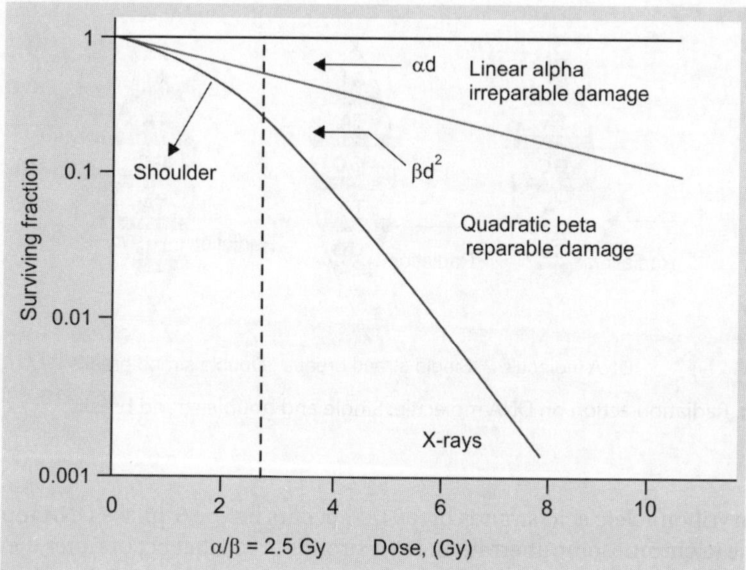

FIG. 2.3: The survival curve and the linear quadratic model for mammalian cells exposed to X-rays. The dose at which the linear and quadratic components are equal is the ratio of alpha/beta.

other by covalent bond. It reduces the distance between two thymine molecules resulting in distortion of the sugar–phosphate backbone.

Deoxyribonucleic acid degradation occurs due to breaks in DNA strand. The break may be either SSB or DSB. If the break is located on one strand, it is referred as SSB. It is easy to repair by taking a template from opposite strand. Oxygen can cause the broken strand becomes per oxidized and prevent it from rejoining. Thus, presence of oxygen potentiates the radiation damage. If two breaks are located on opposite strands, separated by five bases, it is referred as DSB. It is difficult to repair since template from opposite strand is not available for repair. DSB is repaired by homologous recombination (HR) and nonhomologous end joining (NHEJ). If the repair is not proper, it may lead to mutation. This may lead to carcinogenesis through activation of oncogenes, inactivation of tumor suppressor genes, or loss of heterozygosity. A DSB can result in chromosome aberrations. Base damage includes deletion, substitution, and addition to one or both strands of DNA. The loss of change of base is also considered as mutation **(Fig. 2.4)**.

In addition to the above, radiation also causes other damages such as deamination, depurination, oxidation, opening of ring structures, and denaturation. Extent to which the different kinds of molecular lesions affect the cells depends on nature of repair systems present.

The DNA checkpoints monitor the damage at specific points within the cell cycle. It halts the cell cycle to allow time to repair the damage.

Chromosome Aberrations

There are two types of chromosome aberrations namely stable and unstable aberrations. Stable aberration is carried out through number of cell divisions, whereas unstable aberration leads to cell death.

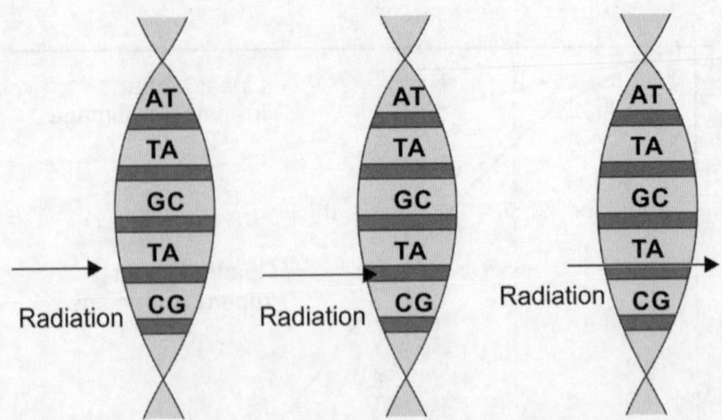

FIG. 2.4: Radiation action on DNA molecule: Single and double strand breaks.

Deoxyribonucleic acid strands break that occurs before S-phase DNA replication gives rise to chromosome aberration. DNA strands break that occurs after the S phase [irradiation of cells in the late interphase (G2)] is called chromatid aberrations. In this, one arm of the sister chromatid is broken.

The unstable chromosome aberrations are: *(i) dicentric, (ii) ring, and (iii) anaphase bridge.* In dicentric, the broken ends of two different chromosomes get united resulting in the formation of dicentric chromosome with two centromeres, hence the name dicentric. In ring aberration, the breaks that occur in both arms of a chromatin get united and appear as ring. Ring and dicentric formation is due to strong force of cohesion between broken ends. In anaphase bridge, the damaged sister chromatids do not separate properly, instead stretch to either pole of the cell. It occurs in late interface and prevents separation of parent into daughter, resulting reproductive death.

Stable chromosome aberrations are: *(i) symmetric translocation and (ii) small interstitial deletion.* In symmetric translocation, break occurs in two different chromosomes at the early interphase (G1) and later broken ends are exchanged and get rejoined. It presents for several years and are passed on to the progeny. This can be easily seen in fluorescent in situ hybridization (FISH) and chromosome painting techniques. In small interstitial deletion, two breaks occur in the same arm of a single chromosome and the sticky ends may rejoin with deletion and loss of DNA. It may lead to malignancy in humans.

The frequency of chromosomal aberrations increases with radiation dose, hence, the magnitude of aberrations is used as an indicator of radiation dose absorbed. Dicentric chromosome aberrations (DCAs) in human lymphocytes are scored and used to estimate radiation dose.

Mutation

Mutation is a change in DNA base sequence that is not recognized by repair enzymes. It has changes in large segment of DNA such as deletion, which encompass more than one gene. There are about 25,000–30,000 genes in human genome, which occupy specific position on the chromosome. The gene has hereditary information, which is coded in the form of specific sequence of bases in DNA. Individual receives two identical genes from his/her parents. In other words, mutation is the change in the information that contained in genes. Muted cell may have normal reproductive capacity but have altered information in one of the gene. Gene mutation may be either dominant or recessive. Dominant means that a single copy of the gene, if mutated, is enough to cause the disease. Recessive means both the copies of the gene need to be mutated to cause the disease. *Huntington's* disease is a common example of an autosomal-dominant genetic disorder.

Radiation can cause mutations both in germ cells and somatic cells. Mutations that occur in somatic cell may lead to cancer induction. Mutations that occur in germ cells (sperm or ova) are passed onto the progeny of the host. Germ cell mutation leads to heritable diseases in the offspring known as genetic mutation.

Radiation Damage in Cells

Radiation damage in mammalian cells is divided *into—(i) lethal damage (LD), (ii) potentially LD (PLD), (iii) sublethal damage (SLD), and (iv) nonlethal damage (NLD).*

The LD is an irreparable damage caused by radiation leads to cell death. Cell fails in reproductive capacity resulting interphase and mitotic death. PLD is lethal under normal conditions, but repair is possible if the postirradiation environment is manipulated. If several hours are allowed between irradiations, cells get repaired. It delays the complex mitosis process and permits DNA damage repair, referred as *rest and recover*. Properly repaired cell continues to function normally, and improper repair leads cell fatality or undergoes mutation.

Sublethal damage is repaired in few hours after irradiation. Repair of SLD is the inherent process by the cell system and supports appearance of shoulder in the survival curve. Repair of SLD is related to radiation quality and dose rate and is seen with low LET radiation. Similarly, repair of SLD is more with low-dose rate compared to high-dose rate radiation. NLD is one in which cell continues to reproduce.

BIODOSIMETRY

In biodosimetry, radiation-absorbed dose is determined by analyzing a biological sample such as blood obtained from the exposed person. It is useful in determining the radiation dose received by a person who is accidentally exposed to high radiation dose (>100 mGy). It helps the exposed individual in assessing the required course of medical management. Various biodosimetric techniques are: *(i) Dicentric Chromosome aberration (DCA) assay, (ii) micronucleus assay, (iii) FISH, (iv) premature chromosome condensation, and (v) γH2AX assay.*

For biological dosimetry purpose, the cell to be assayed should be matured with a long residence time in the body and should be easily obtained from the body. The small lymphocyte present in the blood is highly suitable for this purpose. Generally, the cell is in the stage of cell cycle; hence, it is ideal to collect these cells for biological dosimetry. Though various methods are available, the gold standard for estimation of radiation dose is DCA technique. It is referred as *chromosome aberration analysis (CAA)* and useful in the dose range of 0.1–6 Gy.

Dicentric chromosome aberration assay is based on dicentric scoring in a metaphase spread. This involves many steps with stringent requirements. To perform DCA assay, blood sample is collected within few weeks of whole-body exposure from the exposed individual, and lymphocytes are cultured in growth medium containing antibiotics and phytohemagglutinin (PHA) for 48 hours at 37°C. The PHA is added to stimulate cells to divide. At 45 hours, colcemide is added to arrest the cells at metaphase. At 48 hours, the culture is centrifuged, and the cells are suspended in 0.075 M KCl for 10 minutes to provide hypotonic treatment. The cells are then resuspended in fixative (3:1 methanol:acetic acid). Cells are washed again with the above fixative and the slides are prepared and stained with fluorescence and Giemsa. The cells are then scored for chromosomal aberration analysis. Cells having aberrations such as dicentrics and rings are carefully noted. For biological dosimetry purpose, several hundred cells are scored to get the right estimation of dose. The scoring is studied with a standard dose response curve to estimate the radiation dose.

It is important that the laboratory carrying out the biological dosimetry work must construct its own dose-response curve. The dose-response curve is prepared by exposing in vitro blood samples with different radiation doses. The aberration per cell for each dose is scored. Then, a graph is fitted between absorbed dose (Gy) and aberrations per cell in X- and Y-axis, respectively. The frequency of chromosome aberration is a LQ function of dose for low LET radiation.

MODIFICATION OF RADIATION DAMAGE OR CELL SURVIVAL CURVES

Radiation damage or shape of the survival curve can be modified by the following factors: (i) oxygen, (ii) LET, (iii) dose rate, (iv) dose fractionation, (v) cell cycle stage, (vi) radioprotectors, (vii) radiosensitizers, and (viii) hyperthermia. These are the physical and biological factors influencing cell survival often referred as dose-modifying agents.

Oxygen Effect

Oxygen is a radiosensitizer that can be used to increase cell killing. In the absence of oxygen, cells show resistance to cell killing. The ratio of dose required to bring certain level of damage with oxygen (euoxic) to that without oxygen (anoxic) is called *oxygen enhancement ratio (OER)*. *Barendsen et al.* established the dependence of OER on LET for mammalian cells. Oxygen effect is very important for low LET radiations and it ranges from 2.5 to 3. The OER decreases as LET increases and become 1 for alpha and 1.6 for neutron. Hence, oxygen is important only for low LET radiations. Cells are well oxygenated, if the oxygen tension is about 20–40 mm Hg in human body.

It is believed that tumor consists both oxygenated and hypoxic cells. Since capillaries are far away, it limits diffusion of nutrients and oxygen to the cells deep inside the tumor. Hypoxic cells show high degree of resistance to radiation. Fractionation, hyperbaric oxygen, high LET radiation, hypoxic sensitizer, and hyperthermia can be used to overcome hypoxic cell resistance.

Linear Energy Transfer

The LET is the average energy deposited by the ionizing radiation per unit path length of the medium through which it traverses and is given by the unit keV/μm **(Table 2.1)**. More densely ionizing radiation deposits greater energy along their path than sparingly ionizing radiation (Refer Chapter 1, **Table 1.1**). All radiations can produce same type of biologic effects, but the magnitude of the effect per unit dose differs. In other words, different radiations of equal dose do not produce the same level of biologic response. To evaluate the effectiveness of different radiations, *relative biological effectiveness (RBE)* is used:

$$\text{RBE} = \frac{\text{Dose of high energy X-rays above 200 kV or } ^{60}\text{Co or } ^{137}\text{Cs gamma radiation required to produce certain effect}}{\text{Dose of test radiation required to produce the same effect}} \quad (2.5)$$

Effects include chromosomal mutation, cataract formation and acute lethality, etc.

Relative biological effectiveness increases with LET and reaches maximum at 100 keV/μm and decreases with further increase in LET **(Fig. 2.5)**. Maximum value indicates that the LET required to produce optimum number of ionizations to inactivate the cell and additional energy deposited get wasted. Thus, beyond 100 keV/μm, the RBE decreases with increasing LET due to overkill of cells.

Relative biological effectiveness variation depends not only on LET but also on dose rate, fractionation, temperature, oxygen concentration, pressure, absence of

TABLE 2.1 **The LET of X- and γ-rays and tissue penetration in HVL.**

X- and γ-rays energy (keV)	*LET (keV/μm)*	*HVL (mm) in tissue*	*Source*
80	1.0	38	Diagnostic X-rays
140	1.5	46	^{99m}Tc
364	2.8	65	^{131}I
511	3.5	70	Positron emitters
1,000	5.2	100	^{60}Co

(LET: linear energy transfer)

Courtesy: David J. Dowsett, 2006.

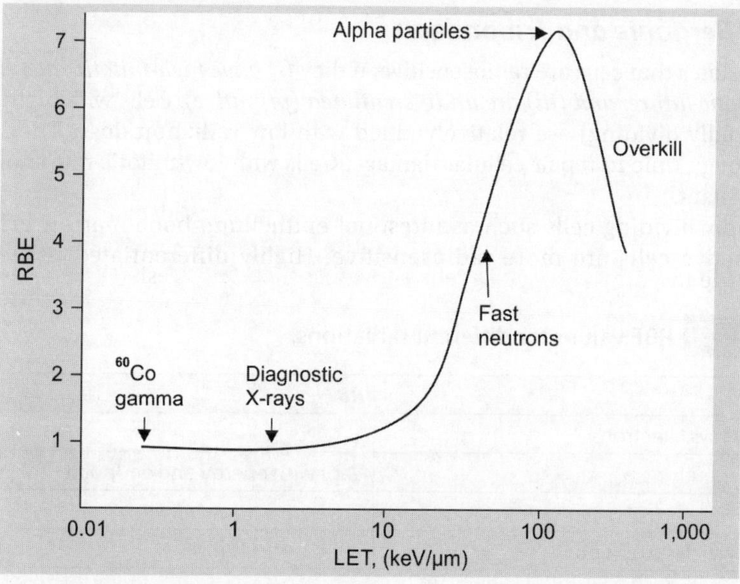

FIG. 2.5: The relation between linear energy transfer and relative biological effectiveness. It is flat initially, then increases with LET and reaches maximum later decreases.

free radicals, and dose distribution within the irradiated material. The specific ionization of 100 ion pairs per micron in water due to X-rays is taken as unity, which is equivalent to LET of 3.5 keV per micron in water. The RBE values of different radiations are different **(Table 2.2)**.

High LET radiations such as carbon ions, negative pion, proton, neutron, and Cf-252 have higher RBE compared to X-rays. The hypoxic cell resistance is much lower and variation of radiosensitivity with cell cycle also smaller for high LET radiations.

Success of high LET radiations in radiotherapy depends upon the *therapeutic gain factor*. It is defined as the ratio of RBE for tumor cells to that of normal tissue. RBE values have been obtained for many tumors, and normal tissues. It is believed that tumor have higher RBE due to the presence of hypoxic cells. In many tumors, the RBE is between that of skin and the intestine. Hence, application of fast neutron in tumor depends on the type of tumor and the normal tissue associated with it.

Carbon ion radiotherapy (CIRT) is practiced in many centers due its highest LET and high RBE (2.5–5). It has Bragg peak and offers clustered damages in DNA. It provides higher dose distribution to the target while reducing dose to organs at risk (OAR). It is suitable for slow-growing tumors with dose escalation.

Cell Cycle

Cell sensitivity to radiation depends on phases of cell cycle due to variation of cell's repair capacity. Most sensitive cells are those in M and late G2 phase, their survival curve is steeper and has no shoulder. Cells in the late S phase are radioresistant and their survival curve is less steep with broader shoulder. Cells in G1 and early S have intermediate sensitivity. An asynchronous cell population is selectively killed in M phase during irradiation. Cells become synchronous after the dose fraction. Position of cells in the second fraction decides the degree of cell kill. To overcome the radiosensitivity variation of cell cycle, fractionation and high LET are used in radiotherapy.

Law of Bergonie and Tribondeau

The law states that cells are radiosensitive, if they *(i) have high-mitotic rate, (ii) have long mitotic future, and (iii) are undifferentiated (primitive).* Cells with high-mitotic rate (rapidly dividing) are relatively killed with low-radiation dose. They do not have enough time to repair cellular damage. Cells with low-mitotic rate show more radioresistant.

Rapidly dividing cells such as intestinal epithelium, bone marrow cells, and reproductive cells are more radiosensitive. Highly differentiated tissues such

TABLE 2.2 RBE values for different radiations.

Particle	*RBE*
X-rays, γ-rays, electrons	1
Thermal neutrons	Vary with energy and endpoint
Protons	2
Heavy particles e.g., alpha	20

(RBE: relative biological effectiveness)
Courtesy: Kelsey CA, 2014.

as muscle and brain are least radiosensitive. Liver has long mitotic future and more sensitive than nerve cells. If a part of liver is cut, cells multiply, and liver is regenerated.

Dose Rate Effect

Survival curves of cells irradiated with low LET radiation at low-dose rate show much lesser steepness compared to that of high-dose rate due to repair of SLD of cells. Variation of effectiveness with dose rate is referred as dose rate effect and found in the range of 1 mGy/min to 1 Gy/min. It is absent at high LET radiation since the damage is less accessible to repair.

In clinical radiotherapy, effective cell killing demands a critical dose rate. In critical dose rate, cells are arrested in mitosis and die while attempting division. Critical dose rate for HeLa cells having cell cycle time of 24 hours is 0.3 Gy/h. Wide range of dose rate is used in radiotherapy, few Gy/min in external radiotherapy and 0.5 Gy/h in brachytherapy. 1–125 seeds use 1.3 Gy/day in seed brachytherapy.

Dose Fractionation

Mammalian cell is characterized by wide shoulder and an exponential region at low doses. Initial shoulder reflects the cell's ability to accumulate some damage before it is killed. The damage below the critical level required for cell killing is called sub lethal dose (SLD). *Elkin and Sutton* had showed the ability of cell to recover from such SLD. A given total dose delivered as single fraction is more effective compared to the same dose delivered in two or more fractions separated by an interval. Following irradiation, cells in M phase are killed and those cells in S phase survive. During the interval between fractions, cell survival increases initially and then decreases and reaches a dip at 6 hours, and again increases. The rise in survival during the first 2 hours is due to repair of SLD. After 2 hours, there is a progression of cells into other phases, which results in a dip in the curve.

Recovery of SLD is possible with dose fractionation techniques. Normal tissue recovers in-between fractions and reduces their damage. Survival curves reappear with shoulder in such fractionation. It is also believed that normal tissue repair is better than tumor cells. Fractionation also helps hypoxic cells to certain extent by redistributing cells in the sensitive phases of the cell cycle. However, its role is limited in high LET radiation. Some tumors have wide shoulder, indicate their ability to accumulate SLD, and perform repairs. It may be reason for failure of radiotherapy in certain cases.

Radioprotector

Chemical compound, which offers protection against radiation, is called radioprotector. It causes vasoconstriction by metabolism and reduces oxygen concentration. Cells become hypoxic and get protected from radiation. Such chemicals include $-NH_2$ and -SH groups, e.g., cysteine. *Dose reduction factor (DRF)* is the ratio of the dose required to produce certain effect with protector to that required to produce the same effect without protector. The maximum DRF that can be obtained is about 1.7.

Radioprotectors scavenge free radicals produced by indirect action and donate hydrogen atom to restore DNA structure. It blocks the proxy radicals formed in the presence of oxygen. However, they are ineffective under high LET radiation. New drugs such as *Cystaphos (WR-638) and Amifostine (WR-2721) are* used in radiotherapy for low toxicity.

Radiosensitizer

Radiosensitizers are compounds that sensitize cells to radiation. There are three groups of sensitizers, namely *(i) DNA base analogous, e.g., 5-bromouridine, (ii) formation of active transient, e.g., iodine compounds, and (iii) modifiers of biochemical process, e.g., DNA synthesis.* Sensitization is increased by the formation of free radicals, which in turn enhance radiation damage. It is believed that sensitizer is not metabolized rapidly in tumor cells; hence, it penetrates deep into the tumor and reaches hypoxic cells and making them sensitive to radiation. Efficiency of sensitization is related to electron affinity of the compounds. Sensitivity is quantified by *sensitizer enhancement ratio* (SER). It is the ratio of the radiation dose without sensitizer to the dose with sensitizer and its range is 2–3.

Hyperthermia

Human cells subjected to >41°C temperature become sensitive to radiation, referred as hyperthermia. Heat sensitizes the cell by interfering with repair process and enhances the radiation damage. *Thermal enhancement ratio (TER)* is the ratio of dose required to produce certain damage with radiation alone to that of with radiation and heat and ranges from 1.3 to 1.6. It sensitizes tumor hypoxic cells more than normal cells. Cells in S phase are selectively killed by heat and eliminate cell cycle sensitivity variation. Low LET radiation with hyperthermia offers advantages of high LET radiation.

HUMAN DATA ON EFFECTS OF RADIATION

Radiation hazards were witnessed by the following events in early days:

- Girls engaged in USA in painting watch and clock dials with luminous paint containing radium resulted in bone irradiation (1920–1930)
- Uranium mine workers exposed to radon gas in a closed environment resulted in lung cancer and received lethal dose (Arizona 1950, New Mexico 1960)
- *Early medical radiation workers*: Radiologists, dentists, and technologists had higher incidence of aplastic anemia and leukemia (1896–1910)
- *Patients injected with contrast agent*: Thorotrast agent resulted in cancer of liver and spleen including angiosarcoma and biliary duct carcinomas (1925–1945)
- Patients who had radium-224 injection for tuberculosis treatment ended with bone cancer.
- Children irradiated with X-rays for benign conditions resulted in benign and malignant tumors (1940, 1950)
- Children of Marshall Island exposed to high level of fallout by atomic bomb test lead to thyroid cancer (1954)
- Atomic bomb explosion on *Hiroshima and Nagasaki*—resulted in solid tumors and leukemia (1945)
- Female patients treated with X-rays for postpartum mastitis and other benign conditions showed incidence of breast cancer
- Patients underwent radiation therapy in spine for ankylosing spondylitis and pain relief treatments resulted in leukemia

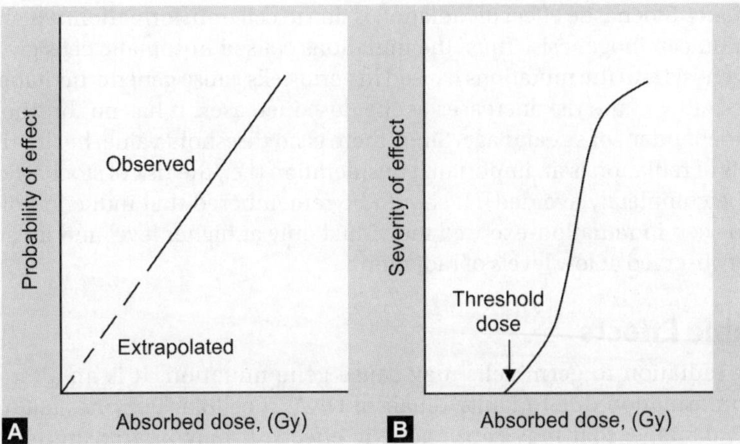

FIGS. 2.6A AND B: Biological effects of radiation: (A) stochastic effect, linear curve without threshold dose, and (B) deterministic effect, quadratic curve with sigmoid and threshold dose.

- Female patients in the *Nova Scotia Sanatorium* had repeated fluoroscopy for pulmonary tuberculosis-increased incidence of breast cancer
- Chernobyl accident had released large amount of radioiodine, which increased the incidence of thyroid cancer in children (1986).

Classification of Radiation Exposure

Radiation exposure can be either chronic or acute exposure based on duration of exposure. Chronic exposure continues to extend over a period from months to years, e.g., low-dose occupational exposure. It does not cause immediate effects to any organ or tissue and the effects may not be observed for many years.

Radiation exposure given in short and finite period (minutes/hours) is called acute exposure, e.g., nuclear reactor accident. It is short-term high-level exposure, which can cause visible changes such as radiation burns, syndrome, and lethality in exposed individuals. An acute dose below 0.1 Gy is unlikely to have any observable effects. An acute dose of 3–5 Gy to whole body has 50% chance of killing the individual. The dose required to cause fatality in 50% of the population within 30/60 days is called $LD_{50/30}$ or $LD_{50/60}$.

Classification of Radiation Effects

The harmful effects of radiation in human body are broadly classified into—(i) stochastic effects and (ii) deterministic effects **(Figs. 2.6A and B)**. Radiation-induced cell killing leads to deterministic effects, whereas cell modification gives stochastic effect. Stochastic effect is further divided into—(i) somatic effects and (ii) hereditary effects. Radiation exposure of somatic cell gives somatic effects, whereas exposure to germ cells leads to hereditary effects.

STOCHASTIC EFFECT

Stochastic effect is the probability of occurrence, which increases with dose, rather than its severity. The dose effect relationship is linear and obey *linear nonthreshold*

(LNT) model. Stochastic effect of radiation is due to cell transformation, which results in radiation carcinogenesis. Thus, the mutations caused in somatic cells give rise to carcinogenesis and the mutations caused in germ cells cause genetic/heritable effect. The probability of the risk increases as the dose increases. It has no threshold dose and is independent of sex and age. Since there is no threshold value, health risk from low levels of radiation is an important consideration (i.e., the risk of stochastic effects cannot be completely avoided). It should be remembered that induction of cancer has been seen in radiation-exposed individual only at higher level and no evidence has been observed at low levels of radiation.

Heritable Effects

Ionizing radiation to germ cells may cause gene mutation. It is an alteration of genetic information due to faulty repair of DNA. If cellular enzymes fail to repair the DNA damage, that may cause genetic effects. It may be transmitted to next generation or in any future generation if reproduction takes place. Radiation-induced genetic effect was first observed by *HJ Muller* (1927) in fruit fly with X-rays. Prevalence of genetic disorders in human population is 70%, but only 10–20% is serious in nature. The doubling dose for human is found to be 1.4–1.8 Gy which could double the frequency of mutations in germ cells.

However, the present knowledge on hereditary effects is limited to laboratory animals. No evidence for increase in hereditary effects or elevated risks were observed in human population exposed to both high and low dose of radiation. Several genetic effects are not observed due to short life span of the individual and liability to reproduce. Only less severe effects are seen in human population because of reproduction. About 30,000 children born to the atomic bomb survivors, exposed to 500 mSv, do not show an increase in the incidence of genetic effect. ICRP-103 (2007) has recommended genetic risk of 0.1% per Sv for workers and 0.2% per Sv for general population, respectively. **Figure 2.7** summarizes both early and late biologic effects due to radiation exposure from 0.001 mSv to 20 Sv.

Radiation Carcinogenesis—Late Somatic Effects

Normal tissues turn into a tumor in steps over a period due to mutation. Mutation results in activation of oncogene, inactivation of tumor suppressor gene, and reduction in the activity of DNA stability genes. As a result, cells undergo transformation and immortalization. It has no threshold for induction of cancer. It has been shown that tobacco and lifestyle play an important role for cancer risk. Genetic and environmental conditions, consumption of alcohol, and exposure to ultraviolet and ionizing radiation are other agents that can increase cancer risk.

Clinically, cancer is a multistep process termed as *initiation, promotion, and progression.* Generally, damaged cell gets repaired and does normal function. Improper repair leads to mutation and is referred as initiation. The mutated cell attains preclinical stage, which is not observable clinically. Viral infection and other physical and chemical agents may promote the cell from preclinical stage to precancer stage. At this stage, it is called minimal cancer but without clinical sign. The promoter need not be a cancer-causing agent. In progression step, precancerous cells converted into cancerous cells with clinically observable signs. Transformed cell produces phenotype clone, evades defense mechanism, and becomes cancer. Cancer cells become metastasis, which may spread to other organs.

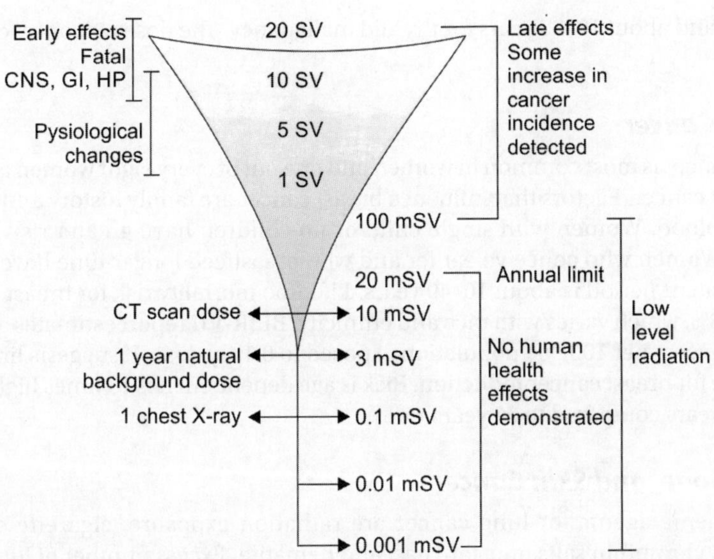

FIG. 2.7: The early and late biologic effects of radiation with dose ranging from 0.001 mSv to 20 SV.

Radiation-induced cancer cannot be differentiated from spontaneous cancer. The risk due to radiation can only be estimated based on the magnitude of exposure. Risk of inducing certain type of cancer is measured by comparing the number of cancers produced in the irradiated population more than those observed in the same size of unirradiated population sample. This is known as risk factor for a specified cancer and is obtained from the population data exposed to high levels of radiation. Since low-dose level dose–effect response is not clear, it is difficult to indicate tumor induction at low doses.

Leukemia

Radiation-induced leukemia is more common since tissue cells are rapidly dividing. It can be acute or chronic with lymphocyte and myeloid form. Acute and chronic myeloid leukemia is reported from >0.2 Sv radiation exposure (Hiroshima and Nagasaki). It can be detected within 1–2 years after exposure, and it reaches a peak after 12 years. It depends upon age at the time of exposure, and it decreases with increase of age. Younger age group is more vulnerable with shorter latent period. BEIR-VII uses LQ model for risk assessment for leukemia as a function of age at exposure. It estimates 70 and 100 leukemia in female and males respectively for an exposure of 0.1 Gy per 100,000 persons with an age distribution equal to US population.

Thyroid Cancer

Thyroid is a sensitive organ, especially in children compared to adults. Women have 2–3 times higher risk than man. Incidence of thyroid cancer is 2% of annual cancer incidence and its mortality rate is 0.2%. Latent period is about 5–35 years for benign nodules and about 10–35 years for thyroid malignancy. The dose response for thyroid is linear.

Breast Cancer

Breast cancer is most common in women and one out of every eight women is affected by breast cancer. Factors that influence breast cancer are family history and estrogen level in blood. Women with single child or no children have greater risk of breast cancer. Women who conceive earlier and who breastfeed longer time have reduced risk. Its latent period is about 10–40 years. Lifetime mortality risk for breast cancer is about 2.8%, which varies with race and ethnicity. BEIR-VII report estimates about 310 breast cancers per 100,000 population exposed to 0.1 Gy dose. It suggests linear dose response for breast cancer induction. Risk is age dependent it is 13 times higher at the age of 5 years compared to 50 years.

Lung, Bone, and Skin Cancer

Carcinogenic agents for lung cancer are radiation exposure, cigarette smoking, asbestos, chromium salts, mustard gas, and hematite. Excess number of lung cancer is reported among uranium miners.

Radiation-induced bone cancer data is minimal. Evidence is available only from patients treated with X-rays and radium watch dial painters exposed to α rays.

Skin cancer includes squamous cell carcinoma and basal cell carcinoma. It can be treated well if detected early. Current safety standard suggests that possibility such skin cancer is rare.

DETERMINISTIC EFFECT

Deterministic effect (nonstochastic) is caused by killing large fraction of cells. Hence, it has threshold dose that depends on radiosensitivity of the cells. Above the threshold dose (>1 Gy) the severity increases with dose. Examples are radiation sickness, sterility, leukopenia, anemia, skin erythema, epilation, skin burns, cataract, and death. It is likely to occur only as the result of radiation accidents and patients irradiated in radiotherapy. It is unlikely in diagnostic radiology, both for patients and occupational workers.

As such, deterministic effects can be completely prevented by limiting the dose levels well below the threshold doses. Time interval between irradiation and the occurrence of deterministic effects is called latent period. It is an indicator for tissue radiosensitivity and inversely proportional to dose. It can be early and late effects.

Early and Late Deterministic Effects

Normal tissues exposed to radiation may manifest deterministic effects as early and late effects. Early effects may appear within few weeks after radiation, whereas late effects appear after month or years. Radiation exposure may lead to loss of function of tissue due to damage of stoma and vasculature and loss of proliferative capacity. These effects can be healed by cellular regeneration and repair process.

Exposure to low levels of radiation over a prolonged period may lead to late somatic effects. Persons who recover from early somatic effects too may develop late somatic effects in life. Late effects are characterized by latent period up to 30 years, e.g., cataract and cancer.

Early Effects on Whole Body

Whole body exposure of dose >1 Gy received in short time may cause *acute radiation sickness or syndrome (ARS).* It starts with symptoms of lack of appetite, nausea, vomiting, and diarrhea followed by headache, fever, and giddiness **(Table 2.3)**. ARSs are classified into:

- Hematopoietic syndrome
- Gastrointestinal syndrome
- Neurovascular syndrome

Hematopoietic syndrome refers to effects on blood and blood-forming organs (<12 Gy). Bone marrow depression results severe anemic conditions and prone to infection. Platelet depletion leads to severe internal bleeding. If bone marrow does not recover within 6–8 hours, death may occur. Lymphocyte counts reach lowest at 48–72 hours. A dose of 2–6 Gy can result life-threatening bone marrow damage.

Gastrointestinal syndromes require a dose of >12–30 Gy to damage the intestinal crypt epithelial cells. Loss of absorption of nutrient, dehydration, loss of weight, severe electrolyte imbalance, and low blood pressure leads to death between 1st and 2nd week. *Neurovascular or central nervous syndrome* occurs at doses >30 Gy. It is due to severe functional damage to the central nervous system. Death may occur within 2 days under coma state.

TABLE 2.3 Early effects due to acute whole-body exposure to low LET radiation.

Dose range	*Effect*
Less than 0.1 Gy	No detectable damage
Above 0.1 Gy	Chromosome aberrations detectable (1–2 dicentrics in 500 cells)
Above 0.5 Gy	Above effect + transient reduction in WBC granulocyte count Temporary sterility in males
Above 1.0 Gy	Above + radiation sickness like loss of appetite, nausea, vomiting, diarrhea (NVD): complete recovery possible at low doses
Above 3.0 Gy	Severity of above effects increases + damage to blood forming organs (bone marrow, spleen, lymph node): death in 4–8 weeks possible (>10%)
3.0–5.0 Gy	All the above with increased severity + anemia, infection, high fever (bone marrow syndrome), about 50% of the exposed persons may die within 60 days ($LD_{50/60}$)
8.0–15.0 Gy	Severity of above effects increases + cells in the gastrointestinal system get severely damaged leading to gastrointestinal syndrome (GIS) such as diarrhea, weight loss, and fever. Death may occur in 1–2 weeks (100%)
Above 10.0 Gy	All the above + manifestation of skin damage
>25 Gy	All the above + severe depression, fatigue, delirium, coma, etc. [central nervous system syndrome (CNS)]. Death occurs in a few hours to days

(LET: AERB: Atomic Energy Regulatory Board; Linear energy transfer)

Courtesy: Atomic Energy Regulatory Board, 2009.

TABLE 2.4 Early effects due to partial body acute exposure with low LET radiation.

Dose	*Region*	*Effect*
0.15 Gy	Testes	Temporary sterility
3.5–6.0 Gy	Testes	Permanent sterility
1.5–2.0 Gy	Ovaries	Temporary sterility
2.5–6.0 Gy	Ovaries	Permanent sterility
3 Gy	Hair follicles	Temporary epilation (fall of hair)
5 Gy	Eye	Cataract (after 5–10 years)
6 Gy	Skin	Skin erythema
10–20 Gy	Skin	Burns, blisters, wounds, necrosis, and permanent hair loss

(LET: linear energy transfer)

Courtesy: Atomic Energy Regulatory Board, 2009.

Effects on Partial Body

Partial body exposure produces only local effects. It may be in the form of sterility, epilation, cataract, skin erythema, burns, blisters, wounds, necrosis, and hair loss **(Table 2.4)**. All the early somatic effects do have a threshold dose, below which they do not occur. Beyond the threshold dose, severity of the effect increases with the dose.

RADIATION EFFECTS ON NORMAL TISSUE AND ORGANS

These are localized organ effects that depend on radiation quality, LET, dose, dose rate, and radiosensitivity of the cell. Organ expresses its response over period with a threshold value. However, these effects can be healed by cellular regeneration and repair process. Important organ effects are skin, blood-forming organs, digestive track, and reproductive systems.

Early Effects of Radiation on Skin

Skin is made up of three layers, namely epidermis, dermis, and subcutaneous tissue. Epidermis consists of dividing cells, which is a target for radiation. Radiation causes erythema, pigmentation, dermatitis, ulceration, necrosis, and malignancy. Erythema and skin burns are most common. Threshold dose for skin is 1 Gy. Dose of 6–10 Gy can cause reddening of skin, >7 Gy can cause loss of hair, and doses of >20 Gy can cause ulceration and necrosis. Skin erythema dose (SED) was used as unit to deliver radiotherapy treatments in early days. It is defined as the X-ray dose required to cause certain degree of erythema within a specified time. The tolerance dose of skin is 60 Gy fractionated over 6–8 weeks.

Skin reactions are severe if the patient is with diabetes mellitus, systemic lupus erythematosus, scleroderma, and homozygosity.

Effects on Blood-forming Organs

The blood-forming organs include bone marrow, spleen, and liver. About 60% of bone marrow lies in pelvis and vertebrae and rest is in ribs, skull, sternum, scapula, and proximal sections of femur and humerus. Bone marrow damage may occur after a threshold dose 3 Gy. Stem cells in blood are radiosensitive which undergo multiplication, maturation, and differentiation without division before becoming mature functional cell. Transient time from stem cells to fully grown functional time varies with circulatory blood components. The cells present in the system include myelocytes, erythroblasts, and megakaryocytes. They mature into polymorphonuclear leukocytes, erythrocytes, and platelets.

A whole-body exposure of 0.3 Gy leads to reduction of lymphocytes, which is most sensitive. A dose of 1 Gy may lead to infection with the symptoms of loss of appetite, nausea, diarrhea, and vomiting. Dose >1 Gy may lead to lymphopenia, granulopenia, thrombopenia, and anemia. A dose of 2 Gy may result in depression of blood counts at 4–5 weeks. A dose of 4–6 Gy may result in temporary raise in granulocytes followed by rapid fall at the end of 1 week. It may result in rapid fall of circulating leukocytes and platelets. If the lymphocytes count falls below 1,200/ mm^3 within 24–48 hours, the prognosis is series, and it falls below 300/mm^3, it may lead to death. Hematopoietic growth factors may be administered to accelerate regeneration of blood cells. Doses >30 Gy may cause aplasia with reduction of stem cells in irradiated volume. Changes in blood counts may exist up to 3 years in patients given fractionated radiotherapy.

Effects on Digestive Track

The radiation exposure to digestive track may affect oral mucosa (tongue, tonsils), esophagus, stomach, small and large intestines. Tongue muscle progresses into fibrosis and fiber atrophy after irradiation. Esophagus contains dividing cells exhibit esophagitis and increased thickness of squamous layer. Desquamation starts at 12th day of irradiation in soft palate and spread to hypopharynx, vallecula, floor of mouth, cheek, etc. Appearance of mucositis and swelling follows in the 3rd week with difficulty in swallowing. The effect is severe during 4th and 5th week. Dysfunction of salivary gland and xerostomia are observed clinically, and symptoms may disappear within 2–4 weeks.

Stomach irradiation causes nausea and vomiting with delayed gastric emptying and epithelial denudement. Ulcer formation is common which leads to bacterial invasion with raise in temperature. Late effects include ulceration (5 months), gastritis (1–12 months), and dysphasia (6 months to 4 years).

Most radiosensitive cells in the intestine are immature stem cells at the base of villi. They become mature cells and migrate to top of the villi and become functional cell in 2 weeks. Its function includes absorption of nutrient from the gut and discharge of waste into the intestine. Small dose may affect enzyme secretion, whereas large dose cause denudation. Patient may have nausea, bloody vomiting, and diarrhea after a dose of 2 Gy. Rectal complication includes diarrhea, proctitis, necrosis, stenosis, and fistula.

Effects on Reproductive System

Radiation exposure can cause tumors, impaired fertility, and hereditary effects. Hereditary effects and cancer induction are stochastic in nature while impaired fertility is deterministic.

Testes contain Sertoli and germinal cells of differing radiosensitivity. Threshold dose for temporary and permanent sterility is 1.5–2 Gy and 2.5–6 Gy, receptively for acute exposure.

The ovary contains oocytes, which decrease with age and reach zero during menopause. Oocytes and ova in the intermediate ovarian follicles are more sensitive. Permanent sterility may occur at 3 Gy of acute exposure, whereas it is 6 Gy for fractionated radiation. Permanent sterility is age dependent and people at the age of 35–40 are more vulnerable than young women.

Effects on Embryo and Fetus

Developing embryo is extremely sensitive to radiation during the first half of the gestation period, as it is characterized by cell proliferation, migration, and differentiation. Gestational period is divided into—(i) preimplantation, (ii) major organogenesis, and (iii) fetal stage **(Fig. 2.8)**. Preimplantation (9–14 days) begins with union of sperm and egg and continues until the zygote is embedded in the uterine wall. Major organogenesis is the period between 2 and 8 weeks (15–50 days). Fetus stage is between 50 and 280 days. Pregnant women exposed to radiation simulate the condition of in utero exposure that will affect the embryo and fetus.

Any radiation damage to the conceptus (conceptus includes the embryo as well as the embryonic part of the placenta and its associated membranes) may result in prenatal death. However, such lethal effects are low if the radiation dose is <100 mGy (ICRP-103). At such low doses, any radiation damage, if occurs, gets repaired. Moreover, these cells are in undifferentiated stage, no congenital anomalies are observed. This is called *all-or-nothing effect* of radiation.

Embryonic malformations include growth retardation, microcephaly, intrauterine death, and growth retardation. Gestation period in humans is shorter than in animals; hence, teratogenic effects are low in humans.

Hiroshima and Nagasaki, Japan data shows that fetus exposed to radiation may have smaller head and brain size, cognitive deficits associated with delayed brain development, behavioral alterations, or reduced intelligence in later part of life at high dose rates.

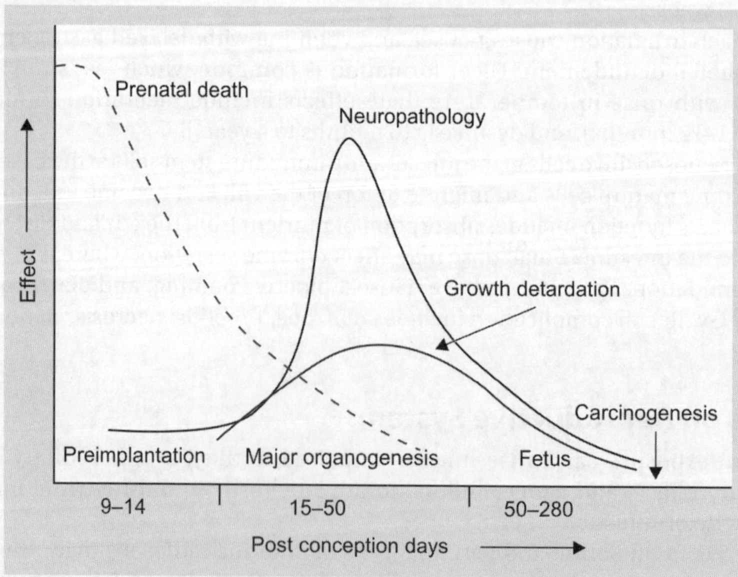

FIG. 2.8: Health effects of radiation exposure in utero at various stages of gestation period.

Risk of mental retardation is about 40% per Sv for high-dose rate exposures. ICRP states mental retardation is a deterministic effect with a threshold dose of 0.1 Sv. At low-dose rate exposures, the intelligence quotient (IQ) reduction is 25 points per Sv. There is also chance of childhood cancer and the ICRP risk estimate is 0.1 per SV. Hence, dose limits are recommended to pregnant women.

RADIOBIOLOGICAL BASIS OF RADIOTHERAPY

Primary methods of treating cancer are surgery, radiotherapy, and chemotherapy. First two are localized treatment and chemotherapy is a systemic treatment that kills cancer cells thorough out the body. Radiotherapy is designed to give maximum damage to tumor cells while reducing the damage to surrounding normal tissues. It is difficult to treat cancer cells without exceeding the normal tissue tolerance. However, rapidly dividing cells are more sensitive to radiation than slowly dividing cells. Fractionated dose kills more cells than a single acute dose. Dose fractionation in radiotherapy can be justified in terms of 4 R's of radiobiology, namely—(i) repair, (ii) repopulation, (iii) redistribution, and (iv) reoxygenation.

Repair

Ability of the cell to recover from radiation damage is called repair. It rejoins broken DNA strands within 15 minutes to 1 hour. It is an intracellular recovery, takes place both in normal and tumor cells. Late reacting normal tissues have greater repair capacity than tumor and early reacting normal cells. Repair depends on the cell type, interfraction time, number of fractions, dose per fraction, and dose rate. It is independent of total dose and overall treatment time.

Fractionation is designed with sufficient time between fractions, so that complete SLD repair is performed. The cells damaged in the first fraction will be repaired before the second fraction. The shape of the survival curve appears with shoulder, which will repeat after each fraction. The survival curves of tumor and normal tissues are well separated. Tumor survival curve is well below that of normal tissue curve.

Repopulation

Repopulation is a proliferation process by which radiation injury is responded. This process takes place in few weeks. Repopulation is important in rapidly proliferating tissue. It is an extracellular recovery and occurs both in normal and tumor cells. The rate of repopulation is higher in tumor cells than normal since tumor has fast dividing cells. Repopulation is getting accelerated in cancer cells after 2–3 weeks. Hence, fraction schedule should be revised after 2–3 weeks for better outcome.

Redistribution

The distribution of cells in the cell cycle is called redistribution. Cells in the M phase are more sensitive, have linear survival curve, referring to minimal repair. Survival curve of cells in S phase exhibits greater shoulder, referring maximum repair. After first fraction, there is abundance of cells in S phase. Thus, radiation-induced partial synchronization is achieved during redistribution. By suitable adjustment of timing, it is possible to fix the cells in most wanted phase at the time of irradiation. They will be killed effectively in the second fraction. Redistribution has little impact in clinical radiotherapy since tumor cells proliferate faster than normal cells.

Reoxygenation

Normal cells are well oxygenated while many cells in tumor are hypoxic. The hypoxic cells are relatively resistant to radiation. During dose fractionation, hypoxic cells get oxygenated due to tumor shrinkage, as they move closer to the vasculature. The cells, which are hypoxic in the earlier fraction, become oxygenated and may be killed in the subsequent fraction. Interfraction time of 24 hours is sufficient to oxygenate hypoxic cells. However, all cancers are not curable with above hypothesis. Reoxygenation is important only with low LET radiation as high LET radiation kills hypoxic cells too.

Conventional and Nonconventional Fractionation Schemes

A variety of fractionation schedules are designed to get the radiobiological advantages: *(i) conventional fraction, (ii) hyperfractionation, (iii) accelerated fractionation, (iv) accelerated hyperfractionation, (v) dynamic fractionation, and (vi) hypofractionation.*

Conventional fractionation consists of 1.8–2.2 Gy per fraction delivered in five fractions per week. A total dose of 60–81 Gy is given in 5–6 weeks. It permits more normal cells to recover from radiation damage than tumor cells.

Hyperfractionation refers to radiation treatment in which the total dose of radiation is divided into small doses and treatments are given more than once a day. Hyperfractionated radiation therapy is given over the same period of time (days or weeks) as standard radiation therapy. It permits normal tissue to recover and reduce repopulation and reoxygenation of tumor cells. It permits dose escalation of about 20–30%.

Accelerated fractionation is defined as reducing the overall duration of a radiotherapy regimen without a significant change in the size of dose per fraction or total dose. This is achieved by giving two or more fractions on some or all of the treatment days. Accelerated fractionation counters repopulation of tumor cells.

Accelerated hyperfractionation combines both hyper- and accelerated fractionation. A dose fraction of 1.5 Gy, 3 fractions per day, 6 hours apart, 7 days a week to a total dose of 54 Gy in 36 fractions over 12 days makes the protocol.

Dynamic fractionation is a dose escalation method to achieve accelerated hyperfractionation. A total dose of 76 Gy is delivered in 5 weeks.

Hypofractionation refers to radiation treatment in which the total dose of radiation is divided into large doses and treatments are given once a day or less often. Hypofractionated radiation therapy is given over a shorter period of time (fewer days or weeks) than standard radiation therapy, e.g.,15 fractions of 2.8 Gy over a period of 3 weeks, making a total dose of 42 Gy. This makes more convenient for the patient as there are fewer appointments to attend.

TIME, DOSE, AND FRACTIONATION MODELS

Various fractionation schemes were established in different clinical centers with considerable difference in treatment and doses. In order to compare the merit of these various fractionations, a common scale is desired. Since normal tissue tolerance is the limiting factor in radiotherapy, it was decided to use the measure of radiation damage to normal tissue for comparison.

Several workers attempted towards this, and various models were evolved. These are called time, dose, and fractionation (TDF) models. *Ellis* proposed the nominal standard dose (NSD) to predict the effective biological dose in terms of dose (d), fraction (N), and overall treatment time (T).

$$NSD = d \times N^{0.65} \times (T/N)^{-0.11} \tag{2.6}$$

where, T/N is a constant. *Orton and Ellis* (1973) developed the TDF from NSD model. Above equation can be made additive by rising power 1/0.65 = 1.54, on both sides of the above equation:

$$TDF \propto NSD^{1.54}, \text{ substituting equation} \tag{2.7}$$

$$TDF = 10^{-3} \times N \times d^{1.54} \times \left(\frac{T}{N}\right)^{-0.17}$$

where, 10^{-3} is a scaling factor to make TDF 100, which corresponds to maximum skin tolerance.

Equation is rewritten by incorporating SI units; that is dose in Gy and t in days.

$$TDF = 1.19 \times N \times d^{1.54} \times \left(\frac{T}{N}\right)^{-0.17} \tag{2.8}$$

The bioeffective doses in TDF units are linearly additive, since TDF is a linear function of N. If there is interruption of radiotherapy treatment, repopulation may occur during the rest period. Ellis proposed a decay factor for giving allowance for such repopulation as:

$$\text{Decay factor} = \left(\frac{T}{T+R}\right)^{0.11} \tag{2.9}$$

where, T is the number of days from starting the course of radiotherapy to interruption and R is the number of days of rest. The overall TDF must be multiplied with the decay factor, to obtain the true TDF value, which compensates for the rest. The greatest advantage of TDF is that it is independent of any specific NSD value and readymade table is available for easy reference. It is also useful in combined treatment involving external beam therapy and brachytherapy.

Worked Example 2.1

Calculate the TDF value for standard external beam treatment of 60 Gy, 2 Gy per fraction delivered in 30 fractions:

Here, N = 30 fractions, d = 2 Gy, and T = 42 days,

$$TDF = 1.19 \times N \times d^{1.54} \times \left(\frac{T}{N}\right)^{-0.17}$$

$$TDF = 1.19 \times 30 \times 2^{1.54} \times \left(\frac{42}{30}\right)^{-0.17}$$

$$= 35.7 \times 2.91 \times 0.9 = 97.65$$

Linear Quadratic Model

This model is derived from the linear quadratic (LQ) cell survival theory, based upon the fundamental mechanism of interaction of radiation with cells, discussed earlier. As per the LQ theory, the survival fraction (S) after N fractions:

$$-\ln S = N(\alpha d + \beta d^2) \tag{2.10}$$

where, d is the dose per fraction in Gy. The above equation accounts only the repair mechanism, not repopulation of cells by the early responding normal tissues. Tumor repopulation is an exponential function of time, and it is given by the equation $N = N_o e^{\lambda T}$, where N is the number of colognes at a time T, and N_o is the initial number of colognes. The λ is a constant related to the potential doubling time of tumor (T_{pot}):

$$\lambda = \frac{0.693}{T_{pot}} \tag{2.11}$$

Then, the survival fraction will be increased by $\frac{0.693}{T_{pot}} \times T$ and the final equation is given by:

$$-\ln S = N(\alpha d + \beta d^2) - \frac{0.693T}{T_{pot}} \tag{2.12}$$

Dividing the entire equation by $-\alpha$, the equation becomes:

$$-\frac{\ln s}{\alpha} = N\left(d + \frac{d^2}{\alpha/\beta}\right) - \frac{0.693\,T}{\alpha T_{pot}} \tag{2.13}$$

Left hand side is called *biologically effective dose (BED)* or *extrapolated response dose* (ERD), which refers to surviving cells per α event following irradiation. Thus, term BED predicts quantitatively the radiation effects and its local control. The final equation is written as (*Barendsen and Fowler*):

$$BED = -\frac{\ln S}{\alpha} = N\left(d + \frac{d^2}{\alpha/\beta}\right) - \frac{0.693T}{\alpha T_{pot}} \tag{2.14}$$

The potential doubling time vary from patient to patient and difficult to determine its value for individual tumors. Hence, it is replaced by a generic repopulation parameter k, which can be determined by clinical data analysis in a group of patients of specific diseases:

$$BED = N\left(d + \frac{d^2}{\alpha/\beta}\right) - k(T - T_k)$$

$$= N \times d\left(1 + \frac{d}{\alpha/\beta}\right) - k(T - T_k) \tag{2.15}$$

where, T_k is the repopulation kick-off time after a radiation treatment, and T is the overall treatment time in days. It is believed that tumor repopulation is negligible up to 21–28 days after the beginning of treatment. Thus, T_k refers to repopulation start up time and it is repopulated at the rate of k Gy per day, where $k = 0$, for $T<T_k$. The overall treatment time is very important for rapidly growing tumors. In head and neck cancer, the local control decreases about 1.4% for each day of prolonged treatment. Similarly, it is about 0.5% per day for carcinoma cervix. The product $N \times d$ refers to total dose (D) and the term $\left(1 + \frac{d}{\alpha/\beta}\right)$ is called relative effectiveness (RE). Hence, the BED is the product of total dose and relative effectiveness ($D \times RE$).

The LQ model is useful for the study of several interesting problems both in external beam radiotherapy and brachytherapy, especially in converting the HDR treatments into LDR equivalent. The BED used in the above discussion is based on the

TABLE 2.5 The α/β ratio for early and late reacting normal tissues, from multifraction experiments.

Early effect	*α/β, Gy*	*Late effects*	*α/β, Gy*
Skin	9–12	Spinal cord	1.7–4.9
Jejunum	6–10	Kidney	1.0–2.4
Colon	10–11	Lung	2.0–6.3
Testis	12–13	Bladder	3.1–7.0
Callus	9–10		

Courtesy: Hall EJ, Giaccia AJ, 2006.

tissue characteristics that again depends on the α/β ratio. This ratio is not a constant and it will vary with tissue types **(Table 2.5)**. *Fowler* (1990) has suggested a α/β value of 10 and 3 for tumor and late reacting normal tissue, respectively. Hence, the BED comparisons should be carried out for tumor, early reacting normal tissue, and late reacting normal tissue separately.

BIBLIOGRAPHY

1. Atomic Energy Regulatory Board. (2009). Workshop on establishment of directorate of radiation safety, AERB, Lecture Notes, 2009. [online] Available from https://www.aerb.gov.in. [Last accessed September, 2022].
2. Bhat NN, Rao BS. Proceedings of national symposium on radiobiology of clinical radiotherapy. Chennai: ICRB; 2018.
3. Board on Radiation Effects Research Division on Earth and Life Studies. BEIR VII: Health Risks from Exposure to Low Levels of Ionizing Radiation, National Academies Press, 500 Fifth Street, NW, Washington DC, 2001;800-624-6242. [online] Available from https://www.philrutherford.com/Radiation_Risk/BEIR/BEIR_VII.pdf. [Last accessed September 2022].
4. Bushberg JT, Seiber JA, Leidholdt EM, Boone JM. The essential physics of medical imaging, 2nd edition. Philadelphia: Lippincott Williams & Wilkins; 2002.
5. Graham DT, Cloke P, Vosper M. Principles of Radiological physics, 5th edition. London: Churchill Livingstone; 2007.
6. Hall EJ, Giaccia AJ. Radiobiology for the Radiologist, 6th edition. Philadelphia: Lippincott Williams & Wilkins; 2006.
7. Kelsey CA, Heintz PH, Sandoval DJ, Chambers GD, Adolphi NL, Paffett KS. Radiation biology of medical imaging. New York: Wiley Blackwell; 2014.
8. Mettler FA, Upton AC. Medical effects of ionizing radiation, 2nd edition. Philadelphia: WB Saunders Co.; 1995.
9. National Research Council, Committee on the biological effects of ionizing radiations. Health effects of exposure to low levels of ionizing radiation (BEIR V). Washington, DC: National Academy Press; 1990.
10. Thayalan K. Handbook of radiobiology. New Delhi: Jaypee Brothers Medical Publisher; 2017.
11. David J. Dowsett, Patrick A. Kenny and R. Eugene Johnston. The Physics of Diagnostic Imaging, 2nd Edition, Hodder Arnold, 2006.

CHAPTER 3

Radiation Protection Standards

INTRODUCTION

Discovery of X-rays, its benefits, and hazards have been discussed in the previous chapter. Radiobiological experiments have improved the knowledge of health effect of radiation and realized the importance of radiation protection. Many national and international bodies have been formed to give advice and recommendations on radiation protection.

United Nations Scientific Committee of the Effects of Atomic Radiations (UNSCEAR) is responsible for advising the General assembly of the United Nations about ionizing radiations. Its reports are used for making policy and estimation of risk in several countries.

International Commission on Radiological Protection (ICRP) and International Atomic Energy Agency (IAEA) are providing required policies and standards for radiation protection. International Commission on Radiological Units and Measurements (ICRU), a sister organization of ICRP, provides standard for radiation measurements, especially units. Basic safety standard (BSS) organ of IAEA, co-sponsored by many international organizations, forms the foundation for radiation protection and safety globally. In India, Division of Radiological Protection (DRP), Bhabha Atomic Research Centre (BARC) was formed in 1952, later transformed as Atomic Energy Regulatory Board (AERB) in 1983.

These bodies issue periodical reports and recommendations on radiation protection aspects of various application of ionizing radiation.

SOURCES OF RADIATION

The sources of radiation are classified as natural and artificial radiation sources (manmade). Public are exposed to secondary particle showers of lower atmosphere and radionuclides of earth, referred as natural radiation. Natural radiation sources include—(i) cosmic rays, (ii) terrestrial radionuclides, and (iii) internal radioisotopes. Artificial sources include—(i) medical exposure, (ii) nuclear weapon testing and radioactive fallout, (iii) occupational exposure, (iv) reactor accident, and (v) consumer products. Annual average dose equivalent is 3 mSv. About 80% of the above exposure arises from natural sources, 20% arises from artificial sources **(Fig. 3.1)**. Terrestrial radiations vary with region, Kerala and northern Iran have high background levels of radiation of 12.5 and 260 mSv/year, respectively.

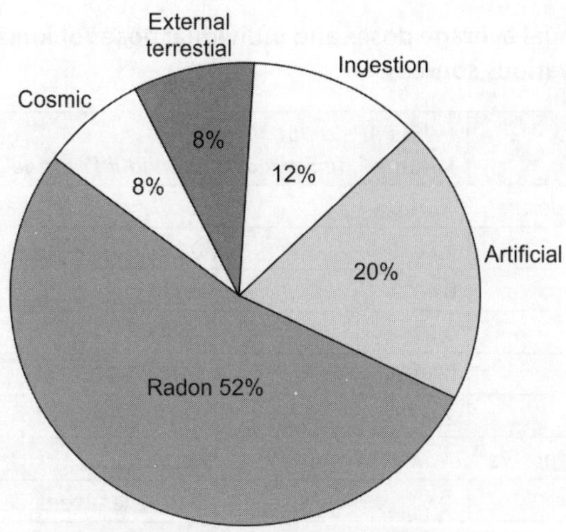

FIG. 3.1: The percentage contribution of various types of man-made sources to the total average effective dose equivalent to the US population.

Natural Radiation Source

Cosmic Rays

Earth is bombarded by high-energy particles originating from outer space that generates secondary particles in the lower atmosphere, referred as cosmic rays. Cosmic rays are energetic protons and alpha particle, which come from the sun and outer space. It is attenuated by earth's magnetic field and by atmosphere, and only small percentage reaches the earth's surface. The magnetic shield diverts most of the radiation around the earth. Earth's atmosphere shields us from most of the remaining radiation that travels to Earth. Cosmic radiation is about 10% of the natural radiation at sea level, and accounts higher at high attitudes. Public are shielded against cosmic rays by an air layer of 10,000 kg/m^2, which is equal to 10 m water thickness.

Cosmic rays are divided based on its origin, energy, and type and flex density. There are three main sources, namely galactic cosmic rays (GCRs), solar cosmic rays (SCRs), and rays from earth's radiation belts (*Van Allen* radiation belts). GCRs arise from sources outside the solar system and its primary energy is about 18^8–10^{20} eV. SCRs are generated near the sun's surface due to magnetic disturbances and originate from solar flares. Van Allen radiation belts are formed by capture protons and electrons by the earth's magnetic field. There are two such belts—one internal at about 3,000 km and an external at about 22,000 km from earth's surface.

Primary cosmic rays are protons (90%) and alpha particles (9%), collide with atmosphere, and produce showers of secondary particles (electrons, muons) and electromagnetic radiations. Part of the secondary cosmic ray particles collides with stable atmospheric nuclei and produces cosmogenic radionuclides such as tritium (^{3}H), beryllium (^{7}Be), carbon (^{14}C), and sodium (^{22}N). However, their contribution to natural background is very little.

Cosmic exposure varies with latitude and altitude. It is minimal at the equator and maximum at the geomagnetic poles (south and north poles). Generally, continental air grafts which fly at about 6,100–12,200 m, the cosmic

TABLE 3.1 Annual average doses and individual doses of ionizing radiation by various sources.

Sources	*UNSCEAR (2008), Volume 1, (mSv/year)*	*Individual's range (mSv/year)*
Natural source of exposure		
Inhalation: Radon	1.26	0.2–10
External terrestrial	0.48	0.3–1
Ingestion	0.29	0.2–1
Cosmic radiation	0.39	0.3–1
Total	2.4	1–13
Artificial source of exposure		
Medical diagnosis	0.6	0 to several tens
Atmospheric nuclear testing	0.005	Possibility of higher doses near test site
Occupational exposure	0.005	≈0–20
Chernobyl accident	0.002	10–150
Nuclear fuel cycle	0.0002	0.02 at 1 km from nuclear reactor site
Total	0.6	
Overall total	*3.0*	*0 to several tens*
(UNSCEAR: United Nations Scientific Committee on the Effects of Atomic Radiation)		

ray exposure doubles in every 1,850 m. The estimated exposure is 4–8 μSv at an altitude of 8–12 km at 50 latitude. In the case of aircrafts flying at 7.5–10 km, cosmic rays account about 3 μSv/h per travel. Apollo astronauts received an average equivalent dose of 2.75 mSv during the lunar mission.

Cosmic ray exposure at ground level is due to muons of energy 1–20 GeV (80%) and electrons (20%) with an average dose rate of 31 nGy/h at sea level. Worldwide, about 4×10^3 million population is exposed with mean annual effective dose of 0.27 mSv at sea level. UNSCEAR's 2008 (2010) global annual dose contribution from various sources of radiations is presented in **Table 3.1**.

Terrestrial Radiations

Terrestrial radionuclides are present on earth since its formation, are called *primordial radionuclides*. Their physical half-lives are comparable to the age of the earth (4.5 billion years). They are present in the rocks in the form of uranium-238, thorium-232, and potassium-40. The geological concentrations of these radionuclides give higher background radiation in some areas. High background sites are present in certain parts of Brazil, Iran, India, and China. Their decay products are the major contributors of terrestrial radiations. Terrestrial radionuclides contribute both—(1) external exposure and (2) internal exposure.

External exposure: External exposure from terrestrial radionuclides accounts an equivalent dose of 0.48 mSv/year.

Internal exposure: Internal exposures occur through inhalation and ingestion and contribute about 1.55 mSv/year to the global population.

- *Inhalation*: Radon (half-life of 3.8 days), a noble gas, moves from earth to air, decays to polonium-218 (half-life of 3 minutes) by alpha emission. The solid decay products are deposited in the tracheobronchial region of lung. It accounts an equivalent dose of 1.26 mSv/year to the bronchial epithelium. Generally, radon concentration is higher in buildings with poor ventilation. The average indoor concentration level is 45 Bq/m^3 and the outdoor level is 7 Bq/m^3.
- *Ingestion*: Ingestion of food and water is another source of internal exposure, and potassium-40 plays a major role and it accounts an equivalent dose of 0.29 mSv/year. It emits beta- and gamma-rays with a half-life of 1.3 billion years and contributes about 0.15 mSv/year. Contribution of radiation exposure from carbon-14, radon-220, lead-210, and polonium-210 is less than that of potassium-40.

Exposure From Artificial Sources

Medical Diagnosis and Therapy

Radiation exposure involves diagnostic radiology, dental exposures, nuclear medicine, and radiotherapy. Medical exposure contributes about 98% of artificial exposures with an annual average effective dose equivalent of 0.6 mSv/year. Globally, about 3.6 billion medical radiation exposures are conducted in a year, causing collective dose of 4.2 million man Sv (UNSCEAR, 2008 survey data). Interventional fluoroscopy and computed tomography are the major contributors. There is an increasing trend in medical exposures globally that is related to increased health benefits to the population.

Medical use of radiation warrants an optimal compromise between clinical utility and radiation dose to patients, staff, and public. Success of radiation protection mainly lies on the education and training of staffs. They should be educated on radiobiology, genetics, risk analysis, methods of reducing radiation dose, decay patterns of radioactivity released in the environment, and absorbing power of different materials to different radiation.

Atmospheric Nuclear Testing

This exposure arises from atmospheric testing of nuclear weapons or bombs and consists of long-lived Carbon-14 (70%) and other radionuclides including ^{3}H, ^{54}Mn, ^{136}Cs, ^{137}Cs, ^{140}Ba, ^{144}Ce, plutonium, and transplutonium elements. It forms 2% of artificial radiation resulting an annual effective dose equivalent of 0.005 mSv, including the highest value of 0.11 mSv in 1963. Such explosions release radioactive products into the atmosphere in turn transported around the world and earth. From 1945 to 1980, about 502 tests were conducted with total yield of 434 metric tons of *trinitrotoluene (TNT)*. After 1963 treaty banning nuclear weapon tests, many underground atomic tests (50 per year) have been conducted globally with much lower yield than atmospheric tests.

Occupational Exposure

The occupational exposures are from uranium mining, military activity, nuclear power operations, aircrews, X-ray and nuclear medicine technologists, and radiologists **(Table 3.2)**, making a total of about 22.8 million workers. Medical

TABLE 3.2 Annual occupational effective dose equivalent (US data).

Category	*Average annual total effective dose equivalent (mSv)*
Uranium miners	12.0
Nuclear power operations	6.0
Airline crews	1.7
X-ray and nuclear medicine technologists	1.0
Radiologists	0.7

workers form 75% of occupational workers. Military activity of production and testing of bombs accounts an effective dose 0.1–0.2 mSv per worker. The estimated annual mean effective dose for airline crews is 2–3 mSv. Workers of nuclear fuel cycle involve an annual effective dose of 1.0 mSv. Annual effective dose to occupational medical workers is about 0.5 mSv. However, interventional radiology exposures may be higher, equal to the regulatory limits. Industrial radiation workers receive an annual effective of 0.3 mSv.

Chernobyl Accident

Chernobyl nuclear power plant accident (1986) occurred in the forrner Soviet Union caused 28 deaths, including 134 acute radiation syndromes. Increased incidence of leukemia and cataract was found in hundreds of recovery workers. Radioactive cloud deposited radioactive material over Soviet Union and Europe, including northern hemisphere in the form of contamination. Thyroid dose from Iodine-125 (^{125}I) was found to be few Gy, whereas whole body dose from ^{137}Cs is few hundred mSv. About 6,000 cases of thyroid cancer were reported in children due to drinking of milk contaminated with ^{125}I. Contaminated areas of Belarus, Russia, and Ukraine reported a dose of about 9 mSv.

Nuclear Fuel Cycle

Nuclear power production involves uranium mining, milling, fuel fabrication, reactor operation, waste storage, transport, and waste disposal. It produces enough residues referred as tailings. About 2 billion tonnes of tailings have been accumulated, which is greater than world uranium production of 2 million tonnes. The annual collective dose is about 50–60 man Sv. In the nuclear fuel cycle, spent fuel is reprocessed to recover uranium and plutonium for reuse. This reprocessing accounts annual collective dose of about 20–30 man Sv. Hazards also arise from nuclear waste, which is stored at surface near the reactor and disposed later. Overall, nuclear power production causes about 200 man Sv, as collective dose due to all operations in which mining dominates.

Consumer Products

Tobacco products such as smoking play a vital role in radiation exposure that causes a dose around 0.36 mSv/year to smokers (USA). Hence, lung receives highest dose equivalent from both smokers (Polonium-210) and nonsmokers (Radon-222). Building materials such as brick, concrete, granite consists of uranium, thorium, and potassium contribute both external and internal exposure as mentioned above. Combustible fuels (coal and natural gas) and consumer products such as smoke alarms (Americium-241), gas lantern mantles (thorium), dental prostheses, certain ceramics, and optical lenses (Uranium) contribute to radiation exposure. To a lesser extent, televisions, wrist watches (tritium and beta emitter), and computer screens account for the above exposures.

Accident Exposures

Radiation accidents may cause early acute health effects or environmental contamination. There were 35 nuclear fuel accidents caused 32 deaths and 61 injuries in employees. Industry faced 80 accidents involving 9 deaths and 120 injuries. Orphan source accidents (34) accounts 42 deaths, including children. Medical accidents mostly come from radiotherapy, and reported 32 accidents involving 46 deaths and 623 injuries.

SYSTEM OF RADIOLOGICAL PROTECTION

Medical diagnosis and treatment is the most useful and peaceful application of ionizing radiation. In this, patient is the direct beneficiary and has no dose limit for medical exposures. All procedures are carried out with sound clinical judgment so that the benefits to the patients always exceed the risk associated with radiation. This involves occupational exposure to radiologists, medical physicists, radiographers, technologists, and nurses.

Principle of Radiation Protection

The objective of radiation protection is to prevent deterministic effects and minimize stochastic effects to occupational workers and public. Doses received by patients during diagnostic procedure should be low. Every effort should be taken to control radiation exposure of people, restrict the probability of loss of control over radiation sources, and mitigate the consequences of any untoward incidences. Radiation safety is concerned with normal operation conditions and as consequence of potential accidental conditions. Such safety is achieved by good work practices under normal working conditions and controlling the exposures by applying the basic principle of *time, distance, and shielding (TDS rules)*. Design of equipment, installation, quality assurance, and good operating procedure will prevent potential exposures. In addition, an effective management system is required to ensure safety. The general principle of radiation safety is based on—(1) justification, (2) optimization, and (3) dose limits.

Justification of Practice

- All exposures either diagnostic or therapeutic shall be undertaken only if the benefit gained outweighs the detriment.
- No practice shall be adopted unless it produces a net positive benefit.

It emphasizes that all applications of radiation should be justified. Total detriment from a proposed practice involving exposure to radiation should be less than the expected benefit. Since deterministic effects exhibit threshold doses, they can be prevented by limiting exposures to levels lower than the threshold doses. However, stochastic effects do not have threshold dose; hence, it is assumed that all radiation doses carry some risk.

Medical exposures need to be justified and the responsibility lies with the medical professional. Justification has three levels as per ICRP (2007). First level believes that medicine does better than harm. Second level specifies the procedure and specific objective. One should justify whether the radiological procedure will improve the diagnosis and offer intended clinical information. Third level refers to application of procedure to individual patient. In this, the consultant and referring physician should verify if the sought information is already available or not, and then justify the procedures by considering all the information based on previous study, alternate procedures, characteristics of individual patient, and expected patient dose. Especially, it is much important in interventional fluoroscopy and neuroradiological procedures.

Optimization

- All exposures, which are justified, shall be undertaken with a minimum possible dose.
- Every effort shall be taken to reduce the dose *as low as reasonably achievable (ALARA)*, taking into account the economic and social considerations.

Its objective is to optimize the risk level and cost of radiation protection. It also makes sure that the individual doses, number of people exposed, and the likelihood of incurring exposures must be kept by ALARA principle. Economic and social factors being considered within restriction, that is the individual patient dose should be subject to dose constraint. Generally, there is no limitation of dose constraint to patient exposures. However, it should be made sure that the doses received by them are commensurate with their medical purpose. Patient can be managed with reference dose levels recommended by ICRP, 1996a, 2001b, and 2007. It is applicable only to diagnostic procedures not for radiotherapy patients, occupational workers, and public. Optimization can be achieved by installation design safety, equipment safety, operational safety, dose constraint, and work practice.

Dose Limits

- The equivalent doses to individuals result from the above practices be subjected to dose equivalent limits.
- These are aimed at ensuring that no individual is expected to radiation risks that are judged to be unacceptable from these practices in normal circumstances.

The effective doses to the individuals shall not exceed the limits recommended by the ICRP. Public who accompanies or visits the patient should receive <1 mSv. Public limit is not applicable to comforters who comfort and care the patients, but 5 mSv per episode is recommended to them. Dose limits can be relaxed to parents of sick children. Special precaution is needed if the patient's partner is pregnant during implant brachytherapy (ICRP 98, 2005). A dose constraint of 0.1–100 mSv is recommended for volunteers used in radiopharmaceutical research (ICRP, 2007).

INTERNATIONAL COMMISSION ON RADIOLOGICAL PROTECTION

In 1915, the *British Roentgen Society* made the first radiation protection recommendations. To regulate the safe use of radiation, the *British X-ray and Radium Protection Committee* was formed (1921) and in 1928, this committee was named as International X-ray and Radium Protection Committee (IXRPC). The first recommendation report came in 1931. Later in the year 1950, it established the maximum tolerance dose in terms of physical units. It was renamed as International Commission on Radiological Protection (ICRP). Radiation units such as roentgen equivalent physical (rep), radiation absorbed dose (rad), and roentgen equivalent man (rem) were defined.

The ICRP is a nonprofit, independent charitable body consisting of experts in radiological protection. Many countries follow its recommendations into polices and regulations. ICRP works closely with its sister concern, International Commission on Radiological Units and Measurements (ICRU). It has official relationship with World Health Organization (WHO) and International Atomic Energy Agency (IAEA).

Earlier Reports

International Commission on Radiological Protection introduced the concept of permissible dose, defined as a dose of ionizing radiation that, in the light of present knowledge, is not expected to cause appreciable bodily injury to a person at any time during his lifetime. The whole body, gonads, and blood-forming organs were considered as critical organs for external radiation. It recommended a permissible dose of 300 mR/week for critical organs including eye, for occupational workers in 1954.

In 1956 report, it emphasized three groups of organs for occupational workers namely—(i) blood-forming organ and gonads, (ii) skin, bone, and thyroid, and (iii) hands, feet, and forearms (1958) and the dose limits are 5, 15, and 80 rem/year, respectively. Limit was also set for single dose; 3 rem/13 weeks for whole body exposure. Concept of doubling dose was introduced; it is the dose of radiation required to induce mutation frequency equal to the spontaneous frequency.

The ICRP-6 and 9 (1962 and 1966) recommended two categories, namely (i) radiation workers and (ii) member of public. For members of public, dose limit was 1/10 of the maximum permissible limits specified for radiation workers, except that for children up to the age of 16 years where annual dose to thyroid is 1.5 rem against earlier limit of 3 rem. The dose to fetus should be limited to about 2 rem. Women of reproductive age should not receive doses in excess of 5 rems in a year. Radiological examinations, if any, should be undertaken within a period of 10 days following menstruation to protect possible embryo.

The epidemiological data on Radium-226 content in the body of radium dial painters and patients treated with radium was the basis for fixing 5 rem/year limit on radiation exposure. ^{226}Ra content of 0.1 μCi uniformly deposited in the human skeleton delivers 5 rem dose per year to the person. Hence, 0.1 μCi of ^{226}Ra is called maximum permissible body burden (MPBB). MPBB is the quantity of radionuclide in the whole body, which, at an equilibrium level or at the end of 50 years of continuous exposure, delivers to the critical organ a dose equivalent rate equal to the maximum permissible for that organ. This approach was abandoned by ICRP-30.

ICRP-26 and 30 Reports

The ICRP-26 (1977) introduced terms such as risk, detriment, and dose equivalent. Risk is a probability that a given individual will incur a deleterious effect because of a dose of radiation. Detriment is a mathematical expectation of the harm incurred from an exposure to radiation considering not only the probability of each type of deleterious effect but the severity of the effects as well. Stochastic and nonstochastic effects were described. Stochastic effects are effects in which the probability of an effect occurring, rather than its severity is a function of dose, without threshold. Nonstochastic effects are those for which the severity of effects varies with dose, and for which a threshold may occur. Dose equivalent (H) is the absorbed dose (D) weighted by quality factor (Q), and other modifying factors (N), and its unit is Sv:

$$H = D \times Q \times N$$

The quality factors are 1, 2.3, 10, and 20 for photons/electrons, thermal neutron, fast neutron/protons/singly charged particle, and doubly charged particle, respectively. Other modifying factor, N is assigned a value of unity.

Working conditions were classified as A and B. Annual exposure limit might exceed 3/10 of the dose equivalent limit in condition A, whereas it is unlikely in condition B. Women of reproductive capacity working under uniform rate of 50 mSv/year, it is unlikely that the embryo could receive more than 5 mSv during first 2 months. Once pregnancy is diagnosed, she should be asked to work in condition B only for the remaining period and it will not exceed 10 mSv so that total dose to embryo would be below 15 mSv. It introduced system of dose limitation, namely (i) justification, (ii) optimization, and (iii) compliance with individual dose equivalent limit.

Annual dose limits are fixed by comparing the level of risk with other safe industry. In industry with high-level safety, the average annual mortality due to occupational hazard does not exceed 10^{-4}. Accidental death in an industry can cause 30 years of average loss of life, whereas a fatal malignancy induced by occupational exposure to radiation would be expected to involve a loss of about 10 years of life, owing to long latency in the development. Commission believed that nonstochastic effects will be prevented, if the annual limit of 50 mSv/year to all tissues except for lenses of the eye to which 150 mSv/year is implemented.

Dose equivalent limit for stochastic effect believes that risk is equal for both uniform and nonuniform whole-body exposure. Lifetime dose to an individual member of the public should not exceed 1 mSv/year. Risk factors for various organs such as gonad, red bone marrow, bone, lungs, thyroid, and breast were recommended.

The report *ICRP-30 (1979)* has provided methodology for calculation of annual effective committed dose equivalent from internally deposited radionuclides. It introduced annual limit of intake (ALI) which is the quantity of radionuclide which taken alone would irradiate a person to the limit set by ICRP for each year of occupational exposures. Derived air concentration (DAC) is the ratio between ALI and the volume of air inhaled by reference man in a working year. The concept of critical organ and MPBB has been abandoned.

ICRP-60 Report

The ICRP-60 (1991) has introduced the basic dosimetric quantities such as radiation-weighting factor, equivalent dose, tissue-weighting factor, and effective dose.

Radiation-weighting Factor

Stochastic effect is based not only on absorbed dose but also on the type and energy of the radiation. Equivalent dose is the product of absorbed dose and radiation-weighting factor. The assigned radiation-weighting factors are 1, 2, 5, and 20 for photons, protons, neutrons (<10 MeV), and alpha particles, respectively.

Tissue-weighting Factors

The relationship between the probability of stochastic effect and equivalent dose depends on the organ or tissue irradiated. The factor, by which the equivalent dose in tissue or organ T is weighted, is called the *tissue-weighting factor* (W_T). It represents the relative contribution of the organ to the total detriment due to these effects resulting from uniform irradiation of the whole body. Effective dose is the product of equivalent dose and tissue-weighting factor. Tissue-weighting factor for various tissues ranges from 0.02 to 0.20. Testes and ovaries have the highest value of 0.20 followed by red bone marrow, colon, lung, and stomach (0.12). Breast, bladder, thyroid, liver, and esophagus have 0.05. Bone surface and skin surface has the lowest value of 0.02. Subsidiary dosimetric quantities such as committed equivalent dose and committed effective dose were also introduced.

Stochastic and Deterministic Effects

Ionizing radiation can cause both deterministic and stochastic effects in irradiated tissue. Deterministic effects should be avoided by setting limits below the threshold. It occurs due to cell killing sufficiently at large doses. Stochastic effects believed to occur even with low doses by modifying the cells that may develop into cancer. Commission uses the term detriment to refer the combination of probability of occurrence of a harmful health effect and a judgment of the severity of that effect.

Dosimetry System and Risk Analysis

The ICRP-60 used DS dosimetry system (DS 86) based on cancer mortality data (1958–1987 report) weighted for nonfatal cancers. It adopted a dose and dose rate reduction effectiveness factor of 2 and multiplicative risk model for risk projection. The genetic risk is 1.3% per Sv for general population and 0.8% per Sv for workers. Total detriment values are 7.3% per Sv for whole population, and 5.6% per Sv for adults.

Dose Limits

The occupational effective dose limit is 20 mSv/year, lens of the eye is 150 mSv, and skin, hands, and feet limits are 500 mSv. (ICRP has determined that for the occupational dose limit, an approximate lifetime dose of 1 Sv is tolerable. This correlates to an annual average dose of 20 mSv. To allow for flexibility, the ICRP also recommended that the dose limit should not exceed 50 mSv in any single year.) Corresponding value for the public is 1 mSv, 15 mSv, and 50 mSv, respectively **(Table 3.3)**. In pregnant women, once pregnancy is confirmed, the conceptus should be protected by applying a supplementary equivalent dose limit to the surface of the women's abdomen (lower trunk) of 2 mSv for the remainder of the pregnancy, (Normally considered equivalent to 1 mSv to the fetus, ICRP-60) and by limiting the intakes of radionuclides to about 1/20 of the ALI. Types of radiation exposure are occupational exposure, medical exposure, and public exposure.

ICRP-103 Report

ICRP-107 (2007) recommendations replace its previous ICRP-60, 1991 recommendations. It updates the radiation- and tissue-weighting factors for equivalent and effective dose quantities. It also updates radiation detriment based on the

TABLE 3.3 Recommended dose limits (ICRP-60, 1991) for planned exposure*.

Exposure condition	*Occupational dose limit (mSv/year)*	*Public limit (mSv/year)*
Effective dose (whole body)	20 mSv/year, averaged over defined periods of 5 years with no more than 50 mSv in any single year	1 mSv/year, a higher value of effective dose is allowed in a single year, provided that the average over 5 years does not exceed 1 mSv/year
Parts of the body (equivalent dose)		
Lens of the eye**	150 mSv/year	50 mSv/year
Skin***	500 mSv/year	50 mSv/year
Hands and feet	500 mSv/year	—

*Effective dose refers to sum of doses from external exposure and committed doses from internal exposures due to intake of radionuclides.

**Occupational and public limit is reduced to 20 mSv and 2 mSv, respectively from 2011 by ICRP-103

***Averaged over areas of no >1 cm^2 regardless of the area exposed. The normal depth is 7.0 mg/cm^2. Limit provides sufficient protection for the skin against stochastic effects. An additional limit is needed for localized exposures to prevent deterministic effects.

Note 1: 1 mSv = 100 mrem

Note 2: Dose limit for women upon declaration of pregnancy is 1 mSv to the fetus. In the case of internal emitter exposures, it is 1/20th of ALI.

Note 3: Dose limits do not apply to medical exposures, to natural sources of radiation, and results of accidental conditions.

(ALI: annual limit of intake; ICRP: International Commission on Radiological Protection)

latest scientific information of biology and physics of radiation. It maintains three fundamental principles of radiological protection, namely justification, optimization, and the application of dose limits. It recognizes planned, emergency, and existing exposure situations. Commission maintains the current individual dose limits for effective dose and equivalent dose from all regulated sources in planned exposure.

Radiation-weighting Factor

Commission assigned radiation-weighting factor of 1, 2, and 20 for photons, protons, and alpha particles, respectively **(Table 1.7, Chapter 1)**. The weighting factor of neutron is a function of neutron energy (2.5–20 MeV). It is for the assessment of stochastic effect only. It believes that deterministic effects may occur when the doses are >1 Gy and there is no threshold for stochastic effects.

Tissue-weighting Factor

Tissue-weighting factor of a tissue refers to fractional harm associated with the stochastic effects of radiation. Fractional detriment of a tissue is the ratio of detriment value of a tissue to overall detriment due to radiation exposure of the whole body. This is often referred as relative detriment. The gender-averaged relative detriment for various organs is given as tissue-weighting factor in the report **(Table 1.8, Chapter 1)**.

14 tissues that have an increase in cancer risk are assigned values from 0.12 to 0.01, whereas 13 tissues where reliable quantitative risk estimate is available are listed as remainder tissues. Important change is the W_T value of breast, from 0.05 (ICRP-60) to 0.12, gonads from 0.2 to 0.08, and remainder from 0.05 to 0.12.

Dosimetry System and Risk Analysis

The use of dosimetry system, DS 02 is based on cancer mortality data (1950–1997) and the dose is slightly higher than DS 86 of ICRP-60. Revised system revealed an increased risk of 48–95% for leukemia and 5–38% for solid tumors. Risk assessment at low doses is done by extrapolation of the risk observed at high-doses to low-doses region, assuming a linear no-threshold (LNT) model. ICRP-103 adopted a dose and dose rate reduction effectiveness factor of two for absorbed doses below 0.2 Gy and from all exposures at dose rates <0.1 Gy/h. There is no such reduction factor for high linear energy transfer (LET) radiation.

The ICRP-107 has estimated a genetic risk of 0.1% per Sv for the working population (18–65 years) and 0.2% per Sv for the public (0–90 years). Comparison of ICRP-103 recommendations with that of ICRP-60 is given in **Table 3.4**. The new risk estimate is five times lower than ICRP-60 values. It emphasizes that at low doses of radiation, the risk of adverse hereditary effects is small compared to the baseline frequencies of genetic diseases in the population.

Detriment

Overall harm due to stochastic effects of radiation is referred as radiation detriment. This is done by assessing the harm due to cancer incidence, mortality, length of life lost if cancer occurs, and the morbidity and sufferings associated with nonfatal cancers. In addition, the risk of genetic disorders and harm arising from them up to the second generation has also been considered in arriving at the detriment.

The present estimate of detriment is based on lethality and life impairment weighted on cancer incidence data. Detriment-adjusted risk coefficients for cancer and hereditary effects combined have been estimated as 5.7% per Sv for whole population, and 4.2% per Sv for adults, respectively. Detriment values of various tissues for working population (18–65) have been given in the form of table. Above detriment values are slightly lower than ICRP-60 estimates. Despite small changes in nominal risk coefficients and distribution, the aggregated detriment values remain close to 5% per Sv. It retained the dose limits recommended by ICRP-60 since the risk estimates did not vary significantly.

Basis of Annual Dose Limit

International Commission on Radiological Protection assumes maximum risk value of 10^{-3} per year in very important industries as acceptable. Dose limits are chosen so that it should be just short of unacceptable or just tolerable. Hence, effective dose limit of 20 mSv may marginally exceed the maximum mortality rate of 10^{-3} per year. This dose limit is based on the evaluation of detriment resulting from a continuous exposure over a working lifetime of 47 years (18–65 years). Variation of the detriment with age of the occupational workers exposed to different 10, 20, 30, and 50 mSv/year is given in the report **(Table 3.5)**. Those exposed to 20 mSv/year, the maximum mortality rate marginally exceeds the value of 10^{-3} per year, only when they attain the age of about 65 years. The aggregate detriment from

TABLE 3.4 Comparison of ICRP-60 and ICRP-103 on dose limits.

Categories of exposure	***ICRP-60, 1991***	***ICRP-103, 2007***
Occupational exposure		
Effective dose	20 mSv average over defined 5 years	20 mSv average over defined 5 years
Lens of the eye	150 mSv/year	20 mSv/year
Skin	500 mSv/year	500 mSv/year
Hands and feet	500 mSv/year	500 mSv/year
Pregnant women	2 mSv to the surface of abdomen or 1 mSv from intake of radionuclides	1 mSv to the embryo/fetus
Public exposure		
Effective dose	1 mSv in a year	1 mSv in a year
Lens of the eye	15 mSv in a year	2 mSv in a year
Skin	50 mSv in a year	50 mSv in a year
Cancer risk	Cancer mortality based on 1958–1987 data	Cancer mortality based on 1950–1997 data
Dosimetry	DS system DS86	DS02 (higher doses)
Risk projection model	Multiplicative risk model	Effective absolute risk (EAR) and effective relative risk (ERR)
DDREF	2	1.5
Genetic risk	• 1.3% Sv^{-1} for general population • 0.8 % Sv^{-1} for worker • Relative contribution to detriment = 18%	• 0.2% Sv^{-1} for general population • 0.1% Sv^{-1} for worker • Relative contribution to detriment = 3 to 4%
Total detriment	• 7.3% Sv^{-1} for whole population • 5.6% Sv^{-1} for adults	• 5.7% Sv^{-1} for whole population • 4.2% Sv^{-1} for adults
(DDREF: dose and dose rate effectiveness factor; ICRP: International Commission on Radiological Protection)		

these exposures is 5% and mean loss of life expectancy at 18 years is 0.5 years. Detriment is calculated assuming low-dose rate exposures and life expectancy of 75 years. This formed the basis of 20 mSv/year for occupational exposures.

Dose Limit

To arrive the public dose limit, an aggregated detriment value of 0.59% as a result of continuous exposure is assumed. Based on this risk level and the variation in natural background radiation levels, ICRP confirmed the public dose limit as 1 mSv/year. Hence, the dose limits remain the same as recommended by ICRP-60, except the lens of eye. Epidemiological studies suggest higher sensitivity of the eye lens; hence, eye lens limit is reduced to 20 mSv/year. Occupational exposure of women who are not pregnant is the same as that of man. If the women are pregnant, the dose limit is

TABLE 3.5 Aggregated detriment due to radiation exposure among workers and members of public.

Annual dose (mSv)	*Fatal cancer (%)*	*Weighted curable*	*Hereditary effects*	*Aggregated detriment (%)*
Worker exposure age from 18 to 65 years				
10	1.8	0.36	0.36	2.5
20	3.6	0.72	0.72	5.0
30	5.3	1.06	1.06	7.4
50	8.6	1.72	1.72	12.0
Public exposure from birth over lifetime				
0.5	0.2	0.04	0.05	0.29
1	0.4	0.08	0.11	0.59
2	0.8	0.16	0.21	1.17
3	1.1	0.22	0.29	1.61
5	2.0	0.40	0.53	2.93
Courtesy: ICRP 103, 2007.				

1 mSv to the fetus for the duration after the declaration of pregnancy to childbirth, considering high sensitivity of the human conceptus. Intake of radionuclides during this period should not exceed 0.05 of ALI. The intent of these two limits for pregnant women is to limit the dose to fetus to about 1 mSv. To give flexibility, the dose limits are averaged over 5 years for both occupational and members of public. If any individual exposure crosses the limits, commission has suggested any special restrictions to the individual. It is left to the decision of the regulatory body.

Categories of Exposure

There are three categories of exposure, namely—(1) occupational exposure, (2) public exposure, and (3) medical exposure to patients. Occupational exposure is defined as all radiation exposure of workers incurred because of their work. It is due to situations that can reasonably be considered as being the responsibility of the operating management. The employer is responsible for the protection of workers and licensee is responsible for the source. Public exposure refers to all exposures of the public other than occupational exposure and medical exposure of patients. It includes natural sources, artificial sources, and embryo and fetus of pregnant workers and the exposure varies widely.

Medical exposure of patient occurs in diagnostic, interventional, and therapeutic procedures. There are wide range of radiological procedures and require proper approach, if it differs from radiological protection. The exposure is intentional that gives direct benefit to the patient. For example, high dose of radiation is used in radiotherapy to treat cancer.

RADIATION RISK

Radiation risk is a probability—that a given individual will incur a deleterious effect because of a dose of radiation. Population risk is divided into—(i) somatic risk, (ii) genetic risk, and (iii) fetal risk. Scientists have developed dose-response models to predict the risk of cancer in human populations due to low-level radiation exposure. Radiation risk to the population can be expressed in terms of—(i) relative risk (RR) and (ii) absolute risk (AR).

Risk Expressions

Relative Risk

Relative risk is the ratio of the cancer incidence in the exposed population to that in general population. For example, an RR of 1.2 predicts a 20% (120/100) increase over the spontaneous rate of cancer incidence.

$$\text{The excess relative risk} = \text{RR} - 1 = 1.2 - 1 = 0.2$$

It gives information about the magnitude of increased risk, not the perspective of the risk in terms of overall health impact. If the natural cancer incidence is 2 per 10,000 and the RR is 4, then radiation-induced cancer risk is 8 per 10,000. A study sample of 10,000 is required to detect the above RR with a statistical confidence of 95% ($p < 0.5$).

Absolute Risk

Another way of expressing risk is absolute risk (AR) and excess absolute risk (EAR). AR is expressed as number of excess cancers cases per 10^4 in a population per Sv per year. For example, if the AR is 4 in 10,000 population, it is expressed as 4×10^{-4} Sv^{-1} y^{-1}. It has minimum latent period of 10 years.

Excess absolute risk is the difference between two ARs, expressed in EAR per unit dose, mostly used in epidemiology study. It is also referred as excess attributable risk. Let us consider a population exposed to 1 Sv radiation having an AR of 90 × 10^{-5}/year. The AR of unexposed population is 20 × 10^{-5}/year. Then the excess AR is the difference between the two ARs: $90 \times 10^{-5} - 20 \times 10^{-5} = 70 \times 10^{-5}$/Sv/year.

Worked Example 3.1

The AR is 4 per 10,000 per Sv per year and the latency period is 10 years. What is the risk of developing cancer in the next 30 years, from a dose of 0.1 Sv?

$$\text{Actual duration} = 30 - 10 = 20 \text{ years}$$

$$\text{Dose} = 0.1 \text{ Sv}$$

$$\text{Risk} = 4 \times 10^{-4}$$

$$\text{Risk of developing cancer} = 20 \text{ y} \times 0.1 \text{ Sv} \times 4 \times 10^{-4}/\text{Sv/y}$$

$$= 8 \times 10^{-4}$$

If 10,000 people are exposed to a dose of 0.1 Sv, eight additional cases of cancer will be seen in that population in the next 30 years.

Dose–Response Models

Dose-response models have been proposed to account the relationship of radiation exposure in humans. It includes—(i) linear nonthreshold, (ii) linear quadratic (LQ), and (iii) linear threshold models. BEIR VII report supports *LNT risk model* **(Fig. 3.2)**. LNT curves are extrapolated from high-dose/dose-rate response obtained from atomic bomb data, Japan. As per the model, the risk of cancer proceeds in a linear fashion at lower doses without a threshold, and even a smallest dose has potential to cause small increase in risk to humans. It addresses health effects of low levels of low

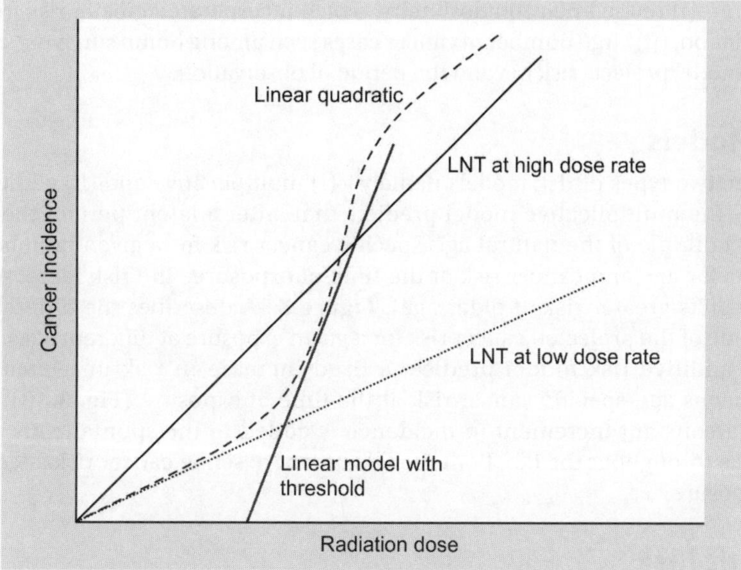

FIG. 3.2: The linear and nonlinear models of radiation effects.
(LNT: linear non-threshold)

LET ionizing radiations such as gamma and X-rays. Even a small dose is not a safe dose, and it will have some biological impact.

Linear curve with threshold supports epidemiological data that some cancer incidences have threshold dose, e.g., skin cancer. However, all radiation-induced cancers do not have threshold. No sufficient evidence is available to accept this model as general hypothesis to access cancer risk.

Linear quadratic dose–response model predicts lower effectiveness for incidence of cancer at lower doses, and that of higher effectiveness at higher doses. At high doses, the curve gets flattened due to substantial cell killing. In analogy to LQ theory of survival curve, the probability of an effect is proportional to sum of linear (αD) and quadratic (βD) components. They represent response to low dose and high dose and high-dose rate effects. The degree of curvature depends on α/β ratio, which can be obtained for different cancers.

Hence, ICRP-99 and BEIR VII recommended LNT hypothesis for general risk estimate. LNT hypothesis with dose and dose rate effectiveness factor (DDREF) for extrapolation from high doses is the basis for radiation protection at low doses and low-dose rates. DDREF is used to convert risk from exposures at high dose and high-dose rate to estimate of risk at low doses. BEIT VII recommended a DDREF of 1.5 to adjust the response observed at high doses to the LNT model curve. It also noted that there is uncertainty in the estimate of DDREF due to inconsistency and imprecision of animal data. LNT model is used to estimate cancer risk for all solid cancers, except leukemia for which LQ model is the better fit. Medical imaging doses and occupational workers doses are low, <100 mSv in which the difference between LNT and LQ model curve is much smaller. The LNT curve represents the extension of linear portion of LQ model. It overestimates the incidence of cancer at lower doses from low LET radiation.

The risk estimates were revised in 1990 after reassessing the Japanese atomic bomb survivors, which resulted an increase in risk estimation. The reasons for the above are—(i) revised neutron dosimetry, which incorporated greater risk from low LET radiation, (ii) large number of cancer cases seen among bomb survivors, and (iii) revised model projects risk beyond the period of observation.

Risk Models

There are two types of risk models namely—(i) multiplicative and (ii) additive risk models. The multiplicative model predicts that, after a latent period, the excess risk is a multiple of the natural age-specific cancer risk for a given population. It accounts for age and cancer risk at the time of exposure. The risk increases with age (predicts greater risk at older age). **Figure 3.3A** describes the differences in magnitude of the projected cancer risk for a given exposure at different ages.

The additive risk model predicts a fixed increase in risk unrelated to the spontaneous age-specific cancer risk at the time of exposure **(Fig. 3.3B)**. In this model, a constant increment in incidence is added to the spontaneous disease incidence throughout the life. Both models do not describe cancer risk adequately, after exposure.

Somatic Risk

Somatic risks may arise from both stochastic and deterministic effects. Radiation may induce both benign and malignant tumors with latent period. Cancer induction is the largest risk of radiation, and it is higher for children than adults. ICRP-103 risk estimate for somatic risk is about 5.5% per Sv for whole population, and 4.1% per Sv for adults. This new risk estimate is nearly five times lower than the ICRP-60 values.

Genetic Risk

Genetic risk is difficult to estimate; hence, mouse-doubling dose and information of human population genetics are used to arrive an estimate. Genetic risk analysis assumes that the—(i) exposed population consists of all ages, and both sexes, and (ii) severe genetic effects in the next two generations.

Genetically significant dose (GSD) is an index to express the radiation-induced mutation in germ cells of a given population. It is the amount of dose required per generation to double spontaneous mutation rate. The spontaneous mutation rate is about 5×10^{-6} per locus, and 15×10^{-4} per gamete for chromosome abnormalities. The doubling dose for humans is estimated as ~1 Gy per generation, which is extrapolated from animal data.

ICRP-103 risk estimate for genetic risk is about 0.2% per Sv for general population, and 0.1% per Sv for workers. This new risk estimate is nearly five times lower than the ICRP-60 values.

Embryo/Fetus Risk

Embryo/Fetus is sensitive during first half of the gestation period. Increased risk of malformation is seen during first 8 weeks and central nervous system (CNS) is highly sensitive during 8–15 weeks of gestation period. Mental retardation is a deterministic effect with threshold dose of 0.1 Sv (ICRP) and is about 40% per Sv for high-dose rate exposures. The embryo risk is about 10% per Sv from 16–25 weeks. In utero X-ray exposure in third trimester will increase childhood cancer risk of the order of 0.1/Sv.

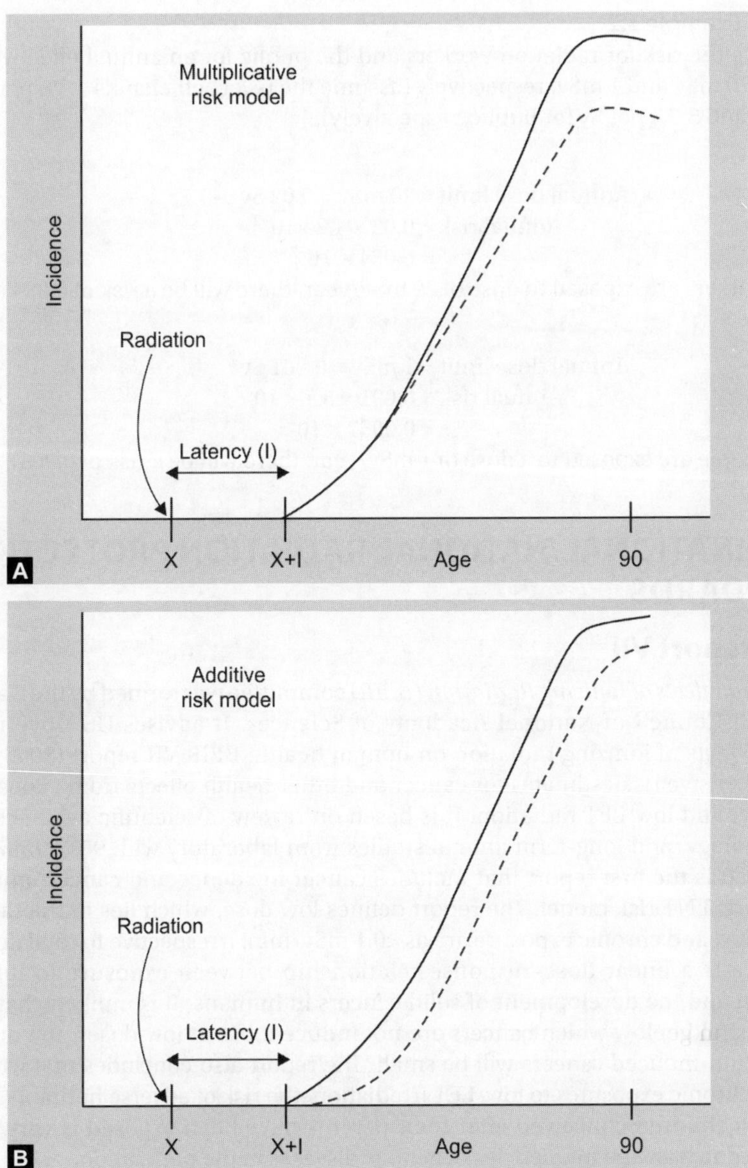

FIGS. 3.3A AND B: (A) Multiplicate model, and (B) Additive model.

However, low doses/dose rates <100 mGy generally carry negligible risk and abortion may be advised, only when doses are >100 mGy. The fetal dose from medical diagnostic procedures rarely exceeds 50 mGy. This will not put the fetus any significant increase in risk for congenital malformation or mental retardation. ICRP estimate for risk of childhood cancer from in utero irradiation is about 0.1 per Sv. This risk is very small for few mSv compared to background risk of 1 in 2,000 live births. The relative incidence of various health effects with radiation exposure in utero at various stages of gestation is shown in **Figure 2.8, Chapter 2**.

Worked Example 3.2

Calculate the risk for radiation workers and the public for an annual effective dose limit of 20 mSv and 1 mSv, respectively (assume the risk coefficient is 4.2% per Sv for worker, and 5.7% per Sv for public, respectively).

Worker:

$$\text{Annual dose limit} = 20 \text{ mSv} = 0.02 \text{ Sv}$$
$$\text{Annual risk} = 0.02 \times 4.2 \times 10^{-2}$$
$$= 0.084 \times 10^{-2}$$

If 100 workers are exposed to dose of 20 mSv/year, there will be a risk of 0.084 or <1.

Public:

$$\text{Annual dose limit} = 1 \text{ mSv} = 0.001 \text{ Sv}$$
$$\text{Annual risk} = 0.001 \times 5.7 \times 10^{-2}$$
$$= 0.0057 \times 10^{-2}$$

If 100 people are exposed to a dose of 1 mSv/year, there will be a risk of 0.0057 or <1.

INTERNATIONAL/NATIONAL RADIATION PROTECTION STANDARDS

BEIR Report VII

Biological Effects of Ionizing Radiation (BEIR) committee was formed by the National Research Council of National Academy of Sciences. It advises US Government on the effects of ionizing radiation on human health. BEIR VII report (2006) gives comprehensive risk estimates for cancer and other health effects from exposure to low dose, and low LET radiation. It is based on review of scientific evidence from epidemiology, and long-term animal studies from laboratory with 95% confidence interval. It is the first report that includes cancer incidence and cancer mortality. It supports LNT risk model. The report defines low dose, which lies in the range of 0–100 mSv, and chronic exposure are as <0.1 mSv/min, irrespective to total dose.

There is a linear dose-response relationship between exposure to ionizing radiation and the development of solid cancers in humans. It is unlikely that there is a threshold below which cancers are not induced, but at low doses, the number of radiation-induced cancers will be small. The report also concludes that with low dose or chronic exposures to low-LET irradiation, the risk of adverse heritable health effects to children conceived after their parents have been exposed is very small, compared to baseline frequencies of genetic diseases in the population.

The BEIT VII attempts to develop risk models for development of cancer in individual, considering his sex and age at exposure. It used data from epidemiological studies to complete the task, e.g., *Atomic-bomb survivor Life Span Study (LSS)*. Its lifetime risk model predicts that approximately one individual in 100 persons would be expected to develop cancer (solid cancer or leukemia) from a dose of 100 mSv. BEIR VII report has given estimate of *lifetime attributable risk (LAR)* incidence of and mortality for all solid cancers and leukemia per 100,000 persons exposed to 100 mSv. It also has given LAR of site-specific cancer incidence for different age at exposure. Other health effects (heart disease and stroke) can occur at higher radiation doses. However, there is no direct evidence of increased risk of noncancers at low doses. The genetic risks are much small compared to spontaneous genetic effects in population.

Basic Safety Standard—IAEA

International Atomic Energy Agency has established an international standard for radiation protection and safety in the form of BSS and published its recommendations as safety series. It was the initiative of IAEA with international and intergovernmental organizations in 1950. The standards are intended for the application and use by government and regulatory authorities who enforce radiation protection on various areas. It includes nuclear facilities, mining and raw material processing, radioactive waste management, use of radiation in industrial, medical and research applications, and decommissioning facilities. Safety standards also support the application of code of contact on the safety and security of radioactive sources, research reactors and international health regulations. It is an international instrument that has legal binding on WHO member states.

The first health and safety measures were approved in 1960 based on ICRP recommendations. First BSS was approved in 1962 and published as IAEA safety series 9, which was later revised in 1967 and 1982. BSS for protection against ionizing radiation and for the safety of radiation sources published as IAEA safety series No 115 in 1996. It is followed by radiation protection and safety of radiation sources, BSS, IAEA safety standard series No GSR part 3, 2014.

International BSS is jointly sponsored by the European Commission (EC), the Food and Agriculture Organization of the United Nations (FAO), the IAEA, the International Labour Organization (ILO), the OECD Nuclear Energy Agency (OECD/NEA), the Pan American Health Organization (PAHO), the United Nations Environment Programme (UNEP), and the World Health Organization (WHO) (the Sponsoring Organizations).

Basic Safety Standard is seen as a global reference for nuclear, radiation protection, radioactive waste, and transport safety. These reports establish safety standard, and guidance about how to implement them. Standards evolve through time and are based on international knowledge and experience. It is used by member states to deliver consistent levels of safety for the protection of workers, public, and the environment. Safety standards are not having binding on member states, and may be adopted by them.

IAEA Safety Standard Series No GSR Part 3, 2014

International Atomic Energy Agency safety standard series No GSR Part 3, on radiation protection and safety of radiation sources: international BSSs, was published in 2014. It supersedes the BSS for protection against ionizing radiation and for the safety of radiation sources published as IAEA safety series No 115 in 1996. This document describes the—(i) general requirements for protection and safety, (ii) planned exposure situations, (iii) emergency exposure situations, and (iv) existing exposure situations. About 52 requirements are recommended under various headlines as described below.

General requirements for protection and safety:

- Application of the principle of radiation protection (1)
- Responsibilities of the government (2)
- Responsibility of the regulatory body (3)
- Responsibility for protection and safety (4)
- Management requirements (5)

Planned exposure situations: Planned exposure situation arises from planned operation of source or from a planned activity that results in exposure due to a source.

It refers to deliberate introduction and operation of sources. It may give rise to both expected and not expected doses. It can be controlled by good design facilities, equipment, and operating procedures, and training. It is expected that exposure of some level does occur in planned exposure situations. The exposure, not expected to occur but occurs due to accident or from an event, is often referred as potential exposure.

Generic requirements:

- Graded approach (6)
- Notification and authorization (7)
- Exemption and clearance (8)
- Responsibilities of registrants and licenses in planned exposure situations (9)
- Justification of practice (10)
- Optimization of protection and safety (11)
- Dose limits (12)
- Safety assessment (13)
- Monitoring for verification of compliance (14)
- Prevention and mitigation of accidents (15)
- Investigations and feedback information on operating experience (16)
- Radiation generators and radioactive sources (17)
- Human imaging using radiation for the purposes other than medical purposes, medical treatment, or biomedical research (18)

Occupational exposure:

- Responsibilities of the regulatory body specific to occupational exposure (19)
- Requirements for monitoring and recording of occupational exposures (20)
- Responsibilities of employers, registrants, and licensees for the protection of workers (21)
- Compliance by workers (22)
- Cooperation between employers and registrants and licensees (23)
- Arrangements under the radiation protection program (24)
- Assessment of occupational exposure and workers' health surveillance (25)
- Information, instruction, and training (26)
- Conditions of service (27)
- Special arrangements for protection and safety for female workers and for persons under 18 years of age undergoing training (28)

Public exposure:

- Responsibilities of the government and the regulatory body specific to public exposure (29)
- Responsibilities of relevant parties specific to public exposure (30)
- Radioactive waste and discharges (31)
- Monitoring and reporting (32)
- Consumer products (33)

Medical exposure:

- Responsibilities of the government specific to medical exposure (34)
- Responsibilities of the regulatory body specific to medical exposure (35)
- Responsibilities of registrants and licensees specific to medical exposure (36)
- Justification of medical exposures (37)
- Optimization of protection and safety (38)
- Pregnant or breastfeeding female patients (39)

- Release of patients after radionuclide therapy (40)
- Unintended and accidental medical exposures (41)
- Reviews and records (42)

Emergency exposure situations: Emergency exposure situations arise as a result of accident, a malicious act or any other unexpected event or series of events. It requires prompt actions to reduce exposures. Preventive measures and mitigatory actions need to be planned to avoid any emergency exposure situation. However, once emergency exposure occurred, only preventive actions can reduce exposure levels.

Generic requirements:
- Emergency management system (43)

Public exposures:
- Preparedness and response for an emergency (44)

Exposure of emergency workers:
- Arrangements for controlling the exposure of emergency workers (45)

Transition from an emergency exposure situation to an existing exposure situation:
- Arrangements for the transition from an emergency exposure situation to an existing exposure situation (46)

Existing exposure situations: Existing exposure situation arises from natural background radiation, exposure due to residual radioactive material that derives from past practices, which is not under the regulatory control or remains after an emergency exposure situation.

Generic requirements:
- Responsibilities of the government specific to existing exposure situations (47)

Public exposures:
- Justification for protective actions and optimization of protection and safety (48)
- Responsibilities for remediation of areas with residual radioactive material (49)
- Public exposure due to radon indoors (50)
- Exposure due to radionuclides in commodities (51)

Occupational exposure:
- Exposure in workplaces (52)

UNSCEAR Recommendations

United Nations Scientific Committee on the Effects of Atomic Radiation (UNSCEAR) was formed by the United Nations in 1955 to collect and evaluate information on the levels and effects of ionizing radiation. It has its headquarters at Vienna, Austria. Its aim is to assess and report levels and effects of exposure to ionizing radiation. It also undertakes broad reviews of the sources of ionizing radiation and effects of that radiation on human health and environment. Several Government and organizations relay the UNSCEAR estimate as the scientific basis to evaluate radiation risk. UNSCEAR has 27 member countries and published 25 reports from inception. Reports of much important are:

- Sources and effects of ionizing radiation, 1996
- Effects of ionizing radiation (Volume 1), 2008

Recent report estimates the background radiation as 3 mSv/year, including 2.4 mSv from natural exposure. It corresponds to annual collective dose of global population is 16 million man Sv.

National Council on Radiation Protection and Measurements

National Council on Radiation Protection and Measurements (NCRP) is a USA-based regulatory organization, formed in 1964. Its mission is to support radiation protection by providing independent scientific analysis, information, and recommendations that represent the consensus of the leading scientists. It has published several recommendations and the latest and useful reports for medical application areas follows:

- *NCRP-147*: Structural shielding design for medical X-ray imaging facilities, 2004
- *NCRP-151*: Structural shielding design and evaluation for megavoltage X- and gamma-ray radiotherapy facilities, 2005

Atomic Energy Regulatory Board

The AERB was constituted on November 15, 1983, by the President of India by exercising the powers conferred by Section 27 of the Atomic Energy Act 1962 (33 of 1962). It is an apex body that regulates the use of ionizing radiation in the country. The AERB is entrusted with the responsibility of developing and implementing appropriate regulatory measures aimed at ensuring radiation safety in applications involving ionizing radiations. The board is fully empowered to lay down standards and frame rules and regulations.

The Chairman AERB is the competent authority, recognized by the Government for enforcing provisions of radiation safety in the use of ionizing radiation. AERB has jurisdiction over all the units of the department of atomic energy and all radiation installations in the country. The mission of the board is to ensure that the use of ionizing radiation and nuclear energy does not cause undue risk to health and environment.

The board covers the safety aspects of all areas of nuclear fuel cycle and use of radiation in medicine, agriculture, industry and research and transport of radioactive materials. The board is assisted by health, safety, and environment group of BARC, viz., Radiological Physics and Advisory Division (RPAD), advisory committees, and task groups.

Major objective of AERB is to develop and publicize specific codes and guides, which will deal with the radiation safety aspects of various applications of radiations. It will also issue authorization related to site, design, manufacture, construction, commissioning, operation, maintenance, and decommissioning and disposal of radioactive sources. Various codes and guides are:

- *AERB safety code No AERB/RF-MED/SC-1 (Rev 1)*: Radiation therapy sources, equipment, and installations, 2011
- *AERB/RF-MED/SC-2 (Rev 2)*: Nuclear medicine facilities, 2011
- *AERB/RF-MED/SC-3 (Rev 2)*: Radiation safety in manufacture, supply, and use of medical diagnostic X-ray equipment, 2016
- *AERB/NRF-TS/SC-1(Rev 1)*: Safe transport of radioactive material, 2016

FACTORS GOVERNING INTERNAL EXPOSURES

Assessment of intake of radionuclides depends on calculation of intake of a radionuclide directly from whole-body countermeasurements. Indirect methods measure radioactivity from urine, feces, and air samples. Biokinetic model is employed to calculate the effective dose from reference dose coefficients recommended by the commission (ICRP 1994b, 1996c). Commission has provided dose coefficients for intakes by inhalation and ingestion for a large number of radionuclides. It relates the intake of a specific radionuclide to the corresponding organ and effective dose committed within specific period. Dose coefficients are specified for members of public and adults and occupational workers.

Alternatively, committed effective dose can be calculated directly from the measurements using functions that relate them to the time of the intake. Measurements may be whole-body or organ content, urine or fecal or environmental samples. Commission provided additional table of dose per unit content as a function of time after the intake.

Radionuclide Concentrations in Air and Water and Contamination Levels

Open radionuclides are used in nuclear medicine; there are possibility of leakage or escape of radioactive gas. The main contaminants of importance in nuclear facility are radioiodine, tritium, fission products, noble gases, etc. Once the effluent is released in the air, the operator has no control and hence cannot escape the consequences arising out of air pollution. The removal of particulate and gaseous contaminants from gaseous effluents is a complex and expensive one. Regulations prescribe the concentrations for such air-borne radioactive material that will lead to annual dose limits **(Table 3.6)**. The assumption is that workers are chronically exposed to 2,000 hour working per year, and breath 2×10^4 mL of air per minute.

Radionuclide concentration in sewage is a matter of concern because it may reach public water supplies. The regulation also prescribes environmental concentrations of radioactivity in air and water, including the concentration of radionuclides disposed of into the sewage water that leads to annual dose limits **(Table 3.7)**. It is based on the assumption that the inhalation and ingestion by the public over a period of 1 year with an average breath of 2×10^4 mL of air per minute and has an annual intake of 7.3×10^7 mL.

TABLE 3.6 **Air concentration that would result annual dose limits to occupational workers.**

Radionuclide	*Air-borne concentration (kBq/mL)*
^{18}F	1.1
^{99m}Tc	2.2
^{125}I	1.1×10^{-3}
^{131}I	7.4×10^{-4}
^{14}C	3.7×10^{-2}
^{133}Xe	3.7

Courtesy: Simon RC et al, 2012.

TABLE 3.7 Air-borne, water, and sewer concentrations that would result annual dose limits for public.

	Environmental concentrations (kBq/mL)		
Radionuclide	***Air***	***Water***	***Sewer concentration (μCi/mL)***
^{18}F	3.7×10^{-3}	2.59×10	2.59×10^{2}
^{99m}Tc	7.4×10^{-3}	3.7×10	3.7×10^{2}
^{125}I	1.1×10^{-5}	7.4×10^{-2}	7.4×10^{-1}
^{131}I	7.4×10^{-6}	3.7×10^{-2}	3.7×10^{-1}
^{14}C	1.1×10^{-4}	1.11	1.11×10
^{133}Xe	1.9×10^{-2}	—	—

Courtesy: Simon RC et al, 2012.

DOSE LIMITS FOR OCCUPATIONAL WORKERS, PUBLIC, COMFORTERS, AND TRAINEES

The ICRP-60 (1991) introduced the concept of permissible dose, defined as a dose of ionizing radiation that, in the light of present knowledge, is not expected to cause appreciable bodily injury to a person at any time during his lifetime as given in **Table 3.3**.

Effective dose limit ensures avoidance of deterministic effect in all body tissues and organs, except skin, which may be subjected to localized exposures. Occupational dose limits exclude exposures from medical procedures and natural background. Actual exposure to diagnostic radiology staff is relatively low, about <1 mSv/year. Dose limits for members of public are generally 10 times lower than those for occupational exposure.

A person may receive radiation dose from external or internal sources. Radionuclides can enter the body through injection, inhalation, wounds, or absorption by skin. The dose limit is same irrespective of the exposure route, internal or external or combination of two. Accumulation of internally deposited radionuclide will depend on their concentration in air, water, rate of intake, and metabolism. Limits are therefore, prescribed in terms *ALI* for different radionuclides.

AERB Dose Limits, Government of India, 2011

Workers

- Effective dose of 20 mSv/year, averaged over consecutive 5 years
- Effective dose of 30 mSv in any year
- Equivalent dose to the lens of the eye is 150 (reduced to 20) mSv in a year
- Equivalent dose to extremities (hand and feet) is 500 mSv in a year
- Equivalent dose to the skin is 500 mSv in a year

Pregnant worker:

Above limits are applicable to female workers also. In case of women worker of reproductive age, equivalent dose limit to embryo/fetus shall be 1 mSv. Once pregnancy has been established, the conceptus shall be protected. Workers shall be monitored by an additional dosimeter worn on the abdomen under lead apron.

[Conceptus shall be protected by applying a supplementary effective dose limit to her abdomen surface (lower trunk) of 2 mSv for the remainder of the pregnancy, which is normally considered equivalent to 1 mSv to the fetus, ICRP-60.] Internal exposures shall be controlled by limiting intakes of radionuclides to about 1/20 of ALI. The employment shall be of such type that it does not carry a probability of high-accidental doses and intakes. Pregnant radiation workers should not be allowed to work in radioiodine therapy ward and in positron emission tomography (PET) facility.

Comforters

Comforters and carers exclude pregnant women, are knowingly and willingly exposed. The dose constraint is 5 mSv per procedure and has no dose limit.

Trainees

Occupational exposures to apprentices and trainees between 16 and 18 years of age shall be controlled the limits are not exceeded.

- The effective dose of 6 mSv in a year
- Equivalent dose to the lens of eye of 50 mSv in a year
- Equivalent dose to extremities (hand and feet) of 150 mSv in a year
- Equivalent dose to the skin of 150 mSv in a year

Note: Apprentices and trainees in radiation facility, if any, shall be of age 16 years only.

Public

The estimated average doses to the relevant members of the public shall not exceed the following limits:

- An effective dose of 1 mSv in a year
- An equivalent dose to the lens of eye of 2 mSv in a year
- An equivalent dose to the skin of 50 mSv in a year

For a variety of reasons, dose limits for the general population are set lower than those for radiation workers. Justifications for this approach include the following:

- Public includes children who might represent a group at increased risk and who may be exposed for their whole lifetime
- It is not the decision or choice of the public that they be exposed
- Public is exposed for their entire lifetime; workers are exposed only during their working lifetime, and presumably only while on the job
- Public may receive no direct benefit from the exposure
- Public is already being exposed to risks in their own occupations
- Public is not subject to the selection, supervision, and monitoring afforded to radiation workers

Dose Limits to Patients

Dose limits are applicable only for radiation workers and not for patients. The decision to use radiation is justified that depends upon individual patient condition. Status of pregnancy should be ascertained in female patients before the diagnostic procedures. In case of doubt, it is better to carry out pregnancy test. She should be informed about the potential effects of radiation and magnitude of risk involved. The procedure is medically indicated, if the risk to the mother of not conducting the procedure is greater than the potential harm to the conceptus. Once the medical procedure is justified, it should be optimized. This means that the conditions should achieve the clinical purpose with appropriate dose.

Procedures involving radioiodine may cause significant risk to the fetus. Guidelines of ICRP-84 (2000c) should be followed in such cases. Cancers of pelvic region cannot be treated by radiotherapy. Cancer site locations that are away from the pelvis can be treated by radiotherapy, by extensive treatment planning and scatter dose calculation. In the event of exposures to the conceptus, termination of pregnancy should not be recommended for doses <100 mGy. If the dose is >100 mGy, termination of pregnancy can be recommended only after ascertaining the importance of pregnancy and based on individual circumstances. Pregnant members of public should not be allowed to visit the radioiodine therapy patients and LDR brachytherapy patients.

BIBLIOGRAPHY

1. BEIR. Health risks from exposures to low levels of ionizing radiation: BEIR VII, National research council of the national academies, NAS. Washington, DC: National Academies Press; 2006.
2. Government of India. (2011). AERB safety code No. AERB/RF-MED/SC-1 (Rev.1): Radiation therapy sources, equipment, and installations. [online] Available from https://www.aerb.gov.in/images/PDF/CodesGuides/RadiationFacility/MedicalApplicationsInvolvingRadiation/4.pdf. [Last accessed September, 2022].
3. International Atomic Energy Agency. (2014). Radiation protection and safety of radiation sources: International basic standards, IAEA safety standard, GSR Part 3. [online] Available from https://www.iaea.org/publications/8930/radiation-protection-and-safety-of-radiation-sources-international-basic-safety-standards. [Last accessed September, 2022].
4. International Commission on Radiation Protection. Recommendations of ICRP. ICRP publication 103. New York: Pergamon press; 2007.
5. International Commission on Radiation Protection. Recommendations of ICRP. ICRP publication 60. New York: Pergamon Press; 1991.
6. Kelsey CA, Heintz PH, Sandoval DJ, Chambers GD, Adolphi NL, Paffett KS. Radiation biology of medical imaging. New York: Wiley Blackwell; 2014.
7. National Council on Radiation Protection and Measurements. Recommendations on limits for exposure to ionizing radiation. NCRP report No.116. Bethesda, MD: National Council on Radiation Protection and Measurements; 1993.
8. UNSCEAR. (2010). Sources and effects of ionizing radiation, 2008, Volume I. [online] Available from http://www.unscear.org/docs/reports/2008/09-86753_Report_2008_GA_Report.pdf. [Last accessed September, 2022].
9. Simon RC, James A. Sorenson, Michael E. Phelps. Physics in Nuclear Medicine, 4th Edition, Elsevier Saunders, 2012.
10. Atomic energy regulatory board, Government of India: http//www.aerb.gov.in.

CHAPTER 4

Radiation Hazards, Evaluation and Control

INTRODUCTION

Application of ionizing radiation always causes some form of hazards. The knowledge of the nature and degree of potential hazard is very vital to take effective control measures. For example, X-ray units and linear accelerators emit radiation only when they are energized. Telecobalt units and open radioisotopes emit radiation all the time. In telecobalt unit, the source is well shielded when it is in *OFF* position, whereas it is adequately shielded during *ON* position, excluding primary beam. The nature and extent of hazard depend on—(1) physical characteristics of the radiation source employed, (2) operation conditions at the place of use of the source, (3) safe handling facilities available, and (4) professional training of the person handling the source. Radiation hazard is divided into—(1) internal hazard and (2) external hazard.

INTERNAL AND EXTERNAL HAZARDS

Internal hazard refers to entry of radioactive material into the living organism. The main sources are—(1) inhalation of contaminated air, (2) ingestion of contaminated food and water, and (3) entry of radionuclide directly in the bloodstream. In telecobalt therapy, internal hazard is rare, since it is a sealed source. Hazard may arise during fire or accident involving melting, evaporation, or dispersal of radionuclide. However, internal hazard is possible in nuclear medicine where open radionuclides are employed.

External hazard arises when the radiation source is outside the body. Diagnostic X-ray units, telecobalt units, sealed sources, and linear accelerators may cause external hazards. X-rays and γ-rays account majority of external hazards since they are highly penetrating. β- and α-radiations take second and third place in terms of external hazards.

Hazard evaluation is necessary to take suitable control measures in radiation areas. Such evaluation starts from radiation equipment design stage. The original equipment manufacturer (OEM) shall ensure that the equipment meets the stipulated safety standards. User of the equipment should also ensure the safety of patients, personnel, and public. It is much important to evaluate hazards under normal working conditions as well as under potential accident conditions, e.g., fire and explosion. The four principal methods by which radiation exposures to persons can be minimized are—(1) time, (2) distance, (3) shielding, and (4) contamination control. Among the three distance is most effective in reducing radiation levels at a point.

APPLICATION OF TIME, DISTANCE, AND SHIELDING

Time

Radiation exposure from a source at a point is directly proportional to the time during which the source is *ON*. Lesser the time spent near the radiation source, lesser will be the radiation dose. As time spent in the radiation field increases, the radiation dose also increases. Hence, the time spent should be minimized in any radiation area. Techniques to minimize time in a radiation field should be recognized or practiced.

All radiation sources do not produce constant exposure rates. Diagnostic X-ray machines typically produce high exposure rates over brief time intervals. For example, chest X-ray produces a skin entrance exposure of 20 mR in 0.05 second, equivalent to 24,000 mR/h. Hence, radiation exposure can be minimized by not energizing the X-ray tube when personnel are nearer to the machine.

Nuclear medicine procedure produces lower exposure rate for extended periods of time. The exposure rate at 1 m from a patient injected with 20 mCi of Technetium-99m (^{99m}Tc), for bone scan, is 1 mR/h. It reduces to 0.5 mR/h after 2 hours, due to decay and urinary excretion by biological half life. Hence, both the knowledge of exposure rate and how it changes over time are important elements in reducing personnel exposures.

The time spent near the radiation source can be minimized by understanding the task to be performed and the suitable equipment required to complete them in short interval with safety. Hence, one must plan and practice the radiation procedure without radiation, and share the essential duties, to reduce radiation exposure. For example, fluoroscopy-screening time should be kept short by using last frame hold facility, in addition to the use of foot switch.

Worked Example 4.1

A radiographer is performing barium examination under fluoroscopy and the equipment is "ON" for 3 minutes for each examination. The radiation level at the location of the radiographer is 100 mR/h. How many such procedures the radiographer can carry out per week?

The annual equivalent dose limit prescribed for the radiographer is (occupational worker):

$$20 \text{ mSv} = 2{,}000 \text{ mrem} \approx 2{,}000 \text{ mR}$$

$$\text{Permitted weekly dose} = 2{,}000 \text{ mR/50 weeks} = 40 \text{ mR}$$

$$\text{Exposure rate at the location of radiographer} = 100 \text{ mR/h}$$

$$= (100/60) \text{ mR/min}$$

$$\text{The exposure in each procedure} = (100 \text{ mR}/60 \text{ min}) \times 3 \text{ min}$$

$$= 5 \text{ mR}$$

Hence, number of procedures the radiographer can associate within 1 week

$$= 40 \text{ mR}/5 \text{ mR} = 8$$

Worked Example 4.2

An operator is handling 10 mCi of Iodine-131 (^{131}I) source with 30 cm tong. Within how much time, the nuclear medicine technician will receive the weekly permissible equivalent dose?

(Assume 1R = 1 rad, $\Gamma_{20} = 2.18$ R-cm^2/mCi-h for ^{131}I)

$$\text{Exposure level at 30 cm from 10 mCi of }^{131}\text{I source} = \frac{2.18 \times 10\ \text{mCi}}{30^2} = 24\ \text{mR/h}$$

Weekly permissible exposure (2,000 mR/50 weeks) = 40 mR

$$\text{Allowed time of work} = \frac{40\ \text{mR}}{24\ \text{mR/h}} = 100\ \text{minutes}$$

Worked Example 4.3

Exposure rate from a source at a point where a service engineer is doing service is 120 mR/h. On an average for how much time the engineer can work at this point without exceeding the equivalent dose limits? (Assume 1 week = 5 days, and 1 year = 50 weeks)

The annual equivalent dose limit prescribed for the engineer is (occupational worker):

$$20\ \text{mSv} = 2{,}000\ \text{mrem} \approx 2{,}000\ \text{mR}$$

$$\text{Permitted weekly dose} = 2{,}000\ \text{mR/50 weeks} = 40\ \text{mR}$$

$$\text{Permitted work per day} = 40\ \text{mR/5 days} = 8\ \text{mR}$$

$$\text{Exposure rate} = 120\ \text{mR/h} = 120/60\ \text{min} = 2\ \text{mR/min}$$

$$\text{Maximum time the engineer can work} = 8/2 = 4\ \text{minutes}$$

Distance

Radiation intensity (exposure rate) from a point source decreases with distance, due to divergence of the beam. It is governed by inverse square law, which states that the exposure rate from a point source of radiation is inversely proportional to the square of the distance of the point from the source. If the exposure rate is X_1 at distance d_1, then the exposure rate X_2 at another distance d_2 is given by:

$$X_2 = X_1 \left(\frac{d_1}{d_2} \right)^2 \tag{4.1}$$

Doubling the distance from the X-ray source decreases the X-ray beam intensity by a factor of 4. If the exposure rate is 100 mR/h at 1 m, then it will be 25 mR/h at 2 m. Larger the distance, lesser will be the radiation dose (refer Chapter 1).

In diagnostic radiology at 1 m from a patient, the scattered radiation is about 0.1–0.15% of the intensity of the primary beam. Hence, all personnel should stand as far away as possible during X-ray procedures. Personnel should stand at least 2 m from the X-ray tube and the patient, and behind the shielded barrier or out of the room, whenever possible.

In nuclear medicine, it is difficult to shield the technologist from the radiation emitted from the patient during patient imaging, and distance is the only primary dose reduction method. The nuclear medicine technologists receive the annual dose mainly by patient positioning and imaging. Hence, imaging rooms should be designed to maximize the distance between the source and control console. Most of the time, the technologists spend their time at the control console for acquisition and image processing. Unshielded radiation sources never be manipulated by hand. Tongs or other handling devices are used to increase the distance between source and hand. A typical exposure rate with distances, for a nuclear medicine facility, is given in **Table 4.1**.

TABLE 4.1 **Exposure Rate with distance in nuclear medicine.**

Radionuclide 10 mCi	*Exposure rate (R/h) at 1 cm*	*Exposure rate (R/h) at 10 cm*
^{67}Ga	7.5	0.075
^{99m}Tc	6.2	0.062
^{123}I	16.3	0.163
^{131}I	21.8	0.218
^{133}Xe	5.3	0.053
^{201}Tl	4.5	0.045
^{18}F	56.6	0.570

Courtesy: Bushberg JT et al., 2012.

Worked Example 4.4

The exposure rate from a fluoroscopic X-ray machine is 5 R/min at 50 cm. What would be the exposure rates at—(1) 40 cm and (2) 60 cm?

1. $X_1 = 5$ R/min, $d_1 = 50$ cm, $d_2 = 40$ cm, $X_2 = ?$

$$X_2 = X_1\left(\frac{d_1}{d_2}\right)^2$$

$$= 5\ \text{R/min}\left(\frac{50}{40}\right)^2 = 7.81\ \text{R/min}$$

2. $X_1 = 5$ R/min, $d_1 = 50$ cm, $d_2 = 60$ cm, $X_2 = ?$

$$X_2 = X_1\left(\frac{d_1}{d_2}\right)^2$$

$$= 5\ \text{R/min}\left(\frac{50}{60}\right)^2 = 3.47\ \text{R/min}$$

Worked Example 4.5

What would be the radiation level at 10 cm from a 5-mCi source Cobalt-60 (^{60}Co)? (Given, $\Gamma = 13$ R-cm^2/mCi-h for ^{60}Co)

Exposure level at 1 cm from 5-mCi ^{60}Co source = $13 \times 5 = 65$ R/h

$X_1 = 65$ R/h, $d_1 = 1$ cm, $d_2 = 10$ cm, $X_2 = ?$

$$X_2 = X_1\left(\frac{d_1}{d_2}\right)^2$$

$$= 65\ \text{R/h}\left(\frac{1\ \text{cm}}{10\ \text{cm}}\right)^2 = 0.65\ \text{R/h} = 650\ \text{mR/h}$$

Worked Example 4.6

What would be the distance required to reduce the radiation level from a 10-mCi ^{192}Ir source to 2 mR/h?

(Given, $\Gamma = 4.69$ R-cm^2/mCi-h for ^{192}Ir)

Exposure rate at 1 cm from 10-mCi ^{192}Ir source = 4.69×10

= 46.9 R/h

= 46,900 mR/h

TABLE 4.2 **HVL values of aluminum and lead for various diagnostic X-ray energies.**

Peak voltage (kV)	*HVL, Aluminum (mm)*	*HVL, lead (mm)*
50	1.57	0.06
70	2.43	0.17
100	3.71	0.27
125	4.71	0.28
150	>5.25	0.30

(HVL: half-value layer; TVL: tenth value layer)

Courtesy: Bushberg JT et al., 2012.

$$X_1 = 46{,}900 \text{ mR/h},\ d_1 = 1 \text{ cm},\ d_2 = ?,\ X_2 = 2 \text{ mR/h}$$

$$X_2 = X_1\left(\frac{d_1}{d_2}\right)^2$$

$$2 \text{ mR/h} = 46{,}900 \text{ mR/h}\left(\frac{1 \text{ cm}}{d_2}\right)^2$$

$$d_2 = 153 \text{ cm or } 1.53 \text{ m}$$

Shielding

When maximum distance and minimum time do not ensure an acceptably low-radiation dose, adequate shielding must be provided, so that radiation beam will be sufficiently attenuated. The material that attenuates the radiation exponentially is called a shield and the shield will reduce exposure to patients, workers, and public. When a photon passes through an absorber of thickness x, both absorption and scattering take place. As a result, transmitted beam will have lesser number of photons:

$$I = I_0 e^{-\mu x} \tag{4.2}$$

where, I is the intensity of transmitted photons, I_0 is the intensity of incident photons, e is the base of natural logarithm, and μ is the linear attenuation coefficient. The attenuation depends on beam energy, nature of the absorber and its density. Based on the linear attenuation coefficient, half-value thickness (HVT) and tenth-value thickness (TVT) can be defined and they can be related by an equation: TVT = 3.32 HVT (refer Chapter 1). **Table 4.2** shows the HVT values for diagnostic X-rays as a function of kV for aluminum and lead.

The shielding type, thickness, and the location are functions of photon energy, number, intensity, source geometry, and exposure rate. Hence, the reduction in intensity depends upon the nature and thickness of the shield and energy of the radiation. Thus thicker the shielding, lesser will be the radiation.

In diagnostic energy range, X-ray attenuation is primarily by photoelectric effect and to some extent, by Compton effect. Photoelectric effect varies with atomic number (Z) and is proportional to Z^3. Hence, one can compare lead (Z = 82) and aluminum (Z = 13) as shielding material for the same thickness (g/cm^2), with their atomic numbers. The reduction in intensity caused by lead over aluminum is given by: $(82/13)^3 \approx 250.3$.

In other words, 1 g/cm^2 of lead will be as effective as 250 g/cm^2 of aluminum. Hence, in many situations, lead is used as shielding material to reduce the volume of shielding. Lead, brick, and concrete are commonly used in medicine for shielding radiation exposure. Lead aprons, gonad shield, lead gloves, lead bricks, and lead glass are also used as shield.

The factors to be considered while determining the amount, and type of shielding are:

- ALARA principle, personnel radiation must be kept As Low As Reasonably Achievable.
- Personnel exposures should not exceed the regulatory limits; this is 20 mSv for occupational workers and 1 mSv for public in India.

INDIVIDUAL AND WORKPLACE MONITORING

Monitoring refers to measurement of dose or contamination for reasons related to assessment of control of radiation exposure or radioactive substances, and the interpretation of the results. Monitoring the workers is the responsibility of registrants and licensees, and employer of the workers, to assess individual doses. In controlled areas, where specific protection measures are required, both individual monitoring and workplace monitoring are required. In supervised areas, where occupational exposure conditions must be kept under review, area monitoring is adequate. Radiation monitoring provides information not only on individual doses but also helps the evaluation of work procedures, information on accidental exposures, information necessary for optimization of protection, and information necessary for medical management.

For personnel monitoring, $CaSO_4$:Dy badges [thermoluminescent dosimeter (TLD)] are used, it is possible to measure X-rays, γ-rays, and β-ray exposures with the help of proper filters Al + Cu and plastic. These badges can measure small doses of 100 μSv with an accuracy of ±10% and can be reused up to 100 cycles. Neutron monitoring is done with CR-39 solid-state detectors. Pocket dosimeter that works on the principle of ionization is used to find out the dose directly. These are calibrated using ^{60}Co or ^{137}Cs source. The above dosimeters are useful in controlled areas when special operations are carried out.

Workplace Monitoring

Workplace monitoring involves measurement of both external and internal dose calculations resulting from exposure to open isotopes. It is carried out by installed and portable area monitors.

Installed area monitors are based on ionization detectors or halogen-quenched Geiger–Müller (GM) detectors. They can detect radiation dose rate in the range of 0.1 μSv/h to 10^5 mSv/h. These monitors are generally installed outside the controlled areas and equipped with audio/visual alarm to give warning when the radiation levels exceed the preset values.

Installed contamination monitors are useful for the measurement of contamination of hands, feet, and clothing of the radiation workers. The use of multiple gas proportional counters provides efficient measurement of α and β radiation doses.

Portable area monitors are useful for radiation survey of the installations and its vicinity. Based on exposure rates measured, the adequacy of radiation protection measures will be judged. If the radiation levels are more than the recommended levels, suitable remedial action must be initiated to ensure adequate protection.

Beta–gamma exposure meters can measure dose rates in the range of few μSv/h to 10 mSv/h. Those with a thin window of 1.7 mg/cm^2 can measure exposures due to α emitters and low-energy photons. GM wide range survey meter has measurement ranges covering μSv/h to 10 mSv/h. This instrument is much suitable for low-level radiation measurements; it is provided with a window, which can measure β exposures. This is rugged and suitable for field use.

Area monitors for environment monitoring are either GM based, or large pressurized argon-filled ionization chambers. They need to be sensitive and should be capable of measuring exposure rates in the range of few nSv/h to 10 mSv/h.

PERSONNEL MONITORING

Radiation exposure must be monitored for both personnel safety and regulatory purposes, and it should be carried out periodically. It should also ensure the safety of personnel, patients, and the public. The Atomic Energy (Radiation Protection) Rules, 2004 (Earlier RPR-1971, Atomic Energy Act, 1962) insist the radiation monitoring as a mandatory one. As per the rules, all radiation workers should be monitored with a suitable radiation-detecting device. There are two types of monitoring, namely—(1) personnel monitoring and (2) area monitoring. Personnel monitoring ensures safety of the personnel, whereas area monitoring ensures the safety of the radiation equipment and the installation.

All personnel who are occupationally exposed to radiation should be monitored regularly. The monitoring frequency is 3 months to ensure uniform rate of personnel dose over the year. Hence, it is aimed to—(1) monitor and control individual doses regularly, to ensure compliance with stipulated dose limits, (2) report and investigate overexposures and recommend necessary remedial measures urgently, and (3) maintain lifetime cumulative dose records of the users of the service. Hence, the radiation received by all the radiation workers during their work should be regularly monitored and a complete up-to-date record of these doses should be maintained.

Requirements of personnel monitoring system are—(1) appropriate range of dose measurement, accuracy, and reliability, (2) response independent of energy and type of radiation or ability to determine the same, (3) minimum fading of signal during the period of use, (4) environmental stability (heat, humidity, and pressure), (5) quick and simple readout system, (6) unaffected by nonionizing radiation, (7) independent of angle incidence, and (8) rugged, light weight, and economical. No such dosimeter satisfying all the above features is available as on date. However, one can be satisfied to some extent by selecting a particular type for a given application.

Monitoring Dosimeters

Personnel monitoring dosimeters are classified into two types, namely passive and active dosimeters. Passive dosimeter store radiation signal and later releases the same for dose analysis, e.g., film badge TLD, OSLD. Active dosimeter receives radiation and gives radiation-induced signal as display of dose or dose rate directly, e.g., pocket dosimeter. Various personnel monitoring systems are—(1) TLD, (2) optically stimulated luminescence dosimeter (OSLD), (3) film badge, (4) pocket dosimeter, and (5) radiophotoluminescent dosimeter (RPL).

Personnel monitoring devices provide—(1) occupational absorbed dose information, (2) assurance that dose limits are not exceeded, and (3) trends in exposure to serve as check on working practice. In India, personnel monitoring program was started in 1959; currently, >160,000 personnel are monitored, including medical, industry, and nuclear facilities. The country-wide personnel monitoring service is offered by private agencies, accredited by *Bhabha Atomic Research Center (BARC)* **(Table 4.3)**.

Thermoluminescent Dosimeter

Thermoluminescent dosimeter is based on the phenomenon of thermoluminescence. When certain materials are heated after radiation exposure, emit light, which is used to measure individual doses from X, β, and γ radiations. It gives much reliable results since no fading is observed under extreme climatic conditions. Typical TLD badge consists of a aluminum (Al) card loaded in a paper wrapper and polythene pouch and kept in a cassette **(Fig. 4.1)**. The cassette has a main body and a slider part. It has a stainless steel Crocodile clip fixed with silver plated eye lets to the slider part, for affixing to the user's clothing.

TLD badge consists of $CaSO_4$:Dy Thermoluminescence (TL) phosphor as detector. The optimized concentration of dopant dysprosium (Dy) is 500 ppm in $CaSO_4$ which

TABLE 4.3 **Accredited personnel monitoring agencies in India.**

State/Region	*Name of the accredited agency*
Andhra Pradesh, Telangana, Tamil Nadu, Karnataka, Kerala, Puducherry, Andaman and Nicobar, and Lakshadweep (Southern Region)	Avanttec Laboratories Pvt Ltd Plot No 17, Arignar Anna Industrial Estate, Mettukuppam, Vanagaram, Chennai, Pin: 600095
Maharashtra, Gujarat, Rajasthan, Goa, Dadra and Nagar Haveli, and Diu (Western Region)	Renentech Laboratory Pvt Ltd C-106, Synthofine Industrial Estate, Off Aarey Road, Goregaon (E), Mumbai, Maharashtra, Pin: 490063
All other states in the central, northern, and Northeastern parts of the country	Ultratech Laboratory Pvt Ltd, Cloth Market, GE Road, Kumhari, Bhilai, Durg, Chhattisgarh, Pin: 490042
All Defense institutions of country	Defense Laboratory, Jodhpur

Courtesy: Atomic Energy Regulatory Board:Website www.aerb.gov.in.

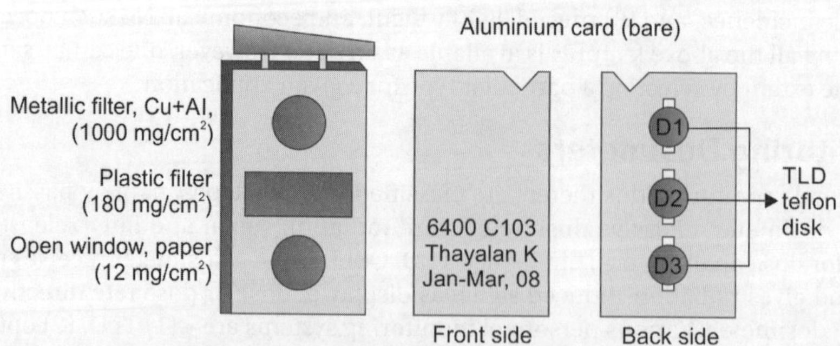

FIG. 4.1: TLD badge Al cards and its holder with filters.

makes it highly sensitive phosphor. It is 40 times more sensitive than LiF:Mg,Ti TLD-100. The response to neutrons is negligible. TL glow curve peak occurs at 220°C and that of Deflon disc is at 230°C. TL response is linear and the glow curve structure remains stable for both low and high LET radiations in the dose range of use. The response and the chemical form of this phosphor are highly stable to climatic conditions. The TLD badge has energy dependent response for photons and beta radiation.

Thermoluminescent Dosimeter Card

Thermoluminescent dosimeter card consists of three $CaSO_4$:Dy Teflon disks of each 0.8-mm thick × 13.3-mm diameter, which are mechanically clipped over three symmetrical circular holes of diameter 12 mm, on a aluminum card (52.5 × 30 × 1 mm). An asymmetric V cut provided at one end of the aluminum card ensures a fixed orientation of card in the TLD cassette. The card is enclosed by a paper wrapper in which user name, service period and service provider name are written. Thickness of this wrapper is 10 mg/cm^2 (size 30 mm width × 105 mm length), and makes measurements equivalent to 10-mm depth below skin surface in cassette. The paper wrapper protects the TLD discs from exposure to light. To protect TLD disks from mishandling, the card along with its wrapper is sealed in a thin polythene pouch (3–4 mg/cm^2 thickness and size of 32 × 60 mm length). The pouch also protects the card from radioactive contamination while working with open sources. Though TL signal fads faster when the card is exposed to bright sun light, exposure to normal room light does not significantly affect the response. However, sunlight exposure will not affect the TLD while it is paper wrapped with polythene pouch.

Thermoluminescent Dosimeter Cassette

Thermoluminescent dosimeter cassette is made of high-impact plastic. There are three filters in the cassette corresponding to each disk namely, Cu + Al, Perspex, and open. The center filter is rectangular whereas top and bottom filters are circular in shape. When the TLD card is inserted properly in the cassette, the first disk (D1) is sandwiched between a pair of filter combination of 1-mm Al × 15.6 mm Dia and Cu (1 thick × 16 mm Dia, 1,000 mg/cm^2), so that Al is facing the radiation. The rectangular copper filter is embedded by molding in the main body whereas a circular copper filter is embedded by molding in slider. Aluminum emblem is fixed by adhesive in the main body and on the slider. Second disk (D2) is sandwiched between a pair of 1.6 mm thick × 25 mm Dia thick plastic filters (180 mg/cm^2). Third disk (D3) is positioned under a circular open window (13.5 Dia). A clip attachment affixes the badge to the users' clothing or to the wrist.

Metallic filter is meant for X and γ radiation, and Perspex is for β radiation. The filters are mainly used to make the TLD disks energy independent. Dose is evaluated and reported in terms of whole body dose and beta dose. Summation of the photon and beta dose is reported as skin dose. The whole body dose is considered to be equivalent to 10 mm depth for photons above 30 keV. After TLD card is read, dose is evaluated by an algorithm (BARC Task Group, 2018). It also permits estimation of photon energy below 200 keV. When the TLD disk is exposed to radiation, the electrons in the crystal lattice are excited and move from valence band to conduction band. There, they get trapped just below the conduction band. The number of electrons in the trap is proportional to the radiation exposure, and thus it stores the absorbed radiation energy in the crystal lattice.

Dose measurements are made by using a TLD reader **(Fig. 4.2)**, which consists of microprocessor-based electronic control circuit, photomultiplier tube (PMT) housing, card transport system, gas heater and temperature control unit, cooling fans and solenoid. The TLD disk is placed in the heater cup or planchet and heated for a reproducible heating cycle. The transport system moves the cards to the reading position whereas the solenoid switches the gas flow ON and OFF. TLD reader provides a programmed heating cycle of the TL dosimeter and senses the instantaneous light emitted by the dosimeter. The electrons return to their ground state with emission of light, which is measured by the PMT. The PMT converts light into an electrical current (signal), which is amplified and measured by a recorder. The reader is calibrated in terms of mR or mSv, so that one can get direct dose estimation. This is done by determining the reader calibration factor (RCF) for a given batch of cards and disc calibration factors (DCF). Daily calibration of service cards is necessary. It requires checking the EHT, light source reading (LSR), N2 gas flow rate, and temperature. Calibration details are available in BARC task group handbook. The disk is annealed and can be used again for personnel monitoring. Both used and unused cards should be annealed under same annealing cycle. It requires a special oven with heater, temperature controller and electrical supply.

Nowadays, widow-based computer-controlled TLD readers are available. They can analyze TLD chips, ribbons, powder, disks, pellets, rods, and microcubes. They display digital glow curve and temperature profile. They can handle one or more planchets at a time either with manual drawer or computer-controlled drawer function. Programmable annealing oven is also available along with the system.

$CaSO_4$:Dy TLD badge can cover a wide range of dose from 50 μSv to 1 Sv with an accuracy of ±10%. Its advantage is high-sensitivity, low-fading, and indigenous production. TLD badges are available as chest badge, wrist badge and head badge and do not provide permanent record. *Lithium fluoride (LiF)* can also be used as TLD phosphor, which has wide dose response range from 10 μSv to 1,000 Sv. Its effective atomic number ($Z = 8.2$) is close to that of tissue and air, energy independent with an accuracy of ±2%.

Guidelines for Using TLD Badge

Thermoluminescent dosimeter badges are used only by radiation workers. Every new radiation worker needs to fill up the *personnel data form (PDF)* and send to BARC-

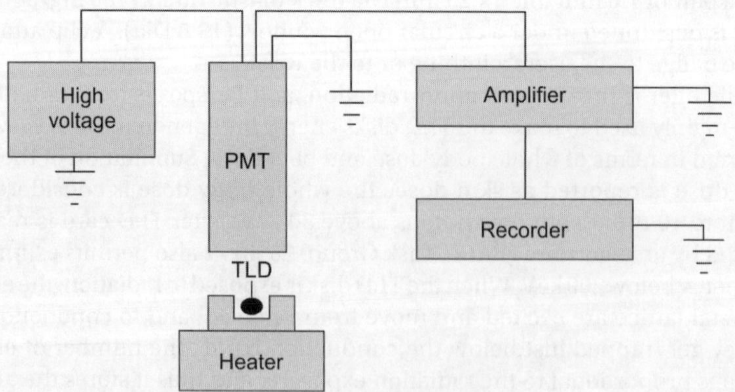

FIG. 4.2: TLD reader to evaluate the radiation dose.

accredited agency. A TLD badge once issued to a person should not be used by any other person. A badge without filter or damaged filter should not be used and be replaced by a new holder. Every radiation worker must ensure that the badge is not left in radiation field or near hot plates, ovens, furnaces, burners, etc. All the used or unused TLD badges should be return, after every service period (quarterly) in one lot to reach 10th of next month. While leaving the hospital premises, workers should deposit their badges in the storage area along with control TLD, which is kept in a radiation-free zone. TLD badge is used to measure radiation dose but does not protect the user from the radiation.

Placement of TLD Badge

Thermoluminescent dosimeter badges are normally worn at chest level (torso) under lead apron, so that it is expected to receive maximum and true whole body radiation exposure. This ensures greater amount of radiation exposure received by most sensitive part of the body. However, lead apron is not indicated for radiotherapy and positron emission tomography-computed tomography (PET-CT) work practice due to high-energy photons. High-energy photons interact through *Compton scattering*, which results in increased dose to the worker. Additional wrist badge is advised for procedures involving brachytherapy, nuclear medicine, source handling, and interventional radiology.

During interventional radiology or cardiology procedure, a collar level dosimeter is used to measure thyroid and eye lens dose. Extremity dosimeter (ring) under the hand gloves is also used as an additional dosimeter. It enables the workers or physician to use their hands nearer to the primary radiation beam. A pregnant radiation worker can wear an additional dosimeter at waist level behind the lead apron, to assess the fetal dose for the remaining period of pregnancy.

Optically Stimulated Luminescence Dosimeter

Optically stimulated luminescence dosimeter (OSLD) is also used as personnel monitoring device, which is replacing film badge and TLD in countries. After radiation exposure, the OSLD is stimulated by a laser light during which light is emitted. Light emission is proportional to the given radiation exposure, which is the principle of OSLD. Emission of light can be plotted graphically, known as *glow curve*. OSL dosimeter consists of thin layer of aluminum oxide (Al_2O_3) as detector **(Fig. 4.3)**. It has three filters, namely—(1) aluminum, (2) tin, and (3) copper.

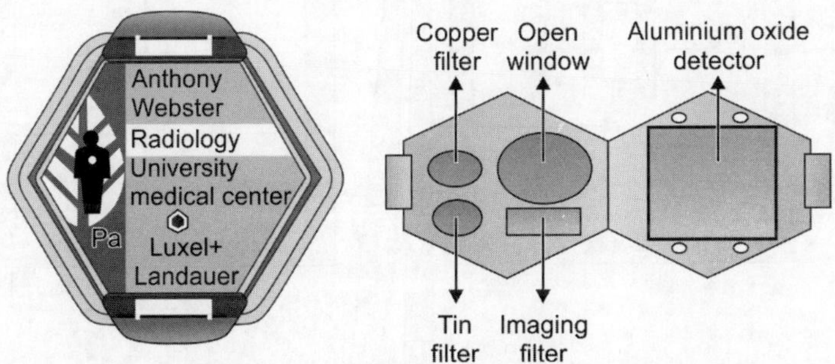

FIG. 4.3: Optically stimulated luminescence dosimeter: (A) OSL Dosimeter; (B) OSL dosimeter composition.

Courtesy: Luxel + Landauer.

Each filter offers small, moderate, and high attenuation to radiation, respectively. During the readout with laser, the area under aluminum filter gives more light, compared to tin and copper. Thus, the luminescence under three filters gives a measure of radiation dose, under three different energies. In other words, high-energy radiation gives luminescence under copper, whereas medium and low energies correspond to tin and aluminum filters, respectively. This kind of energy discrimination is known as *deep (copper), eye (tin),* and *shallow (aluminum),* meaning different penetration depths or different energies.

Optically stimulated luminescence dosimeter can be used up to 1 year; however, it is served as quarterly basis in practice. It can be used to read radiation exposure from 100 μSv to 10 Sv, for X and γ rays, over a useful energy range is 5 keV to 40 MeV. This makes it suitable for use in low-level radiation, especially in medical exposures. The energy and dose range for β is 150 keV to 10 MeV; 100 μSv to 10 Sv, and neutron is 40 keV to 35 MeV; 200 μSv to 250 Sv.

Advantages of OSL dosimeters are—light weight, durable, and simple. It is not affected by heat, moisture, and pressure since it is tamperproof. Reanalysis is possible, if there is error in readout or any dispute. It can be worn for longer periods of time, compared to TLD and film dosimeter. OSL with in-house reader can be used for patient dose measurements. Nowadays, OSLD comes with open filter (bare) facility, to detect dynamic exposures.

Film Badge

Film badge is used to measure external radiation dose of a person from X, β, γ, and thermal neutron radiations. It consists of a *film pack* loaded in a *film holder,* which is made up of plastic with *stainless steel* lining **(Fig. 4.4)**. It can hold one or more photographic films of size 4 × 3 cm², wrapped inside with a light tight *polythene* or paper cover. Generally, the badge has two films—one is slow and the other is fast

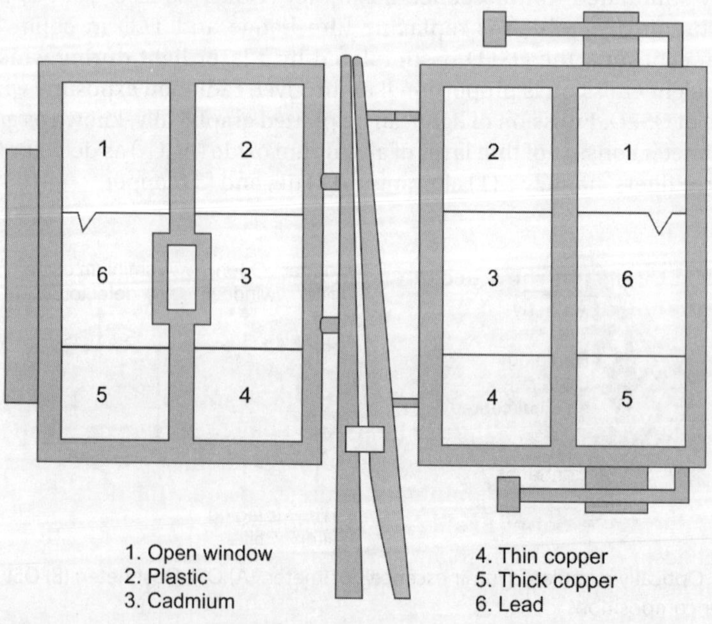

FIG. 4.4: Film badge dosimeter.

and slow film is meant for recording high exposure. The film should be loaded in the film holders so that the flap side of the film pack is always facing the body.

The film holder has six filters namely *open, plastic, cadmium, thin copper, thick copper, and lead.* All the filters have 1-mm thick except thin copper, which is 0.15-mm thick. The filters assess the penetrating power of the radiation and thus permit the energy to be estimated. The filters are fixed on both sides of the holder, to identify type, energy, and penetrating power of incident radiation. Thus, it will identify α, β, *neutron, low-energy X-rays, high-energy X-rays, and* γ*-rays,* over a range of energies from 10 keV to 2 MeV. The emulsion of the film dosimeter is covered by a paper of thickness 20–30 g/cm^2.

There are three types of holders—(1) chest holder, (2) wrist holder, and (3) fore head holder. Film badge is worn compulsorily at chest level. If a lead apron is used, the film badge is worn under the apron at chest level. The film badge worn at the chest level represents the whole-body dose equivalent.

The supply of film is for a period of one calendar month (4 weeks). When the badge is exposed to radiation, it passes through filter and forms latent image in the film. After 4 weeks of use, it is returned for dose computation where the film is processed; optical densities under different filters are measured by a densitometer. Using standard calibration curves, the dose under each filter is evaluated. This standard curve is drawn between log of known radiation exposure and density, under different filters. A control film is always needed to assess background level of radiation. Each institution should keep one film, loaded in a chest holder as control. This control badge should be kept in a cool, dry, and radiation-free area. Monthly dose reports are sent to the individual institutions after processing the film packs. These reports contain monthly doses and up-to-date cumulative doses of the current year. Film badge can be used to measure radiation from 10 μSv to 100 Sv with an accuracy of ±10%.

The doses are reported in mSv and the minimum dose that a film badge can detect is about 0.2 mSv. Advantages of film badge are—(1) it is a permanent record, (2) nature of exposure, types of radiation, and energy can be evaluated, and (3) least expensive device. The film badge has some disadvantages such as fading at high temperatures and humidity, high sensitivity to light, pressure and chemicals, complex dark room procedure, and limited self-life.

The film badges are used only by persons directly working with radiation sources. It is also worth to note that the film badge is used to measure the radiation dose to which the user is exposed.

Pocket Dosimeter

Film and TLD will not show accumulated exposure immediately. In addition to the regular film badges, the radiation doses received by the radiation worker can be assessed by wearing a pocket dosimeter, which gives instantaneous radiation exposure. This is very useful in nonroutine work, in which the radiation levels vary considerably and may be quite hazardous (cardiac catheterization laboratory). The main advantage of pocket dosimeter lies in its ability to provide on the spot/instant check of radiation dose received by the personnel. Suitable protective measures can be undertaken immediately to minimize future exposures. The dose can be read off directly by the person during or after any radiation work.

Pocket dosimeter is an ion chamber with a quartz fiber suspended within an air-filled chamber on a wireframe as shown in the **Figure 4.5**. It has a built-in capacitance, which can be charged by an external potential (charger). The positive charge is placed on the wireframe by means of the charger. The quartz fiber is bent away from the frame due to Coulombic repulsion. This can be visible through an optical lens system upon which an exposure scale is superimposed.

These dosimeters should be fully charged prior to their use so that the initial reading of the dosimeter is set at zero **(Fig. 4.6)**. When exposed to radiation, ion pairs are produced in the air. These ion pairs partially neutralize the positive charge, reducing the Coulombic repulsion and allowing the fiber to move. Hence, the quartz fiber moves closer to the wireframe that can be seen as down range excursion of the hairline fiber on the exposure scale (graticule). The movement of the quartz fiber

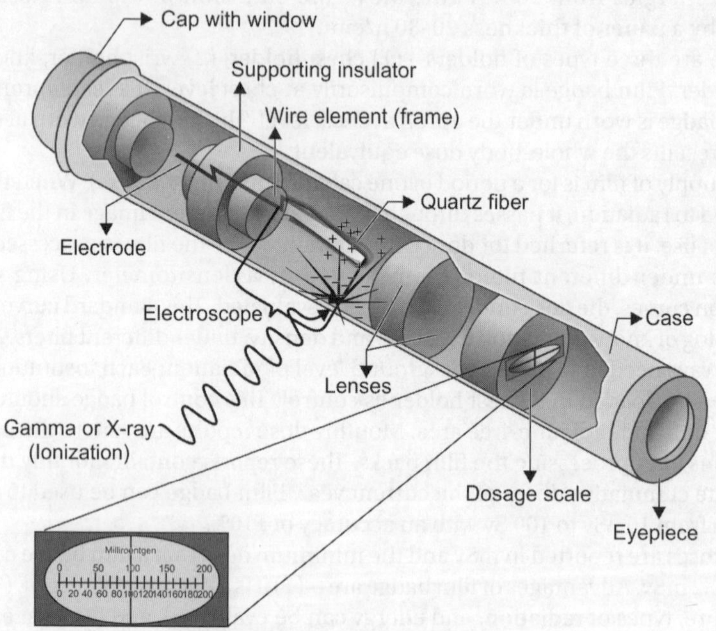

FIG. 4.5: Pocket dosimeter.

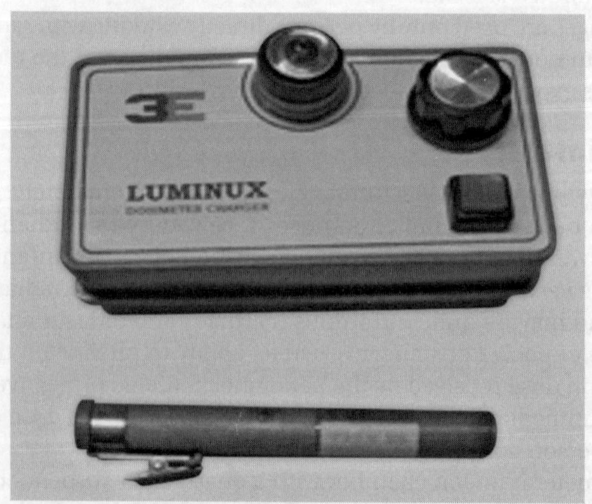

FIG. 4.6: A commercial pocket dosimeter with charger.
Courtesy: Luminex Instruments.

is proportional to the radiation exposure, which is measured in roentgen (R). The roentgen is the unit of exposure = 2.58×10^{-4} C/kg. The dose in air can be calculated from the exposure, where 1-R exposure is equal to 8.76 mGy (0.876 rad) of air dose.

The dosimeter is available in different ranges varying from 0 to 200 mR, 0 to 500 mR, 0 to 5 R, 0 to 20 R, 0 to 200 R, and 0 to 600 R for measurement of X and γ rays. It can detect photon energies from 20 keV to 2 MeV. For personnel monitoring, smallest range of 0–200 mR is generally used. These dosimeters are available both in analog and digital types. Digital dosimeters use either GM tubes or diodes and solid-state electronics. The dose measurement range of pocket dosimeter is 10 μSv to 100 Sv.

The accuracy of the pocket dosimeter is about ±10%. Pocket dosimeter is small and easy to use, and does not provide permanent record. Sudden mechanical shock may result in wrong reading. Hence, these dosimeters should be handled with care to indicate reliable reading of the doses received.

Nowadays, digital pocket dosimeters are available with easy display of instant radiation measurements. Presently, semiconductor diode-based pocket dosimeters with digital display are also available. They have good energy and polar response, with reliable readings, matching to TLD badges. They make loud bleep sounds for every 15–30 minutes on background. The sound becomes more frequent as dose rate increases and becomes continuous sound at high radiation fields. The energy range of these dosimeters is 45 keV to 6 MeV and these are available with mR and μSv display.

Features of Personnel Monitoring Systems

The common problems associated with personnel monitoring dosimeters include—(1) leaving dosimeters in a radiation field, when not worn, (2) radionuclide contamination of the dosimeter, (3) lost or damaged dosimeters, and (4) not wearing the dosimeter while working in radiation. If the body is between the dosimeter and radiation source, the attenuation will cause a significant reduction in exposure. Most of the time, the workers do not remain in fixed geometry, while doing radiation work. As a result, the radiation exposure becomes multidirectional and the recorded value is the average exposure for that individual. It is within ±10–20% of the individual's true exposure. The various types of monitoring systems are summarized in **Table 4.4**.

TABLE 4.4 **Comparison of personnel monitoring systems.**

Dosimeter	*Radiation*	*Range*	*Features*
Film badge	β, γ, X-rays	γ, 0.1–15,000 mSv β, 0.5–10,000 mSv	Permanent record
TLD	β, γ, X-rays	0.01–10^6 mSv	• No permanent record • Patient dosimetry
OSLD	β, γ, X-rays	0.01–10^6 mSv	• Reread dosimeter • Differentiate static and dynamic exposures
Pocket dosimeter	γ, X-rays	0–200 mR 0–500 mR 0–5,000 mR	• Special monitoring • Direct reading

(TLD: thermoluminescent dosimeter; OSL: optically stimulated luminescence)

Courtesy: Bushberg JT et al., 2012.

Use of certain isotopes does not require personnel monitoring systems, especially film dosimeter, e.g., Iodine-125, Iodine-131, Phophorous-32, Strontium-90 and Cobalt-60, if it involves single operation or quantities handled are within few μCi. The α and β rays from the isotopes unable to penetrate the emulsion (20–30 mg/cm^2) of the film dosimeter. Doses below certain level cannot be recorded due to fluctuation in the background and optical density from one film to another.

Overexposure

Radiation worker is said to be overexposure, if he receives a whole-body effective dose of >10 mSv in a quarterly period. An urgent letter will be sent to the institution by Atomic Energy Regulatory Board (AERB) requesting an investigation of overexposure. The Radiological Safety Officer (RSO) of the institution must investigate the causes of the overexposure and submit an elaborate investigation report in the prescribed format to AERB within the stipulated period. The individual also should make a written statement regarding the causes of the overexposure to AERB. This is to take preventive steps to avoid such exposure in future. The AERB will investigate the reported overexposure and the same will be is reported promptly to the institution and the individual.

As per the existing AERB regulatory limits, the effective dose constraint for consecutive 5 years shall be 100 mSv, i.e., average 20 mSv for every year of the sliding 5 years block, the dose limit in any single year should not exceed 30 mSv. If the annual dose limit exceeds the operational limit of 30 mSv, regulator suggests an appropriate period of lay off to the worker from radiation work. All overexposure cases will be examined by the overexposure committee, AERB. About 170 overexposures have been reported up to 2015 in India.

If the radiation exposure exceeds 100 mSv, the worker will be asked to undergo medical examination including complete blood test and chromosome aberration analysis (CAA) by recognized laboratory to confirm the overexposure. It is the only test, which ensures the genuineness of the whole-body exposure measured by the personnel monitoring system. Negative CAA indicates nongenuine of the exposure to the person. If it is not genuine, it may be due to misplacement of badge or wrong storage of badge, etc. Exposure > 250 mSv is ascertained by differential white blood counts immediately after the exposure and two times at the interval of 2 weeks thereafter.

AREA MONITORING

The assessment of radiation levels at different locations in the vicinity of radiation installation is known as area monitoring or radiation survey. These measurements will give an idea about the radiation safety status of the installation. Based on the measurements taken, one could confirm the adequacy or inadequacy of the existing radiation protection status. If radiation levels are higher than the permissible levels, suitable remedial measures can be taken. Instruments used for the above purposes are called radiation survey meters or area monitors. In general, any survey meter/area monitor should consist of two main parts, namely—(1) a device, which detects the radiation and (2) a display system to measure the radiation.

These instruments differ from each other in the medium in which the response takes place and in the method by which the response is detected and quantified. Following are the different types of meters generally used for radiation survey and area monitoring.

- Ionization chamber type (air)
- Geiger–Müller type (neon and halogen gas)
- Scintillation detector type [Solid state, NaI(TI), ZnS(Ag)]

Selection of a particular detector depends upon variety of factors, namely—(1) type of radiation to be detected, (2) quantity to be measured, and (3) response of detector for the energy and type of radiation. They can be used as portable radiation survey meters, capable of measuring radiation count rate in mR/h or μR/h. They are available in the form of vehicle mounted radiation meters, zone monitors and doorway mounted meters, etc.

Ionization Chamber Survey Meter

Ionization chamber usually consists of an outer cylinder (cathode) coated inside with graphite to make it conducts and a central electrode (anode) insulated from the chamber wall **(Figs. 4.7A and B)**. Cylinder is filled either with air or suitable gas, acting as an interacting and detection medium, and a suitable voltage is applied across the electrodes. When the chamber is exposed to radiation, the radiation produces ionization in the gas. Under suitable electric field, positive and negative ions are collected respectively by cathode and anode of the chamber. The movement of ions produces an electric current in the outer electronic circuit of the chamber. The strength of this current is proportional to the number of ionization events caused by

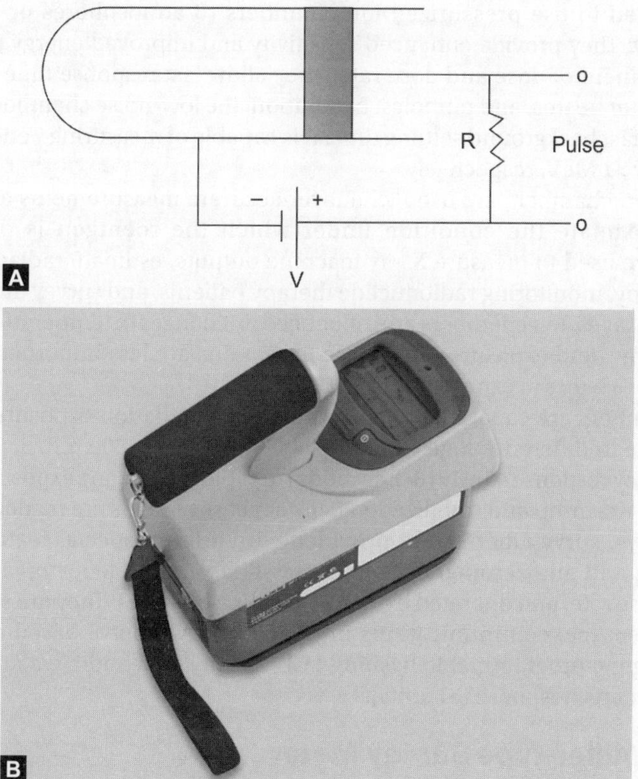

FIGS. 4.7A AND B: (A) Ion chamber principle, (B) Pressurized ion chamber.

Courtesy: Fluke.

the energy absorbed in the air chamber and will serve as a measure for quantifying the exposure/exposure rate or dose/dose rate.

In ionization chamber, the electric field applied is only just sufficient to collect all the primary ions produced by the radiation before they recombine. During this mode, any change in the applied voltage will not affect the number of ionizations produced in the chamber by the radiation. Number of ionizations will be purely dependent on the energy dissipated in the medium. Hence, energy discrimination is possible with ionization chambers for heavily charged particles by pulse height analysis. Since ionization chambers collect only primary ions, electronic amplification of charge is necessary for display purpose. This makes ionization chamber-based instruments somewhat delicate and susceptible to extreme climatic conditions. For X-ray and γ-ray dose measurements, these are operated in current modes. This current is very small (pico-to-nano ampere) and requires very sensitive electrometers for measurement.

Ionization chambers for low-level X-ray monitoring (exposure/exposure rate) are fabricated out of air-equivalent materials (Bakelite, Tufnell) and they can be used over a wide range of energies from 7 keV to 2 MeV. A typical survey meter consists of a 500-cc chamber connected to a battery-operated electrometer and can measure exposure rates from a few mR/h to about 10 R/h. Some of these are provided with an end window of thin Mylar film for β radiation detection.

Ion chambers for radiotherapy are fabricated with phenolic wall material with 200–350-cc chamber volume and operated both in dose and dose rate mode. It is recommended to use pressurized ion chambers (8 atmospheres or 125 psi) for radiotherapy. They provide enhanced sensitivity and improved energy response for the measurement of dose and dose rate. They allow fast response time to radiation leakage, scatter beams, and pinholes. In addition, the low-noise chamber bias supply provides for fast background settling time. It is capable of measuring γ energy >25 keV and β energy >1 MeV, respectively.

Ionization chambers are used whenever accurate measurements are required. They approximate the condition under which the roentgen is defined. Ion chambers are used to measure X-ray machine outputs, estimate radiation levels in brachytherapy, monitoring radionuclide therapy patients, and survey the radioactive material packages. Ion chambers are influenced by changes in temperature, pressure, photon energy, and exposure rate. These limitations are less important in medical applications (5% loss of exposure rate at 10 R/h).

Ion chambers are capable of monitoring higher radiation exposure rate levels, and available in different ranges: 0–5 mR/h, 0–50 mR/h, 0–500 mR/h, 0–5 R/h, and 0–50 R/h. They response slowly (8–2 seconds) to rapidly changing exposure rates and, hence, need warm-up and stabilization before measurements are made.

Nowadays, survey meters are provided with a lot of special features such as autoranging and autozeroing, optional beta slide, simultaneous measurement of dose and dose rate, and operated by two 9V alkaline batteries. They are also provided with check source, communications interface with windows-based excel add-in for data logging, programmable flashing LCD display, and audible alarm with dose equivalent energy response (SI units).

Geiger–Müller-type Survey Meter

In GM survey meter, a higher electric field (500–1,300 V) is applied between the anode and cathode of a chamber, which is filled with a gas of low-electron attachment coefficient (e.g., argon and neon). The electrons produced in the chamber will have sufficient energy to produce secondary and tertiary ionization during their acceleration towards anode. This results in an amplification of ionization events in the chamber. This is known as gas amplification (avalanche), which depends on the nature and the pressure of gas.

In GM counters, use of very thin wire as the anode enables the production of high electric field close to the anode. In addition, the primary avalanche is followed by a successive avalanche due to secondary phenomena (excitation of gas atoms and production of UV photons). Hence, the whole wire is covered by a sheath of electrons. The gas amplification ($\approx 10^8$) is independent of primary ionization (i.e., type and energy of radiation). It cannot be operated beyond the GM region since they continuously discharge.

Geiger–Müller-type instruments are very sensitive and useful for monitoring of low-level radiation, especially in leak testing and radioactive contamination. Since electronic amplification is not necessary, the electronic circuit of GM is very simple, compared to that of ionization chamber. This feature makes the GM-type instruments rugged and less costly. GM counters used for radiation monitoring generally use a mixture of gases (argon, neon, and chlorine/bromine). It detects the presence and provides a semiquantitative estimate of the radiation field magnitude. It provides measurements in counts per minute (CPM). It also provides an approximate measurement of mR/h, since it does not reproduce the conditions under which exposure is defined. However, the relationship between CPM and mR/h is a complicated function of photon energy.

Geiger–Müller counters for X-rays and γ-rays monitoring use copper or chromium cathodes for better efficiency **(Fig. 4.8)**. The primary photons interact with the cathode materials to produce secondary electrons. They show strong dependence in low-photon energies, hence not suitable for pulsed radiation fields. Since GM meters are pulsed in nature, they should be used only in radiation generators that emit continuous X-rays. They should not be used in linear accelerators that emit pulsed X-rays. It is used to indicate radiation, whereas ion chambers are used for precise measurements.

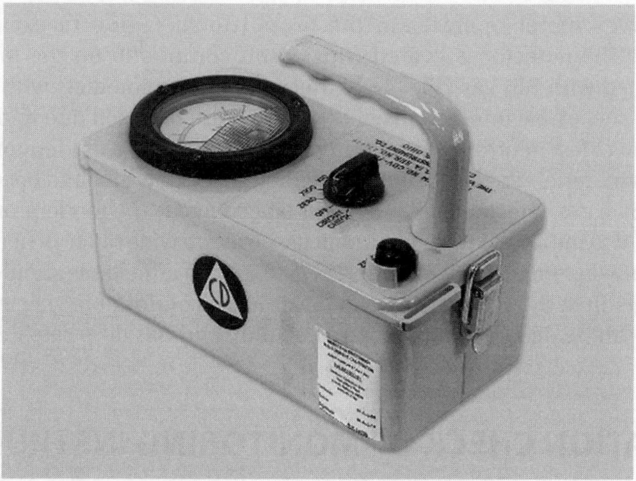

FIG. 4.8: GM type radiation survey meter.
Courtesy: Victoreen.

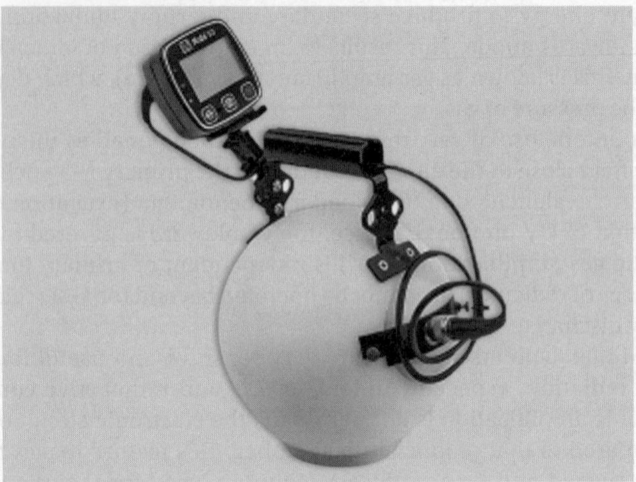

FIG. 4.9: Neutron survey meter.
Courtesy: Ludlum Measurements Inc.

The GM-type meters are mainly used as radioactive contamination monitor with thin window (1.5–2 mg/cm^2) and large surface area. It will respond to α- (> 3MeV), β- (>45 keV), X- and γ-rays (>6 keV) radiations. GM detector is sensitive to particle radiation, but relatively insensitive to γ radiations. It is suitable to measure natural background radiations, which are 50–100 CPM. It is mainly used in nuclear medicine for low-level contamination surveys.

The GM counters have long dead time (100 μs) and result in 20% loss at 100,000 CPM measurements. They should not be used when accurate exposure rates are required, in which count rates are >100. A portable GM survey meter gets paralyzed in very high-radiation field and show zero reading.

Neutron Survey Meter

Neutron survey meter operates in the proportional region to exclude photon background. The detector is coated with boron compound on the inside wall or counter is filled with BF_3 gas **(Fig. 4.9)**. Thermal neutron interacts with ^{10}B by (n,α) reaction and successive interactions of α radiation are detected due to their ionizing ability. To detect fast neutrons, the counter is surrounded by a moderator made up of hydrogenous material. The fast neutrons interact with moderator and become thermal neutrons, which are detected by BF_3 counter placed inside the moderator. The output is proportional to the dose equivalent in soft tissue over a wide range of neutron energy.

It is a lightweight meter (≈4.5 kg) and provided with adjustable shoulder trap. The operator can adjust the viewing angle to maximize a comfortable viewing angle. The display unit can be detached for greater versatility and has dose rate range of 0–100 mSv/h.

CALIBRATION CHECK OF MONITORING INSTRUMENTS

Calibration of Personnel Monitoring Systems

Dosimeters worn on the trunk estimate the whole-body effective dose, whereas wrist and angle dosimeters and finger dosimeters estimate partial body doses. Personnel dose monitors are calibrated in terms of operational quantities with a reference depth of 10 mm for strongly penetrating radiation. The reference depth is 0.07 mm for weekly penetrating radiation. Monitors are irradiated on standardized phantoms to simulate conditions of backscatter in human torso. It needs three phantoms consisting International Commission on Radiation Units and Measurements (ICRU) tissue, which include—(1) slap phantom, (2) pillar phantom, and (3) polymethylmethacrylate (PMMA) rod phantom. If the dosimeter is sensitive to backscattered radiation, calibration in phantom is advised.

Slap phantom represents a human torso of 300 × 300 × 150 mm to calibrate whole-body dosimeters and accounts backscattering of incident radiation. Its front face is provided with water phantom, which consists of 2.5-mm thick PMMA plate, and the other sides are with 10-mm thick. Pillar phantom is a circular cylinder with a diameter of 73 mm and a length of 300 mm. It represents a lower arm or leg, and accounts backscattering of incident radiation to test wrist or angle dosimeters. The circular walls are of 2.5-mm thick, and the end of the walls are of 10-mm thick. The rod phantom is circular with a diameter of 19 mm and a length of 300 mm, represents a finger, and accounts backscattering of incident radiation to test finger dosimeter. If phantoms are used, no correction factors are required.

Calibration of personnel dosimeter involves three steps:

1. Air-kerma in air (K_{air}) is measured in a reference field, using a reference ionization chamber calibrated by a standard laboratory,
2. Reference chamber reading is converted into that of slap phantom at 10 mm (H), by using theoretical values, and
3. The dosimeter is placed at the calibration point and the reading M is obtained.

Then, the ratio (H/M) gives the calibration factor in terms of personnel dose equivalent.

Alternatively, calibration of personnel monitors can be done with radiation quality other than the instrument is intended to measure, provided the calibration condition is same for each dosimeter of same type. Generally, ^{137}Cs, ^{241}Am/Be, and ^{90}Sr/^{90}Y are used as source for photon, neutron, and β calibration, respectively. The secondary standard laboratory assigns a dose equivalent output (mSv) for a given check source along with decay table. The source strength used is about 500 mCi of ^{137}Cs. Using this source, multiple TLD cards are exposed for a known dose of 3 mSv for reader calibration. Later, the cards are read for dose estimation, the read dose, and the decayed output of ^{137}Cs source as on date is compared. The coefficient of variation should be within 5% for new cards or 7.5% for used service cards.

Intercomparison

International Atomic Energy Agency (IAEA), Vienna, Austria, conducted an intercomparison program for personnel monitoring both regional and international levels. Its objective is—(1) to monitor member states, (2) test of the applicability of phantom-related dose equivalent quantities to individual monitoring, and (3) helping to develop an internationally agreed concept of individual monitoring. In involved >21 dosimetry international laboratories and 17 member states in Asia and Oceania region for photon energy of 15 keV to 1.3 MeV.

Calibration of Area Monitors

Radiation survey meter and contamination monitors are calibrated against a reference chamber that is traceable to a national standard. Generally, ion chambers are used as reference for γ radiation and its air kerma in air is determined in a reference field. Then, the dose equivalent at 10 mm (H) of the reference chamber is determined by using theoretical conversion coefficient (h):

$$H = h \times N_R \times M_R$$

Where N_R is the calibration factor of the reference chamber and M_R is the corrected reading of the reference chamber. Radiation quality in which the reference chamber is calibrated should be used for the calibration of the survey meter also. Then, the survey meter to be calibrated is placed at the calibration point and its reading is noted as M. Then, the ratio (H/M) gives the calibration factor in terms of personnel dose equivalent.

Radiation monitors are periodically checked to ensure that they are calibrated correctly. Before each use, an operational check should be made as follows:

- Check the due date of calibration to ensure that calibration date is not exceeded.
- Check the battery to ensure that battery is not dead.
- Source check to ensure that the meter indicates correct radiation field.

BIBLIOGRAPHY

1. Atomic Energy Regulatory Board. (2016). AERB Safety Code No. AERB/RF-MED/SC-3 (Rev.2): Radiation safety in manufacture, supply and use of medical diagnostic X-ray equipment. [online] Available from https://www.aerb.gov.in/images/PDF/RF-MED-SC-3.pdf. [Last accessed October, 2022].
2. Bushberg JT, Seibert JA, Leidholdt EM, Boone JM. The Essential Physics of Medical Imaging, 3rd edition. Philadelphia, PA: Wolters Kluwer/Lippincott Williams & Wilkins; 2012.
3. International Atomic Energy Agency. (2000). Calibration of radiation protection monitoring instruments. Safety reports series No. 16. [online] Available from https://www.iaea.org/publications/5149/calibration-of-radiation-protection-monitoring-instruments. [Last accessed October, 2022].
4. Podgorsak EB. Radiation Oncology Physics: A Handbook for Teachers and Students. Vienna: IAEA; 2005.
5. Rao BS. Radiation protection in medical applications. Proceedings of the National Symposium on Radiobiology of Clinical Radiotherapy. Chennai: IAEA; 2018.
6. Thayalan K. Basic radiological physics, 2nd edition. New Delhi: Jaypee Brothers Medical Publishers; 2017.
7. Bhabha atomic Research Center (BARC) Task group. Hand book on TLD Based personnel monitoring (Rev.1-2018).

CHAPTER 5

Planning a Diagnostic Radiology Facility

INTRODUCTION

Radiological facility in hospital includes diagnostic radiology, nuclear medicine, and radiation therapy. It can be an individual department or combination of all. There are common recommendations to all the departments. However, individual department requires specific recommendations for planning. While planning a radiation facility, consideration should be given to radiation safety, convenience, and economy. Required features are discussed in the following chapters for planning a radiological installation either in diagnostic radiology or nuclear medicine or radiation therapy.

DIAGNOSTIC RADIOLOGY

Diagnostic X-ray facilities include radiography, fluoroscopy, mammography, computed tomography (CT), mobile X-ray, bone mineral densitometry X-ray, and dental units. General-purpose radiography unit employs 50–150 kV_p and directs the beam towards patient and the detector. Barrier that attenuates the primary radiation is referred as primary barrier, e.g., computed radiography (CR) cassette, chest stand bucky, etc. Majority of workload directs the beam towards floor direction. Fluoroscopic units employ 60–120 kV_p, and the detector acts as primary barrier (Image intensifier tube/flat panel detector). Hence, room design needs to consider only secondary radiation. If the unit is provided with both radiography and fluoroscopy, then shielding design depends on workload's share. Interventional facility having multiple X-ray tubes also considers only secondary barrier in shielding design.

Mammography X-ray unit uses 25–35 kV_p and breast support acts as primary barrier. Its room design requires only secondary barrier, and few layers of gypsum are sufficient to provide enough shielding. CT scan employs 80–140 kV_p with a collimated X-ray beam, which is attenuated by the patient and the detector. Nowadays, multidetector CT scans are used, which are efficient in using available radiation. However, amount of scattered radiation per equal scan is not much different from that of single row CT. The only difference is that multidetector CT uses multiple large number scans with multiple rotations. This may demand higher thickness of walls, floor, and ceiling. The secondary scatter is an anisotropic and radiation is higher along the table axis.

Mobile X-ray units require no barrier shielding; only distance needs to be maintained. Distance of 2 m, wearing with lead apron or mobile shield will offer

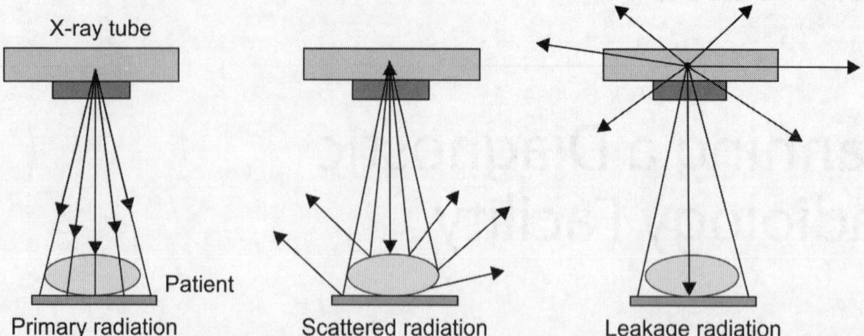

FIG. 5.1: The various sources of exposure, namely primary, scattered and leakage radiations.

enough shielding in such units. Bone mineral densitometer (BMD) is a well-collimated low-intensity X-ray. The scatter is much low, and radiation exposure will not >1 mGy/year at 1 m. Safety requirements of dental units are evaluated by an expert based on the workload and nature of procedures.

SOURCES OF EXPOSURES

The radiations used in medical application appear in two forms, namely—(1) primary radiation, (2) secondary radiation. Secondary radiation consists of scattered and leakage radiation **(Fig. 5.1)**.

Primary Radiation

The radiation passing through an open area defined by a collimator of X-ray tube/radiation source is called primary radiation. It consists of spectrum of radiation, which interacts with patient, grid, table, and detectors. The fluence of the primary is several times greater than the secondary radiation. Mostly primary beam is collimated and restricted to interact with patient only. The amount of primary radiation depends on—(1) output, (2) number of patients per week, and (3) fraction of time the radiation beam is directed towards any location.

Concrete, lead, and steel are used as primary barrier shielding material, depending upon the structural and spatial considerations. For example, concrete is preferred for the construction of walls and ceiling, because it is cheaper. Whenever there is shortage of space, lead and steel can be used as primary barriers.

Scattered Radiation

Scattered radiation arises from patient, tabletop, collimator, or shield. It arises due to interaction of primary radiation with patient or tabletop, causing a portion of the primary radiation to get scattered. It is due to coherent and incoherent scattering process. The fluence of scattered radiation depends on—(1) the volume of the patient irradiated, (2) spectrum of the primary beam, (3) field size, and (4) scattering angle. Scattered radiation must be considered as a separate source, for radiation safety purposes, and, in general, it has low energy. The fluence and quality of the scattered radiation have angular dependence.

In diagnostic radiology, the quality of the scattered radiation is assumed to be same as that of the incident beam. Its magnitude is about 0.1–0.15% of primary at 1 m from patient, for a field area of 20×20 cm^2.

In megavoltage radiations, the ratio of scattered dose to the incident dose is denoted as α, which varies with scatter angle and beam quality. The α is assumed to be 0.1% of the primary for 90° scatter. The maximum energy of the 90° scattered photon is 500 keV. The transmission of the above beam is similar to a 500-kV_p primary beam. The penetrating power of scattered beam is greater at smaller scatter angle, and greater fraction of primary is scattered at smaller angles.

Leakage Radiation

Leakage radiation is the one that emanates from the source housing, other than primary. It is known that X-ray is emitted in all directions. Though X-ray tube is lined with lead, some leakage radiation is transmitted through lead lining. Since it passes through the source housing, its effective energy is very high in diagnostic X-rays. Though it is harder than the primary, it has low intensity relative to the primary. Hence, quality of the leakage radiation is assumed as that of the primary beam.

PLANNING A DIAGNOSTIC X-RAY FACILITY

General Requirements

Location

The rooms housing the diagnostic X-ray units and related equipment should be located as far away as feasible from areas of high occupancy and general traffic, such as maternity and pediatric wards and other departments of the hospital that are not directly related to radiation and its use.

Layout

The layout of rooms in an X-ray department should aim at providing integrated facilities so that handling of X-ray equipment and related operations can be conveniently performed with adequate protection. The doors and passages leading to the X-ray installation should permit safe and easy transport of equipment and nonambulatory patients. The number of doors for entry and windows should be kept minimum. Normally, X-ray room should be provided with only one door.

Unnecessary doors and windows present in an existing room, where X-ray machine is installed, should be bricked off and, if not possible, should be provided with adequate lead lining of 2 mm and kept permanently closed. Whenever lead lining is provided, care should be taken to provide adequate overlapping in the shielding. The darkroom should be so located that the primary X-ray beam cannot be directed on it. A typical layout for a diagnostic X-ray department is shown in **Figure 5.2**.

Room Size

The room housing the X-ray equipment must be spacious enough to permit installation and servicing and operation of equipment with safety and convenience for patients, servicing personnel and operators. It should facilitate the wheeling-in of patients, in and around the couch of the unit. Proper grouping of the rooms comprising the installation should be done bearing in mind their dependence on each other.

The room size must not <18 m^2 for general-purpose radiography and conventional fluoroscopy equipment. Not more than one unit of any type shall be installed

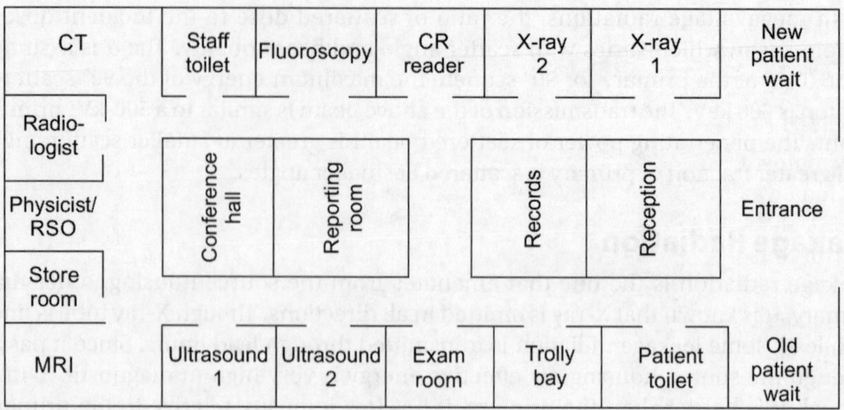

FIG. 5.2: A typical layout of a diagnostic X-ray department.
(CR: computed radiography; RSO: radiation safety officer)

in the same room, and no single dimension of these X-ray rooms shall be <4 m. In mammography, the room size shall be not <10 m^2, and no single dimension of the room shall be <3 m. The size of the room housing the gantry of the CT unit shall not be <25 m^2.

Shielding

Appropriate structural shielding shall be provided for the walls, ceilings, and floors, so that the doses received by the occupational workers and members of public are kept to a minimum and shall not exceed the annual effective doses as prescribed by the competent authority. The current limits are between 20 mSv and 1 mSv for occupational workers and members of public, respectively. The doors of the X-ray room shall provide the same shielding as that of adjacent walls in case persons are likely to be present in front of them when the X-ray unit is energized.

Appropriate shielding must be provided for dark room to ensure that undeveloped X-ray films stored in it will not be exposed to more than an air-kerma rate of 10 μGy/week (about 1.13 mR/week). Thickness equivalent to 2.0-mm lead (15 cm concrete or 23 cm or 9-inch brick walls) with plaster will provide adequate protection outside the X-ray room against both primary and secondary radiation in most of the diagnostic X-ray installation.

Opening and Ventilation

Unshielded openings, if provided in the X-ray room for ventilation/exhaust or natural light, must be located above a height of 2.1 m from the finished floor level/ground outside the X-ray room.

Equipment Layout

The X-ray equipment must be installed in such a way that in normal use, the useful beam is not directed towards control panel, doors, windows, dark room, and areas of high occupancy. The useful beam should preferably be directed towards unoccupied areas and away from the dark room. Sufficient area should be left all around the X-ray table for safe and free movements of equipment/trolley, staff, and service personnel. More than one examination should not be conducted simultaneously in the same room; hence, the installation of more than one X-ray equipment in the same room is discouraged.

Control Panel

In diagnostic X-ray units-operating below 125 kV_p, the control panel should be located away from the primary beam inside a stationery/mobile-protective barrier (MPB). The protective barrier should have sufficient lead equivalence (1.5 mm). Both control console and machine can be housed in the same room.

For equipment operating at 125 kV_p or above, the control panel must be installed in a separate control room located outside but contiguous to the machine room and provided with appropriate shielding, direct viewing window (VW) (1.5-mm lead equivalence) and oral communication facilities between the operator and the patient.

Waiting Area

To avoid crowding of patients and relatives near the entrance door, a waiting area must be provided outside and adjacent to the X-ray room. It should have sufficient area to match the patient workload with toilet facility.

Warning Light and Placard

A suitable warning signal such as the red light must be provided at a conspicuous place outside the X-ray room and kept ON when the X-ray equipment is energized to prevent inadvertent entry of persons not connected with the examination into the diagnostic room. An appropriate warning placard should be posted outside the diagnostic room **(Figs. 5.3A and B)**.

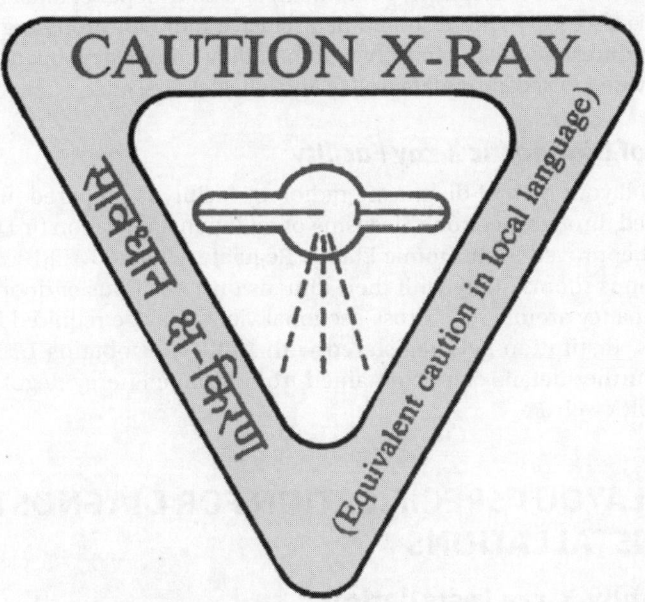

FIG. 5.3A: Placard: X-radiation warning sign.

Courtesy: AERB: www.aerb.gov.in.

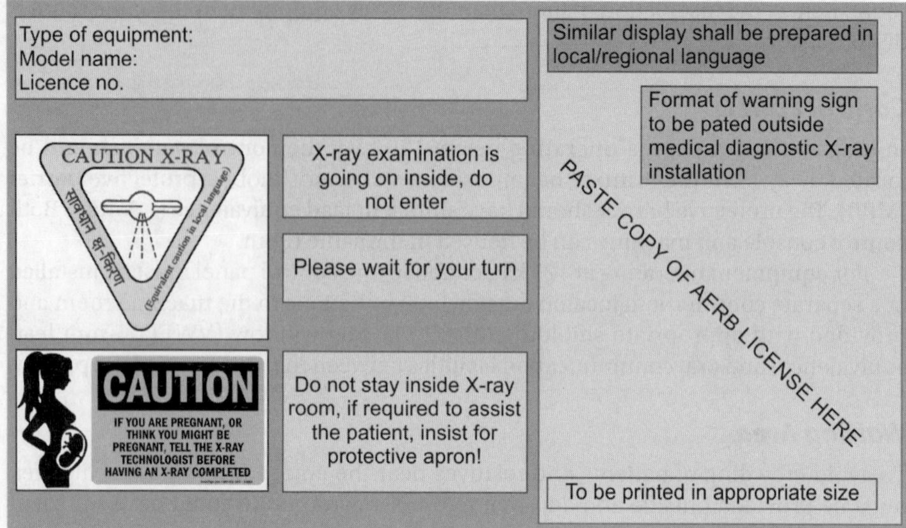

FIG. 5.3B: Warning sign display format as per AERB.

Courtesy: AERB: www.aerb.gov.in.

Other Specifications

The treatment room may be air-conditioned to control temperature, pressure, and humidity. Suitable monitors should be provided to indicate the above parameters. It will ensure long-term, trouble-free, safe operation of the equipment. Spilt AC with sufficient capacity to suit the room size is preferable than window ACs. Suitable electrical interlocks between door, equipment, and control panel must be provided, wherever it is necessary. There should be exclusive room for preparing patients for special procedures, postscan recovery, and handling emergency. In addition, space must be provided to accommodate trolley and wheelchairs, etc.

Approval of Diagnostic X-ray Facility

The site and layout plan of diagnostic radiology facility is prepared in 1:200 scale and submitted through electronic licensing of radiation application (e-LORA) by the user and get approved from Atomic Energy Regulatory Board (AERB). Plan should indicate various rooms along with their dimensions, positions of doors, windows, type of occupancy around, etc. Cross-sectional views may be required for CT scan. Prior to this, institution gets registered with AERB and obtains *Username* and *Password*. Further details can be obtained from Atomic Energy Regulatory Board (AERB) e-LORA website.

MODEL LAYOUT SPECIFICATION FOR DIAGNOSTIC X-RAY INSTALLATIONS

Radiography X-ray Installation

Radiography X-ray units are operated in the range of 50–125 kV_p applied voltage. Objects that are irradiated are considered as primary barriers. Additional shielding

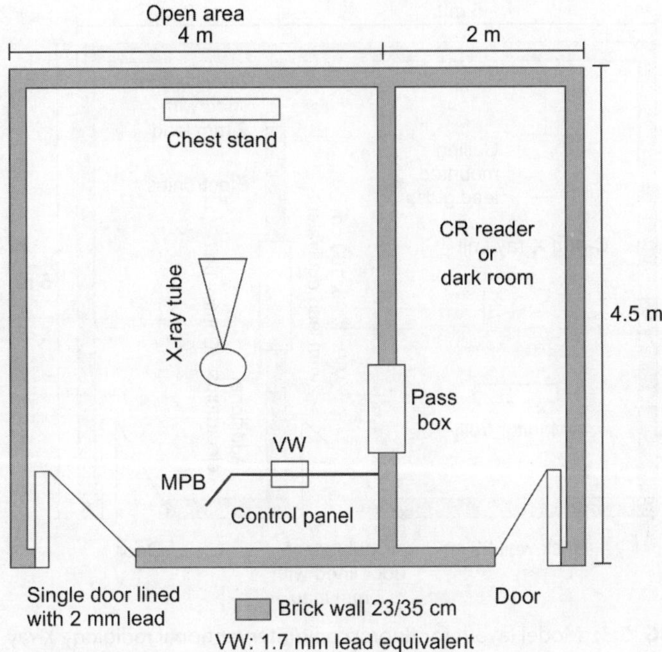

FIG. 5.4: Model layout for a general radiography X-ray.
(CR: computed radiography; MPB: mobile-protective barrier)

must be provided for the wall behind the chest stand. Provisions are made to observe and communicate with the patient on the table. The operator should be in the control area. The shield at the control (protective barrier) must be a permanent/mobile one with 2.1 m height. It should not be used as primary barrier. A viewing window (VW) of suitable size must be there at the control barrier which is centrally placed. Chest stand is positioned away from the control panel or door, preferably on the opposite direction. If dark room is adjacent, lead lined pass-box is provided for easy movement of cassette.

Wall(s) of the X-ray room on which scattered X-ray falls is (are) not <23 cm or 9-inch thickness brick or equivalent, and primary X-ray beam falls is (are) not <35 cm or 14-inch thickness brick or equivalent. The ceiling must have a thickness of concrete (density 2.35 g/cc), not <6 inch or 15 cm. There is a shielding equivalent to at least 23 cm or 9-inch thickness brick or 1.7-mm lead in front of the door(s) and windows of the X-ray room to protect the adjacent areas, either by public or not under possession of the owner of the X-ray room. The density of the normal masonry brick is considered as 1.6 g/cc. A typical model plan is shown in **Figure 5.4** and should have the following specifications:

- *Area*: 18 m^2 (not to scale)
- Mobile-protective barrier of 1.7-mm lead equivalence
- Viewing window glass of 45 × 45 cm^2 size and 1.7-mm lead equivalence
- Window or ventilator (W) at a height of 2.1 m from the finished floor level outside the X-ray room
- Entrance door lead lined with 2.0 mm of lead sheet with proper overlapping at all the joints, and provision of warning light and placard
- Provision of lead apron of 0.25 mm and gonad shield of 0.5 mm lead equivalence

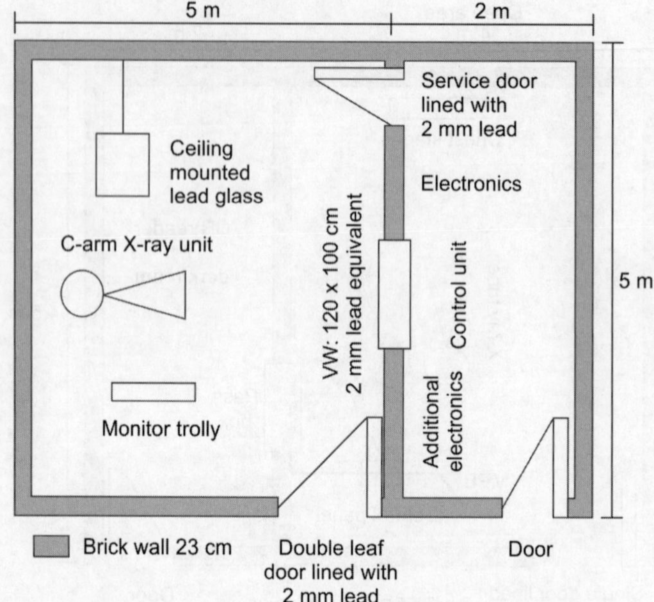

FIG. 5.5: Model layout for fluoroscopy/interventional radiology X-ray.

Fluoroscopy X-ray Installation

Fluoroscopic imaging or interventional radiology/cardiac angiography systems are usually operated at potentials ranging from 60 to 120 kV_p. A primary barrier is incorporated into the fluoroscopic image receptor. Therefore, a protective design for a room containing only a fluoroscopic unit considers only secondary protective barriers against leakage and scattered radiations. However, provisions are made with primary barriers so that the function of the room can be changed later date without the need to add additional shielding. Most modern fluoroscopic X-ray imaging systems also include a radiographic X-ray tube. The shielding requirements for such a room are based on the combined workload of both units. A typical model plan is shown in the **Figure 5.5**.

- *Area*: 7 × 5 = 35 m^2 (not to scale)
- *Viewing window glass*: 120 × 100 cm, 2.0-mm lead equivalence
- Entrance door (double leaf door) and service door are lead lined with 2.0 mm of lead sheet with proper overlapping at all the joints and junctions and provision of warning light and placard
- Walls of minimum 23-cm or 9 inch thickness brick and ceiling of 15 cm concrete
- Provision of lead apron, thyroid shield, and ceiling-mounted lead glass of 0.5-mm lead equivalence

Mammography X-ray Installation

Mammography units are typically operated between 25 and 30 kV_p. The walls are constructed with bricks or gypsum wallboard. Standard gypsum wallboard

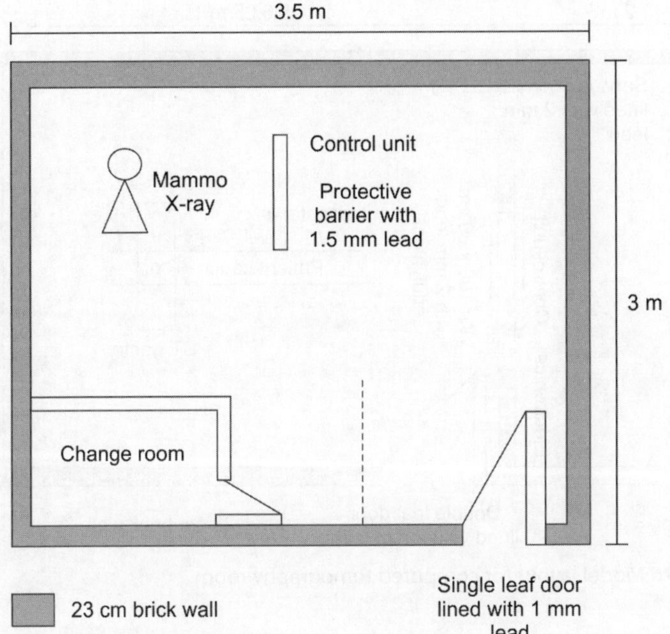

FIG. 5.6: Model layout for mammography X-ray.

construction is usually adequate to shield the walls of mammography room. Gypsum wallboard may contain voids and nonuniform areas. Hence, higher thickness of gypsum wallboard is recommended than that calculated. Adequate protective barrier of lead acrylic or lead glass is incorporated into dedicated mammography units.

Doors need special attention as they offer poor attenuation than brick or gypsum wallboard. Solid core wooden door (5 cm thick) leading to corridors outside a mammography room provides adequate shielding. Standard wooden doors may not be sufficient if the shielded area has significant occupancy. Standard concrete construction provides adequate barriers above and below mammographic facilities. Lead-lined walls and doors are usually not required. A typical model plan is shown in the **Figure 5.6**.

- *Area*: 3 × 3.5 = 10.5 m² (not to scale)
- Window or ventilator (W) at a height of 2.1 m from the finished floor level outside the X-ray room
- Entrance door lead lined with 1.0 mm of lead sheet with proper overlapping at all the joints, and provision of warning light and placard
- Walls of minimum 23-cm thickness brick and ceiling of 15-cm concrete
- Provision of lead glass shield or lead apron of 1.5-mm lead equivalent

Computed Tomography Installation

Computed tomography employs a collimated X-ray fan-beam that is intercepted by the patient and by the detector array. Consequently, only secondary radiation is incident on protective barriers. The operating potential, typically in the range of

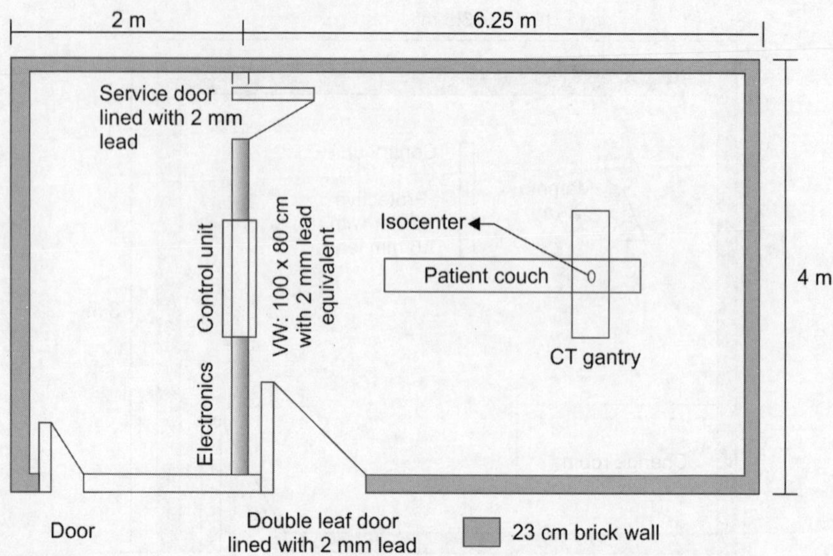

FIG. 5.7: Model layout for computed tomography room.

80–140 kV_p, as well as the workload is much higher than for general radiography or fluoroscopy. Due to the potential for a large amount of secondary radiation, floors, walls, and ceilings need special consideration. Additionally, scattered and leakage radiations from CT systems are not isotropic. The radiation levels in the direction of the gantry are much less than the radiation levels along the axis of the patient table. A typical model plan is shown in the **Figure 5.7**.

- *Area*: 4 × 8.25 = 33 m^2 (not to scale)
- Viewing window glass: 100 × 80 cm with of 2-mm lead equivalence
- Entrance door (double leaf door) and service doors are lead lined with 2-mm lead sheet with proper overlapping at all the joints and junctions, and provision of warning light and placard.
- Walls of minimum 23-cm or 9 inch thickness of brick and ceiling 15-cm of concrete. If the CT scan is housed in the first or second floor, the CT floor thickness should be about 6–8 inch of concrete, to restrict the respective ground floor radiation levels.

Other X-ray Installations

Bone mineral densitometer dose rate at 1 m is less than allowable dose limit for public; hence, no structural shielding is needed even with the smallest room **(Fig. 5.8)**. Dental X-rays use cone-beam CT (CBCT), orthopantomogram (OPG), and intraoral radiography. Normal wall thickness is sufficient to offer protection to such X-ray units and the suggested shielding is recommendary in nature. However, if the installation is not on the ground floor, a 6–8-inch thickness of concrete is required for the ceiling. Mobile C-arm and lithotripsy equipment can be used in operation theater (OT) with normal wall thickness of 9” brick/6” concrete and should have 1.0-mm lead-lined doors/windows.

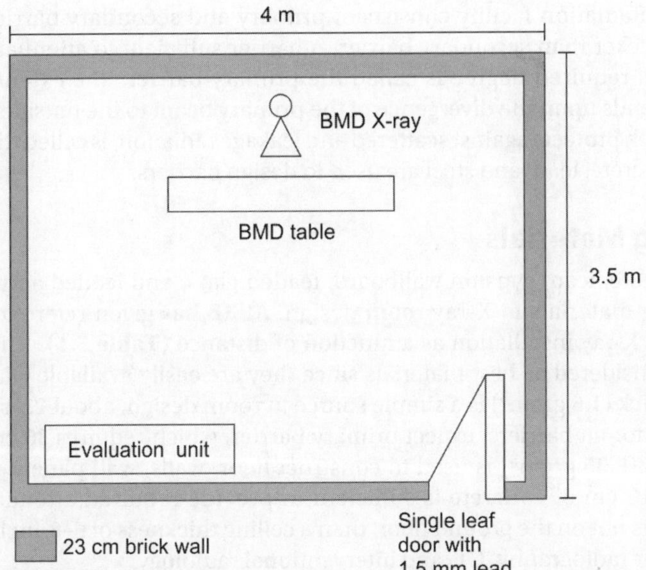

FIG. 5.8: Model payout for bone mineral densitometer.
(BMD: bone mineral densitometer)

DESIGN AND SHIELDING REQUIREMENTS FOR DIAGNOSTIC X-RAY FACILITY

Controlled and Uncontrolled Areas

A controlled area is a limited access area in which the occupational exposure of personnel to radiation is under the supervision of an individual in charge of radiation protection. This implies that access, occupancy, and working conditions are controlled for radiation protection purposes. In facilities that use X-rays for medical imaging, these areas are usually in the immediate areas where X-ray equipment is used, such as X-ray procedure rooms and X-ray control booths or other areas that require control of access, occupancy, and working conditions for radiation protection purposes. The workers in these areas are primarily radiologists and radiographers who are specifically trained in the use of ionizing radiation and whose radiation exposure is usually individually monitored.

Uncontrolled areas for radiation protection purposes are all other areas in the hospital or clinic and the surrounding environment. Uncontrolled areas are those occupied by individuals such as patients, visitors to the facility, and employees who do not work routinely with or around radiation sources. Areas adjacent to but not part of the X-ray facility are also uncontrolled areas.

Protective Barriers

Protective barriers are designed to ensure that the dose equivalent received by any individual does not exceed the applicable maximum permissible value. Barrier should protect all three types of radiation, namely primary, scattered, and leakage radiations. Radiation facility consists of primary and secondary barriers; primary barrier is thicker than secondary barrier. A barrier sufficient to attenuate the useful beam to the required degree is called the primary barrier. The extent of primary barrier depends upon the divergence of the primary beam to the outside barrier. The barrier, which protects against scattered and leakage radiation, is called the secondary barrier. Concrete, lead, and steel are used to design barriers.

Shielding Materials

Brick, concrete, lead, gypsum wallboard, leaded glass, and leaded acrylic are used as shielding materials in X-ray room design. AERB has given reference-shielding material for X-ray installation as a function of distance **(Table 5.1)**. Brick and concrete are considered as best materials since they are easily available with structural strength. Brick (1.6 g/cm^3) is a simple source in room design, about 23-cm thickness is sufficient for all barriers, expect primary barrier, which requires 35 cm. Concrete of thickness (2.35 g/cm^3) is used to construct floor, walls, wall panels, and ceiling. Generally, 15 cm of concrete is sufficient to provide required attenuation. If the installation is not on the ground floor, then a ceiling thickness of 6–8-inch concrete is necessary for radiography, CT, and interventional radiology.

Lead is most preferred due to its high-attenuation properties and low cost. Commercial lead is specified in weight per area (g/cm^2 or lb/ft^2). Generally, 2-mm lead thickness (4.6 lb/ft^2) is sufficient for general radiography X-ray shielding. Though lead is suitable for diagnostic X-ray energy, it has tendency to lose uniformity and requires periodic survey. Lead also possesses serious environmental hazards hence it is discouraged.

Alternative materials such as gypsum wallboard, plate glass, and leaded acrylic are used instead of lead. Gypsum wallboard (sheetrock) of 1 cm is normally recommended at 1.5 m, especially in mammography. Lead glass or leaded acrylic are used with lead equivalent thickness such as 0.5, 1.0, and 1.5 mm. Wall thickness for dental–intraoral radiography is recommendary in nature. Mobile C-arm and lithotripsy X-ray units used in OT should have a wall thickness of 6-inch concrete or 9-inch brick with 1.0-mm lead-lined doors.

TABLE 5.1 **Reference shielding thickness required at 2 m for different X-ray rooms.**

Shielding material	*Dental CBCT/OPG*	*Radiography and fluoroscopy**	*Interventional radiology/Cardiac angiography**	*Computed tomography**
Brick, cm	12	20	23	25
Concrete, cm	8	12	15	15
Steel, cm	—	2.0	2.0	2.5
Lead, cm	0.12	0.15	0.18	0.18
Any other material	1.4 TVT	1.8 TVT	2.0 TVT	2.8 TVT

*Ceiling thickness of concrete of 6–8 inch is adequate.

(AERB: Atomic Energy Regulatory Board; CBCT: cone-beam computed tomography; OPG: orthopantomogram; TVT: tenth-value thickness)

Coutesy: (AERB: www. aerb.gov.in).

Workload, Occupancy Factor, and Use Factor

Workload

Workload (W) is a measure of X-ray tube's use, and it is the time integral of the tube current, over certain period, expressed in mA-min/week. In diagnostic X-ray unit, it is obtained by multiplying the maximum mAs/exposure with beam ON time in min/week (mAs/60). For example, the workload of a hospital with 20 patients per day, three films per patient, and 60 mAs per film is calculated as follows:

W = (20 patients/day) × (5 days/week) × (3 films/patient) × (10 mAs/film) × (1 min/60 s)
= 50 mA-min/week

Higher kV_p settings decrease the workload due to increase of output (mR/mAs), less attenuation in patient, and use of reduced mAs.

Workload Per Patient

National Council on Radiation Protection and Measurement Report No. 147 (NCRP-147) suggested normalized workload per patient (W_{norm}). It conveys the average workload per patient, including various procedures of the patient. The total workload (W_{tot}) is the product of normalized workload, and average number of patients per week (N):

$$W_{tot} = N \times W_{norm} \tag{5.1}$$

This makes the workload as a function of kV_p rather than magnitude of workload. This is much useful to design-shielding thickness since attenuation of radiation by primary barrier depends on kV_p. Workload distribution varies widely, and it is specific to radiography, fluoroscopy, and CT scans **(Table 5.2)**.

The NCRP-49 (1976) describes the structural shielding design and evaluation for medical use of X-rays and γ-rays of energies up to 10 MeV. When the report was made, single-phase generator was in use, the annual dose limit is 100 mrem/year, neglected the image receptor attenuation, and considered low-speed film-combination. Hence, strict adherence of NCRP-49 would result in expensive shielding procedures.

TABLE 5.2 Workload for various diagnostic radiology X-ray units.

Type of X-ray units	*Workload (mA-min/week) for radiation survey*	*Workload (mA-min in 1 hour) for leakage radiation*	*Approximate exposure factors: kV_p, mA, s*
Dental X-rays, OPG/CBCT	150	180*	60–100, 8–20, 1–2 s
Radiography and fluoroscopy (fixed)	400	180	80–100, 50–100, 1–2 s
Mammography	650	40	30–35, 100–200, 1–2 s
Interventional radiology	4,800	180	80–100, 50–100, 1–2 s
CT scan	20,000	500	110–140, 50–100, 1–2 s

*Workload for intraoral X-rays is 20 mA-min/week

(AERB: Atomic Energy Regulatory Board; CBCT: cone-beam computed tomography; OPG: orthopantomogram; CT: computed tomography)

Coutesy: (AERB: www.aerb.gov.in).

TABLE 5.3 **Occupancy factors for diagnostic X-rays.**

Location	*Occupancy level*	*Occupancy factor*
Administrative or clerical offices; laboratories, pharmacies, and other work areas fully occupied by an individual; receptionist areas, attended waiting rooms, children's indoor play areas, adjacent X-ray rooms, film reading areas, nurse's stations, X-ray control rooms	Full	1
Rooms used for patient examinations and treatments	Partial	1/2
Corridors, patient rooms, employee lounges, and staff rest	Partial	1/5
Corridor doors	Partial	1/8
Public toilets, unattended vending areas, storage rooms, outdoor areas with seating, unattended waiting rooms, and patient-holding areas	Occasional	1/20
Outdoor areas with only transient pedestrian or vehicular traffic, unattended parking lots, vehicular drop off areas (unattended), attics, stairways, unattended elevators, and janitor's closets		1/40

(NCRP: National Council on Radiation Protection and Measurements)
Courtesy: NCRP-147, 2015.

TABLE 5.4 **Use factors for primary barrier for a general radiography room.**

Barrier	*Use factor (U)*
Chest image receptor	1
Floor	0.89
Cross-table lateral walls	0.09
Unspecified wall	0.02

(NCRP: National Council on Radiation Protection and Measurements)
Courtesy: NCRP-147, 2015.

Occupancy Factor

Occupancy factor (T) of an area is an average fraction of time (8 h/day) that the individual stays at that area while the X-ray machine is ON. It can be full, partial, and occasional occupancy **(Table 5.3)**. Radiation workers who spent the entire time in controlled areas will have occupancy factor of 1. Occupancy factor modifies the shielding design objective at a point by 1/T or barrier attenuation lowers the radiation level by P/T ratio, where P is effective dose limit.

Use Factor

Use factor (U) is the fraction of the primary beam workload that is directed towards a primary barrier. It depends on the type of X-ray room and orientation of the equipment **(Table 5.4)**. It is estimated for the nature of procedure and the amount of X-ray beam is used in specific orientation. Majority times, the tube is oriented towards the floor to acquire images than other walls.

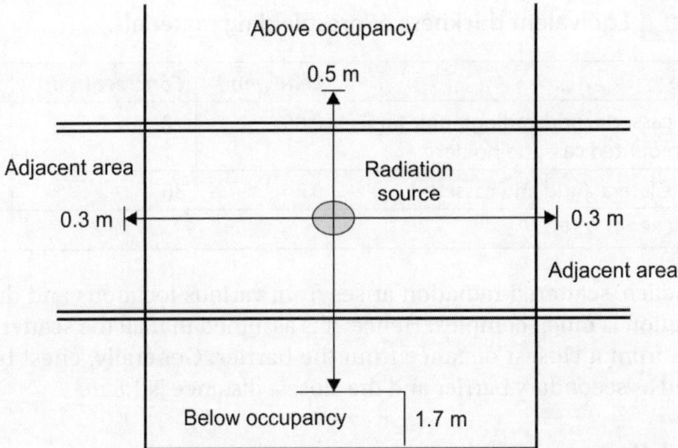

FIG. 5.9: Elevation diagram describes distances to adjacent areas above, and below the X-ray or radiation source for shielding calculation.

Courtesy: NCRP-147, 2015.

Design Limit

Occupational exposure effective dose limit (P) is 20 mSv/year averaged over 5 consecutive years and 30 mSv in any single year. The public dose limit is 1 mSv in a year. It corresponds to effective dose equivalent of 0.4 mSv/week for controlled area (restricted entry) and 0.02 mSv/week for uncontrolled area (assuming 8 hours/day, 5 days/week, and 50 weeks/year).

The NCRP-147 recommends a weekly shielding design limit of 0.1 mGy air-kerma for controlled areas (10 times lesser than NCRP-49). The weekly shielding design limit is 0.02 mGy air-kerma for uncontrolled area. (five times lesser than NCRP-49).

Distance

The NCRP recommends distances (d) to the points of measurement. If the occupancy is below the X-ray/radiation source, sensitive organs of the person below can be assumed not more than 1.7 m above the floor. If the occupancy is above the X-ray/radiation source, the distance can be measured to a point 0.5 m above the floor. Lateral distances to be measured at a point not <0.3 m from far side of a barrier (Fig. 5.9).

Primary and Secondary Barriers

Radiography, fluoroscopy, and dedicated chest X-ray rooms are designed with primary barriers to attenuate the primary beam. It should be made as goal while doing shielding calculation. The unshielded primary air-kerma at a point of interest depends on average number of patients per week, the use factor for the barrier, primary air-kerma per patient at 1 m, and the distance to the point.

Secondary barriers serve to attenuate the unshielded secondary air-kerma from scatter and leakage radiations. All the walls are considered as secondary barrier, excluding primary barriers. Scattered radiation intensity from a patient depends on beam area and scattering angle. Total secondary unshielded air-kerma is calculated from clinical workload distributions at 1 m. It is modified to the point of interest by inverse square law.

TABLE 5.5 Equivalent thickness of preshielding materials.

Hardware	*Lead (mm)*	*Concrete (mm)*	*Steel (mm)*
X-ray film cassette, grid, radiographic table, and wall-mounted cassette holder	0.85	72	7
Cross-table lateral (grid and cassette)	0.3	30	2
Courtesy: NCRP 147, 2015.			

In practice, scattered radiation arises from various locations and distances and the estimation is much complex. Hence, it is assumed that all the scattered radiation originates from a closest distance from the barrier. Generally, chest bucky wall is considered as secondary barrier and the closest distance is 1.5 m.

Preshielding

When a beam is incident on the patient, it is attenuated by the patient, X-ray film cassette, grids, radiographic table, and wall-mounted cassette holder. The attenuation of all the hardware items, excluding the patient attenuation, is referred as preshielding. It is expressed as equivalent thickness of shielding material **(Table 5.5)**. The accepted barrier thickness is given in terms of broad-beam transmission factor (B). It includes both preshielding and additional shielding thickness.

SHIELDING CALCULATION FOR DIAGNOSTIC X-RAY FACILITY

Diagnostic X-ray shielding calculation in earlier days has not accounted the attenuation offered by the X-ray accessories such as cassette/detector, chest bucky, and grid. NCRP-147 addresses this by considering workload, workload distributions, normalized workload per patient, field area, and attenuation of primary by detectors, etc., and incorporated the same as shielding thickness charts. These charts display shielding thickness required for various barriers as function of NT/Pd^2. N is the number of patients per week, T is the occupancy factor, P is the design limit, mGy/week, and d is the distance in meter from the X-ray source to the point of interest.

These charts are drawn between NT/Pd^2 and shielding materials, by assuming specific normalized workloads per patient (W_{norm}). It is provided for radiographic and fluoroscopic rooms, for various shielding materials like lead and concrete. If the site-normalized workload per patient (W_{site}) is different, then the value of NT/Pd^2 is scaled down by $\frac{W_{site}}{W_{norm}}$. A model chart is shown for primary barrier of a radiographic room without preshielding with lead as shielding material **(Fig. 5.10)**. Additional charts are provided for primary radiation, secondary radiation, for both with preshielding, and without preshielding in NCRP-147. It is also available for primary and secondary barriers such as lead and concrete. The graphs with preshielding account beam attenuation of detector, vertical chest bucky, grid, cassette, and other supporting structures. Attenuation offered by the above items may be equivalent to 0.8 mm lead. The cross-table lateral attenuation is equivalent to 0.3 mm lead.

This method requires room's scale drawing, elevation drawing, location of equipment, occupancy factors of adjacent areas, designations of adjacent areas as

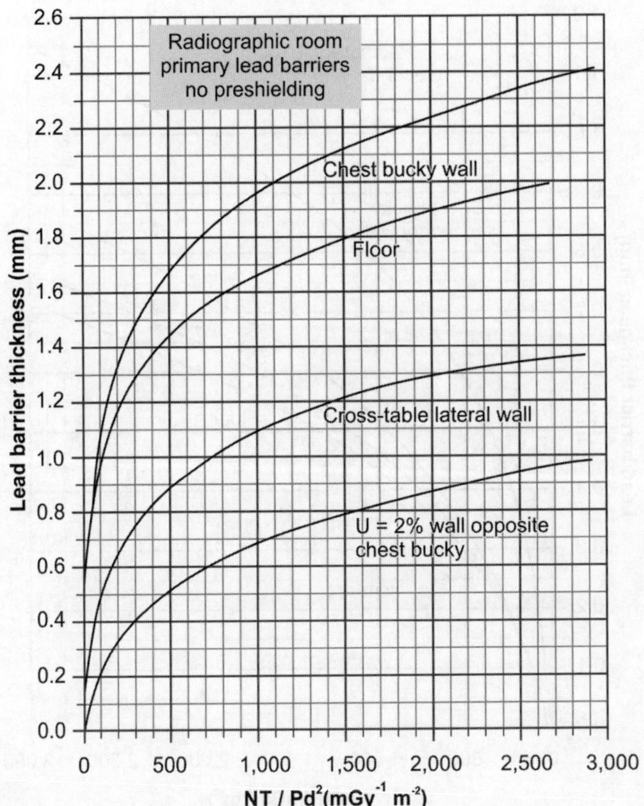

FIG. 5.10: Lead barrier thickness of radiographic room without preshielding as a function of NT/Pd^2 for primary barrier.
Courtesy: NCRP 147, 2015.

controlled and uncontrolled area, distances of adjacent area and average number of patients per week, etc. One should select the chart based on room type and shielding material to be used.

Worked Example 5.1

A radiographic X-ray unit has workload of 100 patients/week. Calculate the—(1) primary barrier thickness at 2.5 m distance, and (2) secondary barrier thickness at 1.5 m distance, using NCRP primary barrier (no-preshielding) chart for lead (T = 1, P = 0.02 mSv/week).

(1) *Primary barrier*:
N = 100 patients/week
P = 0.02 mSv/week
T = 1
d = 2.5 m

$$\frac{NT}{Pd^2} = \frac{100 \times 1}{0.02 \times 2.5^2} = 800 \text{ mGy}^{-1}\text{m}^{-2}$$

Referring the graph for radiographic room—primary lead barrier—without preshielding, using the chest bucky wall curve in **Figure 5.10**, the lead thickness is

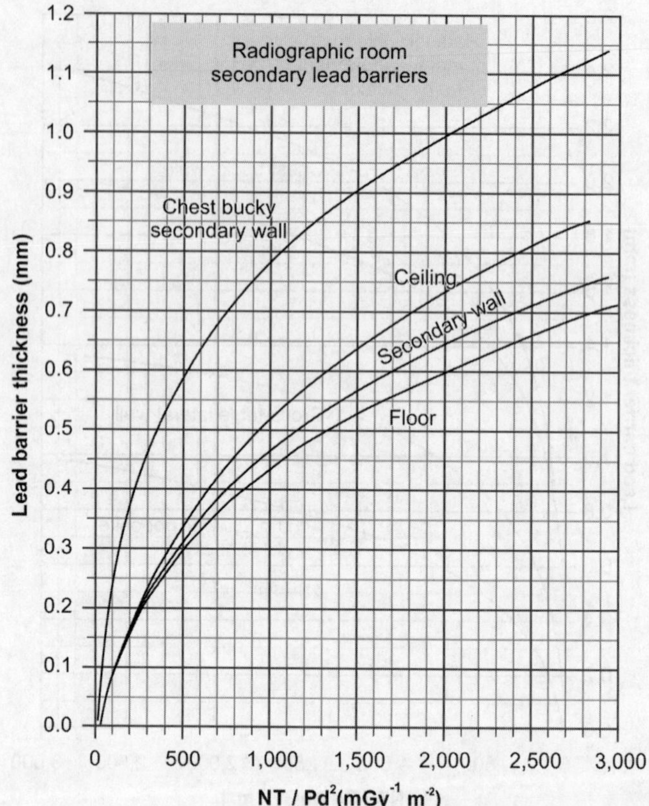

FIG. 5.11: Secondary lead barrier thickness of radiographic room as a function of NT/Pd^2.
Courtesy: NCRP 147, 2015.

1.9 mm or lead thickness of 5 lb/ft^2 should be used. Such shielding should be from finished floor to a height of 2.1 m, with lateral margins of 0.5 m around the image receptor.

(2) *Secondary barrier*:
N = 100 patients/week
P = 0.02 mSv/week
T = 0.2
d = 1.5 m

$$\frac{NT}{Pd^2} = \frac{100 \times 0.2}{0.02 \times 1.5^2} = 444.4\ \text{mGy}^{-1}\text{m}^{-2}$$

Referring the secondary lead barrier chart **(Fig. 5.11)**, the required lead thickness is 0.55 mm. The nearest available lead thickness is 2 lb/ft^2, which is used as secondary barrier.

Alternative Method

The NCRP-147 also provides tabulated data on workload distributions for radiography, fluoroscopy, mammography, and interventional radiology **(Table 5.6)**. This table

TABLE 5.6 Preshielded air-kerma per patient for primary, leakage + scatter for various diagnostic rooms (workload is normalized to primary beam at 1 m) (AAPM TG9 Simpkin 1996a).

Barrier	*Workload (W_{norm}), mA-min per patient*	*Primary (K_p), mGy per patient @1 m*	*Leakage + Scatter (K_{sec}), mGy per patient @1 m*
Radiography (all barriers)	2.5	—	3.4×10^{-2}
Radiography (floor and barriers)	1.9	6.2	2.3×10^{-2}
Radiography (chest bucky)	0.6	2.3	5.5×10^{-3}
Mammography	6.7	—	1.1×10^{-2}
Fluoroscopy (F + R)	13	5.9	3.2×10^{-1}
Cardiac angiography	160	—	2.7
(AAPM: American Association of Physicists in Medicine)			

TABLE 5.7 Secondary transmission factors.

Barrier	*120 kV_p*	*140 kV_p*
Concrete	• $\alpha = 0.0383$ mm^{-1} • $\beta = 0.0142$ mm^{-1} • $\gamma = 0.658$	• $\alpha = 0.0336$ mm^{-1} • $\beta = 0.0122$ mm^{-1} • $\gamma = 0.519$
Lead	• $\alpha = 2.246$ mm^{-1} • $\beta = 5.73$ mm^{-1} • $\gamma = 0.547$	• $\alpha = 2.009$ mm^{-1} • $\beta = 3.99$ mm^{-1} • $\gamma = 0.342$
(NCRP: National Council on Radiation Protection and Measurements) *Coutesy*: (NCRP 147, 2015).		

provides values of unshielded air-kerma (K) per patient at a nominal focus to image distance, for a nominal field size and workload (W). Unshielded kerma is the ratio of the air-kerma behind a barrier thickness to the air-kerma at the same location with no barrier. The data is based on a survey carried out in USA by *Simpkin* (AAPM TG9, 1996a). It is available for primary and scattered plus leakage radiations. These can be used along with transmission equations (*Archer* equation) to determine the required shielding. However, use of transmission equations requires transmission fitting parameters, α, β, and γ, which depend on shielding materials **(Table 5.7)**. Readers shall refer NCRP-147 documents for further details. The transmission is given by:

$$B = \left(\frac{P}{T}\right)\frac{d^2}{KN} \tag{5.2}$$

where, P is the design limit per week, T is the occupancy factor, d is the distance between the radiation source and the point outside the barrier, K is the average unshielded air-kerma per patient at 1 m from the source, and N is the number of patients per week. The above equation can be modified for primary and secondary barrier and including use factor (U) as follows:

$$B_p = \left(\frac{P}{T}\right)\frac{d_P^2}{K_P UN} \tag{5.3}$$

$$B_{sec} = \left(\frac{P}{T}\right)\frac{d_{sec}^2}{K_{sec} N} \tag{5.4}$$

where, K_P is the unshielded primary air-kerma per patient at 1 m from the source and K_{sec} is the unshielded secondary air-kerma per patient at 1 m from the source.

Worked Example 5.2

A radiographic room is handling 125 patient per week. Calculate the primary barrier thickness at 4.1 m considering occupancy, T = 1 and design limit of 0.02 mSv/week. [unshielded primary air-kerma at 1 m is 5.2 mGy per patient, (Refer NCRP-147's **Table 4.5**)].

P = 0.02 mSv/week

T = 1

K = 5.2 mGy/patient

N = 125 patients/week

d = 4.1 m

$$B_p = \left(\frac{P}{T}\right)\frac{d^2}{K_P N}$$

$$= \left(\frac{0.02}{1}\right)\frac{4.1^2}{5.2 \times 125} = 5.1 \times 10^{-4}$$

Referring standard transmission chart, the thickness of concrete is found to be 173 mm (NCRP-147, Appendix B, primary transmission chart). This includes preshielded thickness of hardware items which is equal to 72 mm by referring **Table 5.5**. Hence, actual primary barrier required is = 107 – 72 = 35 mm. In a similar way, the secondary transmission is found. By referring the secondary transmission chart, the secondary barrier thickness is calculated.

SHIELDING CALCULATION FOR COMPUTED TOMOGRAPHY FACILITY

Computed tomography scan is different from other X-ray modalities. The X-ray is mostly attenuated by patient and the detector. Hence, only scattered radiation is considered for shielding calculation. It is operated with 80–140 kV_p and the beam is highly filtered. The workload is much higher and scattered dose distribution is not isotropic (Anisotropic).

Workload for CT Scan

In the case of CT scan, all the walls in the room are secondary barriers, and the detector plays the role of primary barrier. The measured data from an individual CT scan is required to determine the amount of scattered radiation, arising from the gantry. Normally, these measured data are provided as exposure lines per slice for a given mAs from the isocenter of the gantry **(Fig. 5.12)**. Workload of a CT scan is

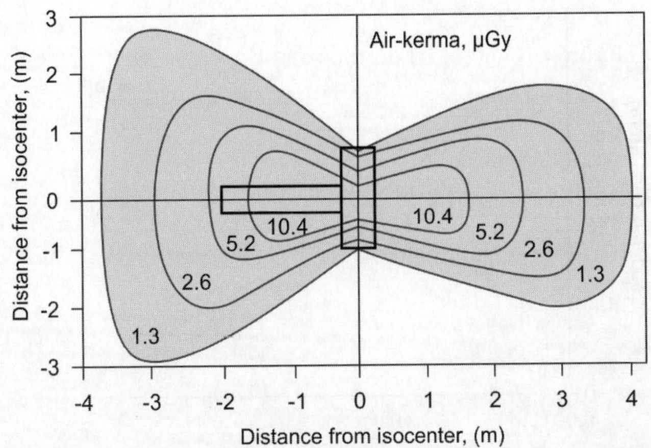

FIG. 5.12: CT scan layout: Secondary radiation distribution from the isocenter in a 32 cm PMMA phantom, measured in air kerma, Gy (140 kV_p, 100 mA, 1 s). Horizontal dose distribution includes both scatter and leakage.

calculated from average number of patients per week, fraction of head verses body scans, and average mAs per patient.

The workload of a head CT scan that has 20 abdominal scans per day, 30 slices per scan with 250 mAs per slice can be calculated as follows (assume 50% of the scans are with contrast, and 50% are without any contrast = 1.5 studies/patient).

Total number of slices = (20 patients/day) × (5 days/week) × (40 slices/study) × (1.5 studies/patient)

$$= 6{,}000 \text{ slices/week}$$

$$W = 6{,}000 \frac{\text{slices}}{\text{week}} \times \frac{200 \text{ mAs}}{\text{slice}} \times \frac{1}{60}$$
$$= 20{,}000 \text{ mA - min/week}$$

Today, helical CT is in use mostly and difficult to estimate number of slices exactly; hence, a workload of 20,000 mA-min per week is used for barrier calculations and area monitoring (AERB). In the case of leakage radiation calculation, it is about 500 mA-min in 1 hour.

Worked Example 5.3

A CT scanner performs 60 head scans and 60 abdomen scans per week using 120 kV_p and produces an average scatter air-kerma of 0.5 mGy/patient at 1 m from the gantry isocenter. Calculate the barrier thickness at 2.5 m from the gantry isocenter. (Assume T = 0.2, P = 0.02 mSv/week).

P = 0.02 mSv/week
T = 0.2
d = 2.5 m
N = 60 + 60 = 120 patients/week
K = 0.5 mGy/patient at 1 m

$$B = \left(\frac{P}{T}\right)\frac{d^2}{KN} = \left(\frac{0.02}{0.2}\right)\frac{2.5^2}{0.5 \times 120} = 0.01$$

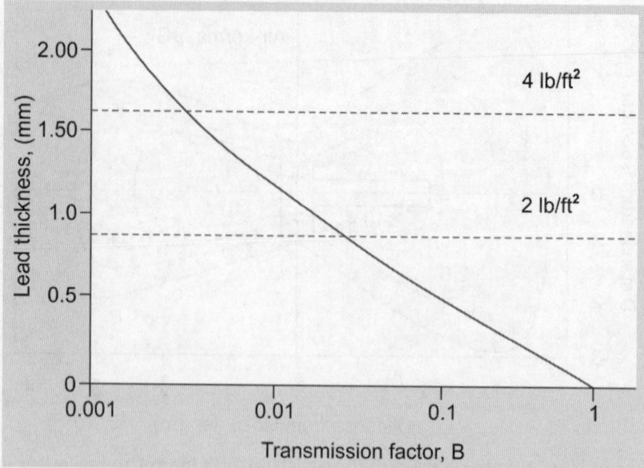

FIG. 5.13: Lead thickness versus transmission factor for secondary radiation in computed tomography operated at 120 kV_p (NCRP 147).

Referring the transmission chart **(Fig. 5.13)**, the required lead thickness for the transmission of 0.01 is 1.25 mm. This is >2 lb/ft^2, so it requires 4 lb/ft^2 = 1.58-mm lead thickness. The transmission and barrier thickness of other walls, ceiling, and floor can be calculated similarly. In the case of floor and ceiling, the concrete chart is used instead of lead.

Dose Length Product Method

National Council on Radiation Protection and Measurement uses dose length product (DLP) or CTDI for the calculation of CT workload. DLP of all the head and body scans done in a year are collected and then average scattered kerma is determined using different constants of proportionality. NCRP recommends 0.09 μGy/mGy-cm for head scans and 0.36 μGy/mGy-cm for body scans. If considerable number of repeat examination or contrast study is there, then DLP is multiplied by a factor of 1.4. The scatter fraction/cm at 1 m from a head or body phantom:

$$K_{head} = 9 \times 10^{-5}\ cm^{-1}$$
$$K_{body} = 3 \times 10^{-4} cm^{-1}$$

The total air-kerma from scatter and leakage at 1 m is calculated as follows:

$$K_{sec}\ (head) = K_{head} \times DLP \times 1.4 \tag{5.5}$$

$$K_{sec}\ (body) = 1.2 \times K_{body} \times DLP \times 1.4 \tag{5.6}$$

The factor 1.2 corrects for repeated examinations with contrast agents. The transmission can be obtained as given below.

Worked Example 5.4

A CT scan conducts 50 head and 75 body examinations per week. The DLP for head examination is 1,200 mGy-cm and body average is 550 mGy-cm from NCRP data.

Calculate the total scatter at a point which is at 2.5 m from the scan plane, applying public radiation limit and assuming full occupancy (T = 1).
DLP head = 1,200 mGy-cm
DLP body average = 550 mGy-cm
N = 50 (head)
N = 75 (body)
d = 2.5 m, P = 0.02 mSv/week

$$K_{sec}\text{ (head)} = K_{head} \times \text{DLP} \times 1.4$$
$$= 9 \times 10^{-5}\text{ cm}^{-1} \times 1{,}200 \times 50 \times 1.4 \times \frac{1}{2.5^2}$$
$$= 1.2\text{ mGy/week @ of } 0.024\text{ mGy per procedure}$$

$$K_{sec}\text{ (body)} = 1.2 \times K_{body} \times \text{DLP} \times 1.4$$
$$= 1.2 \times 3 \times 10^{-4} \times 550 \times 75 \times 1.4 \times \frac{1}{2.5^2}$$
$$= 3.32\text{ mGy/week @ } 0.044\text{ mGy per procedure}$$

Total scatter kerma = 1.2 + 3.32 = 4.52 mGy/week

$$\text{Transmission factor} = \frac{0.02}{4.52} = 0.0044$$

Referring the chart **(Fig. 5.13)**, the required lead thickness for the transmission of 0.0044 is about 1.6 mm. Similarly, it can be calculated to different barrier distances, design limits, and occupancy.

BIBLIOGRAPHY

1. Atomic Energy Regulatory Board. (2016). AERB safety code No. AERB/RF-MED/SC-3 (Rev. 2): Radiation safety in manufacture, supply and use of medical diagnostic X-ray equipment. [online] Available from https://www.aerb.gov.in/images/PDF/RF-MED-SC-3.pdf. [Last accessed October, 2022].
2. Bushberg JT, Seibert JA, Leidholdt EM, Boone JM. The essential physics of medical imaging, 3rd edition. Philadelphia, PA: Wolters Kluwer/Lippincott Williams & Wilkins; 2012.
3. Dance DR. Diagnostic Radiology Physics: A Handbook for Teachers and Students. Vienna, Austria: International Atomic Energy Agency; 2014.
4. National Council on Radiation Protection and Measurements. Structural shielding design for medical X-ray imaging facilities. National council on radiation protection and measurements (NCRP), report No. 147, Bethesda, 2015. [online] Available from https://eva.fcien.udelar.edu.uy/pluginfile.php/10700/mod_resource/content/1/NCRP%20Report%20No.%20147.pdf. [Last accessed October, 2022].
5. Thayalan K. Basic radiological physics, 2nd edition. New Delhi: Jaypee brothers Medical Publishers; 2017.
6. Atomic Energy Regulatory Board (AERB) website :https://www.aerb.gov.in.

CHAPTER 6

Quality Assurance in Diagnostic Radiology

INTRODUCTION

Quality assurance (QA) is a set of procedures carried out in an equipment to verify manufacturer's specifications. In medical use of radiation, QA policies are helpful to maintain the quality of patient care. It is designed specific to an equipment to meet the standards. Professional organizations such as American College of Radiology (ACR) and the American Association of Physicists in Medicine (AAPM) have recommended QA programs for radiological practice. Atomic Energy Regulatory Board (AERB) has recommended set of QA procedure for diagnostic X-ray units.

The objective of QA is achieving good quality images with patient care. It is organized as a program that includes staff training, standard equipment, and facility. Its implementation involves administrative, clinical, physical, and technical aspects. The following paragraphs will explain the QA procedures related to diagnostic radiology.

QUALITY ASSURANCE

The goal of QA in diagnostic radiology is to obtain optimal image with minimum radiation dose and at minimum cost. To achieve the above goal, systematic QA programs are to be developed and implemented in all diagnostic X-ray facilities. This will enable us to monitor periodically the performance of the X-ray unit.

A radiological image may be good to look, due to proper density and positioning. If it does not reveal anatomic details, then its image quality is not assured. The radiologists may not be able to extract diagnostic information from the radiograph, which may lead to repeat examination (retake). Retakes result in unnecessary radiation dose to patients, staff, and public, and increase the workload and cost. The parameters, which affect the image quality, are:

- Applied tube potential (kV_p)
- Tube current (mA)
- Time of exposure (s)
- Focal spot size, filtration
- Contact between film and screen
- Focus-to-film distance (FFD)
- Beam alignment, congruence of optical and radiation field
- Film processing and viewing conditions, etc.

The QA program begins with performance evaluation tests of the X-ray unit at the manufacturing site, followed by acceptance tests after the installation is completed.

Then QA tests are carried out at regular intervals or after every major repair often referred as quality control (QC). The reasons to test the imaging equipment are:

- To observe the equipment performance at installation whether it is meeting vendors' specifications.
- Later test ensures that it is currently working as well as it did at the time of installation.
- To determine that repairs or modifications have improved recent improper performance.

Every QA program involves the following steps: (1) performing the QA tests **(Table 6.1)**, (2) recording the results, (3) analyzing the result, (4) take corrective and preventive measures, and (5) repeating the QA again. QA tests require specific tools for the measurement **(Table 6.2)**. AERB recommended QA test at least once in 2 years and after any repairs that have radiation safety implications. However, institution can have their own protocol to carry out tests based on the nature of equipment and its use.

TABLE 6.1 Various QA tests to be performed for diagnostic X-ray equipments.

Radiography/fluoroscopy (C-arm/Interventional radiology)	*Mammography*	*CT scan*	*Dental X-ray*
Congruence of radiation and optical field	Accuracy of operating potential/ accuracy of timer	Radiation profile width/slice thickness	Accuracy of operating potential/ accuracy of timer
Central beam alignment	Linearity of mA/mAs loading stations	Measurement of operating potential	Linearity of mA loading stations
Effective focal spot measurement	Total filtration and aluminum equivalence of the compression device	Timer accuracy	Reproducibility of radiation output
Accuracy of operating potential (kV_p)	Reproducibility of radiation output	Measurement of mAs linearity	Low-contrast sensitivity
Accuracy of irradiation time	Radiation leakage at 5 cm from the external surface of the X-ray tube housing	Output consistency	High-contrast sensitivity
Total filtration	Imaging performance evaluation	Measurement of computed tomography dose index (CTDI)	Tube housing leakage
Linearity of mA/mAs loading stations		Low-contrast resolution	

Continued

Continued

Radiography/fluoroscopy (C-arm/Interventional radiology)	***Mammography***	***CT scan***	***Dental X-ray***
Output consistency		High-contrast resolution	
Low-contrast sensitivity		Radiation leakage levels from X-ray tube housing at 1 m from the focus	
High-contrast sensitivity			
Exposure rate at tabletop			
Tube housing leakage			

(CT: computed tomography; QA: quality assurance)

TABLE 6.2 QA tests, their frequency, and tools required.

Test	***Frequency***	***Test tool***
kV_p	Once in 2 years	kV_p meter
Timer	Once in 3 months	Spinning top/Timer meter and dose-measuring meter
Output, mR/mAs	Monthly	Dose-measuring meter
Inherent filtration	Once in 3 months	Dose-measuring meter, and aluminum absorbers
Focal spot size	Once in a year	Focal spot test tool with nonscreen film cassette
Central beam alignment	Once in 2 months	Beam alignment test tool with screen film cassette
Congruence of radiation and optical field	Once in 2 months	Collimator test tool with screen film cassette
Low- and high-contrast sensitivity	Once in 2 years	Contrast test tool
Exposure at tabletop	Once in 2 years	Pocket dosimeter
Tube housing leakage	Once in 2 years	Radiation survey meter
Grid alignment	Annually and whenever film density appears nonuniform	Grid alignment test tool

(QA: quality assurance)

QUALITY ASSURANCE TEST FOR RADIOGRAPHY/ FLUOROSCOPIC X-RAY EQUIPMENT

The QA tests are applicable to radiography, radiography and fluoroscopy, C-arm, interventional radiology, and cardiology (cath lab) equipment. For radiography units, low-contrast sensitivity, high-contrast sensitivity, and exposure rate at tabletop tests are not applicable. In the case of C-arm, interventional radiology and cardiology, congruence of radiation and optical field, central beam alignment, and effective focal spot measurement tests are not applicable. Respective QA format is available in AERB website: www.aerb.gov.in

Congruence of Radiation and Optical Fields

The optical field in the X-ray equipment is used for defining the radiation field and to limit the same only to the area of clinical interest on the patient. If the optical field and radiation field are not congruent, the area of clinical interest may be missed in the radiograph leading to retake and unnecessary radiation to patients.

The collimator test tool is used for testing the congruence of optical and radiation fields. This test tool consists of a fiberglass board of size 24 cm × 27 cm with a rectangular area 20 cm × 16 cm marked on it by coating of X-ray opaque material. This rectangular area is divided into four equal segments by two graduated perpendicular bisectors. Two concentric circles of radii 4 mm and 8 mm are engraved in the center, which enable the use of this test tool in conjunction with the beam alignment test tool.

To carry out the test, the table is kept horizontal with the help of a spirit level. A screen type cassette, loaded with a medium-speed X-ray film, is placed on the table. The collimator test tool is kept above a screen type cassette **(Fig. 6.1A)**. FFD is kept as 100 cm, to obtain the shift of fields directly in terms of percentage of FFD. The light field is adjusted to coincide with the rectangular area marked on the test tool. The film is then exposed under suitable kV_p (60) and mAs and developed.

From the radiograph, the shift along the individual directions (X, X′, Y, and Y′) between the edges of optical and radiation fields is measured **(Fig. 6.1B)**. It should be

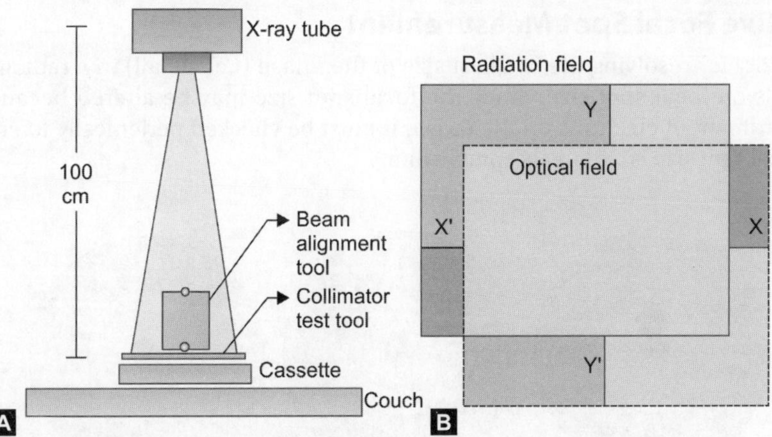

FIGS. 6.1A AND B: (A) Beam alignment and collimator test tool, (B) Congruence of optical and radiation fields.

within 2% of FFD. Sum of the shifts of the optical and radiation fields along horizontal and perpendicular directions for X + X′ and Y + Y′ dimensions is also measured and expressed in percentage of FFD.

- Tolerance should be within 2% of FFD.

Central Beam Alignment

If the X-ray beam is not perpendicular to the image receptor, the image may be distorted. This may result in loss of minute details. If grid is used, the distortion will be magnified resulting in total loss of minute details. The beam alignment can be tested using a beam alignment test tool.

The test tool consists of a transparent acrylic cylinder of inner diameter 6.3 cm, outer diameter 7.5 cm, and length 15.2 cm. Acrylic circular disks, each of 6-mm thickness, are fastened on both sides of the cylinder. Stainless steel balls of diameter 1.6 mm are coaxially fixed at the center of both these disks.

Beam alignment test is usually carried out simultaneously along with the test for congruence of optical and radiation field. To do this, two concentric circles of radii 4 mm and 8 mm are engraved in the center of the collimator test tool. The procedure for the congruence of optical and radiation field is repeated. The beam alignment test tool is kept on the collimator test tool such a way that the stainless steel ball of the lower side of the tool is just above the center collimator test tool as shown in **Figure 6.1A**. The film is exposed to 100 kV_p and 60 mAs and processed.

If the beam alignment is perfect, the image of the top ball will merge with the image of the ball at bottom. The deviation of beam from the perpendicular is determined from the location of the image of the top steel ball in the circles in the radiograph. The image of the two steel balls on the radiograph is observed to evaluate tilt in the central beam. If the images of the two steel balls overlap, the central ray of the beam is within 0.5° **(Figs. 6.2A to C)**. If the image of the top ball falls within the image of the inner circle, the central ray lies within 1.5° from the perpendicular. If it falls between the images of inner and outer circles, the central ray is within 1.5–3° from the perpendicular.

- Tolerance limit for the central beam alignment is 1.5°.

Effective Focal Spot Measurement

The ability for resolving the smallest size of the image (i.e., detail) in a radiograph depends on focal spot size. Since the focal spot size may be altered because of bombardment of electrons on the target, it must be checked periodically to ensure that focal spot size is within acceptable limits.

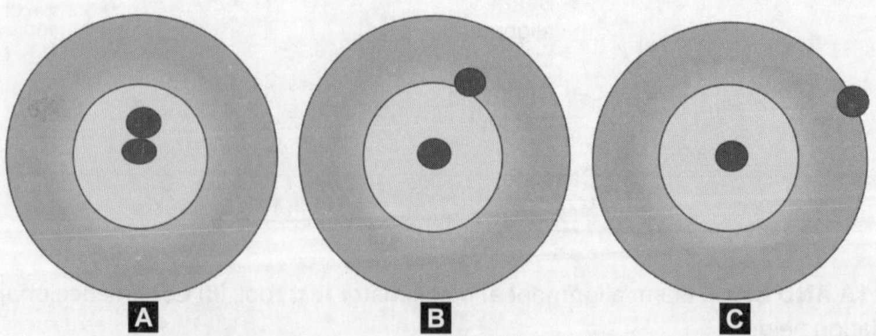

FIGS. 6.2A TO C: Beam alignment test tool and interpretation of image of the two steel balls.

Focal spot size is evaluated using the focal spot test tool based on the principle of minimum resolution. Bar/hole test pattern is employed for evaluating focal spot by minimum resolution. At minimum resolution, the edge gradient (penumbra) of one pattern of the pair images overlaps with the image of other and the images of both the patterns of the pair cannot be resolved separately. In this condition, the focal spot size (f) is related with line width and magnification (M) as follows:

$$f = \left[\frac{M}{M-1}\right] \times \text{line width}$$

The test tool consists of an acrylic hollow cylinder of about 6.0-cm diameter and 15-cm height. An acrylic circular disk is fastened on one end of the cylinder. Bar patterns engraved on tungsten plate are mounted on this circular disk. The bar test pattern consists of 12 groups of lines (slits) of sizes gradually reducing in dimensions. Each group consists of six lines arranged such that a subgroup of three parallel lines is perpendicular to the other subgroup. The sizes and spacing of the slits in these groups decrease by steps of 16% from 0.84 line pair/mm to 5.6 line pair/mm.

The focal spot size values quoted in the reference **Table 6.3** are computed for a magnification of 4/3. This magnification is achieved by maintaining the FFD as 60 cm so that the test tool kept on the image receptor will have test pattern at 45 cm from the focus (60–15 cm, which is the length of test tool). Magnification is calculated as the ratio between FFD and focus-to-object distance (60/45 = 4/3).

To carry out the test, the focal spot test tool is placed on a nonscreen cassette loaded with film. The FFD is kept at 60 cm **(Fig. 6.3)**. Non-screen technique is necessary to avoid blurring of images of test pattern. The tool is placed over the cassette so that the vertical patterns are within the anode to cathode direction. The film is exposed and processed. The bar pattern on the radiograph is observed and the smallest group in which all six bars (both vertical and horizontal) are clearly resolved is identified. Minimum resolvable line pair size and the corresponding focal spot size can be obtained from **Table 6.3**. The vertical and horizontal groups give vertical and horizontal dimensions of the focal spot.

TABLE 6.3 Effective focal spot size of for a magnification of 4/3.

Smallest group resolved	*lp/mm*	*Effective focal spot size (mm)*
1	0.84	4.3
2	1.00	3.7
3	1.19	3.1
4	1.14	2.6
5	1.68	2.2
6	2.00	1.8
7	2.38	1.5
8	2.83	1.3
9	3.36	1.1
10	4.00	0.9
11	4.76	0.8
12	5.66	0.7

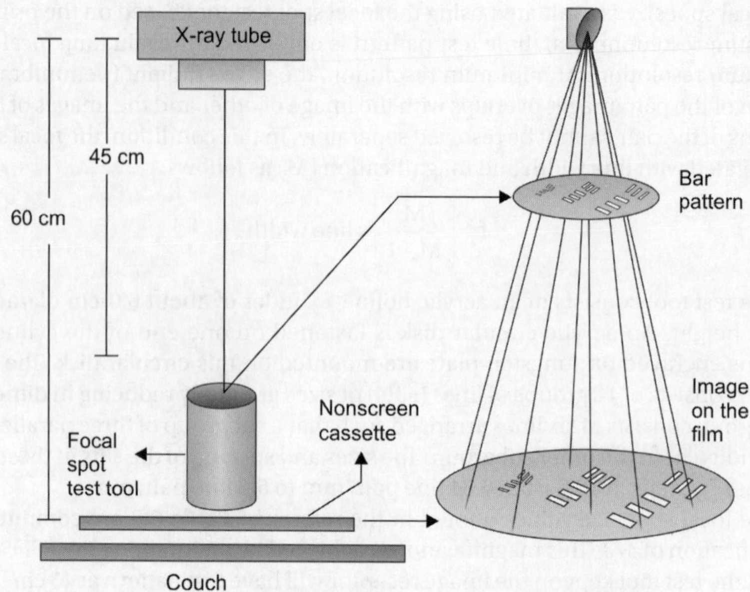

FIG. 6.3: Bar test pattern for testing focal spot size and its image.

The test is done for both small and large focal spot of the X-ray machine, if provided. If f is the focal spot size in mm, then tolerance values for different focal spot sizes are:

- +0.5 f for f < 0.8 mm
- +0.4 f for 0.8 ≤ f ≤ 1.5 mm
- +0.3 f for f > 1.5 mm

Accuracy of Operating Potential (kV_p) and Accuracy of Time

The applied kilovoltage (kV_p) affects the quality and quantity of X-rays reaching the image receptor. This in turn influences the contrast and density of the radiograph. If there is variation in the kV_p setting, it will affect the image quality of the radiograph. Hence, it is necessary to check the kV_p settings periodically.

This can be done by using a kV_p meter or all in QA tool. The all-in-one QA tool employs two solid-state detectors with different beam hardening filters **(Fig. 6.4)**. When exposed to radiation, the ratio of the signals produced by these detectors will be proportional to the peak tube voltage. A ratio circuit either with an analog digital circuit (ADC) or a microprocessor software system displays the peak kilovoltage, digitally corresponding to a particular ratio of either analog or digital signals. This method is instantaneous and direct reading. Corrections for beam filtration should be applied if necessary. In addition, the all-in-one tool gives dose, dose rate, pulses, pulse rate, exposure time and integrated dose length product (DLP) in a single exposure.

The beam is centered on the marked area on the top surface of the kV_p meter or all in one QA tool. In the later, both kV_p and timer accuracy can be done in single measurement. Focus-to-detector distance (FDD) is kept as 100 cm. Routinely used mA station is selected, for a set kV_p, and time and the unit are energized. The kV_p and the time are measured and recorded. Similarly, measurements are taken for five different kV_p and time settings. Then, a minimum/lower mA station is selected, and

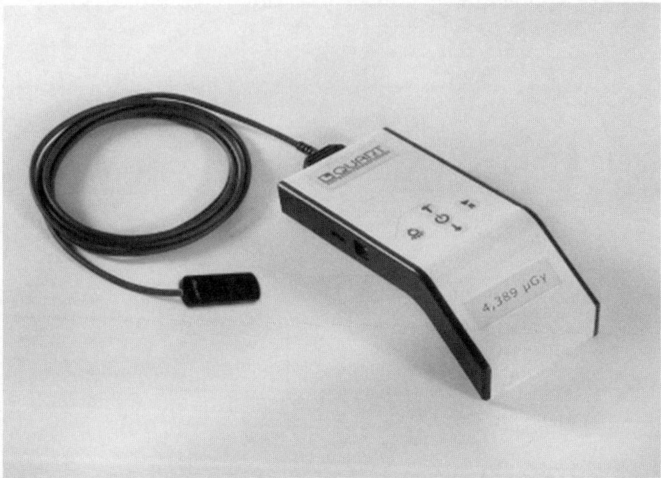

FIG. 6.4: All-in-one QA tool for diagnostic radiology.
Courtesy: Meditronix Corporation, India.

measurements are repeated. Next, maximum/higher mA station is selected, and all the measurements are repeated. Average of the measured values of kV_p and time is found. The variation between the set kV_p and the measured kV_p is found. Similarly, the difference between the set time and measured time is found.

- Tolerance for kV_p is ±5 kV_p
- *Tolerance for timer is given by % error*: ±10%

Accuracy of Time by Spinning Top

If the exposure time set on the diagnostic X-ray unit is not optimal, the radiograph can be underexposed or overexposed. This may lead to repeat examinations. Hence, there is a need to test the timer of the X-ray unit periodically. The manual spinning top (for single-phase half-wave and full-wave rectified systems only) and motorized synchronous tops (for single-phase, three-phase, and high-frequency systems) can be used to test the accuracy of the timer.

Spinning top consists of a rotating circular brass plate with a small rectangular portion cut (hole) at its periphery **(Fig. 6.5)**. Since the rectangular cut portion is moving with the brass plate, the film receives exposure only when X-ray pulses are produced. Production of X-ray pulses depends upon the rectification of the X-ray unit. A single-phase half-wave rectified system produces 50 pulses/second, and therefore 50 X-ray pulses are generated per second. The time taken for one pulse is 0.02 second (1 s/50). If it is a single-phase full-wave rectified unit, it will produce 100 X-ray pulses per second and the time taken for each pulse is 0.01 second. Hence, for a set time of 0.5 seconds, the half-wave and full-wave rectified unit emits 25 and 50 pulses, respectively.

To check the timer, the spinning top is placed on a cassette loaded with film. For a set time, the unit is energized while the top is rotating. The experiment is repeated to cover the entire range of the timer. The pulses passing through the hole of the circular plate produce equally spaced rectangular density patterns on the film. The spacing between the patterns depends upon the speed of rotation of the spinning top. Exposure time is determined by dividing the number of density patterns produced on the film by the pulses per second:

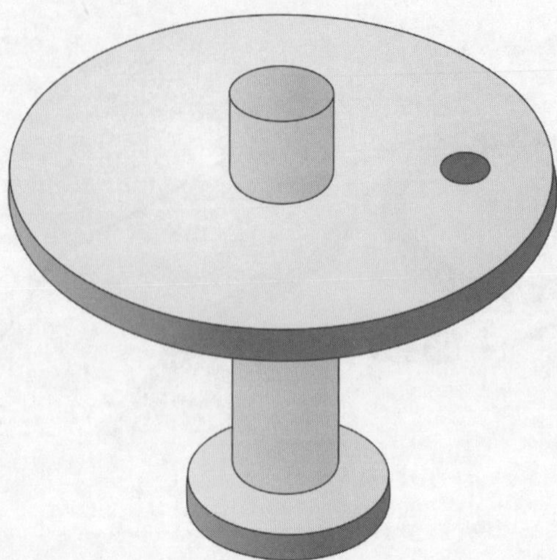

FIG. 6.5: Spinning top test tool.

$$\text{Time} = \text{Number of density patterns on the film/Pulse frequency}$$

In the case of three-phase and high-frequency units, synchronous spinning tops are used. These units produce density patterns, which may appear as an arc of continuous trace of density. Counting the density patterns may not be possible. In such cases, the angle subtended by the arc at the center of the image of the circular plate is measured with a protractor. The exposure time is calculated as the ratio of angle subtended by the arc to the total angle (360°). The speed of rotation (typically one rotation per second) of the disk is suitably selected.

Nowadays, meters incorporating solid-state detectors are available for the measurement of exposure time. For half-wave and full-wave X-ray units, the number of pulses obtained from one of the solid-state detectors is counted and displayed. In three-phase and high-frequency X-ray units, the output from the detector in connected to an input circuit of a crystal oscillator. The gated output of the oscillator is counted and displayed digitally.

- Tolerance for timer is given by % error: ±10%

Total Filtration

All diagnostic X-ray units must have fitted with a minimum thickness of filter to cut off low-energy components from X-ray beam. The low-energy X-rays do not contribute to the image formation but give unnecessary patient exposure. If the filtration is too high, image contrast will be reduced. Therefore, the total filtration provided for the X-ray tube shall be optimum for patient safety and image quality. For this purpose, regulatory bodies recommend total filtration requirement for X-ray machines for different maximum rated tube potentials. Atomic Energy Regulatory Board recommends the total filtration requirements of X-ray diagnostic equipment **(Table 6.4)**.

Total filtration includes the inherent filtration and the added filtration. Hence, total filtration evaluation is necessary to verify whether the added filtration is adequate or not. Total filtration of the X-ray tube is evaluated by determining the half-value thickness (HVT) of the beam by using a pocket dosimeter or all-in-one QA tool. The HVT is measured for the maximum operating potential of the tube.

The pocket dosimeter is kept at the center of radiation field of area 20 cm × 20 cm at a distance 100 cm from the target. For a given kV_p and mAs, the dosimeter is exposed without any absorber and the reading is noted. The measurement is repeated, and the average is obtained. An aluminum filter of 0.5 mm is interposed (at the collimator level) and the measurements are repeated. Similar measurements are repeated for aluminum filters of thickness 1, 1.5, 2, 3, 4, and 5 mm **(Fig. 6.6A)**.

Transmission curve of the X-ray beam can be plotted on a graph sheet between absorber thickness and measured dosimeter readings **(Fig. 6.6B)**. The absorber thickness for 50% transmission will be HVT of the X-ray beam. Total aluminum filtration (All mm) at maximum kV_p is determined from HVT **(Tables 6.5 and 6.6)**. Total filtration required is:

- 1.5 mm Al for $kV_p \leq 70$

TABLE 6.4 **Filter specification for diagnostic X-ray units.**

Maximum rated tube potential (kV_p)	***Minimum total filtration (mm Al)***
Less than 70	1.5
70 to and including 100	2.0
Above 100	2.5

TABLE 6.5 **HVT as a function of filtration and tube potential (single-phase generators).**

Total filtration (mm Al)	***Peak potential (kV_p)***									
	30	***40***	***50***	***60***	***70***	***80***	***90***	***100***	***110***	***120***
	Half-value thickness (mm Al)									
0.5	0.36	0.47	0.58	0.67	0.76	0.84	0.92	1.00	1.08	1.16
1.0	0.55	0.78	0.95	1.08	1.21	1.33	1.46	1.58	1.70	1.82
1.5	0.78	1.04	1.25	1.42	1.59	1.75	1.90	2.08	2.25	2.42
2.0	0.92	1.22	1.49	1.70	1.90	2.10	2.28	2.48	2.70	2.90
2.5	1.02	1.38	1.69	1.95	2.16	2.37	2.58	2.82	3.06	3.30
3.0		1.49	1.87	2.16	2.40	2.62	2.86	3.12	3.38	3.65
3.5		1.58	2.00	2.34	2.60	2.86	3.12	3.40	3.68	3.95
(HVT: half-value thickness)										

TABLE 6.6 **HVT as a function of filtration and tube potential (three-phase generators).**

Total filtration (mm Al)	***Peak potential (kV_p)***								
	60	***70***	***80***	***90***	***100***	***110***	***120***	***130***	***140***
	HVT (mm Al)								
2.5	2.2	2.4	2.7	3.1	3.3	3.6	4.0		
3.0	2.3	2.6	3.0	3.3	3.6	4.0	4.3	4.6	5.0
3.5	2.6	2.9	3.2	3.6	3.9	4.3	4.6		
(HVT: half-value thickness)									

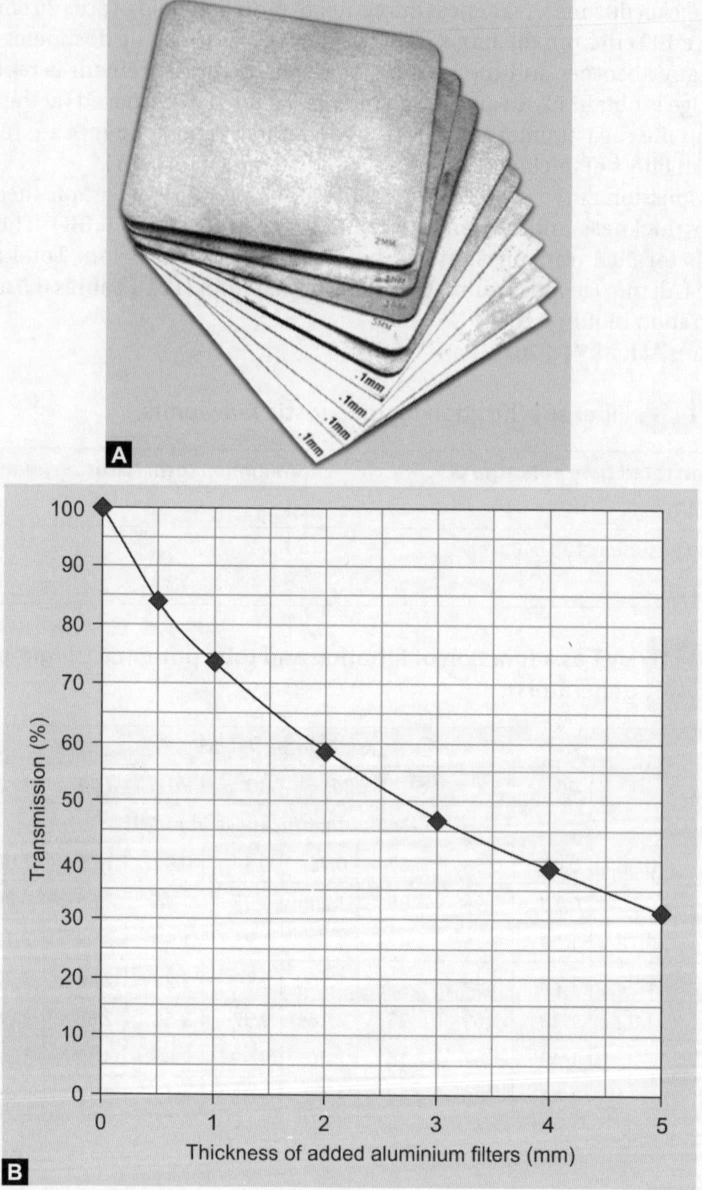

FIGS. 6.6A AND B: Quality assurance test for filter: (A) Aluminum plates, (B) transmission curve to find HVL.

- 2.0 mm Al for $kV_p \leq 100$
- 2.5 mm Al for $kV_p > 100$

Linearity of mA/mAs Loading Stations

The linearity of mA can be tested by measuring the radiation output of the machine. A pocket dosimeter and charger or all-in-one QA tool is used to measure the radiation output.

The charged pocket dosimeter is kept at the center of the radiation field of area 20 cm × 20 cm at a distance 100 cm from the focus. For a fixed kV_p (say 100) and time, an available mA station is selected. The tube is energized, and radiation output is measured in μGy by the dosimeter. The measurements are repeated three times to eliminate statistical variations and the average is obtained. Similar measurements are made by keeping the kV_p and time as constant, for another two mA stations. For each set of measurement, μGy/mAs = X is calculated. From this, the coefficient of linearity (CoL) is obtained as follows:

$$\text{CoL} = \frac{X_{max} - X_{min}}{X_{max} + X_{min}}$$

The CoL is <0.1.

Output Consistency

To test the radiation output consistency or reproducibility, the pocket dosimeter or all-in-one QA tool is used. The charged pocket dosimeter is kept at the center of field size 20 cm × 20 cm at a distance 100 cm from the focus. For a fixed mA and time (mAs), an available kV_p station (say, 70 kV_p) is selected and the tube is energized. The dosimeter reading is noted, and the measurements are repeated five times. Average of the five-dosimeter reading is obtained and mR/mAs ratio is noted as X. Similar measurements are made for one more kV_p ($n = 2$), by keeping the mAs constant. The consistency at each kV_p station is checked by evaluating the coefficient of variation (CoV):

$$\text{CoV} = \frac{1}{X} \times \left[\Sigma \frac{(X_i - X)^2}{n-1} \right]^{\frac{1}{2}}$$

$$\text{CoV} = \underline{\qquad\qquad} \text{ for 70 } kV_p$$

$$\text{CoV} = \underline{\qquad\qquad} \text{ for 80 } kV_p$$

The CoV should be < 0.05.

Low-contrast Sensitivity

To test the low-contrast sensitivity, low-contrast resolution test phantom is used. The phantom is positioned in the radiation field and exposed with suitable kV_p and mAs. Diameter of the smallest size hole clearly resolved on the monitor is found.

- *Recommended performance standard is*: 3.0-mm hole pattern must be resolved.

High-contrast Sensitivity

High-contrast resolution test phantom (wire mesh lines or bar strips/pattern) is used for high-contrast sensitivity test. The test tool is positioned and is exposed with suitable kV_p and mAs. Numbers of mesh lines or bar strips that are resolved on the monitor (lp/mm) are noted.

- *Recommended performance standard is*:
  - 1.5 lp/mm for bar pattern
  - 30 lp/inch for wire mesh lines

Exposure Rate at Tabletop

A pocket dosimeter/all-in-one QA tool is kept on the table, below the center of image intensifier (II) tube or flat panel radiation field. Focus to tabletop distance is kept as

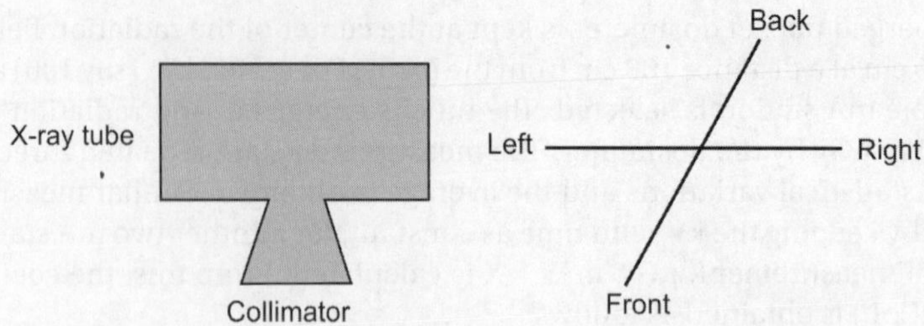

FIG. 6.7: X-ray tube housing leakage test measurements.

30 cm. The tube is energized with maximum kV_p and mAs with and without automatic exposure control (AEC). Meter reading is noted in cGy/min. Two more readings are taken, and the average is found.

Tolerance limits are:

- Exposure rate without AEC mode ≤5 cGy/min
- Exposure rate with AEC mode ≤10 cGy/min

Tube Housing Leakage

Tube housing radiation leakage measurement is carried with an ionization radiation survey meter. For checking the leakage radiation, the collimator of the tube housing is fully closed, and the tube is energized at maximum kV_p, normal mA and time of 1 second. The focus to film distance (FFD) is kept as 100 cm. The operating time should be greater than the time constant of the survey meter. The exposure rate at 1.0 m from the focus is measured at different locations as follows **(Fig. 6.7)**:

- Left (anode side)
- Right (cathode side)
- Front
- Back
- Top from the tube housing
- Collimator

From the maximum leakage rate (mR/h = X) for both tube housing and collimator, leakage in 1 hour is computed by assuming workload as 180 mA-min in 1 hour. The maximum radiation leakage at 1 m is calculated as follows:

$$\text{Maximum leakage} = \frac{180\ \text{mA - min in 1 hour} \times \text{Maximum}\ \frac{\text{mR}}{\text{h}}\ \text{measured}}{60 \times \text{mA used}}$$

Maximum radiation leakage from tube housing: _____ mR in 1 hour
Maximum radiation leakage from tube collimator: _____ mR in 1 hour

- Tolerance limit of leakage radiation at 1 m from the focus should be < 115 mR in 1 hour.

Leakage Limits

The leakage radiation through the protective tube housing in any direction, averaged over an area not >100 cm^2 with no linear dimension >20 cm, shall not exceed an air-kerma of 1 mGy (115 mR) in 1 hour at a distance of 1.0 m from the target when the tube is operating at the maximum rated kV_p and for the maximum rated current at that kV_p. This is applicable to all X-ray units except mammography and dental units [AERB/RF-MED/SC-3 (Rev. 2)].

Radiation Protection Survey of the Installation

To carry out radiation survey, a survey meter with valid calibration certificate and a phantom is required. Layout of the scanner is drawn in a paper and various locations are noted. A water phantom is placed in the radiation field, and the unit is energized with suitable exposure parameters of kV_p (80–100), mA (50–100), and exposure time (1–2 s). Maximum radiation levels in mR/h or μGy/h are measured at various locations:

- Control console/operator position
- Outside patient entrance door
- Behind windows, if any
- Patient waiting area

The workload of 400 mA-min/week is usually taken for calculation, whereas 4,800 mA-min/week is used for interventional radiology units. The maximum radiation level per week is calculated as follows:

$$\text{Maximum radiation level/week (mR/week)} = \frac{\text{Workload in } \dfrac{\text{mA-min}}{\text{week}} \times \text{maximum radiation measured, mR/h}}{60 \times \text{mA used for survey measurement}}$$

- *Permissible limit*: For location of radiation worker: 20 mSv in a year (40 mR/week)
  For location of member of public: 1 mSv in a year (2 mR/week)

QUALITY ASSURANCE TEST MAMMOGRAPHY X-RAY UNIT

Accuracy of Operating Potential/Accuracy of Timer

The beam is centered on the upper surface of the kV_p meter or all-in-one QA tool. In the later, both kV_p and timer accuracy can be done in single measurement. FDD is kept as 65 cm. One mA station is selected for set kV_p and time, and the unit is energized. kV_p and time are measured from the meter and noted. Three more kV_p and time are set for the same mA and the meter readings are noted. The whole process is repeated for another mA station and corresponding readings are measured. Average of the measured values of kV_p and time is found. Variation between the set kV_p and the measured average kV_p is found. Same way the difference between the set time and measured time is found:

- Tolerance for kV_p: ±1 kV_p
- Tolerance for timer: % error: ±10%

Linearity of mA/mAs Loading Stations

The charged pocket dosimeter/all-in-one QA tool is kept at the center of the radiation field at a distance of 65 cm from the focus. For a fixed kV_p and time, an available mA station is selected. The tube is energized and radiation output is measured in μGy by the meter. The measurements are repeated two times to eliminate statistical variations and the average is obtained. Similar measurements are made for two more mA stations by keeping the kV_p and time constant. For each set of measurement, μGy/mAs = X is calculated. From this, the CoL is obtained:

$$\text{CoL} = \frac{X_{max} - X_{min}}{X_{max} + X_{min}}$$

Tolerance: CoL < 0.1

Total Filtration and Aluminum Equivalence of the Compression Device

Total filtration of the X-ray tube is evaluated by determining the HVT of the beam by using a pocket dosimeter/all-in-one QA tool. The HVT is measured for the maximum operating potential of the tube.

A pocket dosimeter is kept at the center of radiation field at a distance of 65 cm from the target. For a given kV_p and mAs, the dosimeter is exposed without any absorber, but with compression device and the reading is noted. The measurement is repeated, and the average is obtained. An aluminum filter of 0.1 mm is interposed (at the collimator level) and the measurements are repeated. Similar measurements are repeated for aluminum filters of thickness 0.2, 0.3, 0.4, and 0.5 mm along with compression device. Transmission curve of the X-ray beam is plotted on a graph between the absorber thickness and measured dosimeter readings. The absorber thickness for 50% transmission will be the HVT of the X-ray beam. The measured values are recorded as follows:

(The unit may have any one of the combination of target and windows: Mo target with Be or Rh window/Rh target with Rh window/W target with Al or Rh window)

Added filter thickness: _____ mm molybdenum

HVT of the unit is: _____ mm of Al for ____ kV_p

Recommended tolerance values:

- First HVT at 30 $kV_p \geq 0.3$-mm Al
- First HVT at 40 $kV_p \geq 0.4$-mm Al
- First HVT at 50 $kV_p \geq 0.5$-mm Al

Reproducibility of Radiation Output

Pocket dosimeter/all-in-one QA tool is kept at the center of field size at a distance of 65 cm from the focus. For a fixed mA and time (mAs), an available kV_p station is selected and the tube is energized. The dosimeter reading is noted in µGy, and the measurements are repeated three times. Average of the three-dosimeter reading is obtained and the ratio, µGy/mAs is noted as X. Similar measurements are made for one more kV_p, by keeping the mAs constant. The consistency at each kV_p station is checked by evaluating the CoV:

$$\text{CoV} = \frac{1}{X} \times \left[\Sigma \frac{(X_i - X)^2}{n-1} \right]^{\frac{1}{2}}$$

Tolerance: CoV < 0.05

Radiation Leakage at 5 cm from the External Surface of X-ray Tube Housing

For checking the leakage radiation, the collimator of the tube housing is fully closed, and the tube is energized at maximum kV_p and normal mAs. The operating time should be greater than the time constant of the survey meter. The exposure rate at 5 cm from the external surface of the tube housing is measured at different locations:

- Left (anode side)
- Right (cathode side)
- Front
- Back
- Top

Maximum radiation leakage at 5 cm from the external surface of the tube housing is calculated with a workload of 40 mA-min in 1 hour as follows:

$$\text{Maximum leakage} = \frac{40\text{ mA - min in 1 h} \times \text{Maximum}\dfrac{\text{mR}}{\text{h}}\text{measured}}{60 \times \text{mA used}}$$

The results are recorded as follows:
Maximum radiation leakage from tube housing: ____mGy in 1 hour

Leakage limit: The leakage radiation averaged over an area of 10 cm^2, with no linear dimension >20 cm and located at 5 cm from any point on the external surface of the X-ray tube housing does not exceed 0.02 mGy in 1 hour.

- *Tolerance*: <0.02 mGy in 1 hour

Imaging Performance Evaluation

Mammography requires careful optimization of technique and equipment. Even a small change in equipment performance, film processing, patient setup, or film viewing conditions can decrease the sensitivity of mammography. Hence, good performance testing is necessary by a suitable phantom to determine baseline values and to monitor with periodic QC testing.

Mammography test phantom can be used to optimize imaging techniques. It simulates the radiographic characteristics of compressed breast tissues and contains components that models breast and disease pattern in the phantom image. Phantom consists of an acrylic block, a wax insert, and an acrylic disk attached to the top of the phantom. It is intended to mimic the attenuation characteristics of a standard breast of 4.2 cm, compressed breast thickness of 50% adipose, and 50% glandular tissue composition. The wax insert contains six cylindrical nylon fibers of decreasing diameter, five simulated calcification groups (Al_2O_3) of decreasing size, and five low-contrast disks of decreasing diameter and thickness that simulates masses **(Figs. 6.8A to C)**.

Identification of the smallest objects of each type, which are visible in the phantom image, indicates system performance. As per the recommendation, at least four fibers, three microcalcification groups, and three masses must be clearly visible, at an average glandular dose of <3 mGy. The optical density at the center of the phantom image must be at least 1.2. In addition, the compression needs to be calibrated and the AEC device must be checked.

Radiation Protection Survey of the Installation

To carry out radiation survey, a survey meter with valid calibration certificate and a phantom is required. Layout of the scanner is drawn in a paper and various locations are noted. Breast phantom is placed in the unit, and it is energized with suitable exposure parameters of applied kV$_p$ (30–35), applied mA (100–200), and exposure time (1–2 s). Maximum radiation levels in mR/h are measured at various locations:

- Control console/operator position
- Outside patient entrance door
- Behind windows, if any
- Patient waiting area

Workload of 650 mA-min/week is taken for calculation. The maximum radiation level per week is calculated as follows:

$$\begin{array}{l}\text{Maximum radiation}\\ \text{level/week (mR/week)}\end{array} = \frac{\text{Workload in}\dfrac{\text{mA - min}}{\text{week}} \times \text{maximum radiation measured,}\dfrac{\text{mR}}{\text{h}}}{60 \times \text{mA used for survey measurement}}$$

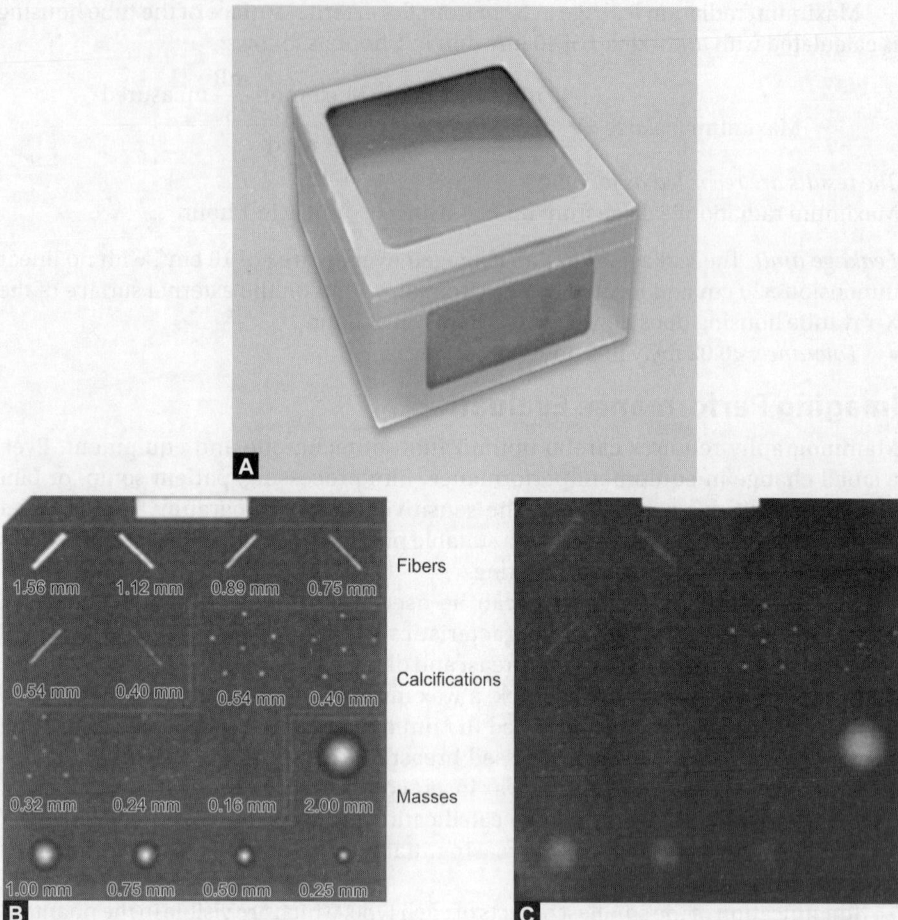

FIGS. 6.8A TO C: Mammography phantom consists of wax insert containing 6 nylon fiber group, 5 aluminum oxide peck groups, and 5 disc of mass lesions (clockwise): (A) Phantom, (B) Wax insert and (C) Phantom image.
Courtesy: Dr Kamakshi Memorial Hospital P Ltd, Chennai.

- *Permissible limit*: For location of radiation worker: 20 mSv in a year (40 mR/week) For location of member of public: 1 mSv in a year (2 mR/week)

QUALITY ASSURANCE FOR COMPUTED TOMOGRAPHY

Mechanical Tests

Mechanical test includes—(1) alignment of table to gantry, (2) gantry tilt, (3) laser alignment, (4) table alignment and positional accuracy, (5) axial patient position accuracy, and (6) radiation profile width/slice thickness.

Alignment of Table to Gantry

Congruence between gantry midline and table midline is checked using plumb line.

- Tolerance should be within ±5 mm.

Gantry Tilt

An X-ray film is held vertically by wrapping in an envelope and Perspex block at the gantry end of the patient table. It is parallel to the Sagittal plane and intersects the scan and coronal planes at right angles. Three axial exposures are made in the same film for—(1) zero gantry tilt, (2) superior gantry tilt, and (3) inferior gantry tilt. After processing the film, the + and – angles between the scan planes at maximum gantry tilt relative to zero gantry position are found. These superior and inferior tilt angles from zero position should be equal.

- Difference between set and measured gantry angle should be within ±2°.

Alternatively, align the laser test QC device with gantry lasers. It is also aligned with vertical side gantry lasers over the full range of vertical couch travel. It can be achieved by moving the table up and down. The gantry is tilted to one direction and returned to the vertical position. The gantry is tilted in the opposite direction and returned to the vertical position.

- Alignment of laser QC device with vertical side gantry lasers should be within ±1° for both directions.

Laser Alignment

Laser alignment QC device containing two pegs (rod) is used to do the test. It is to check the gantry lasers and room alignment lasers are properly aligned with CT gantry and table. It is much important if the CT image is used for radiotherapy simulation. The QC device is placed centrally on the table and aligned with the sides of the table. It is positioned using the gantry lasers orthogonal to the long-axis of the table (Z). The alignment of room lasers is (walls and ceiling) tested relative to the gantry lasers. A CT scan is performed with 1-mm slice thickness, which demonstrates holes in the test device. The holes from left to right should be similar on visual inspection.

- Tolerance limit for alignment is ±1 mm.

Table Alignment and Positional Accuracy

To check the degree of couch movement indicated on the gantry with actual distance travelled, a ruler is placed along the length of the table. A load of about 70–80 kg is placed on the table to mimic patient weight. Initial table position is noted, and the table is moved with increment of 1, 2, 3, 4, and 5 cm, away and toward the gantry. Difference between the set gantry display and actual distance travelled is measured.

- Tolerance should be within ±1 mm.

However, helical CT or CT used for radiotherapy application requires the following procedure. Laser alignment QC test tool is positioned at the extreme end/top of the table using gantry lasers. Weight of 70–80 kg is evenly distributed on the table to mimic patient weight. CT scan of 1-mm slice width is obtained by scan projection radiography (SPR) mode. Then the QC device is positioned at the extreme end/bottom of the table and scan is repeated. The image is visually inspected, and the position of the horizontal holes in the image is measured by the curser.

- Tolerance should be within ±1 mm.

To test the accuracy and reproducibility of table indexing, a ruler is placed centrally along the long-axis of the table. An initial table position is chosen (arbitrary) and a load of 70 kg is evenly distributed on the table. Table is manually set with different increments from the reference position; say 1, 2, 3, 4, and 5 cm, respectively.

At the same time, the couch increments are measured correspondingly by computer control. The difference between the manual and computer control couch position is measured.

- Tolerance should be within ±1 mm.

To test scout scan accuracy, the laser alignment QC test tool is positioned along the long axis of the table as well as at the table center. The first peg position of the device is aligned with gantry lasers at the starting point if scout image. Using the scout image, 1-mm slice is directly set on both peg position in the device. CT scan is performed so that both pegs in the device are imaged. The distance between the centers of pegs is measured in the image. The two CT slices should be centered over the holes of each peg.

- Tolerance should be within 25 cm ±1 mm.

Axial Patient Position Accuracy

An envelope-wrapped film is placed flat on the table and illuminated by external scan light. The position of the light is marked by pinpricks on the film envelope and the table is moved to the scan plane. The internal light will coincide with the mark on the film envelope if the distance between the internal and external light is correct. Internal and external laser light alignment is measured.

- Tolerance should be within ±2 mm.

Radiation Profile Width/Slice Thickness

A nonscreen cassette is used to obtain dose profiles for this study. The film is positioned at the isocenter in air for each slice width setting. A given kV_p (100) and mAs (100) are selected, and the film is exposed for a slice thickness of 1 mm. After developing the film, density profile is obtained either by scanning microdensitometer or measured by a ruler. For greater accuracy, calibration curves can be used to convert optical density into dose profile. This is repeated for 2-mm and 3-mm slice thicknesses, etc. From the density profile, the profile width, i.e., full-width-at-half-maximum (FWHM) is found for each slice thickness.

Alternatively, Catphan phantom can be used which contains metal inserts/rods inclined at an angle to the imaging plane **(Figs. 6.9A and B)**. The thickness of the metal insert should not be greater than the nominal slice thickness. Greater thickness may interfere with submillimeter slice studies in multislice CT scans. The phantom is scanned, and axial mode measurements are made in the image to estimate slice thickness.

Tolerance:

- *Slice thickness < 1 mm*: 0.5 mm
- *Slice thickness 1–2 mm*: ±50%
- *Slice thickness > 2 mm*: ±1 mm

Measurement of Operating Potential

All-in-one QA tool or kV_p meter is used to study the operating potential. For set kV_p and mA loading station, CT is energized and the kV_p is measured. Without changing the kV_p, two more mA stations are selected and corresponding kV_p is measured. Whole measurements are repeated for three more kV_p settings.

- *Tolerance*: ±2 kV_p.

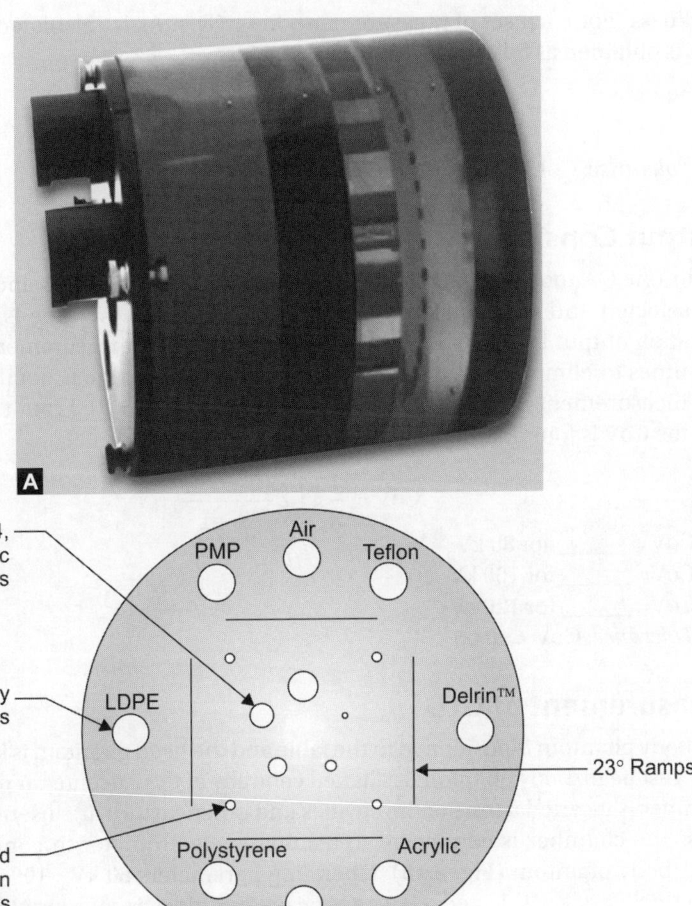

FIGS. 6.9A AND B: Catphan phantom with metal inserts.

Courtesy: The Phantom Laboratory, USA.

Timer Accuracy

All-in-one QA tool is used to study the timer accuracy. For a set time, kV_p, and mA, CT is energized, and the observed time is noted. Without changing kV_p and mA setting, two more readings are observed for corresponding set time. From the set and observed time, the % error is calculated.

- *Tolerance*: Error < ±10%

Measurement of mAs Linearity

All-in-one QA tool is kept at the center of the radiation field. The kV_p and slice thickness are selected and kept constant. For a set mAs, the tube is energized, and radiation output is measured in μGy by the meter. The measurements are repeated three times to eliminate statistical variations and the average is obtained. Similar measurements are made for two more mAs setting without changing the kV_p and slice thickness. For each set of measurement, X = μGy/mAs is calculated. From this, the CoL is obtained as follows:

$$\text{CoL} = \frac{X_{max} - X_{min}}{X_{max} + X_{min}}$$

- *Tolerance*: CoL: < ±0.1

Output Consistency

All-in-one QA tool is kept at the center of field of view. The mAs and slice thickness are selected and kept constant. For a set kV_p (say 80), the tube is energized, and radiation output is measured in μGy by the meter. The measurements are repeated five times to eliminate statistical variations and the average is obtained in μGy (X). The measurements are repeated for 100 and 120 kV_p ($n = 3$). From the mean output (X), the CoV is found:

$$\text{CoV} = \frac{1}{X} \times \left[\Sigma \frac{(X_i - X)^2}{n-1} \right]^{\frac{1}{2}}$$

- CoV = ______ for 80 kV_p
- CoV= ______ for 100 kV_p
- CoV= ______ for 120 kV_p
- *Tolerance*: CoV < ±0.05

Measurement of CTDI

The body phantom is positioned in the table and the head phantom is kept on the head rest. Test head/body phantom is aligned centrally at the isocenter. A pencil ionization chamber is inserted in one of the cavities and other cavities are inserted with Perspex rods. The chamber is connected to a suitable electrometer in conjunction with a head/body phantom **(Fig. 6.10)**. Operating parameters 80 kV_p, 100 mAs for a given slice thickness are selected. CT is energized and dose is measured in axial ($CTDI_c$) and four peripheral cavities of the head phantom in mGy/mAs. Since peripheral dose is measured at four cavities, its mean value ($CTDI_p$) is found for head phantom.

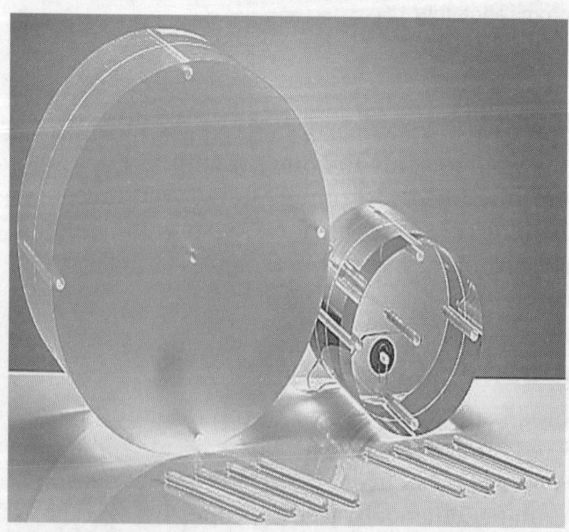

FIG. 6.10: ACR accredited PMMA Phantom for CTDI measurement.
(ACR: American College of Radiology)

Then, the kV_p is changed to 100, and 120 with same mAs and slice thickness and the measurements are repeated. This procedure is repeated for the body phantom and the axial ($CTDI_c$) and mean peripheral dose ($CTDI_p$) values are obtained as before. Results are recorded and weighted CTDI ($CTDI_w$) is calculated as follows in mGy/mAs:

$CTDI_c$ for head phantom: ____ mGy/mAs
$CTDI_p$ for head phantom: ____ mGy/mAs
$CTDI_c$ for body phantom: ____ mGy/mAs
$CTDI_p$ for body phantom: ____ mGy/mAs

$$CTDI_w \text{ for head} = \frac{1}{3}\, CTDI_c + \frac{2}{3}\, CTDI_p$$

$$CTDI_w \text{ for body} = \frac{1}{3}\, CTDI_c + \frac{2}{3}\, CTDI_p$$

- *Tolerance*: ±20% of the quoted value (expected)
  ±40% of the quoted value (maximum)

Low-contrast Resolution

A low-contrast resolution test phantom is positioned in the field of view. A given kV_p, mA, and the exposure time (s) are set on the scanner. The phantom is exposed for a given window width and slice thickness. The resolution is measured from the phantom in mm and the percentage of contrast difference is calculated as follows **(Fig. 6.11A)**:

Low-contrast resolution ___ mm at ___% contrast difference

- *Tolerance*: 5.0 mm at 1% contrast difference (minimum)
  2.5 mm at 0.5% contrast difference (expected).

High-contrast Resolution

A high-contrast resolution test phantom is positioned in the field of view. A given kV_p, mA and the exposure time (s) are set on the scanner. The phantom is exposed for a given window width, using a high-resolution algorithm. The size of the smallest resolvable bar/hole pattern is found in mm or lp/cm and the percentage of contrast difference is calculated as follows **(Fig. 6.11B)**:

Size of the smallest resolvable bar/hole phantom ___ mm or ___ lp/cm

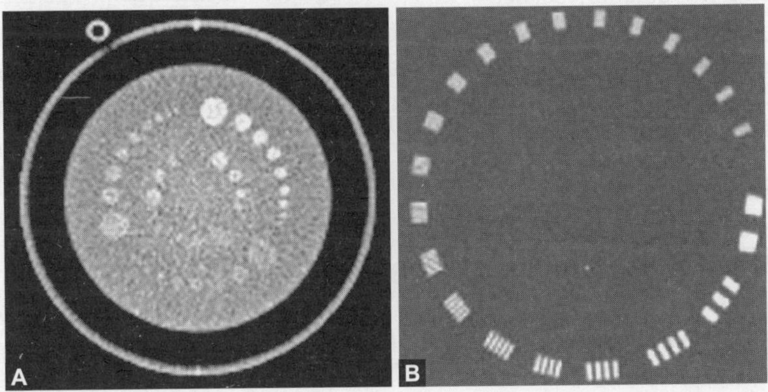

FIGS. 6.11A AND B: Catphan phantom images: (A) low contrast insert image, (B) high contrast insert image.

Courtesy: The Phantom Laboratory, USA.

- *Tolerance*: At 10% contrast difference, the size of the bar/hole pattern that could be resolvable should be 1.6 mm or 3.12 lp/cm.
  Expected high-contrast resolution: 0.8 mm or 6.25 lp/cm

Total Filtration

All-in-one QA tool is kept at the center of radiation field. Exposure parameters of maximum kV_p, mA, and exposure time (s) are selected. The dosimeter is exposed without any absorber and the reading is noted. The measurement is repeated, and the average is obtained. An aluminum filter of 0.5 mm is interposed (at the collimator level) and the measurements are taken. Similar measurements are repeated for aluminum (Al) filters of thickness 1, 1.5, 2, 3, 4, and 5 mm.

Transmission curve of the X-ray beam is plotted on a graph sheet between the absorber thickness and measured dosimeter readings. The absorber thickness for 50% transmission will be the HVT of the X-ray beam. Total filtration measured at maximum kV_p in mm of Al is found.

- Tolerance for total filtration is: 2.5 mm Al for $kV_p > 100$.

Radiation Leakage Levels from X-ray Tube Housing for Leakage Measurement

Tube housing radiation leakage measurement is carried with an ionization type radiation survey meter. For checking the leakage radiation, the collimator of the tube housing is fully closed, and the tube is energized at its maximum kV_p, normal mA, and exposure time of 1 second. The operating time should be greater than the time constant of the survey meter. The exposure rate at 1.0 from the focus is measured at different locations:

- Front (cathode)
- Back (anode)
- Left from the tube housing
- Right from the tube housing

From maximum leakage rate (X = mR/h) for tube housing, leakage in 1 hour is computed by assuming workload as 500 mA-min in 1 hour. The maximum radiation leakage at 1 m is calculated as follows:

$$\text{Maximum radiation leakage} = \frac{500\ \text{mA - min in 1 h} \times \text{Maximum} \frac{\text{mR}}{\text{h}} \text{measured}}{60 \times \text{mA used for measurement}}$$

Maximum radiation leakage from tube housing: ___ mR in 1 hour and maximum radiation leakage at 1 m from the focus for a workload of 500 mA-min in 1 hour is ____ mR in 1 hour is found.

- *Recommended upper limit*: Leakage radiation at 1 m from the focus should be < 115 mR in 1 hour.

Radiation Protection Survey of the Installation

To carry out radiation survey, a survey meter with valid calibration certificate and a phantom is required. Layout of the scanner is drawn in a paper and various locations are noted. Head phantom is fixed in the CT scanner, and CT is energized with suitable exposure parameters of kV_p (110–140), mA (50–100), and exposure time (1–2 s). Maximum radiation levels in mR/h are measured at various locations:

- Control console/operator position
- Outside patient entrance door
- Behind windows, if any
- Patient waiting area

A workload of 20,000 mA-min/week is taken for calculation. The maximum radiation level per week is calculated as follows:

$$\text{Maximum radiation level/week (mR/week)} = \frac{\text{Workload in } \dfrac{\text{mA-min}}{\text{week}} \times \text{maximum radiation measured, } \dfrac{\text{mR}}{\text{h}}}{60 \times \text{mA used for survey measurement}}$$

- *Permissible limit*: For location of radiation worker: 20 mSv in a year (40 mR/week)
  For location of member of public: 1 mSv in a year (2 mR/week)

BIBLIOGRAPHY

1. Atomic Energy Regulatory Board (AERB). Radiation safety training module: Diagnostic radiology quality assurance test for computed tomography equipment. [online] Available from https://www.aerb.gov.in/images/PDF/DiagnosticRadiology/QUALITY-ASSURANCE---COMPUTED-TOMOGRAPHY.pdf. [Last accessed October, 2022].
2. Atomic Energy Regulatory Board. Lecture notes, Workshop on establishment of directorate of radiation safety. Mumbai: Atomic Energy Regulatory Board; 2009.
3. International Atomic Energy Agency. (2009). Quality assurance for PET and PET/CT systems. IAEA human health series No. 1. [online] Available from https://www-pub.iaea.org/MTCD/Publications/PDF/Pub1393_web.pdf. [Last accessed October, 2022].
4. International Atomic Energy Agency. (2012). Quality assurance program for computed tomography: diagnostic and therapy applications. IAEA Human Health Series No.19. [online] Available from https://www-pub.iaea.org/MTCD/Publications/PDF/Pub1557_web.pdf. [Last accessed October, 2022].
5. Thayalan K. The Physics of Radiology and Imaging. New Delhi: Jaypee Brothers Medical Publishers; 2014.

CHAPTER 7

Radiation Protection and Safety in Diagnostic Radiology

INTRODUCTION

The personnel working in diagnostic radiology departments should receive exposures well below the regulatory limits on the lines of ALARA (As Low As Reasonably Achievable) principle. Hence, training, equipment, and work practices are so designed to minimize time with radiation sources. Maximize the distance between the worker and radiation sources and provide appropriate shielding. Hence, sufficient protective devices should be provided to the personnel. In addition, there are certain personnel requirements, responsibilities, to be adhered to achieve complete radiological safety. This safety should cover all the personnel including staffs, patients, and the public. Personnel protection requirements vary with nature of radiological examination such as radiography, fluoroscopy, mammography, and computed tomography (CT).

EQUIPMENT AND PERIPHERALS

Patient dose can be reduced by selecting optimal equipment and its peripherals. Constant potential/high-frequency generator can reduce the dose significantly. The couch used with the X-ray equipment shall not have attenuation of >1.2-mm aluminum (Al) equivalent. The couch shall have markings in the center for patient positioning.

Other requirements are, use of fast screen-film combination *(e.g., rare earth, 400 speed for pediatric)*, low attenuation *(e.g., carbon fiber)* materials for cassette front, antiscatter grid interspacing and tabletops, including grid removal, etc.

Tube Voltage (kV_p)

Increasing the kV_p results in greater transmission of X-rays through the patient. This means that the absorption is lesser in the patient even though the exposure/mAs is higher. The best way to reduce patient dose is reduction of mAs. This will reduce the image contrast due to higher effective energy of the X-ray beam. Hence, one must balance between patient dose and image contrast. As a rule of thumb, patient exposure can be reduced by using a higher kV_p and lower mAs.

Filtration

A filter is a metallic sheet introduced in the path of the X-ray beam to reduce patient dose. Diagnostic X-rays consists of both low- and high-energy X-rays. The low-energy X-rays are absorbed in the first few centimeters of tissue by increasing skin dose. The high-energy X-rays transmit through the patient and contribute to image formation. Filtration can remove selectively low-energy X-rays, and thereby reducing patient's dose and skin injuries. As filtration is increased, the beam become hardened and decreases the image contrast. Filtration also decreases tube output hence an optimal filtration is required for each X-ray unit (refer Chapter 6 for more details).

Control Panel

The control panel/operation switch must be located at a minimum distance of 3 m from the X-ray tube. In mobile X-ray unit, the cable length shall not be <2 m.

Carbon Fiber Materials

Use of carbon fiber materials in patient support, antiscatter grids, and cassette front, in place of conventional materials, allows transmission of larger proportion of the X-ray beam. At 80 kV_p, the use of carbon fiber material reduces skin dose significantly. The overall reduction of absorbed dose in the skin of the patient facing the X-ray tube, from the combined use of carbon fiber materials in patient supports, antiscatter grids, and radiographic cassettes, is in the range of about 30–50%. If the X-ray tube voltage is not changed, the percentage reductions in absorbed dose in deeper tissues will be similar.

Image Receptors

The speed of the image receptor determines the number of X-ray photons necessary to produce an optimal image signal. This is directly related to the patient dose. Higher speed (400) system requires less exposure to produce the same optical density and decreases the patient dose. Faster film increases the quantum mottle and faster screen (thick) decreases the spatial resolution. Thus, higher speed film-screen reduces the patient dose, but limit the image quality.

Computed radiography (CR) uses photostimulable storage phosphor (PSP) detectors, and the digital radiography (DR) receptors have wide latitude. These systems allow postprocessing methods, to manipulate image density for optimal viewing. They compensate for under- or overexposure and reduce retakes. Underexposed images are associated with high-quantum mottle and poor contrast resolution. Overexposed images contribute higher patient dose. The PSP receptor system is equivalent to 200-speed screen-film system in terms of quantum mottle and noise for adult abdomen and chest radiography. In the case of extremity imaging, CR should be used at higher exposure levels (e.g., speed 75–100), whereas in pediatric imaging increased speed (e.g., 400) is recommended.

Conventional screen-film has inherent safety feature. If high kV_p is used, the film becomes over dark, thereby increasing the patient dose. One can easily identify this and carry out necessary remedial measures. In digital image receptors, one cannot notice this adverse effect on image quality since it is adjusted in postprocessing. Therefore, higher patient exposures may go unnoticed. Hence, digital image receptors require strict quality assurance check.

TABLE 7.1 Specification for protective devices.

Protective devices	*Lead equivalent (mm)*
Lead aprons	0.25
Lead gloves/Protective goggles	0.25
Gonad/Thyroid shield	0.25
Couch-hanging lead flaps	0.5
Ceiling-suspended lead glass	0.5
Mobile-protective barrier (MPB)	1.5
Lead glass viewing window	1.5
Protective door	1.7
Pass box	2.0
Temporary film storage	2.0

PROTECTIVE DEVICES

Personnel protection may be achieved by using several protective devices and adopting good work practices. These devices should include lead apron, thyroid shield, lead gloves, gonad shield, lead glass, ceiling-mounted lead glass, etc., especially in radiography and fluoroscopy imaging. Specification of the protective devices is given in **Table 7.1**.

Lead Apron

The lead apron should have a lead equivalent thickness of 0.25–0.5 mm. Usually, it is made up of rubber material to provide flexibility and handling **(Fig. 7.1A)**. Aprons protect the torso of the body and are available in wrap around designs. It is to protect the backside when the worker is exposed to scattered radiation. Attenuation offered by the lead apron is as follows:

- *0.25 mm*: >90% scattered radiation is attenuated.
- *0.5 mm*: 95–99% scattered radiation is attenuated.

Though higher thickness aprons offer greater protection, it weighs 50–100% more than the 0.25-mm thickness which is a great matter of concern in fluoroscopy. The weight of the apron becomes the limiting factor in the ability of the radiologist and other workers to complete the investigation. There are some designs (Skirt-vest) which put much weight on the hips instead of shoulders. Lead aprons do not cover the arms, lower legs, the head and neck, thyroid, and eyes. Nowadays, lightweight lead aprons are available.

Lead Gloves, Lead Glass, and Ceiling-mounted Lead Shield

Protective gloves made up of 0.25-mm lead thickness may offer protection to the hands **(Fig. 7.1B)**. Lead glasses attenuate X-rays about 30–70%, depending upon the content of the lead. Hence, weight is a major concern in lead glasses. Normal lead glasses used in the hospital may offer 20% attenuation. Lead glass of 2-mm lead equivalent is used in mobile-protective barrier, CT scan, and cardiac catheterization laboratories (cath lab) at control consoles as viewing window. Lead flaps of 0.5-mm lead equivalent is used in C-arm and interventional radiology X-ray units. Lead glass or leaded acrylic shields are transparent and often provide greater attenuation than lead aprons.

Ceiling-mounted glasses are used in cardiac cath lab and interventional imaging radiology procedures **(Fig. 7.1C)**. It is counterbalanced and easily positioned to a specific location and height. These devices can be placed between patient and the personnel in the room.

Organ Shields: Thyroid Shield and Gonad Shield

Whenever required, suitable shielding material should be used to shield the organs of interest or critical organs. For example, when limb (hand) is X-rayed, lead apron may be provided to the patient. Personnel can wear thyroid shield and lead glasses for protection in the imaging room. The thyroid shield **(Fig. 7.2A)** is made up of lead and wraps around the person's neck. It offers protection like that of lead apron.

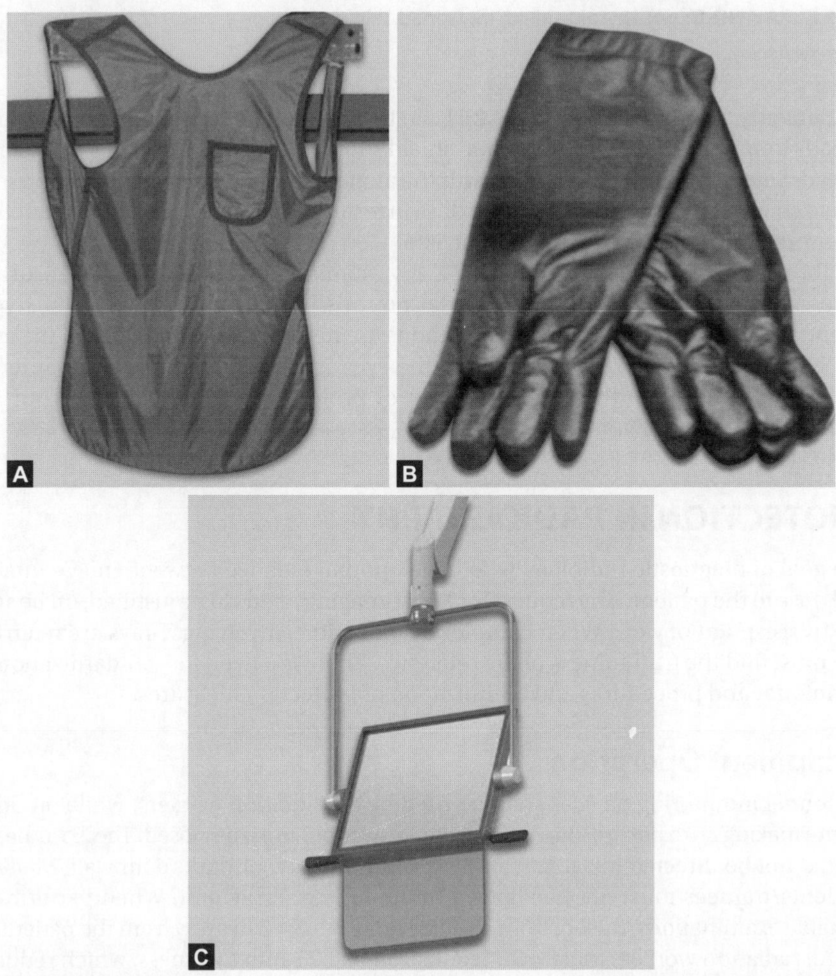

FIGS. 7.1A TO C: (A) Lead apron, (B) Lead gloves, and (C) Ceiling mounted lead glass shield and flaps.

Courtesy: Kenex Electro-medical.

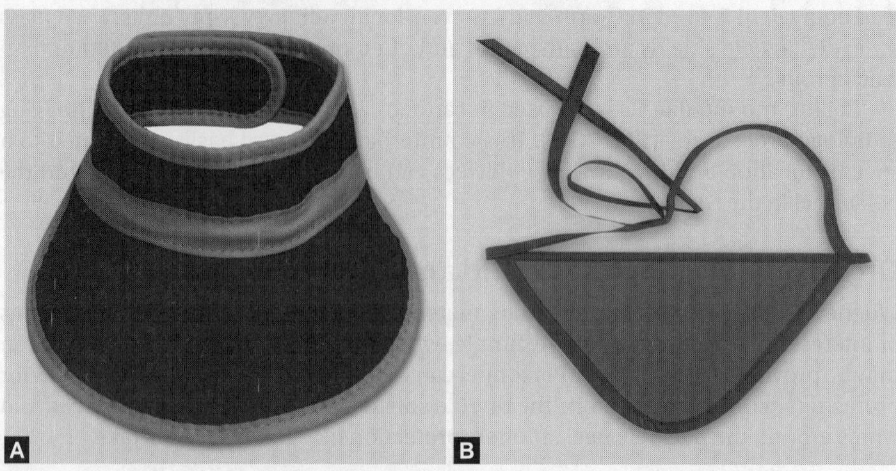

FIGS. 7.2A AND B: (A) Thyroid shield; (B) Gonad shield.
Courtesy: AmRay.

Similarly, gonadal shield **(Fig. 7.2B)** can be provided to the patient to protect the gonads from primary beam. The gonad shield should have a lead thickness of 0.5 mm of lead. Shields should not interfere with the anatomy under investigation. The use of gonad shield can reduce the absorbed dose in testes by up to 95%, while the reduction of absorbed in the ovaries can be about 50%.

The eyes should be shielded during X-ray examinations involving high-absorbed doses in the eyes, such as conventional petrous bone tomography. This is very important when multiple X-ray examinations are needed. Absorbed dose in the eyes can be reduced by 50–75% by shielding the eyes. The use of the posterior–anterior projection rather than the anterior–posterior projection can reduce the absorbed dose in the eyes by 95%.

PROTECTION IN RADIOGRAPHY

The goal of diagnostic radiology is to have optimal balance between image quality and dose to the patient. Any request for X-ray imaging needs to be justified, on benefit versus risk point of view. When complex examinations involving X-rays are referred, one must find the truthfulness of the reference. There is a need for standardization of techniques and procedures and optimization of protection measures.

Equipment Operation

Personnel monitoring devices shall be used by all radiation workers, while on duty. Before making an exposure, the doors of the X-ray room must be closed. The X-ray beam should not be directed towards windows, control panel, or dark room wall. Medical students/trainees must not be allowed to operate an X-ray unit. When performing portable examinations, the operator should stand at least 2 m away from the patient.

All radiation workers must wear lead apron of 0.25-mm thickness, which reduces radiation exposure by a factor of about 10. Use of leaded glass, lead gloves must be encouraged in fluoroscopy type of work. Repeat X-rays must be avoided to reduce patient dose. Gonad shield, eye shield, and thyroid shields should be used, to protect the patient organ, during radiography.

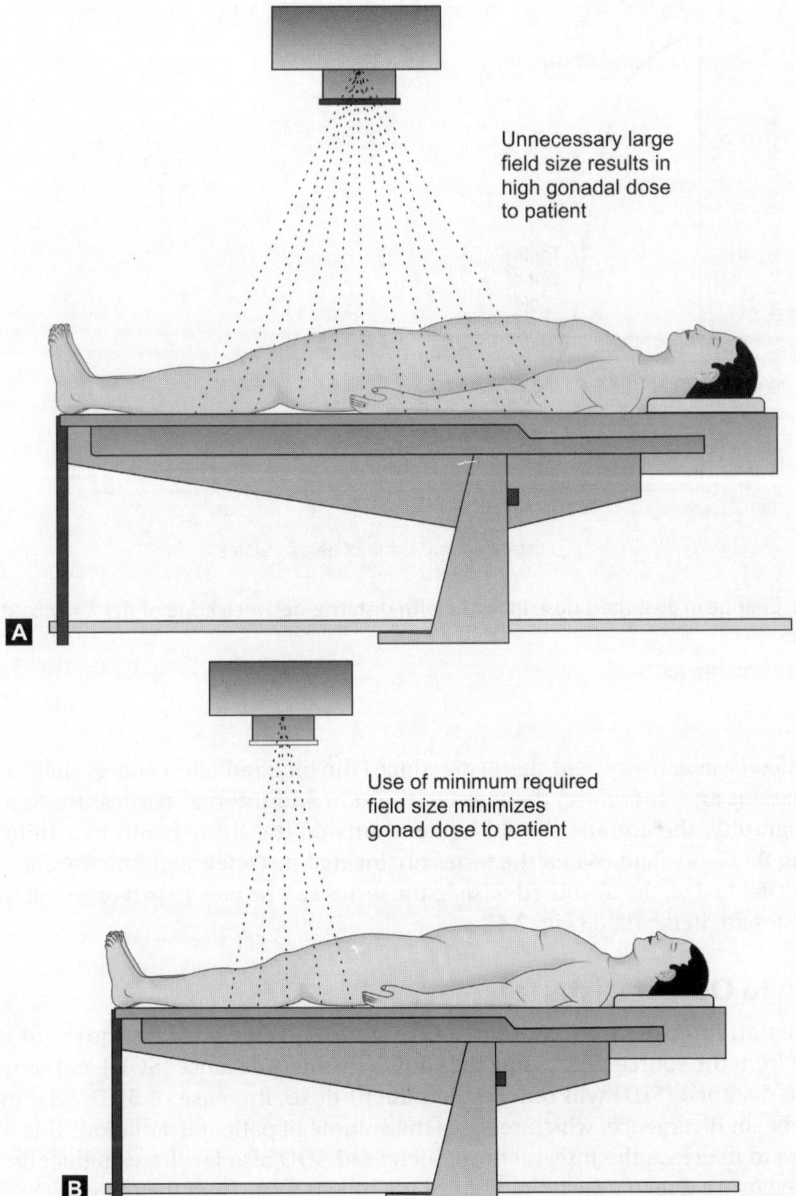

FIGS. 7.3A AND B: Field size and dose reduction, (A) Uncollimated beam; (B) Collimated beam to reduce gonad dose.

Courtesy: Safety aspects in diagnostic radiology, 1989.

Field Area

Reduction of field size by collimation is another important dose reduction technique. Hence, minimal field size to cover the patient volume is sufficient. Field size reduction reduces the scatter thereby reducing the dose to adjacent organs. The scatter incident on the detector also decreases, resulting an improved image contrast. Hence, the rule of thumb is use of smallest possible field size just sufficient to cover the anatomy with good collimation **(Figs. 7.3A and B)**.

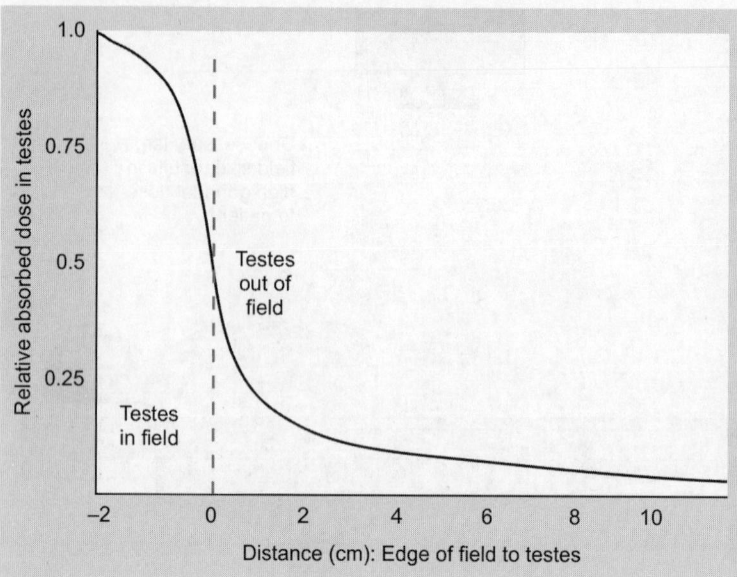

FIG. 7.4: Change in absorbed dose in testes with distance between edge of the X-ray field and testes.

Courtesy: Parthasarthy KS.

The decrease in X-ray field size also reduces the total radiation energy delivered to the patient and, therefore, the mass of the skin and internal tissues irradiated. In radiography, the gonads should be kept outside the X-ray beam by carefully adjusting the X-ray field. When the testes are located just a few centimeters outside the X-ray field edge, the absorbed dose in the testes can be one-fourth or less of that when testes are in the field **(Fig. 7.4)**.

Source to Object Distance

The radiation intensity from a point source varies inversely as the square of the distance from the source. Increasing the source to object distance (SOD) and source to image distance (SID) will reduce the patient dose. Increase of SOD/SID ratio reduces beam divergence, which reduces the volume of patient irradiation. This will enable us to decrease the integral dose. Increased SOD also facilitates reduction of patient exposure due to tube leakage since the tube is away from the patient. On the other hand, decrease of SOD increases the radiation intensity sharply at the surface of the patient **(Fig. 7.5)**.

In radiography with stationary X-ray equipment, the SID is normally 100 cm. When the SID is <100 cm, the quality of the diagnostic information becomes poorer, therefore, longer SID has clinical advantages. Chest radiography should be performed with a SID of at least 180 cm to keep the magnification unity. The SOD should be not <45 cm in radiography. In the case of C-arm units, fixed SID is used; therefore, increase of SOD is the only way of reducing patient dose. Hence, in fluoroscopy minimum distance between source and the patient must be not <30 cm.

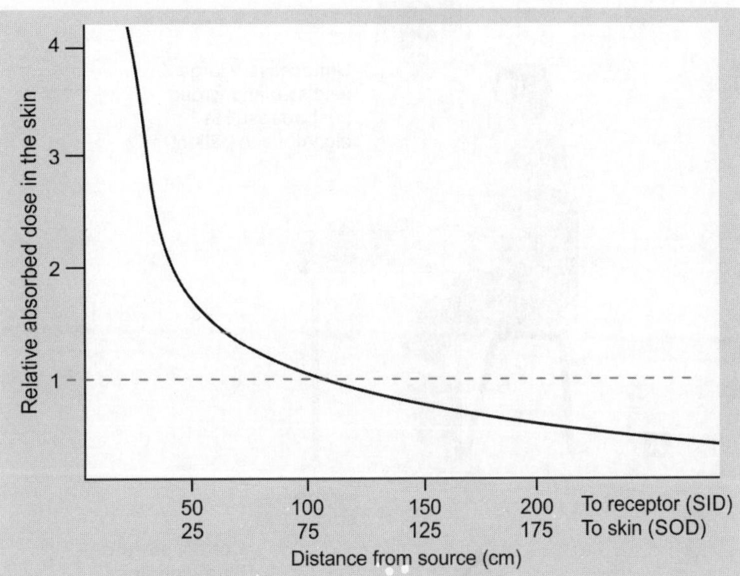

FIG. 7.5: Dependence of absorbed dose in the skin on the distance from the X-ray source; the skin to image receptor distance is constant at 25 cm.

Courtesy: Parthasarathy KS.

Patient Positioning and Motion

The collimator is adjusted to exclude radiosensitive organs such as gonads, breast, and eyes **(Figs. 7.6A and B)**. Gonad shield is used wherever necessary. Patient motion is a matter of concern in diagnostic imaging. It may cause motion artifacts, which may increase repeat X-rays. This will increase the patient dose. To reduce patient motion, (1) short exposure times, (2) use of immobilization or sedation, (3) entertainment or distracting devices should be applied and adopted. Immobilization devices (mechanical supporting or restraining devices) shall be used to prevent movement of children during exposure.

Occupancy in the Room

Only persons whose presence is necessary should be in the imaging room during the exposure. Overcrowding should be avoided. All such persons must be protected with lead aprons/shields.

Assistance to Patients

Holding of children or infirm patients for X-ray examination shall be done only by an adult relative or escort of the patient. Hospital personnel should not hold the patients during imaging procedure. No person should routinely hold patients during diagnostic examinations, certainly not those who are pregnant or under the age of 18 years. Such persons shall be provided with protective aprons and gloves. The X-ray film should not be held by hand. In no instance shall the holder's body be in the useful beam, and should be as far away from the primary beam as possible.

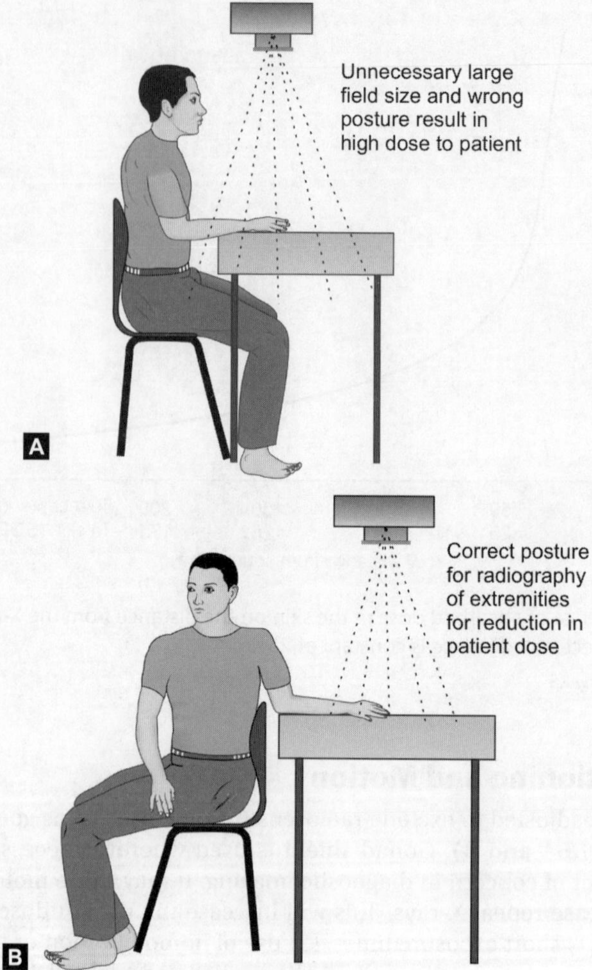

FIGS. 7.6A AND B: (A) Wrong positioning, and (B) Correct positioning.

Courtesy: Safety aspects of diagnostic radiology, 1989.

Repeat Examinations

Repeat X-ray examination is a matter of concern in diagnostic radiology. Reduction of repeat films can also reduce patient dose significantly. Hence, the film reject rate due to all causes should be kept below 5%. Proper instruction to the patient, checking the factors before exposure, proper darkroom procedure, and periodic maintenance of automatic processors may also help to reduce repeat X-rays and patient dose.

Requirements for Operational Safety

- Always wear personnel monitoring thermoluminescent dosimeter (TLD) badge at chest level under the lead apron
- Always stand behind the protective barrier while operating X-ray equipment. It protects X-ray technologist(s) from scattered radiation emitted from patient during X-ray imaging.

- Avoid self-holding of the patient for X-ray imaging. If needed, ask the patient's relative to assist the patient by providing him a lead apron.
- The parent or relatives or escort are provided with protective aprons and instructions when there is a need to position and hold the children or infirm patients during X-ray examinations
- Collimator (diaphragm) is used to limit the X-ray field size to the area of interest, which is just sufficient to cover the anatomy of the patient.
- Ensure that patients/relatives/staffs do not crowd the X-ray room. Only the patient whose radiological examination is to be carried out shall be allowed in the room.
- Ensure that X-ray room door(s) is closed during X-ray imaging.
- Operate the mobile X-ray equipment by extending the control cable, so that 2 m distance is ensured between equipment and technologist.
- Always wear lead-protective apron during mobile X-ray imaging.
- During use of portable X-ray equipment, ensure that X-ray tube is immobilized on the stand and film cassette shall not be held in hand by any person.

X-ray Technologist Responsibilities

- Only qualified X-ray technologists will be allowed to handle X-ray equipment.
- Do not direct the X-ray beam at the windows of the room or towards the control panel or dark room wall.
- Gonad shield must be used on patients whenever appropriate, and the field size must be adjusted to the minimum size.
- Medical students/trainees must not be allowed to operate an X-ray unit.
- Storage of undeveloped X-ray films and personnel monitoring device must be kept in areas protected from radiation.
- Technologists must wear lead apron; it reduces radiation exposure by a factor of about 10.
- Each equipment must have a separate logbook, which provides information about the equipment manufacturer, model, serial number, date of purchase, cost, repair details, down time, etc.

Safe Work Practice for Dose Reduction in General Radiography

Diagnostic X-ray contributes the highest radiation dose to the patients. The radiation dose received by a patient is specified in terms of entrance surface or skin dose (ESD). Effective dose in general radiography ranges from 0.1 to 1 mSv. ESD for chest radiograph is 0.1 to 0.2 mGy and for abdominal radiograph is 0.7 mGy. The ESD increases with short focus to skin distance. The patient exposure is proportional to mAs and kV_p squared, and inversely related to the square of the distance from the focal spot. A rule of thumb is that a technique of 100 kV_p and 100 mAs produces an exposure of about 1 R at a distance of 1 m. Hence, optimal technique must be used to reduce patient dose. The following are the important steps, which will protect the patient from radiation dose:

- Any X-ray examination should be prescribed only after a critical evaluation of the patient's condition, to avoid unnecessary exposures.
- Transfer of radiographs from one institution to another should be encouraged to avoid repeat examinations.
- A new diagnostic X-ray equipment must not be used unless quality assurance tests have been performed satisfactorily.

- No fluoroscopic or CT examination should be conducted, if the required information can be obtained from radiography.
- All efforts shall be made to keep the patient dose as low as technically achievable.
- Radiological examination of the lower abdomen and pelvis of a pregnant woman or women of reproductive age must be conducted only when considered essential. It should be carried out only, if her last menstrual period (LMP) is within 28 days.
- In all other X-ray examinations, the abdomen and the pelvis must be covered with a protective shield.
- Gonad shield, eye shield, and thyroid shields should be used, to protect the patient organ.
- Repeat X-rays must be avoided to reduce patient dose.
- Use of rare earth-intensifying screens will reduce the patient dose significantly.
- Records of all radiological examinations should be maintained. Reports and radiographs should be given to the patient for future reference.

PROTECTION IN MAMMOGRAPHY

Mammography X-ray system consists of cassette carrier, focal spot selector, and compression device, in addition to general radiography tube specification. Multiple focal spots and targets are provided. The unit should indicate the selection of focal spot and target prior to exposure. Compression device must be flat and parallel to the breast support. Its edges are smooth and bend upwards so that it is comfortable to the patient and shall not appear on the image. Compression shall be released after the end of the exposure. X-ray tube should have filter as follows:

- *Mammography*:
  - Be 1 mm + Mo 0.03 mm (Mo target)
  - Be 1 mm + Rh 0.025 mm (Rh target)

In mammography, Mo target with Mo/Rh filter and Rh target with Rh filter are commonly used. Mo cannot be used as filter with Rh targets in mammography X-ray tubes.

Special viewing boxes are needed for mammography since films are exposed to high optical densities. Films should be viewed in high luminance view boxes with low ambient light. View box of luminance of 3,000 cd/m^2 is usually recommended. Film-masking provision is made available to mask areas beyond the mammography image border. It will help to identify low-contrast regions. Microcalcifications can be viewed with the help of magnifying lens.

Radiation Dose

Mammography involves low kV_p X-rays hence, photoelectric absorption mostly accounts the radiation dose. Low-energy scatter also contributes to the radiation dose to the tissue which depends on—(1) tissue thickness, (2) X-ray beam quality, and (3) detector sensitivity. The effective dose to the patient in mammography is of the order of 0.4 mSv.

Tissue compression lowers the radiation dose, by minimizing the photon scatter especially the low-energy scatter. If efficient screen-film systems are used, then lesser photon density is enough to give optimal image. This will reduce radiation dose to the patient. The nature of anode material and filter also influences the patient dose.

Choice of carbon fiber grid and cassette will also reduce radiation dose. To improve the film sensitivity, longer developing time and higher developer temperature are recommended.

Radiation dose can induce cancer in the breast, which is the main risk in mammography. Glandular tissue is the site for carcinogenesis hence, mean glandular dose (MGD) is considered as dose index to evaluate risk. The glandular dose varies with depth, beam quality, breast thickness, and optical density of the image. Since the glandular tissue is lying at different depths, the dose also varies; hence, measurement is difficult. MGD is estimated as follows:

$$\text{MGD} = \text{K} \times \text{p} \times \text{g}$$

Where K is the entrance surface dose (ESD) in air-kerma, p and g are the conversion values for a given half-value layer (HVL) of the beam. For example, if the HVL of the mammography beam is 0.3 mm, then the corresponding p and g values are 1.10 and 183 mGy/Gy, respectively. The ESD decreases with increase of kV_p but reduces the subject contrast. The acceptable level of ESD is about 5–6 mGy and the corresponding MGD is:

$$= \text{K} \times \text{p} \times \text{g}$$
$$= 5 \times 10^{-3}\ \text{Gy} \times 1.10 \times 183\ \text{mGy/Gy}$$
$$= 1.0\ \text{mGy}$$

The upper limit of MGD is 3 mGy. The ESD can be measured by keeping a standard breast phantom.

PROTECTION IN DENTAL X-RAYS

Dental X-ray equipment includes—(1) intraoral radiography (IOPA) (2) panoramic radiography (OPG), (3) cephalometry, and (4) cone beam computed tomography (CBCT). Intraoral radiography are further divided into bitewing, periapical and occlusal radiography. The dental X-ray units may be fixed, mobile and portable (handheld) units.

X-ray tube housing for dental (IOPA) X-ray equipment shall be so constructed that leakage radiation through the protective tube housing in any direction, averaged over an area not >100 cm^2 with no linear dimension >20 cm, shall not exceed an air-kerma of 0.25 mGy in 1 hour at a distance of 1.0 m from the X-ray target when the tube is operating at the maximum rated kV_p and for the maximum rated current at that kV_p.

All dental equipment shall be provided with suitable collimation and shielding features such that the radiosensitive organs, i.e., the eye and thyroid are not exposed to the primary beam. The collimation/cone shall provide the same degree of radiation shielding as specified for X-ray tube housing. The collimation shall be such that the primary radiation beam is fully intercepted by the image receptor at the maximum focal spot to image receptor distance.

Equipment selection is much vital in dental radiography. In intraoral X-rays, focus to film distance must be 20 cm for 60 kV_p and it is 30 cm for above 70 kV_p and the effective focal spot range is 0.4 to 0.7 mm. This is applicable also to panoramic cephalometric X-ray units. CBCT X-ray units shall have FOV of 6 cm × 6 cm with nominal focal spot size of 0.5 mm. They are operated with 70–120 kV_p (10–150 mAs).

In OPG and dental CBCT, the face-positioning device shall be provided to limit the minimum focal spot to skin distance, not <15 cm. Tube locking is provided so that beam is not directed outside the image receptor. Cassette carrier is interlocked so that the exposure is not possible unless the film cassette is in the cassette. The effective dose in dental X-rays is of the order of 0.005–0.01 mSv.

Safe Work Practice in Dental Radiography

- New dental X-ray equipment shall not be used unless quality assurance tests are performed satisfactorily.
- The direct beam must not irradiate any person other than the patient.
- Dental film should be fixed in position/held by the patient. It should never be held by the dentist worker.
- The staff must keep away from the patient, during exposure to avoid scattered radiation, i.e., 1 m at least. If the workload exceeds 1,800 mAs a week, a protective apron should be worn.
- Patient should be protected with protective apron of 0.25 mm pb equivalent to cover the whole trunk.
- The X-ray beam size should be restricted by suitable cylindrical cones to the minimum aperture appropriate to the examination. Specifications for dental cones are:
    - *50–60* kV_p: 10 cm
    - *60–75* kV_p: 20 cm
    - *Above 75* kV_p: 30 cm
- Radiological examinations should not be made in the absence of clear-cut clinical indications.
- Extensive or repeated X-ray examinations of children or pregnant women should not be undertaken without considerable forethought.
- Justification and imaging guidelines for pediatric and pregnant patients
- Optimization of radiation protection of individuals undergoing medical exposures
- Diagnostic reference levels should be established.
- Carers and comforters and volunteers of biomedical research should be protected
- Management of unintended and accidental medical exposures

PROTECTION IN FLUOROSCOPY

Fluoroscopy imaging contributes large portion of dose in medical imaging (18%) due to continuous X-ray production and real-time image output. Though the exposure technique is moderate (3 mA, 80 kV_p), the examination ON time extends from minute to hours with 7.5–15 frames/s. Cineangiography studies employ high exposure rates of 175–600 mGy/min with short exposure times. Some systems have turbo mode where the exposure rate may exceed up to 175 mGy/min; hence, such mode should be used judiciously. Patient dose also depends upon the angulation of the beam through the patient. Exposure rates are greater in lateral examination than that of anteroposterior. For example, a fluoroscopy imaging involves a technique of, 2 mA, 80 kV_p, 10 minutes ON time, delivers an exposure of 60 mGy at 1 m. The skin entrance exposure at 30 cm will be:

$$= (100/30)^2 \times 60$$
$$= 667 \text{ mGy}$$

TABLE 7.2 **Average effective doses for diagnostic X-ray procedures.**

Examination	*Dose (mSv)*
Dexa scan	0.001
Dental X-rays	0.01
Mammogram	0.4
Chest X-rays	0.1
Abdomen X-ray	0.7
Lumbar spine	1.5
Interventional cardiology (angiogram and angioplasty)	1–100
Chest CT	7.0
Abdomen CT	8.0

(AERB: Atomic Energy Regulatory Board; CT: computed tomography).

Courtesy: AERB data, 2017.

Thus, in fluoroscopy, the skin entrance dose is higher. Patient's entrance air-kerma rate depends on beam angulation through the patient. The air-kerma rate increases with thickness of the patient. The entrance exposures of various imaging systems such as radiography, fluoroscopy, and CT scan are given in **Table 7.2** [Atomic Energy Regulatory Board (AERB)].

Several X-ray-induced injuries have been reported in interventional procedures including, percutaneous transluminal coronary angioplasty, radiofrequency cardiac catheter ablation, vascular embolization, transjugular intrahepatic portosystemic shunt placement and percutaneous endovascular reconstruction, etc. Physician and technologist training play a vital role in such procedures.

Equipment Specification in Fluoroscopy

Equipment with conventional fluoroscopy is provided with protective lead glass of 2-mm lead equivalence up to 100 kV_p. Lead equivalence shall be increased at the rate 0.01 mm per kV_p. Bucky slot shall be provided with protective flaps of 0.5-mm lead equivalence. X-ray tube and fluorescent screen should be rigidly aligned so that both move synchronously.

The focus to tabletop distance shall not be <30 cm. The patient entrance dose is limited to a maximum of 10 cGy/min with automatic exposure control (AEC) and 5 cGy/min without AEC. Equipment shall have a cumulative timer and its range shall not exceed 5 minutes. X-ray tube is provided with multiple focal spots (0.3, 0.6, and 1.2 mm) to handle adult and pediatric patients. Image intensifiers (II) are available in different sizes (4.5, 9, and 12 inch) and proper selection of intensifier Image size to match a specific institution is very important.

The image intensifier has wide dynamic range and the entrance exposure is controlled by light limiting aperture or electronic of the subsequent detector (e.g., TV, camera). Entrance exposure is 1 μR per image in fluoroscopy, and 4 μR per image for digital subtraction angiography (DSA). Any reduction in exposure is limited by quantum mottle.

Dose Reduction in Fluoroscopy

The most important method of dose reduction in fluoroscopy is to limit the beam ON time, by using short burst of exposures. One can also use the last image-hold facility, to view the image even after the exposure. This will reduce the fluoroscopy time by 50–80% in many procedures. Pulsed fluoroscopy reduces dose by allowing frame rates lesser than real time. It may be used along with digital image memory to reduce patient dose. This is a suitable technique in patients where higher temporal resolution is not required.

Use of optimal image intensifier system (conversion gain, high-contrast ratio, spatial resolution, and contrast sensitivity) can also reduce the patient dose. Reducing the field size by collimation will also reduce the integral dose. Maintaining much distance between the X-ray tube and patient will also reduce the skin dose. Though magnification technique improves spatial resolution, it also increases the patient dose and hence used sparingly.

Dose–area–product (DAP) meter should be used to measure the patient dose in fluoroscopy **(Fig. 7.7)**. It is provided with every fluoroscopy machine. DAP is the product of absorbed dose and exposure area, expressed in Gym^2 or $mGycm^2$. It quantifies not only the dose within the radiation field but also the area of the tissue irradiated. It will correlate with the total energy imparted to the patient, which is related to the effective dose and overall cancer risk.

Dose–area–product meter is a radiolucent ionization chamber fixed across the primary beam permanently, beyond the collimator. It consists of ionization chamber, which intercepts the radiation field. Factors such as kV_p, mA, exposure time (s), and area can be changed to suit individual patients. The ionization signal generated is proportional to the beam area. The area irradiated increases with square of the distance whereas the radiation intensity decreases as per inverse square law. Therefore, the product of intensity and area is independent of distance from the source. For example, a $10 \times 10 = 100$ cm^2 area with an entrance exposure of 2 mGy may yield a DAP of 200 $mGycm^2$ (100×2).

If the DAP meter is calibrated with field size, SOD, source to detector distance (SDD), and collimation, real-time display of patient dose can help the physician to modify the procedure to minimize skin injuries. It is easy to identify the patient who may be at risk due to radiation. Regulation requires recording of DAP meter value for each patient. Hence, physician training plays an important role in dose reduction methods.

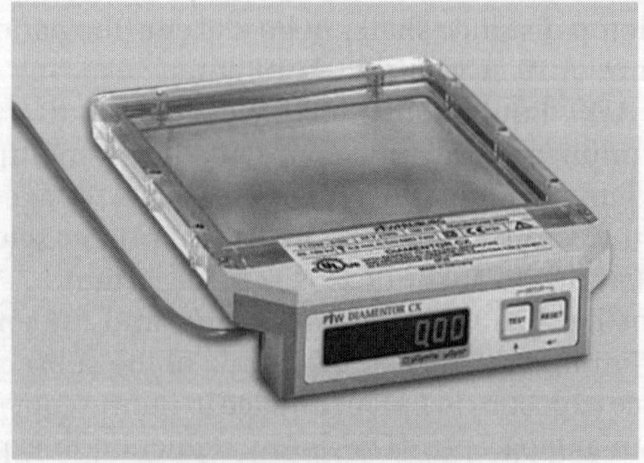

FIG. 7.7: Dose area product (DAP) meter.
Courtesy: PTW/Medical equipment and service solutions.

In fluoroscopy units, X-ray tube is beneath the couch and the scattered radiation levels are higher. It is two to three times higher at the X-ray tube level than that of at tabletop level and is 50% lesser at II tube level. Couch hanging lead flaps may reduce this radiation considerably. An operator positioned at 3 feet from the beam entrance area will receive 0.1% of the patient's ESD.

Nowadays, flat panel systems are used that have advantage of large size, less bulky, absence of image distortion, and high detective quantum efficiency (DQE) at moderate-to-high incident air-kerma rate (IAKR). However, flat panel systems suffer from high levels of electronic noise, especially at low IAKR. Typical IAKR values are 15–40 μGy/min.

Requirements for Operational Safety

Since interventional procedures involve angiography and angioplasty procedures. It causes higher radiation exposures of 1–100 mSv, all the personnel involved in the procedure should address the following for operational safety:

- Use of lead apron, couch flaps, lead gloves, and ceiling suspended lead screen must be encouraged in fluoroscopy type of work. Advisable is skirt type lead apron to distribute weight.
- Wearing of personnel monitoring TLD chest badge while at work. Additional wrist badge for procedures requiring hands close to primary beam
- Imaging system should be positioned as close to the patient surface as possible
- Personnel themselves in opposite to the X-ray tube during oblique orientation
- During C-arm procedures, standing on the side of the image intensifier is safest because there is more scatter produced at the entrance surface side of the patient.
- Keep the table height as high as comfortable possible for the operator
- During fluoroscopy, workers should not be there in the room if not necessary
- Restriction of X-ray beam size (collimation) to being as small as necessary for the clinical purpose
- Preventive maintenance and periodic QA of equipment
- Updating with the current regulatory requirements

Safe Work Practice for Dose Reduction in Fluoroscopy

Fluoroscopy imaging time is higher, and it may vary from 1–3 to 15 min for an interventional procedure. Therefore, the radiation dose is higher for both patient and the operator. High-radiation exposure may induce skin erythema. Hence, the skin entrance dose should not exceed 50 mGy/min to the patient. It will vary with kV_p and patient thickness. Higher the kV_p and lesser the patient thickness, lesser the radiation dose to the patient. A typical fluoroscopy examination may give a dose of 10–30 mGy/min. 1-minute fluoroscopy screening at the rate of 50 mGy/min dose rate is equal to 15 pelvis radiographs. Dose reduction to the patient may be achieved by the following:

- Selection of suitable exposure factors (kV_p, mA), e.g., higher kV_p (>60) is much effective in dose reduction
- Time of exposure must be shorter
- Keep patient's extremities out of the beam
- Minimize use of steep angles of the X-ray beam
- Minimize the use of cine mode
- Magnification technique should be avoided or kept lower
- Antiscatter grid should be removed when imaging small patients of thin body parts

- Use of low-frame rate, especially in DSA
- Use low-dose rate pulsed fluoroscopy
- Use heavy X-ray beam filtration
- Use of lower-dose ABC options
- Use of last frame hold features
- Use of high kV_p technique
- Use frame averaging and pulsed fluoroscopy
- Use the largest FOV suitable for the given clinical study
- Utilize radiation only when imaging is necessary to support clinical care
- Vary the imaging beam angle to minimize exposure to any one skin area
- Monitor radiation dose in real time to assess patient risk/benefit during the procedure
- Direction of X-ray beam should be far away from the fetus, if pregnant women are examined.

PROTECTION IN COMPUTED TOMOGRAPHY

Computed tomography (CT) is a valuable and lifesaving imaging tool in medical imaging. It is a major contributor of patient dose. It performs 8% diagnostic issues, but provides 48% of the population's collective dose **(Fig. 7.8)**. Most CT scanners use fixed kV_p and mAs regardless of patient size. CT scan image never looks like overexposed or underexposed as in radiographs. There is a tendency to use tube current-time (mAs) without any changes. Such patients often exposed to excessive radiation. Image quality also changes with noise and graininess based on body habitus. Generally,

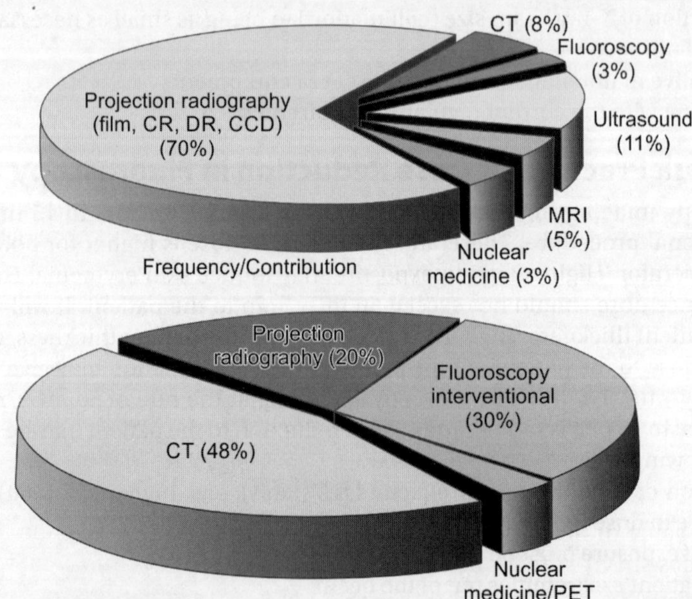

FIG. 7.8: Frequency distribution of medical imaging and patient radiation dose in percentage. (CR: computed radiography; DR: digital radiography; CCD: charge coupled device; PET: positron emission tomography).
Courtesy: David J Dowsett et al, 2006.

large-size patient is given increased mAs to avoid excessive noise. The patient dose in CT depends on applied kV_p, mA, tube rotation time, pitch, and filter.

Hence, manufacturers implemented CT dose management procedures as per ALARA principle. It is based on tube current modulation as a function of tube rotation angle and axial position on the patient. It will compensate attenuation variations along the beam path through the patient. Some scanners use scout scan as localizer or measure the transmitted radiation to determine mA. Automatic tube current modulations compensate the thickness variation in torso of body from AP to lateral projections, which will reduce the patient dose without reducing image quality. However, one must be aware of noise involved in such techniques. Alternatively, iterative reconstruction can be used to reduce the dose.

Various modulation methods are—(1) angular tube current modulation, (2) longitudinal tube current modulation, (3) angular-longitudinal tube current modulation, and (4) AEC. AEC system modulates tube current in *x*, *y*, and *z* axes in which acceptable level of noise is varied according to patient size, anatomical region, and diagnostic task. AEC method of current modulation has an edge over other methods.

Radiation Dose in CT

In CT scan, volume of tissue is irradiated at all angles and dose distribution is more homogeneous. Patient dose is uniform in head scan, whereas it is nonuniform in abdomen scan. Absorbed dose varies between center and periphery region of the body. Patient skin dose may be higher (20–40 mGy) than at body center. Effective dose (E) in CT scan is calculated from the computed tomography dose index (CTDI) which is measured in a specific phantom with 10-cm ion chamber, both at the periphery and center. From the measured values, CTDI weighted ($CTDI_w$) and CTDI volume ($CTDI_{vol}$) can be obtained:

$$CTDI_w = \frac{2}{3(CTDI_{peri})} + \frac{1}{3(CTDI_{cent})}$$

$$CTDI_{vol} = \frac{CTDI_w}{Pitch}$$

Modern scanners display $CTDI_{vol}$ and dose length product (DLP), which gives information about amount of radiation given to the patient. Typical values $CTDI_{vol}$ of head torso and brain perfusion studies are 80, 50, and 600, respectively. DLP is related to scan length (L):

$$DLP = CTDI_{vol} \times L$$

The effective radiation dose (E) is proportional DLP and the slope of E/DLP is called k factor or E_{DLP} (mSv/mGy-cm):

$$E = k \times DLP \tag{7.1}$$

The k value of head, neck, chest, abdomen, and pelvis is given in **Table 7.3**. Effective dose in CT scan for head, chest, and abdomen is 1–2 mSv, 7 mSv, and 8–10 mSv, respectively.

Computed tomography radiation dose will not produce deterministic effects but may increase cancer-induced risk (Stochastic effects). Typical CT scan effective doses vary from 2 to 20 mSv for head to abdomens. Multiple CT scan involving contrast may increase patient dose. CT exposure to pregnant women may get a

TABLE 7.3 Conversion factors, k values (adults) for dose length product—CT dosimetry.

Age	*kV$_p$*	*Head*	*Neck*	*Chest*	*Abdomen*	*Pelvis*
Adult:	*Male*					
	80	0.0017	0.005	0.0107	0.0132	0.01
	100	0.0018	0.0049	0.0104	0.0132	0.0099
	120	0.0018	0.0049	0.0105	0.0134	0.01
	140	0.0018	0.005	0.0107	0.0134	0.0102
	Female					
	80	0.0019	0.0055	0.0188	0.017	0.0157
	100	0.002	0.0053	0.0183	0.017	0.0155
	120	0.002	0.0053	0.0185	0.0173	0.0157
	140	0.002	0.0055	0.0188	0.0173	0.016

Courtesy: ICRP-103, 2007.

fetus dose of about 10–15 mGy, which may be permitted with clinical intent. Multidetector computed tomography (MDCT) radiation dose is same as that of axial CT scans. Generally, CT scan dose is higher than radiographic X-rays. A thoracic CT scan (chest) is equal to about 100 conventional X-rays in terms of radiation dose.

The $CTDI_{vol}$, DLP, and radiation dose structured report (RDSR) are displayed before the scan, which will help the technologist to know the dose levels. Notification value is a dose metric of individual scan or series of study. It can be set to values higher than the diagnostic reference level (DRL). Alert value is the cumulative dose metric of the entire study, which can be set in the scanner. FDA alert value is 1 Gy for $CTDI_{vol}$.

Many CT systems calculate the CT air-kerma index (C_a) and air-kerma length product (PKL) during the scan and display on the console monitor. CT volume (C_{vol}) is the ratio of the CT air-kerma index and pitch factor. The PKL is the product of CT air-kerma index and scanning length. The C_a is measured in air on a polymethylmethacrylate (PMMA) phantom for head and body. Tables are available with ratio of organ dose to air-kerma in the axis of rotation for 1 mAs. Once C_a is known, it is multiplied by mAs and conversion coefficients to estimate organ doses. Alternatively, if kV_p and mAs are known, dose can be calculated from beam calibration data that is C_a and C_{vol} values.

Optimization of Radiation Dose in CT

Optimized imaging protocol is one in which mAs is adjudged so that the image noise level is within acceptable limits. Selection of thin slices leads to reduction of tissue volume. Smaller voxels experience lesser number of photons per voxel leading to noise. Hence, dose is increased (higher mA) to maintain same noise. Thin slice exhibits less partial volume effects, which are beneficial in high-contrast tissue. As the number of slices increases, the absorbed dose per unit mass remains the same but the total energy imported is higher in higher slice patients. Tissues of high-tissue contrast require low dose without reduction in diagnostic image quality (lung, bone, and renal stone protocol).

Obese patients may require higher dose hence, kV_p of 140 can be used and suitable abdominal protocols can be created for such patients. Low kV_p can increase the visibility of contrast medium in angiography or brain perfusion studies. This can be achieved at a tube voltage of 80–100 kV_p. Protocols are compared with optimized protocols of same model CT scanner. Increasing the pitch does reduce the dose if other parameters are same. However, it limits spatial resolution (image quality) in the axial direction and increases noise. CT system will increase mA and dose to maintain the same image quality.

Safe Work Practice for Dose Reduction in CT

- Use of optimal X-ray beam filtration
- Use of X-ray beam collimation and FOV
- X-ray tube current modulation and adoption for patient body habitus
- Ensure body imaging protocols do not use automatic mA modulation techniques
- Peak voltage optimization
- Scan only the z-axis for the required length
- Avoid radiation directly to the eyes
- Use iterative reconstruction, if possible
- Improved detection system efficiency
- Use of noise reduction algorithms
- Increased pitch or table increment (increase the effective slice thickness)
- Use of pediatric protocols
- Reducing the number of multiple scans with contrast material
- Create low-dose protocols (chest, kidney stone)
- Only scan the contrast phases necessary for diagnosis and vary mA according to contrast phase
- Ensure $CTDI_{vol}$ does not exceeds 0.5 Gy in brain perfusion study

PROTECTION IN PEDIATRIC IMAGING

Children have higher radiation sensitivity than adults and have a longer life expectancy (larger window to express radiation damage). Radiological examinations in infants and children are increasing. Pediatric radiological procedure should be individually planned, and projections should be limited to what is necessary for diagnosis. Therefore, imaging techniques that do not use ionizing radiation should always be considered as an alternative.

Children are more vulnerable to the late somatic effects and genetic effects of radiation than adults (epidemiologic study). The children receive higher dose when adult settings are used. Children are 10 times more sensitive to radiation than adults and girls are more sensitive than boys. The risk for developing a radiation-related cancer can be several times higher for a young child compared with an adult exposed to an identical technique. Radiation risks in children are a public health issue. Hence, one must examine the following issues before carryout the imaging:

- Justification of requested examinations
- Vetting of referrals for complex examinations
- Standardization of techniques and procedures
- Optimization of protection measures

Pediatric Radiography

Equipment and Peripherals

The selection of equipment-associated peripherals should suit the pediatric imaging work, so that the radiation dose will be lesser. Fast screen-film combination, e.g., rare earth, 400 speed and low attenuation, e.g., carbon fiber materials for cassette fronts for pediatric reduce dose. Digital radiography gives lesser dose than film-screen radiography. CT and fluoroscopy offer higher dose. Using the same adult technique to pediatrics leads to higher radiation dose. Hence, examination-specific protocols are required. Use of constant potential/high-frequency generator is beneficial to children. Patient motion should be avoided during examinations under radiation. To fulfill this, one can adopt the following—(1) short exposure times, (2) incorporation of entertainment, or distracting devices, and (3) immobilization or sedation of the patient **(Fig. 7.9)**.

Dose Reduction Methods in Pediatric Radiography

- Higher kV_p and lower mAs
- Use of increased filtration
- Employ increased SOD
- Posterior-anterior projections in female patients
- Antiscatter grids are normally not required in pediatric radiography as the gain in image quality does not justify the increase in patient dose, except in children in their teens and when the body build is such as to increase scatter
- Good image detail is achieved by maintaining a balance between the use of a small focal spot size and a short exposure time
- High-speed screen-film combinations should be used wherever possible to enable reduction in radiation exposure and exposure time, as the reduced resolution obtained is comparatively insignificant for the majority of clinical indications

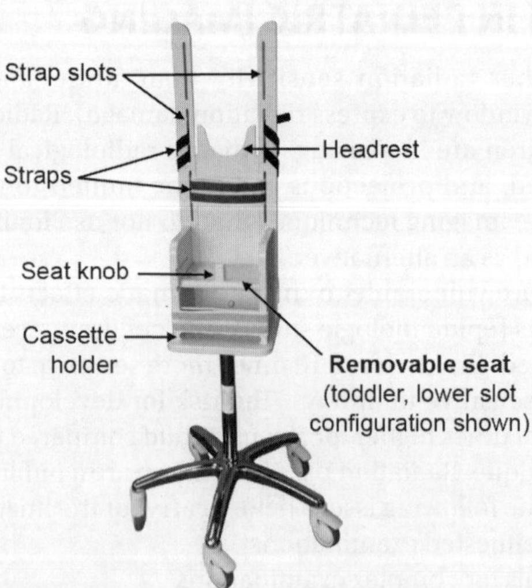

FIG. 7.9: Immobilization of child during chest radiography.
Courtesy: Universal Medical, Inc. USA.

- The use of AEC is generally not appropriate in children as the sensors (size and geometry) are normally designed for adult patients. Instead, exposure charts corresponding to radiographic technique, patient thickness in the X-ray beam and presence or absence of anti-scatter grid are much safer and easier to use.
- The radiation beam should be limited using collimation
- Shielding devices (gonads, thyroid, and lens) should be appropriately positioned to be efficient for protecting the tissues for which they are placed and to avoid unnecessary repeat examinations.
- Immobilization, when required, should be provided by specialized devices, if possible.

Pediatric Fluoroscopy

Fluoroscopy offers much higher dose to the children than radiography imaging. Hence, optimal selection of equipment and specialized techniques are very much essential. The image intensifier should have diameter of 4.5 in (11 cm). X-ray generator should have range of mAs from 0.1 to 6, so that one can have varying techniques from 100 mA × 1 ms to 800 mA × 7 ms. This is suitable for imaging children having weight from 3–140 kg at 65–75 kV_p. The X-ray tube should have at least two focal spots namely 0.3 mm (3–4 years child), and 0.6 mm (8 years children). Cine frame rate should be >60 fps. Typical values of ESD per radiograph and DAP for common pediatric fluoroscopy examinations are given in **Table 7.4**.

Dose Reduction Methods in Pediatric Fluoroscopy

- Patient should be positioned as close as possible to the image intensifier.
- The X-ray tube should be as far away as possible from the patient table to avoid excessive skin dose.
- Lowest frame rate is acceptable and last-image-hold facility should be used.

TABLE 7.4 Typical entrance surface dose (ESD) per radiograph and dose area product (DAP) for common pediatric fluoroscopy examinations (RPOP, IAEA).

	Age				
Examination	***0***	***1***	***5***	***10***	***15***
	Entrance surface dose (μGy)				
Abdomen AP	110	340	590	860	2010
Chest PA/AP	60	80	110	70	110
Pelvis AP	170	350	510	650	1,300
Skull AP	—	600	1,250	—	—
Skull LAT	—	340	580	—	—
	Dose area product (mGycm^2)				
MCU	430	810	940	1,640	3,410
Barium meal	760	1,610	1,620	3,190	5,670
Barium swallow	560	1,150	1,010	2,400	3,170

(AP: anteroposterior; IAEA: International Atomic Energy Agency; LAT: lateral; PA: posteroanterior; ESD: entrance surface dose)

- Some centers prefer to set a "floor" (a kV_p) below which the system will not go, such as 70 kV_p for pediatric patients and 80 kV_p for adults.
- Additional copper filtration also reduces patient dose.

Pediatric Computed Tomography

Computed tomography and interventional procedures are high-dose procedures in radiology and yield higher individual patient doses than other radiological procedures. The patient dose in CT is an important issue for children as reports suggest that in some centers, the exposure factors used for scanning children are the same as for adults. This problem is relatively lesser in interventional procedures as the machine, on the basis of body thickness falling in the X-ray beam, automatically adjusts factors in most modern equipment. CT scanning contributes most collective dose from radiographic exposures due to the increasing use of this modality.

Computed tomography scans are increasingly used in pediatric imaging. Mostly fixed kV_p and mAs, regardless of patient size, are used. Fixed techniques in CT may lead to unnecessary patient dose, e.g., neonatal, children. About 7 million CT examinations are performed annually on children in US. CT in children has increased about eight-fold since 1980, with annual growth of about 10% per year. Children receive higher doses than necessary when adult settings are used. The effective dose from single pediatric CT ranges from 1–30 mSv, and one-third of the children have three scans, which will triple the cancer risk. There is no need for these large doses and CT settings can be reduced significantly without losing the image quality. Hence, children should not be scanned using adult techniques and pediatric CT protocol or dose reduction methods should be made available.

To reduce the dose, technical chart (tube current) can be made for each CT scan (**Table 7.5**). The chart displays various body diameter and % of mAs required. It is

TABLE 7.5 **Technique chart, 120 kV_p, 300 mAs, and 32 cm diameter patient for dose reduction.**

Patient diameter (cm)	*% mAs*	*mAs*
14	0.3	1
16	0.6	2
18	1.2	4
20	2.2	7 (43% dose↓)
22	4.2	13
24	7.9	24
26	15	45
28	28	85
30	53	160
32	100	300
34	188	564
36	352	1,058
38	661	1,983
40	1,237	3,712

Courtesy: Jerold T Bush Berg et al, 2012.

prepared with 120 kV_p, 300 mAs, 5 mm slice and pitch 1, for creating a good-quality image of a 32 cm torso. From the chart, one can infer that a 30 cm patient requires about half of the mAs (160) to produce the same quality of image. For a 20 cm patient, only 7 mAs is required, which reduces the patient dose by 43%. Thus, the technical chart is very useful to reduce patient dose, with proper selection of mAs for each patient. However, it is not possible to maintain constant image noise overall patient sizes, since CT cannot achieve extremely low and high mAs values.

Dose Reduction Methods in Pediatric CT

As per American College of Radiology (ACR) CT Accreditation program, using the PMMA phantom, the $CTDI_{vol}$ can be calculated. For an adult body and head, it is about 25 mGy and 75 mGy, respectively. Taking these as baseline data, dose reduction factors (RF) can be obtained **(Tables 7.6 and 7.7)**. Tables present RF for pediatric abdomen and thorax and head, respectively:

$$\text{Pediatric mAs} = \text{Baseline data} \times \text{RF}$$

Worked Example 7.1

An adult thorax is examined at a technique of 120 kV_p, 0.5 seconds scan time, 200 mA, pitch = 1, and FOV = 35 cm. What is the appropriate pediatric technique for a 5-year-old thorax at a pitch of 1?

TABLE 7.6 Patient thickness, age, and RF for pediatric CT in abdomen and thorax.

PA thick (cm)	*Age*	*Abdomen RF*	*Thorax RF*
9	Newborn	0.43	0.42
12	1	0.51	0.49
14	5	0.59	0.57
16	10	0.66	0.64
19	15	0.76	0.74
22	S adult	0.90	0.82
25	M adult	Baseline	Baseline
31	L adult	1.25	1.16

(CT: computed tomography; PA: posteroanterior; RF: reduction factor highlight)

TABLE 7.7 Patient thickness, age, and RF for pediatric CT in head.

PA thick (cm)	*Age*	*Pediatric CT, head mAs RF*
12	Newborn	0.74
16	1	0.86
17	5	0.93
19	M adult	Baseline

(CT: computed tomography; PA: posteroanterior; RF: reduction factor)

From **Table 7.6**, the RF for 5-year-old thorax is 0.57, then—

$$\text{Pediatric mA} = \text{Baseline} \times \text{RF}$$
$$= 200 \text{ mA} \times 0.57 = 144 \text{ mA}$$

Worked Example 7.2

An adult head is examined in a CT technique of 140 kV_p, 0.5 seconds scan time, 400 mA, pitch = 1, and FOV = 25 cm. What is the appropriate technique for a 1-year-old child head?

From **Table 7.7**, the RF for a 1-year-old head is 0.86, then—

$$\text{Pediatric mA} = \text{Baseline} \times \text{RF}$$
$$= 400 \text{ mA} \times 0.86 = 344 \text{ mA}$$

In general, a head examination with adult protocol (200 mAs) may give 23–49 mGy organ dose in brain. If the mAs is adjusted to 100 and dose becomes 11–25 mGy. Similarly, the abdomen dose reduces from 21–43 to 5–11 mGy, if the mAs is adjusted as shown in **Table 7.8**.

The following are the general methods of dose reduction in pediatric CT:

- Every CT examination is justified and inappropriate referrals are eliminated.
- Number of multiple scans with contrast media must be reduced
- Information about previous procedures are collected from the patient.
- Alternative approaches like ultrasound or MRI must be considered.
- Information may be provided to the patient in accordance with national standards.
- Justification needs to be included in the clinical audit.

Dose Reduction Methods in Pediatric Chest CT

- Image quality in CT is generally more than what is required for confident diagnosis. Awareness on this can help in significant reduction in patient dose.
- Radiologists and physicians should be aware that images with low noise, even if they do not look very crisp, may provide the diagnostic information.
- mAs reduction at defined kV_p has been used with success by many center and is the most efficient method of dose management in children as also in adults. There is lack of consensus on kV_p reduction in CT examination.
- Many authors suggest using 100–200 mAs settings for high-resolution chest CT in children. However, reliable diagnostic studies can be obtained using much lower mAs. In cooperative children who can breathhold, as low as 34 mAs can be used, whereas 50 mAs for noncooperative children.
- Whenever radiosensitive tissues such as breast and thyroid fall within the exposed area, they should be shielded. Breast anlage (primordium or the first rudiment

TABLE 7.8 Typical CT pediatric organ and effective doses with normal and adjusted mAs for head and abdomen examinations.

Exam	*Organ*	*Organ dose (mGy)*	*Effective dose (mGy)*
Head (200 mAs)	Brain	23–49	1.8–3.8
Head (100 mAs, adjusted)	Brain	11–25	0.9–1.9
Abdomen (200 mAs)	Stomach	21–43	11–24
Abdomen (50 mAs adjusted)	Stomach	5–11	6–12

Courtesy: IAEA, 2012.

of the breast, the underdeveloped tissue) protection using, for example, 2-mm thick bismuth-coated latex shielding reduces the dose to the breast anlage by approximately 40%.

- Recent technology developments include automatic tube current modulation where the tube current is adjusted according to thickness and density of tissues to maintain a constant level of image noise.

Dose Reduction Methods in Pediatric Abdominal CT

Strategies should include obtaining only necessary CT examinations. MRI and US should take priority. If possible, the examination should be tailored to answer the specific question asked by the referring clinician, for example, pelvic scanning is not always necessary when an abdominal scan is requested, and it may be possible to curtail follow-up CT examination to a specific organ. In addition, imaging parameters such as kV_p and mAs need to be adjusted for patient size. Size-based tables for abdominal multidetector CT and body CT angiography in children are available. In one study, children were classified by colors based on weight and this was shown to significantly reduce scanning errors in settings for pediatric MDCT.

Recent technology developments include automatic tube current modulation where the tube current is adjusted according to thickness and density of tissues to maintain a constant level of image noise. Finally, the use of multiphase scanning should be curtailed as much as possible.

PREGNANCY AND DIAGNOSTIC RADIOLOGY

Whenever diagnostic examination is prescribed, the risk of mother being exposed by not doing the procedure should be greater than the risk of potential harm to the fetus. Most of the radiological examinations involve low doses of radiation; hence, there is no restriction in examinations. Radiation doses are unlikely to cause risk of causing fetal death, malformation, or impairment of mental development. Dose limits do not apply to patients undergoing radiological investigations. The examination area may be either away from the radiation field or within the radiation field. If the fetus comes in the direct beam, methods of reducing the fetus dose should be followed. As per International Commission on Radiological Protection (ICRP-84), certain precautions are required in terms of—(1) before irradiation, (2) during irradiation, and (3) after irradiation.

Before Irradiation

Before the radiological examination, it is to be ascertained whether the—(1) patient is pregnant, (2) fetus is in the direct beam, and (3) procedure is relatively high dose. Any women of reproductive age are considered pregnant, when the menstrual period is overdue or missed, excluding hysterectomy or tubal ligation in patients. Advisory notice should be posted at several places as follows:

"If it possible that you might be pregnant, notify the physician or radiographer/ technician before your X-ray examination."

Since diagnostic dose is mostly <50 mGy, pregnancy test is generally not prescribed, However, it may be necessary in high-dose fluoroscopy examination of abdomen or pelvis. Once pregnancy or possibility of pregnancy is confirmed, the radiologist should be informed. He should take suitable measures to keep the dose minimum without compromising image quality.

When the fetus is in the direct beam, it is important to know the procedure is whether low dose or high dose. If it is high-dose procedure, alternative examinations such as ultrasonogram should be suggested. If it is not possible, the stage of gestation, fetus dose, medical indication, and the risk of delaying the examination should be analyzed and shared with referring physician.

Chest X-ray and pelvimetry are two vital procedures for maternal women. WHO recommends no routine chest X-ray during pregnancy, unless a case of silent chest disease (1992). Pelvimetry provides only limited information about pelvic measurements. It should be taken in rare occasions only with clear reasons (WHO, 1999). Of course, ultrasonogram provides required pelvimetry information more effectively.

During Irradiation

X-ray examination of chest, skull, and extremities, which are remote from the fetus, can be done safely at any time, with collimation and routine shielding. Risk of not making the diagnosis creates greater risk than the radiation risk.

When the X-ray examination involving fetus in the direct beam as in abdomen or pelvis, it can be delayed. Not undertaking such examination should provide lesser risk to the fetus. If X-ray examination is performed, enough care should be taken to minimize fetus dose. An alteration of techniques should not reduce image quality. Collimation, high kV_p, removal of grid, and reducing number radiographs are beneficial to the fetus.

Pelvic fluoroscopy such as barium enema gives high doses of about 3–7 mGy. Longer imaging time, double-contrast barium enema may double the radiation dose. If fluoroscopic time exceeds 7 minutes, the dose may approach even 50 mGy. Whenever high-dose procedures are done, parameters such as kV_p, dose rate, exposure time, DAP, grid use, imaging geometry, and projections are recorded to permit subsequent fetal dose estimate.

Computed tomography scan of the uterus causes a fetal dose of 10–40 mGy. Since it is a collimated beam, it is easy to limit the area of interest rather than scanning the entire abdomen.

After Irradiation

Pregnant women exposure can lead to apprehension about possible of fetal effects. It may lead to delay or withheld further diagnostic examinations or termination of pregnancy. Since the dose is <100 mGy, the risk is much low, and termination of pregnancy is not required.

No fetal dose estimation is required in low-dose procedures, whereas it is required in CT and fluoroscopy. The radiation risk depends on fetal dose and gestational age. Determination of embryo/fetus dose from plain X-ray films of abdomen or pelvis radiography is much difficult. Generally, mean skin exposure per film is calculated first then organ dose at depth is estimated. Mean dose of ovaries is often taken as approximate fetal doses.

Countrywide survey data indicates that diagnostic doses vary by a factor of 30 or more for same examination. Factors such as kV_p, waveform, filter, grid, film and screen combination, film processing, etc. are responsible for the variation of doses.

Against the belief, digital fluoroscopy offers high doses than conventional fluoroscopy. Hence, calculation of fetal dose is required if the dose is >10 mGy. Fetal dose depends on patient thickness, distension of bladder, and uterus shape. Fetus-absorbed dose is uniform at early stage, as the fetus grows, the dose is less uniform. Estimation of dose in fluoroscopy is also difficult that requires exposure time, beam movement, and location of the beam. Generally, duration of conceptus in the primary beam is uncertain since the beam is moving. Pulsed fluoroscopy, magnification mode, grid use, etc. influence dose in fluoroscopy.

Ten-day Rule and its Present Status

Ten-day rule was postulated by ICRP for woman of reproductive age. It states that—"whenever possible, one should confine the radiological examination of the lower abdomen and pelvis to the 10-day interval following the onset of menstruation." The original proposal was for 14 days, but this was reduced to 10 days to account for the variability of the human menstrual cycle. In most situations, there is growing evidence that a strict adherence to the "ten-day rule" may be unnecessarily restrictive. When the number of cells in the conceptus is small and their nature is not yet specialized, the effect of damage to these cells is most likely to take the form of failure to implant, or of an undetectable death of the conceptus; malformations are unlikely or very rare. Since organogenesis starts 3–5 weeks postconception, it was felt that radiation exposure in early pregnancy could not result in malformation.

The main risk is that of abortion if the radiation exposure results in death of the conceptus. It requires a fetal dose of >100 mGy for this to occur. Based on this, it was suggested to do away with the 10-day rule and replace it with a 28-day rule. This means that radiological examination, if so justified, can be carried throughout the cycle until a period is missed. Thus, the focus is shifted to a missed period and the possibility of pregnancy. If there is a missed period, a female should be considered pregnant unless proved otherwise. In such a situation, every care should be taken to explore other methods of getting needed information by using nonradiological examinations.

Termination of Pregnancy after Radiation Exposure

According to ICRP-84, termination of pregnancy at fetal doses of <100 mGy is not justified based upon radiation risk. At fetal doses between 100 and 500 mGy, the decision should be based upon the individual circumstances.

The issue of pregnancy termination is undoubtedly managed differently around the world. It is complicated by individual ethical, moral, and religious beliefs as well as perhaps being subject to laws or regulations at a local or national level. This complicated issue involves much more than radiation protection considerations and requires the provision of counseling for the patient and her partner.

At fetal doses >500 mGy, there can be significant fetal damage, the magnitude and type of which are a function of dose and stage of pregnancy. Many believe that this dose can cause sterility in the exposed individual, but really it is not so. The gonads are radiosensitive organs in the human body. The threshold radiation dose for permanent sterility in men is 3.5–6 Gy, and for women 2.5–6 Gy for acute doses. As diagnostic X-ray examinations involve small doses, they imply no risk of sterility.

Pregnancy and Abdomen CT Scan

Occasionally, a patient will not be aware of a pregnancy at the time of an X-ray examination and will naturally be very concerned when the pregnancy becomes known. In such cases, the radiation dose to the fetus/conceptus should be estimated, but only by a medical physicist/radiation safety specialist experienced in dosimetry. The patient can then be better advised as to the potential risk involved. In many cases, there is little risk, as the irradiation will have occurred in the first 3 weeks following conception. In a few cases, the conceptus will be older and the dose involved may be considerable. It is, however, extremely rare for the dose to be high enough to warrant advising the patient to consider terminating the pregnancy.

If a calculation of radiation dose is required to advise the patient, the radiographic factors should be noted if known. Some assumptions may be made in the dosimetry, but it is best to use actual data. The patient's date of conception or date of LMP should also be determined.

Pregnancy and Cardiac Catheterization

There will be many situations where the benefit of performing the procedure is much greater than any small possible harm that might arise from the radiation exposure. However, as always with any medical exposure, each procedure must be clinically justified. Once justified, due care is taken to optimize how the procedure is performed to minimize radiation exposure to the fetus, consistent with achieving the desired clinical outcome. The radiation exposure to fetus predominantly arises from scattered radiation within the patient. Some of the main methods for minimizing the dose to the fetus include:

- Restricting the X-ray beam size to being as small as is necessary for the clinical purpose
- Choosing the direction of the primary beam so that it is as far away from the fetus as possible
- Selecting appropriate exposure factors
- Ensuring that the overall exposure time is as small as possible

For well-performed procedures, estimated fetal doses are typically quite small, and well below the level of concern for radiation effects. As a final comment, putting a lead apron on the table to cut down any primary beam from the X-ray tube reaching the fetus has very little effect, but it can be reassuring to the patient and staff. It is recommended, provided the use of the apron does not compromise the performance of the procedure.

Counseling of Patients

Patients who have received diagnostic studies while pregnant are often alarmed because of emotional perceptions surrounding radiation. The health professionals should advise patients about the steps that will be taken for risk assessment and provide appropriate information regarding the risk associated with diagnostic (and therapeutic) radiation exposure during pregnancy. The following points should be considered:

- It is unlikely that radiation from diagnostic radiological examinations will result in any deleterious effects on the child, but the possibility of a radiation-induced effect cannot be entirely ruled out.
- The patient should be counseled that the risk assessment is being done not because there is reason to believe there is great risk in her circumstance but because it is one of the precautions normally taken whenever a pregnant woman receives certain diagnostic studies. (*Note*: This applies only to diagnostic studies. The risk from therapeutic studies may be severe, such as fetal thyroid ablation.)

- Each case must be assessed according to the gestational age when exposed and the radiation levels received by the conceptus from each exposure.
- A precise fetal dose assessment requires numerous pieces of information about the X-ray system, the examinations conducted, the patient size, etc. Therefore, "typical" fetal dose numbers should be used with the understanding that there may be a significant difference between the "typical" dose numbers and the dose numbers resulting from an actual dose assessment.
- The dose evaluation may take up to a week to complete.
- When all the information is acquired, the radiation risk will be assessed and will be reviewed along with other possible risks of pregnancy so that the physician, the patient, and other involved persons understand the circumstances and can thus make a reasonable decision regarding the management of the pregnancy.

Other Factors

Identification of the patient, female patient of reproductive age, and determination of pregnancy status is necessary before performing any kind of imaging. Elimination of screening X-ray examinations can significantly reduce population dose. Yearly dental check-up with X-ray examinations should be avoided. Use of high-speed films or DR systems in dental X-ray imaging can reduce patient dose. Mammography examination should not be used as a screening procedure in patients with age <35–40 unless there is a familial history of breast cancer.

The repeat X-ray examinations range from 1–15%. This number will be higher in—(1) training centers, due to lack of experience, and (2) mobile X-rays (chest, lumbar spine, thoracic spine, kidneys, ureter, bladder, and abdomens), due to proper positioning difficulty. Lack of AEC may also increase the repeat X-rays and technique chart of various examinations should be posted at the control panel. This will enable the technologist to select correct radiographic technique. The retakes are monitored periodically, and suitable action must be taken to improve image quality.

Improperly loaded cassettes, excessive fog due to light leak or poor film storage conditions, processor artifacts due to dirty components or contaminated chemicals, uncalibrated X-ray unit, or improper imaging techniques can also increase the retakes. A periodic quality assurance program to test the performance of the X-ray unit, image receptors, and film processing systems is necessary.

Effects on Radiation Exposure in Utero (ICRP-84)

It is unlikely that radiation from diagnostic radiological examinations will result in any deleterious effects on the child, but the possibility of a radiation-induced effect cannot be entirely ruled out. The effects of exposure to radiation on the conceptus depend on the time of exposure with respect to the date of conception and the amount of absorbed dose.

Prenatal doses from most properly done diagnostic procedures present no measurable increase in the risk of prenatal death, malformation, or the impairment of mental development over the background incidence of these entities. Higher doses, such as those involved in therapeutic procedures, can, however, result in significant fetal harm.

There are radiation-related risks throughout pregnancy that are related to the stage of pregnancy and the fetal absorbed dose. Radiation risks are most significant during organogenesis and the early fetal period, somewhat less in the second-trimester, and least in the third-trimester.

Central nervous system (CNS) is sensitive to radiation and associated with malformation in low LET radiation <250 mGy. A dose of >500 mGy may cause intrauterine growth retardation and CNS damage during the 7–13 weeks. A dose of >1,000 mGy may reduce IQ by 30 points that lead to severe mental retardation during 8–16 weeks of gestational age.

Radiation has been shown to cause leukemia and many types of cancer in both adults and children. Throughout most of pregnancy, the embryo/fetus is assumed to be at about the same risk for potential carcinogenic effects of radiation as are children. Typical effective doses to the conceptus from diagnostic procedures and CT scan are given in **Tables 7.9 and 7.10**.

TABLE 7.9 **Approximate conceptus doses from diagnostic procedures.**

Diagnostic procedure	*Conceptus dose (mGy)*
Cervical spine (AP, LAT)	<0.001
Extremities	<0.001
Abdomen (21 cm) Abdomen (33 cm)	1.0 3.0
Chest (PA, LAT)	0.002
Thoracic spine (AP, LAT)	0.003
Lumbar spine (AP, LAT)	1.0
Limited IVP (21 cm)	6.0
Fluoroscopy: Small bowel study (6 min, 20 digital spot images)	7.0
Fluoroscopy: Double-contrast barium enema study (4 min, 12 digital spot images)	7.0

(AP: anteroposterior; IVP: intravenous pyelography; LAT: lateral; PA: posteroanterior)

Courtesy: McCollough CH et al, 2007.

TABLE 7.10 **The conceptus doses from single CT scan.**

Examination	*Conceptus dose (mGy)*
Head CT	0
Cheat CT	0.2
CT angiogram of coronary arteries	0.1
Abdomen CT	4.0
Abdomen/Pelvis	25
CT angiography of aorta (Chest through pelvis)	34

(CT: computed tomography)

Courtesy: McCollough CH et al, 2006.

Continuation of Work of a Pregnant Employee in X-ray Department

A pregnant worker can continue working in an X-ray department as long as there is reasonable assurance that the fetal dose can be kept <1 mGy during pregnancy. It is important to ensure that pregnant women are not subjected to unnecessary discrimination. There are responsibilities for both the worker and the employer. First responsibility for the protection of the conceptus lies with the woman herself, who should declare her pregnancy to management as soon as the condition is confirmed. The ICRP-84 recommends the following:

- Restricting the dose to the conceptus does not mean that it is necessary for pregnant women to avoid work with radiation or radioactive materials completely, or that they must be prevented from entering or working in designated radiation areas. It does, however, imply that the employer should carefully review the exposure conditions of pregnant women. Their working conditions should be such that the probability of high accidental doses and radionuclide intakes is insignificant.
- When a medical radiation worker is known to be pregnant, there are three options that are often considered in medical radiation facilities—(1) no change in assigned working duties, (2) change to another area where the radiation exposure may be lower, or (3) change to a job that has essentially no radiation exposure. There is no single correct answer for all situations, and in certain countries, there may even be specific regulations. It is desirable to have a discussion with the employee. The worker should be informed of the potential risks, local policies, and recommended dose limits.
- Change to a position where there is no radiation exposure is sometimes requested by pregnant workers who realize that risks may be small but do not wish to accept any increased risk. The employer may also arrange for this to avoid future difficulties in case the employee delivers a child with a spontaneous congenital abnormality (which occurs at a rate of about three in every 100 births). This approach is not required on a radiation protection basis, and it obviously depends on the facility being sufficiently large and flexibility to easily fill the vacated position.
- Changing to a position that may have lower ambient exposure is also a possibility. In diagnostic radiology, this may involve transferring a technician from fluoroscopy to CT scanning or radiography or some other area where there is less scattered radiation to workers. An ethical consideration is involved in the above two alternatives since another worker will have to incur additional radiation exposure because a coworker became pregnant.
- There are many situations in which the worker wishes to continue doing the same job, or the employer may depend on her to continue in the same job to maintain the level of patient care that the work unit is customarily able to provide. From a radiation protection point of view, this is perfectly acceptable providing the fetal dose can be reasonably accurately estimated and falls within the recommended limit of 1 mGy fetal dose after the pregnancy is declared. It would be reasonable to evaluate the work environment to provide assurance that high-dose accidents are unlikely.
- The recommended dose limit applies to the fetal dose, and it is not directly comparable to the dose measured on a personal dosimeter. A personal dosimeter worn by diagnostic radiology workers may overestimate fetal dose by about a factor of 10 or more. If the dosimeter has been worn outside a lead apron, the measured dose is likely to be about 100 times higher than the fetal dose. Workers

in nuclear medicine and radiation therapy usually do not wear lead aprons and are exposed to higher photon energies. Despite this, fetal doses are not likely to exceed 25% of the personal dosimeter measurement.

- Finally, factors other than radiation exposure should be considered in evaluating pregnant workers' activities. In a medical setting, there are often requirements for lifting patients and for stooping or bending below knee level. There are several national groups that have established nonradiation-related guidelines for such activities at various stages of pregnancy.
- Occasionally, there are situations where family members provide essential medical care, either in the hospital or at home, to patients who have received radionuclides. In such circumstances, public dose limits do not apply to the family member. Efforts should optimally be directed at not involving females who are or may potentially be pregnant. If it is essential to involve the help of a pregnant female, it should be done in such a way that the fetal dose from this involvement does not exceed 1 mGy.

Chance of Approaching the Dose Limits of Exposure

Radiation doses to occupationally exposed staffs working with radiological equipment are generally low and it is unlikely that the equivalent dose limit recommended by ICRP will be approached. However, for some fluoroscopic examinations, there is a potential for higher radiation doses to staffs. During interventional radiology procedures, particular radiation protection problems arise from the extended fluoroscopy times and from the use of certain radiological equipment, which may not have lead rubber-protective curtains. Consequently, the implications of the ICRP recommendations on the radiation exposure of the fetus of staff performing fluoroscopy procedures should be assessed.

RADIATION SAFETY OF PATIENTS (AERB SAFETY CODE)

Radiation safety of patients is ensured by compliance to requirements given in this safety code. Though medical exposures have no "dose limits", all referring physicians, doctors, and X-ray technologists should be aware of radiation protection aspects such as justification and optimization of radiation exposure of patients. For ensuring radiation protection during medical exposures, the hospital/center should—(1) set and follow the standard exposure protocols for adult as well as pediatric patients as per the image quality required for clinical diagnosis; (2) have in place a quality control protocol which should ensure the right procedure to the right patient and correct reporting. The quality control protocol should be reviewed periodically; and (3) provide the patient, dose records for future reference.

For patients who are pregnant or likely to be pregnant, the following aspects should be considered in addition to the above—(1) a woman presenting herself for X-ray examination should be asked about the possibility of pregnancy, (2) radiography of areas away from the fetus such as chest, skull, extremities should be carried out with proper beam limitation and shielding of abdomen and with low-dose protocols.

Pediatric patients: The following practices are deemed unjustified and should be avoided—(1) following adult exposure protocols for children, (2) using AEC systems in imported equipment, which are not customized to Indian population before use,

(3) radiographs taken by unqualified personnel, (4) not considering alternate means of diagnosis (MRI, USG, etc.), (5) not asking for previous X-ray records, for the same ailment, (6) expecting best quality images, even if there is no additional gain in terms of diagnosis.

In addition to the requirements mentioned, for pediatric patients, the following measures should be followed—(1) X-ray beam should be carefully collimated to the area of interest, excluding other regions, especially gonads, breast, thyroid, and eyes, (2) antiscatter grid should be used judiciously for children, when high-image quality is of prime concern, (3) for the desired X-ray tube current and time product (mAs), should use shortest exposure time, and (4) additional filters if provided by design should be used.

Radiation Safety of Personnel

- The operator shall avoid routine holding of patients without using protective aprons
- Ensure holding of children or infirm patients for X-ray examination shall be done by a person wearing lead aprons.
- Always wear protective apron while operating mobile/portable X-ray equipment.
- Use design provided protective ceiling suspended screens and table curtains/ flaps.
- Use personnel monitoring services (TLD badges) as per the guidelines issued by accredited laboratories and regulatory body

Interventional procedures constitute higher radiation exposure to the physicians and allied medical professionals, since the procedures are lengthy, complex, and carried out at proximity to radiation field. Hence, all personnel associated with the use of the interventional radiology/C-arm/fluoroscopy equipment shall:

- Use design provided protective ceiling suspended screens and table curtains/ flaps.
- Position the imaging system as close to the patient surface, as possible.
- In oblique orientation, position themselves opposite to the X-ray tube.

BIBLIOGRAPHY

1. Atomic Energy Regulatory Board (AERB): www.aerb.gov.in
2. Atomic Energy Regulatory Board. (2016). AERB safety Code No. AERB/RF-MED/SC-3 (Rev. 2): Radiation safety in manufacture, supply and use of medical diagnostic X-ray equipment, 2016. [online] Available from https://www.aerb.gov.in/images/PDF/RF-MED-SC-3.pdf. [Last accessed October, 2022].
3. David J. Dowsett, Patrick A. Kenny and R. Eugene Johnston. The physics of diagnostic imaging, Hodder Arnold, 2006.
4. International Atomic Energy Agency. (2012). Radiation protection in pediatric radiology. Safety reports series No. 71, IAEA, 2012. [online] Available from https://www-pub.iaea.org/MTCD/Publications/PDF/Pub1543_web.pdf. [Last accessed October, 2022].
5. International commission on radiological protection (2000). Pregnancy and Medical Radiation. ICRP Publication 84. [online] Available from https://www.icrp.org/publication.asp?id=icrp%20publication%2084#:~:text=Abstract%20%2D%20ICRP%20Publication%2084%20concerns,exposed%20to%20radiation%20each%20year. [Last accessed October, 2022].

6. McCollough CH, Bruesewitz MR, Kofler JM Jr. CT dose reduction and dose management tools: Overview of available options. Radiographics. 2006;26:503-12.
7. McCollough CH, Schueler BA, Atwell TD, Braun NN, Regner DM, Brown DL, et al. Radiation exposure and pregnancy: When should we be concerned? Radiographics. 2007;27:909-18.
8. Parthasarthy KS. Protection of the patient in Diagnostic radiology, Summary of the current ICRP principles, AERB.
9. Safety aspects in diagnostic radiology, Division of radiological protection, BARC,1989.
10. Thayalan K. Basic radiological physics, 2nd edition. New Delhi: Jaypee Brothers Medical Publishers (P) Ltd.; 2017.
11. Bushberg JT, Seibert JA, Leidholdt EM, Boone JM. The essential physics of medical imaging, 3rd edition. Philadelphia, PA: Wolters Kluwer/Lippincott Williams & Wilkins; 2012.

CHAPTER 8

Planning a Nuclear Medicine Facility

INTRODUCTION

Nuclear medicine has both diagnostic and therapeutic application. Hence, patient related to above services should be handled separately. Non-radioactive areas must be separated from radioactive areas. Areas of high activity and contamination shall be demarcated by physical barriers. The active rooms, wards, and areas of source storage and handling shall be marked with radiation symbol and legend denoting the identification of active area and presence of radiation hazards. Active areas shall be arranged in increasing order of the activity with entrance provided at the lowest active area.

Incoming and outgoing radioisotopes are handled separately without any chance of mixing. Based on safety, easy maintenance, durability, and sanitation, the high-tech healthcare environment is addressed. A proper balance between technological and human factor is required.

In general, nuclear medicine facility consists of: (1) reception area, (2) radiopharmaceutical administration, (3) hot waiting areas, (4) diagnostic imaging rooms, (5) toilets, (6) radioactive waste collection room, and (7) therapy rooms **(Fig. 8.1)**.

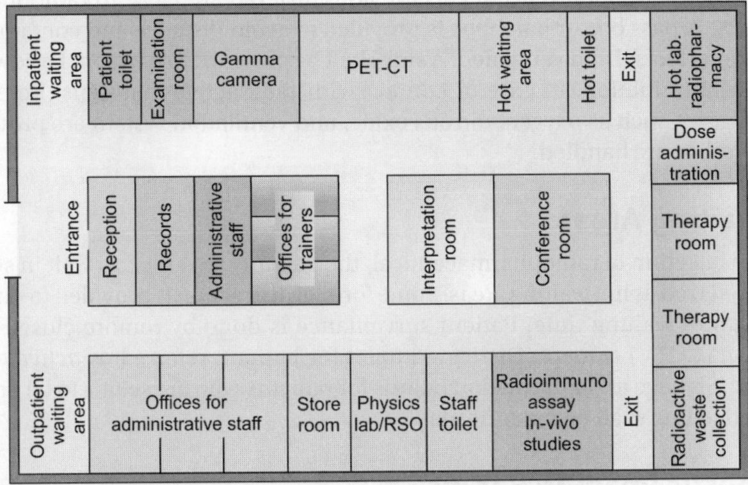

FIG. 8.1: Model floor plan for a full pledged nuclear medicine facility.
Courtesy: IAEA Human health series No. 37, 2020.

GENERAL REQUIREMENTS

Planning a nuclear medicine facility should have nearby airport access for transport of radioactive isotopes from inland and abroad. In local production of short-lived isotopes, reliable delivery must be ensured. Reliable method of transport is essential for consistent supply and delivery. Stable electricity and uninterrupted power supply (UPS) are essential.

Location

Location of the nuclear medicine facility should be chosen that it is away from general patient ward, source of intense radiation, and public occupancy areas. It is close to the related facilities such as general patient and reception area, UPS room, and change room. Fire hazard potential should be minimum in the area chosen. The location of the installation or facilities are made, so that the possibilities for spread of both surface and air bone contamination are minimal.

The location should be chosen that the minimum expenditure on shielding, radiation levels can be effectively maintained with permissible limits in the immediate vicinity. If the facility is located near the plot boundary, a distance of 3 m is maintained between external walls of the facility and plot boundary for any contingency in future. The facility should not be in residential buildings.

Reception Area

The reception should control the patient access to the operation area where radioactivity is used. Standard signage should be displayed prominently to identify areas of radioactivity. The signage should include for possibility of pregnant and breastfeeding patients. The doors must be closed with restricted entry. Only authorized staffs and patients are permitted.

Radiopharmaceutical Administered Rooms

Rooms where radiopharmaceuticals are administered are close to radiopharmacy laboratory. A pass box or hatchbox is provided to avoid distance and contamination and it is interlocked and ventilated. A sink shall be provided to frequent handwashing and decontamination, in case of contact with radioactive materials. Emergency medical gases such as oxygen, nitrous oxide, and ventilation system are provided, if radioaerosols, are handled.

Hot Waiting Areas

After the injection of radiopharmaceutical, the patients are asked to wait in separate rooms, referred as hot waiting areas. Some form of distraction is provided to minimize the length of waiting time. Patient surveillance is done by remote closed-circuit television (CCTV) camera. Dedicated toilet for patient, referred as *active toilet*, is provided. Signage and information boards for patients who are seems to be pregnant or breastfeeding shall be made available.

Diagnostic Imaging Rooms

Rooms to house equipment such as gamma camera, single-photon emission computerized tomography (SPECT)/computed tomography (CT) and positron emission tomography (PET)/CT should have sufficient area and infrastructure facility. Modern scanners may weight 2,500 kg and centered over area of 1 m^2. Hence, floors should be leveled accurately to avoid any misalignment. Floor trenches for electrical and signal cables and video system for monitoring patients are required. In addition, ventilation system, chiller, and reconstruction computer facility should be made available. Additional space for stretcher movement, collimator cart movement, and maintenance are provided. Manufacturer's installation instructions should be followed.

Toilets

Patient and staffs should have separate toilet facilities. A dedicated active toilet is available for patients who had radiopharmaceutical injection. In addition to normal toilet for staffs, one additional toilet is made available for decontamination purpose, whenever arises. It includes sink, eye washing, and shower-bathing facility.

Radioactive Waste Collection Room

A dedicated waste collection room is required for short-term storage before disposal. The room must have secure door, adequate lighting, an electrical system with high degree of protection, containment against flooding, and fire extinguishing system.

Therapy Rooms

Isolation wards shall be provided for patients undergoing nuclear medicine therapy requiring hospitalization. Mostly, it is provided along with general ward such as oncology wards for easy nursing. However, some specific requirements are there for therapy rooms. The access to the rooms is controlled and remote CCTV camera is used for patient surveillance. Discharge of the rooms from the toilet is collected and their release to the general sewage system is delayed sufficiently (delay tank) to permit radioactive decay of the isotope. In case of volatile radionuclides such as iodine-131, special ventilation system is required as per the regulation. Plumbing shall provide direct flow of liquid effluents from active areas directly to the delay tank. Effluent lines and delay tank shall be leak proof and corrosion resistant. Rooms' structural shield must be sufficient as per regulation. A room for temporary collection of radioactive waste is also required.

Air-conditioning

Air-conditioning is essential to maintain a clean, dust-free, and dry environment for electronic instruments that are sensitive to heat and moisture changes; high humidity is bad for electronic components, causing corrosion as well as current leakage. Instruments must be housed in an air-conditioned environment, and a dehumidifier may be needed to maintain humidity at about 50%.

Warning Light and Placard

A suitable warning signal such as the red light must be provided at a conspicuous place outside the room and kept ON when the unit is in use, to prevent entry of persons not connected with the examination or treatment. An appropriate warning placard must also be posted outside the room's entrance or door **(Figs. 8.2A and B)**.

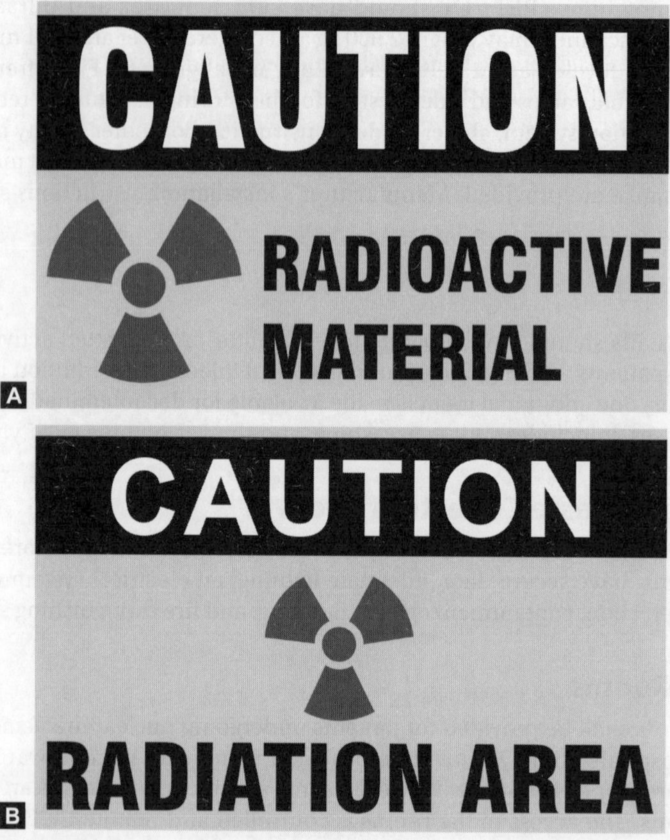

FIGS. 8.2A AND B: (A) Placard for storage and transport containers, (B) Placard for radiation areas/rooms with trefoil symbol. ***(For color version, see Plate 1)***

Approval of Nuclear Medicine Laboratory

The site and layout plan of nuclear medicine facility in 1:200 scale is prepared and submitted through e-Licensing of Radiation Applications (e-LORA) and gets approved from Atomic Energy Regulatory Board (AERB). Plan should indicate various rooms along with their dimensions, positions of doors, windows, exhausts, along with fume hoods, workbenches, sinks and occupancies around it including ceiling and below the floor, if any. Prior to this, institution get registered with AERB and obtain USERNAME and PASSWORD. For additional details, visit the site AERB e-LORA: *www.aerb.gov.in.*

CATEGORIZATION OF LABORATORIES

The level of nuclear medicine services is categorized according to the service it handles. The term level refers to complexity of procedure it involves. There are three levels in diagnostic nuclear medicine facility and two levels in therapy nuclear medicine. Academic institution or general hospital where there is a need for a comprehensive clinical nuclear medicine service, human resource development and research program uses all the services including diagnostic and therapeutic.

Diagnostic Nuclear Medicine Level 1

This level provides basic and general nuclear medicine services. It may be the first in the locality and is suitable for basic primary and secondary healthcare infrastructure services. It is relatively simple in instrumentation with modest infrastructure, and lowest staffing levels.

Diagnostic Nuclear Medicine Level 2

This will offer specialized diagnostic nuclear medicine imaging including cardiac and oncological investigations in addition to the level 1 service. More complex equipment, infrastructure, and human resources may be required, e.g., tomographic capability and quantification.

Diagnostic Nuclear Medicine Level 3

This facility would operate at the highest level, using complex equipment such as hybrid SPECT/CT cameras to perform specialized investigations. This is the most resource-intensive level.

Therapeutic Nuclear Medicine Level 1

This level provides outpatient services to administer a limited amount of radioactivity to patients. Relatively modest support about patient isolation and waste management is required.

Therapeutic Nuclear Medicine Level 2

This level provides for inpatient treatment. The infrastructure will include a designated isolation facility, where patients can remain for the necessary period following administration of high-activity radionuclide treatment. Appropriate radiation monitoring equipment and protected waste storage areas are essential. Staff must be trained to administer high-radionuclide activities safely.

GENERAL GUIDELINES ON FINISHES AND SYSTEMS

Floor

Floors should be welded seam sheet flooring with an integral base in all radiation areas—radiopharmacy, administration room, hot waiting room, diagnostic imaging room, radioactive waste storage room, exercise and stress testing room, and other laboratories.

Ceiling

Ceilings are made generally with lay-in acoustic tiles. Procedure and treatment rooms are made with lay-in acoustic ceiling tiles with a washable sprayed plastic finish. Radiopharmaceutical laboratory should have pharma grade ceiling, in plastic laminate or aluminum, welded and sanitizable.

Walls and Protection

Generally, walls should be easily cleanable and decontaminable. Corridor and nonspecific areas are made with walls that have corner card. Floor tiles can be used to cover corners. This will prevent damage from cart and stretcher movement. Imaging and administration room's walls where specific risk of contamination is possible should be easily washable and decontaminable. Radiopharmaceutical laboratory walls may be covered with pharma grade walls or decontaminable epoxy painting, depending upon the type of laboratory. It can be done with decontaminable epoxy painting. All room corners should be made rounded.

Doors

Radiopharmacy room and radioactive waste storage rooms are provided with secured doors. The access can be through two doors interlocked or between a filter/changing room, depending upon the laboratory level. Scanning rooms must have interlocked doors. Other rooms need no special requirements except an easy cleaning and decontamination. In imaging room, system to control access interlocked to the status of the equipment is not required.

Security Access Control

Security and access control is required to the nuclear medicine facility main area. Radiopharmacy area, source storage rooms, and sensitive data storage area should have restricted entry. Mostly access will be granted by authorized staff.

Heating, Ventilation, and Air-conditioning

Heating, ventilation, and air-conditioning (HVAC) system is required to control possibility of radioactive contamination to the staff and environment from unsealed sources. While handling radiopharmaceuticals, microbiological contamination is possible which should be prevented. Hence, the importance of HVAC system than shielding requirements should be planned at the starting level.

Ventilation system shall be of once-through type with unidirectional airflow. Air is directed to flow from less risk areas of contamination to that of high-risk areas. High-risk areas pressure should be kept low compared that of low risk. Radiopharmacy laboratory is excluded from this and needs specific arrangements. The air coming from outside is filtered to reduce dust and particle. The position of the outside air intake should prevent possibility of recirculation of exhaust air. The exhaust air must be expelled to outside through suitable filters. For example, it can be let out directly to open area after passing through charcoal and high-efficiency particle activity (HEPA) filters.

In areas where hot cells and fume hoods are installed, dedicated exhaust system is provided for each device. Supply air diffusers are positioned as far as away from air inlets and cell doors. HVAC routing through shielding needs special care as per regulation.

Power Supply

Modern scanners require dedicated power supply with adequate power. SPECT gamma camera requires 3–4 kWh, whereas a PET/CT requires 90 kWh and about 20 kWh continuous power supply demand. UPS and generator should support

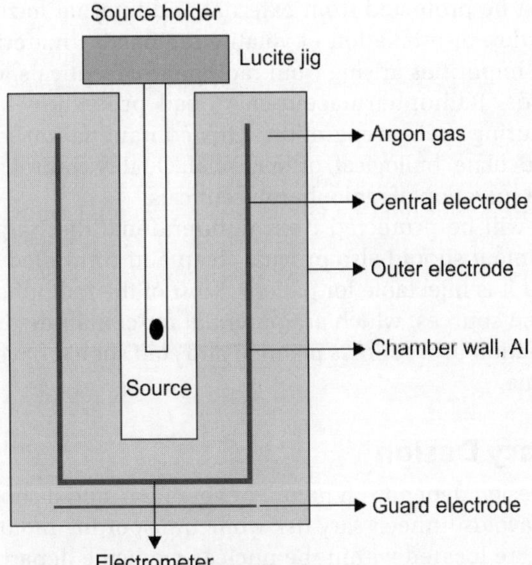

FIG. 8.3: Isotope calibrator.

electric power supply for smooth operation of equipment. This is useful to patient safety and equipment protection. Power lines to other subsystems such as imaging workstations, reconstruction servers, picture archiving and communicating systems (PACS), and radiological information system (RIS) are also required.

Other Essential Requirements

- There should be an adequate supply of lead containers and shielding lead bricks.
- Remote handling devices are desirable.
- *An isotope dose calibrator*: Gas-filled detectors and semiconductor detector systems **(Fig. 8.3)**.
- A fixed zone monitor to display radiation status in that area.
- A portable beta gamma survey meter and contamination monitor. This can be ionization chamber or GM detector type.
- In-house transport container to transport radioisotopes.

RADIOPHARMACY DESIGN AND RADIOPHARMACEUTICAL PREPARATION

Radiopharmaceuticals are medicinal products containing shot-lived radioisotopes and follow local regulation. Range of radiopharmacy varies that based on clinical demand and decision on prepare or purchase. Hence, it requires adequate staffs, facility, operating system, quality system, and equipment necessary to provide radiopharmaceutical of desired quality and safety for patient administration. Radiopharmaceuticals that are injected intravenously should be prepared aseptically to give sterile injections. Standard quality control procedures are in place and secured place for receipt and storage of radioactive material and waste is required. Laboratories should offer safety to the operator, radiopharmaceutical, and the environment. Risk assessment is essential before starting the service or any new procedure.

Operator must be protected from external and internal hazards arising from unintended injection or inhalation of volatile radioactive materials or gas. There may be chemical impurities arising from radiopharmaceuticals, which may cause biological hazards. Radiopharmaceuticals need protection from unintended contamination during their preparation. This contamination may be chemical, radionuclide, particulate, biological, or microbial. Quality control should access the risk and for safe preparation of radiopharmaceuticals.

Environment will be protected from unintentional discharge of radioactive material. Environment should also provide clean and controlled space for aseptic dispensing so that it is injectable for patient. Most of the radiopharmaceuticals are unsealed and open sources, which are potential for contamination and spillages. Clear decontamination procedure is planned and staff should have enough training to perform the same.

Radiopharmacy Design

Radiopharmacy design depends on nature of operation, and it should allow orderly flow of work and avoids unnecessary risk while transporting radioisotopes. Mostly, radiopharmacies are located within the nuclear medicine department and access only by authorized personnel. Its site should be located close to the main facility and relation with other facility with proper shielding as per regulation. It should be away from gamma cameras, patient waiting areas, and offices. It is also important to consider whether there are working areas above or below the radiopharmacy laboratory to avoid unnecessary radiation exposure to people working in those areas. Hot laboratories and radioactive storage areas should be located away from other busy work areas such as public corridors, secretarial offices and away from imaging and low-level counting rooms. Radiopharmacy should have restricted access for security reasons and have lock and key facility. Wash basins and sinks should be made available where unsealed radioactive materials are handled. It is advisable to have elbow or foot-operated taps for sinks in hot laboratories.

All surfaces of walls, floors, ceiling, benches, tables, and seats should be smooth, impervious, and nonabsorbent and allow easy cleaning and decontamination. It should be free from cracks and crevices and covered with nonporous, leak-proof, and nonreactive material, which are easily washable. Floor surfaces, ceiling, and benches should be continuous, nonshedding, easily cleanable, and covered to the wall to prevent accumulation of dirt and contamination. This is much vital on radiation safety point of view and provides environment to handle sterile products for patient administration. Floor, benches, and other work surfaces should be strong and sturdy to bear the weight of lead shielding. Its tabletop should have a smooth laminated finish. The radiation levels outside the laboratory should be within the permissible levels. Technetium-^{99m}Tc) generator should be kept under lock surrounded by shielding material. A good radiopharmaceutical practice of preparation and dispensing is in place to meet the national regulation.

Storage areas will be necessary for radioactive materials as well as for non-radioactive components used in radiopharmaceutical preparation. These areas will need suitable shielding, and depending on the type of product being prepared, a refrigerator and freezer may also be required. A typical radiopharmacy layout is shown in **Figure 8.4**. Laboratory is designed so that there is separate storage of glassware and work tools (tongs, stirring devices), not used with radioactive materials to avoid unnecessary contamination or mixture with similar items used with radioactive preparations.

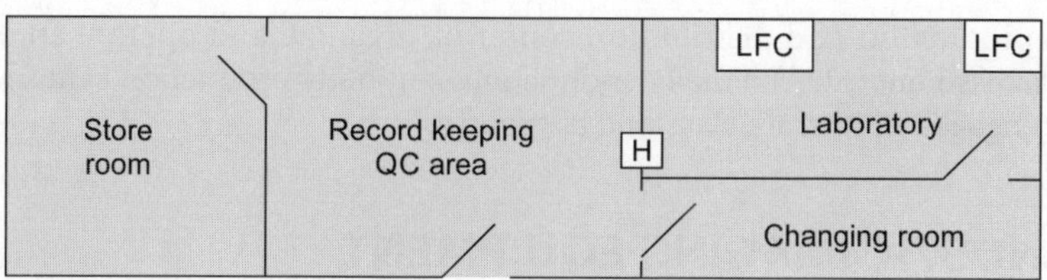

FIG. 8.4: Model of basic radiopharmacy facility.
(LFC: Laminar flow cabinet; QC: quality control; H: Hatchway)

The radiopharmacy needs to be equipped with at least one isotope calibrator so that all activity can be measured accurately. In addition, a reference source (e.g., ^{137}Cs) will be necessary to ensure continuing reliability of the calibrator. Since radiopharmacies will be handling unsealed sources of radioactivity, contamination monitors will be required to check for any radioactivity that may have been spilt.

In Vitro and Radioimmunoassay

The design and structure of the building can affect the quality of a radioimmunoassay (RIA) center. Premises should generally provide working conditions that are hygienic and spacious. A patient reception area with a waiting room and an area for taking blood samples should be available. The reception area should be equipped with a couch, resuscitation trolley, and other special facilities. It is essential to reserve an area for recordkeeping and sorting and labeling of samples.

Floors and benchtop should be smooth and of nonabsorbent material to facilitate cleaning and decontamination in the event of chemical or radioactive spillage. Sinks should be conveniently located at each workbench. A separate wash basin, labeled to this effect, should be reserved for washing of hands of laboratory personnel, with its use prohibited for any other purpose. The washing-up area for glassware, used RIA tubes, and reusable pipette tips should have one or two large sinks and a drying oven.

A storage room for buffer chemicals, solvents, test tubes, and other consumables is provided. A laboratory preparing its own tracers using imported ^{125}I sodium iodide would need a "hot" laboratory with sufficient space to accommodate a fume cupboard, fraction collector and/or high-performance liquid chromatography (HPLC) system, as well as a refrigerator to store stock solutions of radioactive material. The areas designated for assays are separated from those reserved for other activities such as patient reception, recordkeeping, and computing.

Types of Radioimmunoassay Laboratories

Radioimmunoassay laboratories are graded based on nature and scope of activity. A grade 1 laboratory is a basic one using reagents, whether obtained in bulk or as commercial kits, from an outside source, with minimal production of reagents confined to standards and quality control material for the simpler analytes. A grade 2 laboratory would similarly use primary reagents obtained from elsewhere but, in addition, produce its own tracers, at least for selected procedures, using ^{125}I produced elsewhere in the country or obtained from abroad.

A laboratory which can produce polyclonal antibodies, in addition to grade 1 and 2 facility falls into grade 3. A grade 3 laboratory could serve as a national or regional reagent production and distribution center or organize and operate an external quality assessment (EQA). Finally, monoclonal antibody production centers, if they are also engaged in RIA, are classified as group 4.

DIAGNOSTIC IMAGING EQUIPMENT

An in vivo diagnostic imaging facility needs optimal space, equipment, and manpower. The nature and number of equipment required depend on the volume of the service. The design and planning should address many factors including radiation safety. The minimum requirements are: (1) counting systems for uptake measurements, (2) gamma camera, (3) positron emission tomography, and (4) hybrid imaging systems like SPECT-CT,PET-CT and PET-MRI.

Counting Systems for Uptake Measurements

Counting system is required for uptake measurements of thyroid function and other in vitro and diagnostic studies. This includes NaI:Tl well counter, liquid scintillation counter, and in vivo counting systems **(Fig. 8.5)**. Gamma counting systems are based on two types of detectors, namely (1) NaI:Tl or CsI:Tl, (2) CdTe or CZT crystals. It includes probes for thyroid uptake study, probe for sentinel lymph node detection. NaI:Tl or CsI:Tl is used in thyroid study and detects ^{131}I, ^{123}I, and ^{99m}Tc photons. It requires lead shielding around the unit to shield environmental radiation. CdTe or CZT crystals are used as portable intraoperative radiation detection probe. Its features include energy resolution and counting efficiency or sensitivity.

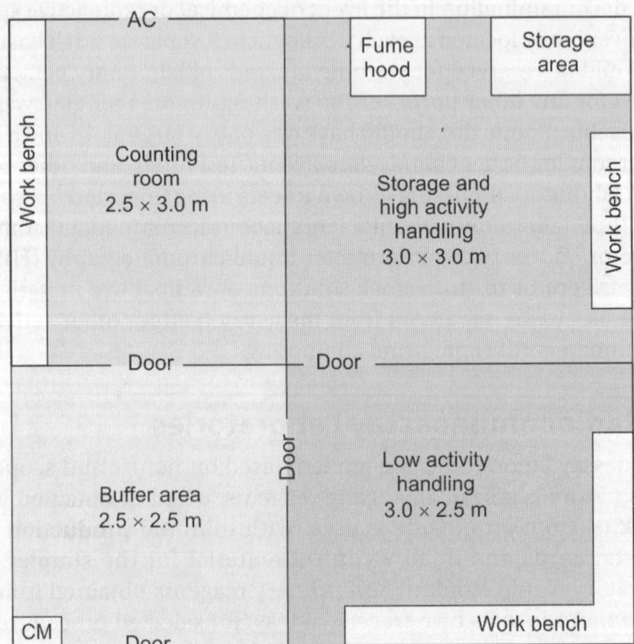

FIG. 8.5: Typical plan of a radioisotope laboratory.

(AC: air conditioner; CM: contamination monitor)

Note: Windows or exhaust to be provided as per requirement

Gamma Camera

A gamma camera is provided with computer and appropriate clinically proven software. It is a device that gives 2D planar images by detecting gamma rays emitted from the radiopharmaceutical administered to the patient. It is capable of tracing in vivo a functional, biochemical, or molecular process. Inorganic crystals such as NI(Tl) or CsI(Tl) are used as crystal with photomultiplier tubes (PMTs). It may contain one or more heads and collimators. Reasonable ranges of collimators are parallel holes collimator, pinholes collimator, diverging collimator, and converging collimator.

Positron Emission Tomography

Patients injected with positron radioisotopes such as Fluorine-18 emit two gamma rays of each energy 511 keV due to positron annihilation within the tumor or pathology site. Detection of annihilation coincidence of photon is useful to reconstruct axial tomography images similar to that of a CT scan. It has a ring gantry with Lu_2SiO_5:Ce (LSO) or $Bi_4Ge_3O_{12}$ (BGO) as detectors with PMTs. Advantage of PET system over SPECT is improved spatial resolution, statistical quality, and quantitative analysis accuracy. Since it does not require mechanical collimator, its image formation process is different from SPECT. Another advantage is to quantify the physiological process in-vivo.

Hybrid Imaging Systems

Positron emission tomography system is offering functional information without anatomical details such as density and tissue composition. CT scan provides required anatomical information with high-spatial resolution, even though the functional information is poor. Hence, emission scanners are combined with CT or MRI scanners, namely SPECT-CT, PET-CT, and PET-MRI to achieve both metabolic and functional, as well as anatomical information.

The SPECT-CT imaging is done in close sequence while the patient is in the same bed; almost, it is equal to simultaneous imaging. CT data is used for attenuation correction of SPECT images, and to display of metabolic data. It allows efficient, simultaneous navigation in function and anatomy. Since two images are obtained in different resolution, the SPECT images need to be scaled down to match voxel sizes. Role of SPECT-CT is rapidly increasing and becomes gold standard in conventional nuclear imaging.

In PET-CT, the patient is in the same bed position and images are acquired by sequential imaging, and the final image is fused and displayed **(Fig. 8.6)**. It gives accurately aligned anatomical and functional images in a single imaging session. In addition, CT provides attenuation correction for PET systems. The temporal and spatial difference between the two sets of images is neglected. It also quantifies the value of standardized uptake value (SUV) at the point of interest. PET-CT becomes a major tool in cancer detection and treatment follow-up. It has application in oncology and nuclear cardiology. It offers fast acquisition and high throughput of patients.

The PET-MRI system offers anatomical and functional information with excellent soft tissue contrast. Integration of systems is more complex and silicon photomultipliers are used instead of PMT, which can operate in the presence of magnetic field. This made the system for simultaneous acquisition in contrast to PET-CT. Segmentation method is used to carry out attenuation correction. Though it uses advanced iterative reconstruction algorithm, it overestimates the SUV values, compared to PET-CT.

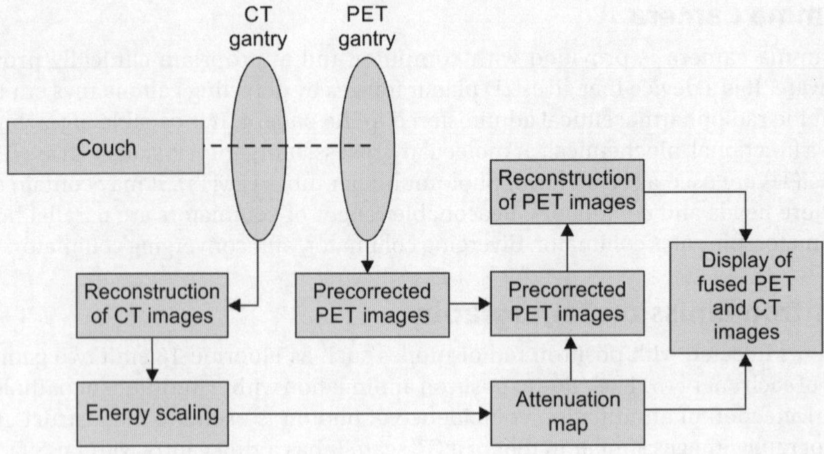

FIG. 8.6: PET-CT functional diagram.

Model Layout Specification for Nuclear Imaging Rooms

Imaging rooms should be at least as large as given in the manufacturer's recommendations, but preferably larger to accommodate patients on stretchers. A larger area provides a more pleasant working environment and reduces the risk of radiation to staff. In some hospitals, rooms should have double glazed and insulated windows to avoid the buildup of dust. Tight fitting oversize doors and efficient heating, air-conditioning, and humidity control units are also required. All rooms should have their own separate power supply and stabilizers and be equipped with hand wash basins with hot and cold running water. An intercom and/or telephone are important for facilitating communication.

- *Land area*: 150–160 m^2 (not to scale)
- *Ceiling height*: 3 m
- *Entrance door*: Double door with placard and warning light

However, land area varies with composition of equipment and service offered. Wall construction material and thickness depend on the equipment, either gamma camera or PET-CT or combination of both. It needs to be calculated based on the workload, isotope, nature of occupation around, and activity handled per week. Facilities using Ge-68/Ga-68 generator will require a hot laboratory of area of 12 m^2. However, an alternative place must be identified in the hot laboratory for storage of decayed Ge-68/Ga-68 generators. Model layouts are shown in **Figures 8.7 and 8.8**.

In general, facility should have rooms for gamma camera/PET-CT, radioactive storage, radiopharmacy, dose administration, postadministration waiting, active toilet, decontamination, and radioactive waste storage. In addition, rooms for physician, technologist, reception, records, etc., are provided. All the walls/partitions of the PET facility should be made of concrete only, the thickness of which will depend on the required workload. Normal brick (9″ or 23 cm) design may be sufficient for gamma camera, whereas PET-CT requires about 23 cm of concrete for walls and ceiling.

Decontamination room is optional. Active toilet may be used for personnel decontamination by providing a shower and wash basin. Radioactive waste storage room for PET facility is optional. Fume hood to be installed, if required.

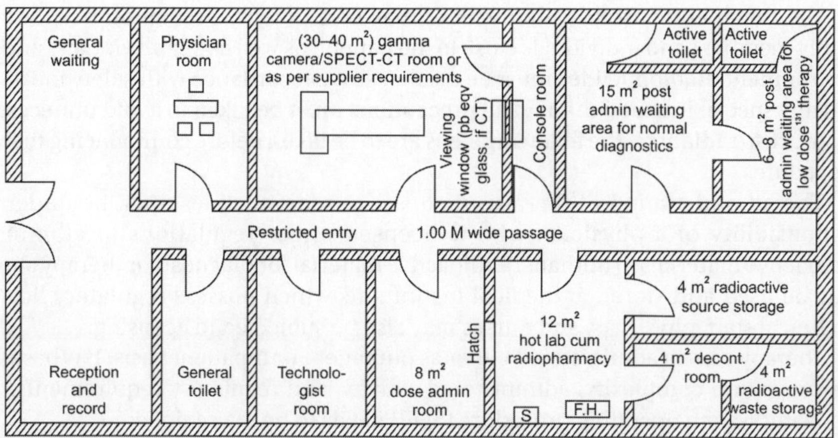

FIG. 8.7: Model layout of nuclear medicine in vivo imaging facility—total area 150–160 m^2.
(FH: fume hood; S: sink)
Courtesy: AERB: website: https://www.aerb.gov.in.

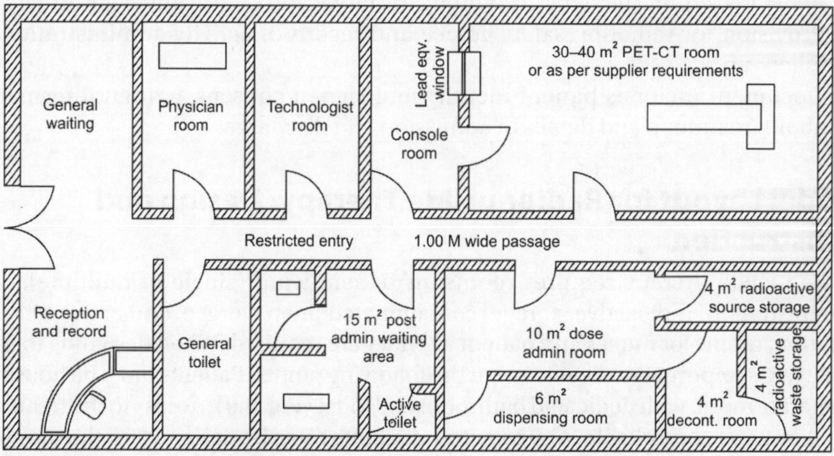

FIG. 8.8: Model layout of PET-CT in vivo imaging facility—total area 150–160 m^2.
Courtesy: AERB: website: https://www.aerb.gov.in.

RADIONUCLIDE THERAPY

Iodine-131 (sodium iodide, NaI) is commonly used for the treatment of thyroid cancer and hyperthyroidism. It is available in the form of liquid and capsules. Phosphorus-32 (sodium phosphate) in colloidal form is used for the treatment of polycythemia vera and some leukemia as well as palliation in metastases of bone. Strontium-89 and samarium-153 lexidronam are used to treat intractable pain from metastatic bone disease. Iodine-131 and yttrium-90 are monoclonal antibodies used to treat non-Hodgkin's lymphomas.

Iodine-131, once administered, is secreted in all body fluids including urine, saliva, and perspiration. Hence, patient requires hospital admission in some cases. It is better to admit patients before the administration of ^{131}I. Radioactive contamination is possible with floor, bed, mattress, light switch, toilet, and telephone, which should be covered with plastic or absorbent-plastic backed paper.

The therapeutic use of radionuclides may be a potential radiation risk for both family members and individuals close to the patient, as well as health workers and the environment. Radionuclides must be used in strict accordance with safety measures and any special instructions, and all precautions must be taken to avoid unnecessary exposure to radiation. The following steps are to be taken before commencing therapy procedures.

The administration of therapeutic doses of radionuclides must be under the responsibility of a physician who is licensed under regulations to administer radioactive materials to humans. Radioactive material for diagnosis or therapy should only be used and stored at medical institutions which possess regulatory license. Technical staff, physicists, and nurses may also be subjected to licensing.

Therapy can be administered either as outpatient or inpatient basis. It is based on the procedure complexity, administered activity, and regulatory requirements. The following system operating procedure (SOP) needs to be maintained:

- Therapy is indicated based on clinical history, histological report, concomitant treatment, hormonal status, and possible medical interaction.
- Pregnancy test of the patient
- Information regarding breastfeeding
- Activity is administered by accounting the target and critical organ absorbed dose
- Provision for radiation safety advice and record of activity administration for follow-up
- Document includes patient identity and signed consent, written information about treatment, and details of admission and discharge.

Model Layout for Radionuclide Therapy: Design and Construction

Radionuclide therapy requires rooms for patient ward (single or multiple), dose administration, radioactive storage, contaminated linen storage, and active toilet. In addition, rooms for nurses and patient attender are required. When designing therapy facility, it is important to bear in mind the following points: Patients must be housed in a separate room, with dedicated bathroom and toilet **(Fig. 8.9)**. Access to the treatment room must be controllable. Any required shielding must be designed for the proposed floor plan in the eventuality of pregnant patients in adjacent rooms. All the walls/partitions of the facility should be made of concrete only, the thickness of which will depend on the area of the room, position of the bed, and the occupancies all around. The ducting line of the fume hood should be shown in the plan, and decontamination room is optional. The active toilet may be used for personnel decontamination by providing a shower and wash basin. Also, the plumbing and ducting line from the isolation ward to the delay tank is to be shown clearly **(Fig. 8.10)**.

It is both easier and less costly to design a facility correctly from the start than to modify it later. Close cooperation between the nuclear medicine staff and architects and builders is vital. If an existing space is to be modified, it may be necessary to determine experimentally the adequacy of walls and floors as radiation shields. If any building work is to be performed, a regular inspection of work in progress is advisable to ensure adherence to agreed plans and specifications.

It should be noted that: (1) brick walls often have inadequate mortar joints, which can be a shielding problem, and (2) flooring should be free of open joints and sealed to the walls, a fact often forgotten by builders.

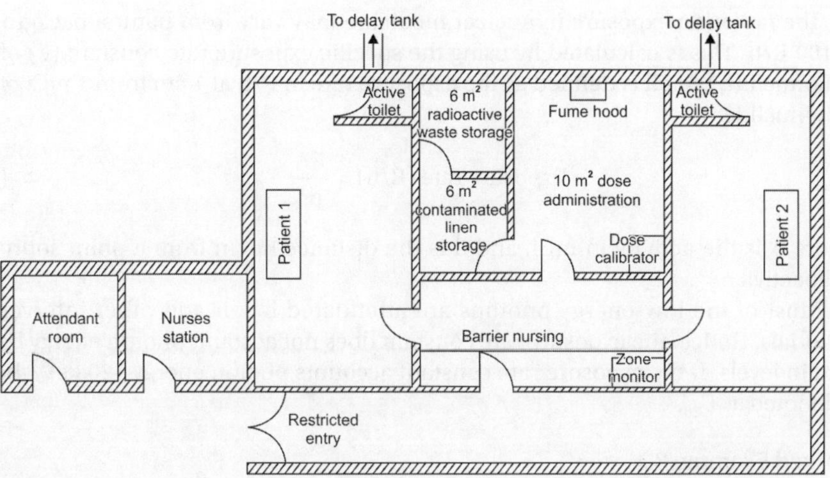

FIG. 8.9: Model layout plan for two bedded isolation ward for with large dose Iodine therapy.
Courtesy: AERB: website: https://www.aerb.gov.in.

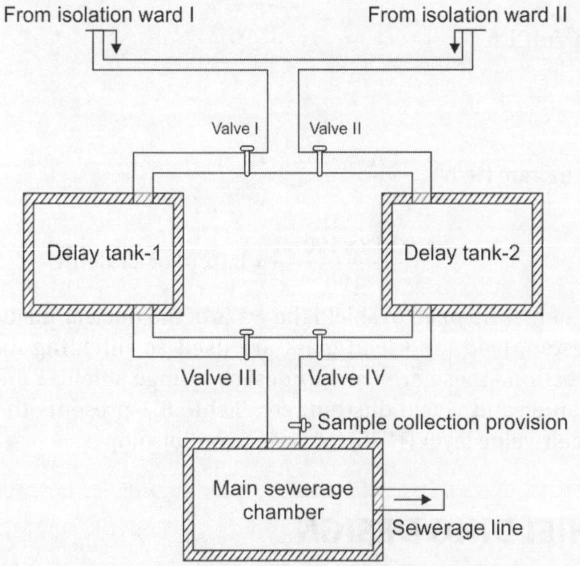

FIG. 8.10: Dual delay tank system for collection and safe disposal of radioactive waste from iodine therapy isolation ward (capacity of the delay tank for a single patient is 3000 liters each).
Courtesy: AERB: website: https://www.aerb.gov.in.

DESIGN AND SHIELDING REQUIREMENTS FOR MEDICAL RADIOISOTOPE LABORATORIES

Nuclear medicine uses liquid isotopes for imaging and therapeutic purpose. Generally, tungsten, lead, lead glass, and leaded acrylic are used as shield for vials and syringes. Syringe shield reduces hand exposure by a factor of 100 during dose preparation and administration. Radiopharmaceutical laboratory uses leaded glass and acrylic shields. Lead pigs, L-bench, isotope storage, and transport lead container are routinely used. Though lead apron and lead gloves are often used, they have limited use in nuclear medicine.

The radiation exposure in nuclear medicine may vary from natural background to 100 R/h. This is calculated by using the specific exposure rate constant (Γ) of the radionuclide, which is defined as the exposure rate in R/h at 1 cm from 1 mCi of the radionuclide.

$$\text{Exposure rate (R/h)} = \frac{\Gamma A}{d^2} \tag{8.1}$$

where A is the activity in mCi, and d is the distance in cm from a point source of radioactivity.

Most of the low-energy photons are attenuated by air and other intervening materials. Hence, the exposure rate constant does not account photon energy below certain levels. If the exposure rate constant accounts photon energy >20 keV, then it is denoted as Γ_{20}.

Worked Example 8.1

A vial contains 100 mCi of ^{131}I having a Γ_{20} = 2.18 R-cm²/mCi-h. What will be the exposure at 100 cm, if a nursing staff sits for 1 hour?

A = 100 mCi

Γ_{20} = 2.18 R-cm²/mCi-h

d = 100 cm

Time = 1 hour

$$\text{Exposure rate (R/h)} = \frac{\Gamma A}{d^2}$$

$$= \frac{2.18 \times 100 \times 1}{100^2} = 0.0218 \text{ or } 21.8 \text{ mR}$$

In general, there is no need to shield the walls of the nuclear medicine laboratory. However, tungsten, lead, and lead glass are used as shielding materials to give personnel protection. These are used to design syringe shield, L-bench, lead pigs, transport container and waste dustbin, etc. **Table 8.1** presents the exposure rate constants and half-value layer (HVL) for various radioisotopes.

PET-CT SHIELDING DESIGN

The PET-CT role is increasing nowadays in clinical application. It is a hybrid machine, which has both PET and helical CT scan. The common radioisotope used in PET is ^{18}F and its energy is 511 keV with a gamma ray constant of 5.66 R-cm²/mCi-h. Its patient dose rate constant is 0.092 μSvm²/MBqh (AAPM-TG 108). Peoples need to be protected are technologists, nurses, facility employees (radiation and nonradiation workers), and public. The areas that should be considered during shielding calculation are radionuclide storage and disposal, radiopharmaceutical administration, uptake room, control console, active toilet, and surrounding areas. The factors influencing radiation protection are radionuclide, procedure protocol, dose rate from the patient, and the facility layout. Shielding design requires determination of transmission first, then referring standard graphs, barrier thickness can be estimated. Shielding is required if transmission factor (B) < 1, and no shielding is necessary, if B > 1. The transmission (B) is given by the relation:

TABLE 8.1 **Exposure rate constants and half-value layer for various radionuclides.**

Radionuclide	Γ_{20} *(R-cm²/mCi-h)**	*Air-kerma rate constant (μSv.m²/GBq.h)*	*Half-value layer, Lead (mm)*
^{125}I	1.47	34.6	0.02
^{131}I	2.18	51.3	3.0
^{99}Mo	1.47	34.6	7.0
^{99m}Tc	0.62	14.6	0.3
^{67}Ga	0.75	17.7	1.0
^{201}Tl	0.45	10.6	0.2
^{51}Cr	0.18	4.24	1.7
^{111}In	3.2	75.4	1.0
^{133}Xe	0.53	12.5	0.2
^{18}F	5.66	135	3.9
^{11}C, ^{13}N, ^{15}O	5.85	139	3.9

*Multiplied by 23.69 will yield air-kerma rate constant in μGy.m²/GBq.h

Courtesy: Bushberg JT et al, 2012.

$$B = \frac{K \times P \times d^2}{T \times N_W \times A_o \times t'} \tag{8.2}$$

where K is a constant that depends on the units used (10.9 or 12.8),
P is the design limit in μSv per week.
d is the distance from the source to barrier in meter
T is the occupancy factor
N_w is the number of patients per week
A_o is the administered activity, in MBq
t′ is the time that varies with uptake time and imaging time

(1). *Uptake room calculation*:
K = 10.9 for uptake room calculation

$$t' = t_U \times R_{tU} \tag{8.3}$$

where t_U is the time between dose administration and imaging, referred as uptake time in hour, usually takes 30–60 minutes, and R_{tU} is the dose reduction factor over time t_U and it is obtained from:

$$R_{tU} = 1.443 \times \frac{T_{1/2}}{t_U} \times \left[1 - \exp\left(-0.693\frac{t_U}{T_{1/2}}\right)\right] \tag{8.4}$$

where $T_{1/2}$ is the half-life of the radioisotope, $R_{tU} = 0.83$, if $t_U = 60$ minutes, and R_{tU} accounts the decay during the uptake time, t_U.

(2). *Imaging room calculation*:
K = 12.8, for imaging

$$t' = F_U \times t_1 \times R_{t1} \tag{8.5}$$

where F_U is uptake time decay factor in μSv, obtained from the relation:

$$F_U = \exp\left(-0.693\frac{t_U}{T_{1/2}}\right) = 0.68,\text{ for } t_U = 60 \text{ minutes} \tag{8.6}$$

t_I is the imaging time in hours, usually 15–30 minutes, and R_{tI} is the dose reduction factor over imaging time tI and obtained from the relation:

$$R_{tI} = 1.443 \times \frac{T_{1/2}}{t_I} \times \left[1 - \exp\left(-0.693\frac{t_I}{T_{1/2}}\right)\right] \tag{8.7}$$

= 0.91 for t_I = 30 min, and 0.95, t_I = 15 min. R_{tI} accounts for decay during the imaging time, t_I.

Worked Example 8.2

A patient is administered 555 MBq of ^{18}F with workload of 40 patients per week and the uptake time is 1 hour. What is the transmission factor, B for an uncontrolled area (T = 1), at a point 4 m from the patient chair in the uptake room?

K = 10.9,

P = 20 μSv/week

N_W = 40 patients/week

d = 4 m,

T = 1

A_o = 555 MBq, t_U = 1 hour

$$t' = t_U \times R_{tU} = 1 \times R_{tU} = 1 \times 0.83 = 0.83 \text{ (by equation 8.3)}$$

$$B = \frac{K \times P \times d^2}{T \times N_W \times A_o \times t'}$$

$$= \frac{10.9 \times 20 \times 4^2}{1 \times 40 \times 555 \times 0.83} = 0.189$$

Referring **Table 8.2**, the thickness required in lead is 12 mm or 16 cm concrete for the transmission.

Worked Example 8.3

A patient is administered 555 MBq of ^{18}F with a workload of 60 patients per week. The uptake time is 60 minutes and the average imaging time is 30 minutes. What is weekly dose equivalent to a point 3 m from the patient during PET scanning? (Dose rate constant for ^{18}F is 0.092 μSvm²/MBqh)

K = 12.8,

P = 20 μSv/week

N_W = 60 patients/week

d = 3 m

A_o = 555 MBq

t_U = 60 min = 1 h

t_I = 0.5 hours

$$t' = F_U \times t_I \times R_{tI} = 0.68 \times 0.5 \times 0.91 = 0.309 \text{ (by equation 8.5, 8.6 and 8.7)}$$

$$\text{Dose equivalent at 3 m} = \frac{\text{Dose rate constant} \times N_W \times A_o \times 0.85 \times t'}{d^2}$$

$$= \frac{0.092 \times 60 \times 555 \times 0.85^* \times 0.309}{3^2} = 89.4\ \mu\text{Sv}$$

TABLE 8.2 **Broad-beam transmission factors for 511 keV in lead (mm), concrete (cm), and iron (cm).**

*Thickness**	*Lead (mm)*	*Concrete (cm)*	*Iron (cm)*
0	1.0	1.0	1.0
1	0.8912	0.9583	0.7484
2	0.7873	0.9088	0.5325
3	0.6905	0.8519	0.3614
4	0.6021	0.7889	0.2353
5	0.5227	0.7218	0.1479
6	0.4522	0.6528	0.0905
8	0.3362	0.5180	0.0319
10	0.2485	0.3987	0.0107
12	0.1831	0.3008	0.0035
14	0.1347	0.2243	0.0011
16	0.0990	0.1662	0.0004
18	0.0728	0.1227	0.0001
20	0.0535	0.0904	—

*Before the start of PET scan, the patient empties the bladder hence only 0.85% activity remains in the patient.

Courtesy: AAPM TG 108.

Worked Example 8.4

A patient is administered 555 MBq of ^{18}F with a workload of 40 patients per week. The floor-to-floor distance is 4 m. The uptake time is 60 minutes, and the average imaging time is 15 minutes. How much shielding is required for an uncontrolled room below the PET-CT room?

$K = 12.8$,

$P = 20\ \mu Sv/week$

$N_W = 40$ patients/week

$d = (d + 1) - 1.7 = (4 + 1) - 1.7 = 3.3$ m

$A_o = 555$ MBq,

$F_U = 0.68$ (by equation 8.6)

$R_{t1} = 0.95$ for $t_1 = 15$ minutes, $t_U = 1$ hour

$$t' = F_U \times t_1 \times R_{t1} = 0.68 \times 0.95 = 0.646 \text{ (by equation 8.5)}$$

$$B = \frac{K \times P \times d^2}{T \times N_W \times A_o \times t'}$$

$$= \frac{12.8 \times 20 \times 3.3^2}{1 \times 40 \times 555 \times 0.85 \times 0.646} = 0.228$$

Referring **Table 8.2**, the thickness required in lead is 12 mm or 14 cm concrete for the transmission. If the room of interest is in upper floor, then the distance $d = (d - 1) +$

0.5 m. If it is adjacent room, d = d + 0.3 m. PET-CT can handle 12 patients per day in 8-hour duty, so that 60 patients can be scanned per week to a maximum.

Alternate method:

$$\text{Weekly dose} = 0.092\,\frac{\mu\text{Sv m}^2}{\text{MBq.h}} \times 40 \times 555\text{MBq} \times 1 \times 0.85 \times \frac{0.646}{3.3^2}$$

$$= 102.98\ \mu\text{Sv}$$

Transmission factor: 20 µSV/102.98 µSV = 0.194

From **Table 8.2**, the thickness of lead required is 12 mm and that of concrete is 15 cm.

Worked Example 8.5

A patient is administered 555 MBq of F-18 with a workload of 40 patient/week. The floor-to-floor to distance is 4 m. The uptake time is 60 minutes, and the average imaging time is 15 minutes. How much shielding is required for an uncontrolled room above the PET-CT room?

$$K = 12.8,\ P = 20\ \mu\text{Sv/week}$$

$$N_W = 40\ \text{patient/week}$$

$$d = (d - 1) + 0.5 = (4 - 1) + 0.5 = 3.5\ \text{m}$$

$$A_o = 555\ \text{MBq},\ F_U = 0.68$$

$$R_{tI} = 0.95\ \text{for}\ t_I = 15\ \text{minutes}$$

$$t' = F_U \times t_I \times R_{tI} = 0.68 \times 0.95 = 0.646$$

$$B = \frac{K \times P \times d^2}{T \times N_W \times A_o \times t'}$$

$$= \frac{12.8 \times 20 \times 3.5^2}{1 \times 40 \times 555 \times 0.85 \times 0.646} = 0.257$$

Referring the **Table 8.2**, the thickness required in lead is about 10 mm or 14 cm concrete for the transmission.

BIBLIOGRAPHY

1. Atomic Energy Regulatory Board. Nuclear medicine facilities: AERB Safety code No: AERB/RF-MED/SC-2 (Rev. 2), 2011. [online] Available from https://www.aerb.gov.in/images/PDF/CodesGuides/RadiationFacility/MedicalApplicationsInvolvingRadiation/3.pdf. [Last accessed October, 2022].
2. Bushberg JT, Seibert JA, Leidholdt EM Jr, Boone JM. The essential physics of medical imaging, 3rd edition. Philadelphia, PA: Wolters Kluwer/Lippincott Williams & Wilkins; 2012.
3. Cherry SR, Sorenson JA, Phelps ME. Physics in nuclear medicine, 4th edition. Philadelphia, PA: Elsevier Saunders; 2012.
4. International Atomic Energy Agency. Nuclear medicine resources manual, IAEA Human health series No. 37, Vienna, 2020. [online] Available from https://www.iaea.org/publications/13391/nuclear-medicine-resources-manual-2020-edition. [Last accessed October, 2022].
5. Madsen et al. AAPM Task Group 108: PET and PET/CT shielding. Med Phys. 2006;33(1):4-15.
6. Atomic Energy Regulatory Board (AERB), website: https://www.aerb.gov.in

CHAPTER 9

Quality Assurance in Nuclear Medicine

INTRODUCTION

Quality assurance (QA) is a set of procedures carried out in an equipment to verify manufacturer's specifications. In medical use of radiation, QA policies are helpful to maintain the quality of patient care. It is designed specific to an equipment to meet international standards. If it is done during the installations of an equipment, it is referred as acceptance testing. Acceptance testing meant for initial evaluation of an equipment performance. It also establishes baseline data for that equipment to compare with future test data. QA tests performed on the equipment later are referred as quality control (QC). It is to verify that the system is working within the limits of initial evaluation or baseline data.

Quality assurance in nuclear medicine is essential to ensure that the equipment is always performing to its specifications. The type of QA program and acceptance testing guidelines vary with type of equipment and country. However, the Joint Commission on the Accreditation of Healthcare Organizations (JCAHO), United States (US) and the National Electrical Manufacturers Association (NEMA) guidelines form the basis for most of the QA tests. Additional information can be obtained from International Atomic Energy Agency (IAEA) human health series and American Association of Physicists in Medicine (AAPM) task group reports as listed in the reference.

Quality assurance tests are performed initially during the acceptance testing and commissioning. QC tests are repeated as annual, quarterly, weekly, and daily basis. Sources required are point source, line source, and sheet flood sources of radionuclides, namely: ^{99m}Tc, ^{57}Co, ^{201}Tl, ^{123}I, ^{67}Ga, ^{131}I, and Indium (^{111}In). Required phantoms are quadrant bar phantom and single-photon emission computed tomography (SPECT) phantom with lead pot and lead mask. Proper energy and energy windows of radionuclide must be used as in **Table 9.1**. All the measurements must be taken under same conditions such as clinical studies. AERB recommended (1) QA tests for gamma camera/SPECT and (2) positron emission tomography (PET) and PET/CT are discussed in the following paragraphs.

TABLE 9.1 **Energy and energy window of radionuclides.**

Radionuclide	*Gamma energy level (keV)*	*Energy window (%)*
^{201}Tl	70,167	20
^{133}Xe	81	20
^{57}Co	122	20
^{99m}Tc	140	15/20
^{123}I	159	20
^{67}Ga	94,184,296	20
^{111}In	171,247	20
^{131}I	364	20

(*Source*: AAPM TG-177).

QUALITY ASSURANCE FOR GAMMA CAMERA

Quality assurance of gamma camera and SPECT consists of the following tests. All the tests are carried out as per IAEA human health series 6, 2009 and AAPM task group 177, 2019 recommendations **(Box 9.1)**.

Centering of Pulse Height Analysis Window

Aim is to test all preset pulse height analysis (PHA) windows and ensures that it properly centered for various clinical radionuclides. A point source of 10 MBq with source mounting system and lead mask are required.

After removing the collimator, the source on the mounting system is aligned with the head. Lead mask is positioned centrally on the crystal housing. Default energy and window width for the radionuclide are set. Observe the display and inspect whether the said photopeak is centered in the window settings. If not, center the photopeak manually over the window width. Peak value that properly centers the photopeak is noted. This can be repeated for other radionuclides.

If the system is not having pulse height spectrum, manually set correct energy of radionuclides with narrow window (5%). Check maximum counts at the correct energy level or record the energy at maximum count level.

Tolerance: Visual observation

Intrinsic Flood Field Uniformity

Aim of the test is to count density variation over the camera's useful field of view (UFOV) without collimator. A point source of Technetium-99m (Tc) of activity 10–20 MBq is required. QA frequency is acceptance testing—annual and daily.

After removing the collimator, the head is rotated towards the point source. Source is placed on a gypsum wallboard and centered over the detector UFOV. A lead mask is positioned centrally on the crystal housing, or the source is placed on a lead shield with copper attenuating plates and suspended in air. The distance between the detector and point source is kept as 5 × UFOV. This will give 2% lesser count rate at detector edge than its center. Lower distance requires software correction for nonuniform illumination. Acquire flood images with 10 million counts for matrix size

Box 9.1: Recommended QA tests for gamma camera/SPECT.

Parameter

- Centering of PHA window
- Intrinsic flood field uniformity
- Extrinsic flood field uniformity
- Intrinsic flood field uniformity through narrowed and asymmetric (off-centered) PHA windows
- Intrinsic spatial resolution and spatial linearity
- Extrinsic spatial resolution
- System planar sensitivity
- Collimator hole angulation
- Intrinsic count rate performance and dead time with and without scatter medium
- Maximum count rate
- Multiple window spatial registration (MWSR)
- Detector dead shielding leakage
- Scan speed energy resolution
- Energy resolution

SPECT scanner

- Pixel size (x and y direction)
- Integral tomography uniformity
- Tomographic resolution in air (x and y direction)
- Center of rotation offset and alignment axes
- Slice thickness at the center of the field of view
- Variations of uniformity of sensitivity with angle
- Alignment (registration calibration SPECT/CT)

Note: QA part of CT component same as diagnostic CT, refer Chapter 6, Quality Assurance in Diagnostic Radiology. Additional test includes alignment of table to gantry, accuracy of gantry tilt, and table indexing accuracy.

(CT: computed tomography; PHA: pulse height analysis; QA: quality assurance; SPECT: single-photon emission computed tomography)

of 256 × 256 or larger. The required number of counts depends upon purpose of the test and vendor's protocol.

Hard copy of the image is obtained and visually inspected for nonuniformities and reported. Alternatively, quantitative analysis of flood images can be done with software help. Integral uniformity (IU) and differential uniformity (DU) in UFOV and central field of view (CFOV) can be deduced. Acquired flood images are compressed to 64 × 64 matrix before analysis. Vendor provides software for automatic analysis.

Tolerance is ±10% of the reference value.

Extrinsic Flood Flow Uniformity

To test the systems uniformity of the camera, including the collimator defects. All the parallel-hole collimators are tested with planar sheet source. Other multi-hole collimator may also be tested. Flood source of ^{99m}Tc is used for acceptance testing and annual test, whereas ^{57}Co flood source is used for daily checking. QA frequency is acceptance testing—annual and quarterly.

Collimator to be tested is mounted on the head so that head is vertically facing upward. The planar sheet source is kept on the collimator directly. For parallel-hole collimator, a 15-cm gap is allowed which enables the dual detector system to acquire counts simultaneously. The observed count rate of parallel-hole collimator is independent of distance. Vendor's PHA window is centered on the photopeak. Image acquisition is made with matrix size of 256 × 256 or larger. Acquire 10 million counts for acceptance testing, and 5 million counts for routine testing.

Image is inspected visually for any nonuniformity such as variations in brightness or density. Collimator defects may appear as singular areas of nonuniformity. No structural pattern is seen expect in high-energy collimators, which is due to ability of the detector to resolve thick septa in areas between photomultiplier tubes (PMTs). It is not usually considered as PMT pattern. Quantitative analysis of the image is performed to obtain IU over the UFOV. This can be achieved automatically by software's assistance. Reports include IU of UFOV, collimator defects, or visible PMT pattern. Acquired flood images are compressed to 64 × 64 matrix before analysis.

Tolerance is ±10% of the reference value.

Intrinsic Flood Field Uniformity through Narrowed and Asymmetric (Off-centered) PHA Windows

Aim is to test the gamma camera for PMT imbalance or decoupling and crystal hydration through narrowed and asymmetric PHA windows. Flood source required is ^{99m}Tc and arrange the system as earlier in Intrinsic Flood Field Uniformity test. QA frequency is acceptance testing and annual.

Set 15/20 PHA window on the photopeak, acquire images on the display with suitable counts, and record hard copy of an image. Repeat the same for 10% of the PHA window (126 and 154 keV) and acquire flood field images for each detector. Set 10% PHA window asymmetrically over lower half of the photopeak (126–140 keV), which should acquire counts only from the lower half of the photopeak. Set 10% PHA window asymmetrically over upper half of the photopeak (140–154 keV). This should acquire only from the upper half of the photopeak.

Images are inspected visually for unusual pattern of nonuniformities at narrower PHA windows. Quantitative values of uniformity are also obtained with software help. All PMTs are identified, if a single or multiple PMTs are visibly different, it refers to tube imbalance or decoupling. If multiple hot spots are seen, it refers to crystal dehydration.

Tolerance: Visual observation

Intrinsic Spatial Resolution and Spatial Linearity

Aim of the test is to measure intrinsic spatial resolution and spatial linearity of the gamma camera without collimator. ^{99m}Tc line/point source, slit phantom, or quadrant bar phantom are required **(Fig. 9.1)**. QA frequency is acceptance testing—annual and weekly.

Spatial resolution is a measure of sharpness and detail of gamma camera, which is measured by the width of line spread function (LSF). LSF is obtained by plotting the count density profile orthogonally across the line source image. The resolution achievable by the detector and the electronics, excluding the blurring caused by the collimator, is called intrinsic special resolution. It is limited by two factors, namely: (1) multiple scattering of gamma photons within the detector, and (2) statistical

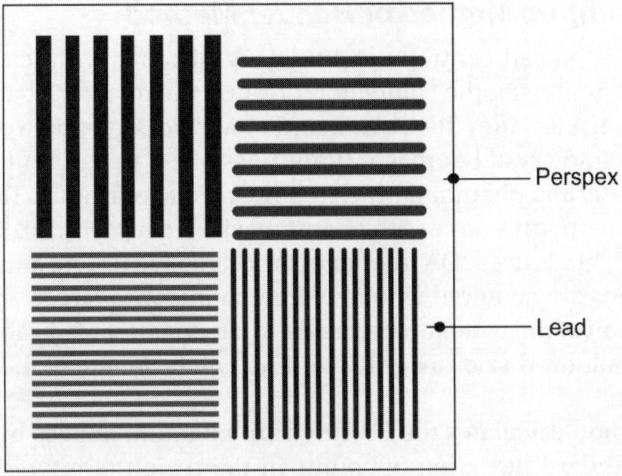

FIG. 9.1: Quardrant bar phantom.

Courtesy: IAEA human health series No. 6.

fluctuation in the distribution of light photons among PMT from one scintillation event to the next. Spatial resolution may vary across the field of view (FOV).

Spatial resolution is specified at width of the LSF at half height referred as full width at half maximum (FWHM). Full width at tenth maximum (FWTM) is also specified which is a measure of contrast loses. Another method of measuring resolution is by using quadrant bar phantom of bar widths 2, 3, 3.5, and 4 mm. It consists of four different panels of parallel bars of decreasing size and spacing to cover the UFOV. The bar width of the smallest quadrant should be half of the expected spatial resolution.

Spatial linearity refers to the ability of gamma camera to locate acquired events accurately. Nonlinearity is measured as deviation between true and imaged line source locations in mm.

Slit Phantom Method

After removing the collimator, the slit phantom is attached. Position the slit phantom close to the crystal face and 2–3 mm thick cardboard is kept between the phantom and crystal. Point source of activity 200–400 MBq of ^{99m}Tc is placed centrally at 4 × UFOV distance. QA frequency is acceptance testing and annual.

Camera zoom factor and matrix size are so chosen that the pixel size perpendicular to the slit is <0.2 FWHM. Acquire minimum of 250 counts per pixel at the peak location of the slit in the image. Hard copy of the image is obtained.

For spatial resolution analysis, obtain LSF on the computer display by placing a wide profile (30 mm) orthogonally across on each slit image. Minimum of 1,500 counts at the peak location of LSF profile is required. If the pixel size is >0.2 FWHM, peak values are obtained from the parabolic fit of three largest counts of the LSF peak. Linear interpolation is used to half-maximum position on either side of the LSF peak. A 30 mm separation between the slit can be used to check pixel calibration.

For spatial linearity, inspect images of the slit for nonlinearity. Bending of line images around the PMT refers to loss of tube balance. Results are reported as no nonlinearity or <1 or >1 mm.

Tolerance: ≤1 or ≤1.05 mm of the reference value.

Quadrant Phantom Method or Hander Method

A point source is placed centrally at 4 × UFOV distance with lead mask without collimator. After removing the collimator, position the quadrant bar phantom close to the crystal face. A 2–3 mm thick cardboard or acrylic is kept between the phantom and crystal to avoid crystal damage. If not possible, a gap of up to 2.5 cm is kept between the crystal and phantom, which require no magnification. The magnification factor for a 2 meter point source with phantom with 2 cm gap is 1.013. A point source of 40–200 MBq ^{99m}Tc is used. QA frequency is acceptance testing annual and weekly.

Digital images are acquired with 5 million counts with largest matrix size. Pixel size should be half of the width of the smallest bar. Smallest resolvable bar is visually inspected. A quadrant is said to be visible, if half of the length of the bar is observed at that quadrant.

Hander method calculates the FWHM from phantom images by comparing the average and standard deviation of counts in the region of interest (ROI). Hence, circular ROI is drawn over a visible quadrant with a bar size that best matches the expected FWHM. ROI is centered in the quadrant as largest as possible excluding the edges. FWHM is calculated by using ROI analysis tool (AAPM TG-177). Average pixel values and standard deviation are reported.

For spatial linearity, inspect images of the phantom for nonlinearity. Bar patterns should be straight and without distortions. Bending of bar images around the PMT refers to loss of tube balance. Results are reported as no nonlinearity or <1 or >1 mm.

Tolerance: ≤1 mm or ≤1.05 of the reference value.

Extrinsic Spatial Resolution and Spatial Linearity

Aim is to test the system spatial resolution of the camera with installed collimator. It is measured with a line source in air at 10 cm from the collimator face. It is done for each parallel hole low-energy collimator. Line source containing activity of 200–400 MBq of ^{99m}Tc or ^{57}Co source of similar activity, and quadrant bar phantom is required. Former is used with low-energy collimator, whereas later is used for medium- and high-energy collimators. QA frequency is acceptance testing—annual and weekly.

The collimator to be tested is attached to the head. The line source is placed parallel at 10 cm away from the collimator face, and perpendicular to the axis of measurement. Separate images are obtained along x-axis and y-axis. Matrix size and zoom factor are chosen so that digital resolution perpendicular to the capillary tube is <1/5 of expected FWHM. Acquisition is continued until the peak count in the image exceeds 500 counts.

When quadrant bar phantom is used, it is placed directly on the face of low-energy collimator. Then a ^{57}Co sheet source is placed on it. High-resolution matrix is chosen so that pixel width should be half of the smallest bar width. Acquire two images per detector by rotating the phantom to 90° or 180° during imaging. Each image should contain at least 5 million counts.

For spatial resolution analysis, obtain LSF on the computer display by placing a wide profile (30 mm) orthogonally across on each slit images. Profiles are drawn at several locations spanning the detector FOV. Peak LSF value is found by parabolic fit with three largest counts of the LSF peak. Linear interpolation is used to identify half-maximum position on either side of the LSF peak. In the case of bar phantom images, visually identify the smallest resolvable bars. A quadrant is said to be visible, if half of the length of the bar is visible at that quadrant.

For spatial linearity, the line source or bar pattern is inspected visually for nonlinearity. Bar patterns should be straight and without distortions. Bending of bar images around the PMT refers to loss of tube balance. Results are reported as no nonlinearity or <1 or >1 mm.

Tolerance spatial resolution: ≤1.05 of the reference value.
Tolerance spatial linearity: ≤1.05 of the reference value.

Extrinsic Planar Sensitivity

Aim is to test the planar sensitivity of the gamma camera. It is measured in counts per minute per activity (CPM/kBq). A disk source of ^{99m}Tc of known activity is required. Frequency of QA is acceptance testing and annual.

The source is centered in the UFOV by means of a low-attenuation source holder (cardboard box), at a constant distance (say 10 cm). Activity is measured with low-energy parallel hole collimator under low attenuation and scattering conditions. Acquisition is made for 1 minute for a given matrix size. It is repeated for all detector, radionuclide, and collimator combination. The time of assay and time of imaging are noted. Background counts are obtained for the same matrix size for 1 min.

Total counts with source and background are obtained for each detector, radionuclide, and collimator combination. The entire matrix is used to get total counts, instead of ROI. Decay and background corrections are applied. System sensitivity is calculated for each detector, radionuclide, and collimator combination. In the case of multihead camera, ratio of the sensitivity to other is found in terms of percentage.

Tolerance for planar sensitivity is ±10% of reference value.

Collimator Hole Angulation

Aim is to test the septal alignment and hole angulation for all parallel hole collimators. A point source containing 200–320 MBq activity of ^{99m}Tc is required. QA frequency is acceptance testing.

Collimator to be tested is mounted on the head and the head is turned towards a wall. A point source with holder is placed near the wall at 2.5 m from the collimator face. Source is properly aligned to the center of the collimator. Image is acquired to a preset level of 5×10^6 counts with default PHA and maximum matrix size. The test is repeated by keeping the point source at four additional locations on the collimator. Each location should be about halfway to the edge of the FOV. It is repeated for all parallel hole collimators.

Image is visually inspected with maximum matrix size display. The shape of the point source is noted. Image at the center may appear symmetrical and round. The hole angulation or collimator defects may appear as streaks or severely distorted shape.

Tolerance for collimator hole angulation is ±10% of reference value.

Intrinsic Count Rate Performance

Aim is to measure count loss (20%) due to dead time of the camera at high-count rates. Count rate is plotted as a function of source activity. The maximum count rate and the count rate at which 20% count loss occurs are identified. QA frequency is acceptance testing and annual.

Various methods of measurements are suggested, and two-source method is explained below. It can be done both intrinsically and extrinsically. Two-point sources of 2 MBq activity of ^{99m}Tc is required, assuming each source makes count loss of about 10%, while the observed count rate is 80,000–100,000 counts per second (cps). Source activity depends on the detector size and distance.

For intrinsic test, remove the collimator from the head and turn the head horizontally. Position the lead mask on the crystal housing with default PHA window. (1) One of the sources is kept in air near the central axis of the detector at 30 cm distance from the detector to minimize scatter. Larger FOV camera requires low activity while low-energy high-resolution collimator (LEHR) camera needs higher activity. It is measured for each detector in multiple detector system. A static image is acquired for 10 seconds.

(2) The second source is suspended beside the first source without interfering the view of the first. Second static image is taken for 10 seconds. (3) After removing the first source, third static image is acquired with only with second source. (4) Remove the second source, record the background count, and count rate for the same time. The whole procedure is repeated by reversing the order of the source.

All data set net counts rate is corrected for background. Pulse pair resolving time or dead time (τ) in microsecond is calculated using paralyzable formula for each set of data:

$$\tau = \frac{2R_{12}}{(R_1 + R_2)^2} \times \ln \frac{(R_1 + R_2)}{R_{12}}$$

where R_1 are R_2 the net count rate for sources 1 and 2 respectively, and R_{12} count rate of both sources 1 and 2. Input count rate (ICR) for 20% count loss ($R_{-20\%}$) is calculated as follows:

$$R_{-20\%} = \frac{1}{\tau} \times \ln\left(\frac{10}{8}\right) = \frac{0.2331}{\tau}$$

Output count rate (OCR) for 20% count loss ($C_{-20\%}$) is calculated as follows:

$$C_{-20\%} = 0.8 \times R_{-20\%}$$

Tolerance of dead time is ±10% and input count rate is ±10% of reference.

Maximum Count Rate

The aim is to test the maximum count rate of the scanner. A point source of 40 MBq of ^{99m}Tc, movable stand, and lead mask are required. QA frequency is acceptance testing and annual.

Remove the collimator from the head and turn the head horizontally. Position the lead mask on the crystal housing with default PHA window. The source on the movable stand is kept at large distance in air and positioned along the central axis of the detector. Count rates are recorded as the source is moving progressively towards the detector. The count rate increases, reaches a maximum, and then decreases. Measurements should be taken quickly to avoid overestimation. The maximum count rate is recorded and compared with vendors reference value.

Tolerance: ±20% of the reference value.

Multiple Energy Window Spatial Registration

The aim is to test the accuracy of gamma camera's position events as a function of energy. A point source of multiple energy such as ^{67}Ga: 93 keV, 184 keV, and 300 keV is required. Each photopeak is imaged with separate energy window. The source is kept in 6 mm thick lead vial having a circular aperture of 5 mm at the bottom. Alternatively, five-point sources in an unshielded plastic vial can be placed, so that one source at the center and remaining four sources on the corners of the FOV on a parallel hole collimator. QA frequency is acceptance testing and annual.

Position the source directly on the crystal without collimator or on the low-energy parallel hole collimator. Source is imaged for nine positions, one at the center, four points on the x-axis, and four points on the y-axis. The off-axis points are 0.4 and 0.8 times of the distance from the center to edge of UFOV on both x+, x–, y+, and y- directions. Acquisition of image is done for every energy window of 20%. Center the PHA window at 93 keV, 184 keV, and 300 keV photopeak, if three energy windows are available. Point sources are imaged until the peak pixel count reaches a minimum of 1,000 counts.

Line profiles of 5–10 pixel wide are drawn on x and y directions for each of the point sources on the acquired image. The profile is centered on the point source and of short length and has odd number of pixels to include half maximum of peak counts on either side of the photopeak. The centroid of counts for each point source is calculated in mm. Displacements for each energy window are compared with reference value.

Tolerance: ≤1.10% of reference value.

Detector Head Shielding Leakage

The aim is to test detector head leakage so that it should response only to incident radiation that passes through the collimator. Point sources of activity of 4 MBq of ^{99m}Tc are required. QA frequency is during acceptance testing.

Collimator suitable to the gamma energy of the source is mounted on the camera head with default PHA window. Sources are positioned consequently at 12 locations around the detector head shielding. It is also found in locations of cable exit and shield joints. Counts are recorded for each site for a preset time of 100 seconds. The source is positioned in the FOV at 10 cm from face of the collimator. Counts are recorded for the same 100 seconds. Remove the source and record the background counts.

Maximum count when the sources are around the detector head is obtained. Similarly, counts when the source transmits through the collimator are noted. Ratio of the two counts gives the percentage of leakage of the head.

Tolerance: ≤1.10% of reference value.

Scan Speed

The aim is to check the correct speed of electronic window and nonuniformities of scan speed. A flood source of ^{99m}Tc or ^{57}Co is required. If line source is used, the length of the source should cover the lateral field view completely when it is positioned perpendicular to the direction of scan. QA frequency is during acceptance testing.

The flood source is fixed to the collimator. A default PHA window is centered on the photopeak and counts rate <20,000 counts/s is obtained. Whole body scans are performed with different speed.

Scans are inspected visually for intensity variations. Longitudinal profiles are drawn through the middle of digital image. If it is a two-pass system, two longitudinal profiles are drawn. The intensity of the profile should be smooth or flat. Profile intensity fluctuation of >5% requires rectification.

Tolerance: ≤1.05% of reference value.

Energy Resolution

The aim is to measure the energy resolution of the gamma camera by measuring FWHM of the energy peak. A point source of ^{99m}Tc of energy 140 keV is used. Energy resolution of other radionuclides, keV per channel, and different detectors also be tested. Frequency of QA is acceptance testing and annual.

Using the point source, intrinsic energy spectrum is obtained such as uniformity imaging. It ensures that each PMT is illuminated uniformly. Acquisition is made by either (1) stored spectrum and (2) manual spectrum method. In the former method, acquisition is made with smallest keV per channel available, so that peak channel should have 10,000 counts. The FWHM is obtained by using vendor's software.

In the manual spectrum method, series of measurement of the counts are made in a narrow 2% energy window. Center of the energy window is shifted across the range of energies that span the photo peak of the radionuclide. Record the counts for fixed time, so that maximum of 10,000 counts are obtained at the spectrum peak.

In energy spectrum, locate the energy on either side of the photopeak that has half of the counts at the spectrum peak. Interpolation between energy points on the spectral curve is used to identify peak, peak count, and half-maximum counts. FWHM is computed as % of the energy peak for ^{99m}Tc source.

Those cameras which do not have facility to store energy spectrum, energy resolution is obtained from the display. Change the energy window width until the energy window intersects the half maximum count level on each side of the energy peak. It gives approximate FWHM values of that of previous methods. It is referred as *nonstored spectrum method.*

During acceptance testing, two radionuclides (^{99m}Tc, ^{57}Co) are used and two-energy spectra are acquired. In that case, peak channel location is used to calculate keV per channel. It ensures proper energy scaling per channel.

Tolerance: ≤1.05% of reference value.

QUALITY ASSURANCE FOR SPECT SYSTEM

Pixel Size (x and y Direction)

The aim is to determine the absolute pixel size of all matrix sizes for tomographic reconstruction. One or two-point sources and a ruler are required. QA frequency is during acceptance testing.

The point source is placed on the camera along the x-axis, 5 cm from the edge of one side FOV. Static acquisition of 50,000 counts is made with 256 × 256 and 512 × 512 matrix size. One planar image is acquired without zoom. Point source is moved horizontally in x-axis to a position 5 cm away from the other edge of the FOV. Acquisition is repeated and one planar image is obtained. Whole test is repeated by keeping the source in y-axis as above. It may be also tested for all clinical tomographic zoom conditions.

Center of gravity of the point sources is calculated along x (COGX) and y (COGY) directions, for each raw projection of image. From the observations, distance between the positions of each of the pair of point sources is calculated. Pixel size (mm) is obtained by dividing the distance between point sources by corresponding distance in pixels (Refer IAEA, Human Health Series 6, 2009 for calculation details).

Tolerance: ≤1.05% of reference value.

Integral Tomographic Uniformity

The aim is to test tomographic uniformity of the SPECT system. A tomographic uniformity phantom filled with 200–400 MBq of ^{99m}Tc is required. It is usually done after planar uniformity test. QA frequency is acceptance testing and half yearly.

The phantom is placed with its center at least within 2 cm of the axis of rotation. The center axis of the phantom is parallel to the axis of rotation. Acquisition is made for different angles with matrix of 64 × 64 or 128 × 128 and 1 million counts per slice. A 10-cm phantom may collect 10 million total counts or 2.4 lakhs counts per angle position. After performing uniformity correction, reconstruct the data with ramp filter. Attenuation and scatter correction is applied, if necessary.

The images of phantom are inspected at various transaxial positions as per NEMA guidelines. Place five pixels thick profile about the center of the image and estimate the height ring artefacts by measuring their contrast relative to surroundings. The minimum or maximum value at the location of ring artefact is identified ($C_{max/min}$). Obtain two values beyond the edges of the artefacts along the profile and find the average values (C_{ave}).

$$\text{Contrast} = \frac{C_{max/min} - C_{ave}}{C_{max/min} + C_{ave}}$$

The absolute value of contrast is the ratio between difference in values and sum of the values. Repeat for all other transaxial slices in the phantom and get the absolute value of contrast. The average of five slices about the central slice in the phantom gives the central value. The edge value is obtained by averaging 3 cm on the profile centered, 2 cm from the observed edge.

Tolerance: Integral tomographic uniformity—10.7–18.8%.

Tomographic Resolution in Air

The aim is to test the tomographic resolution in air. It ensures that the reconstruction process is not degraded by either tomographic acquisition or reconstruction. A point source of ^{99m}Tc is required. QA frequency is acceptance testing and half yearly.

The point source is placed in air within 1 cm of the center of rotation. Acquisition is made for different angles, by keeping the radius of rotation as 15 cm to achieve 10,000 counts per view. Data is reconstructed with ramp filter. Static planar acquisition is made with same matrix size. Repeat the test by keeping the point source 8 cm off axis. Repeat the test by keeping the point source at the axis of rotation, but close to the edge of FOV.

Profile is drawn through the reconstructed image of the point source. Calculate the FWHM both in vertical and horizontal directions. FWHM of the planar image in the horizontal direction is also calculated.

Tolerance: ≤1.10 of reference value.

Center of Rotation Offset and Alignment Axes

To test the center of rotation offset, alignment of the camera y-axis and head tilt with respect to the axis of rotation. The center of gravity of point source is found by angle by angle to find the center of rotation. ^{99m}Tc point source with provision to suspend in air within FOV and a computer system are required. QA frequency is acceptance testing, and weekly or quarterly.

The head is aligned parallel to the axis of rotation with sprit level, a point source is suspended in air so that it is within: (1) 2 cm of the axis of rotation and (2) 2 cm of the center of FOV. Tomographic acquisition is made with 10,000 counts per angular position over 32 angles. Keep the point source at 10 cm radial distance away from the center of rotation and repeat acquisition. Keep the point source along the axis of rotation, but away from the central slice, and repeat the entire process. Repeat this test by keeping the point source at the edge of the FOV in the opposite direction. Whole procedure is repeated for opposite rotation of the camera. If earlier test is clockwise, this should be done in anticlockwise direction.

Generally, data is analyzed by using vendor's software or IAEA human series 6, 2009. The center of gravity of the point source along x and y direction is found for each angular position, then position of the center of rotation is estimated. These values are converted into mm by using known pixel values of the camera. It is performed for each head, if it is multiheaded SPECT scanner.

Tolerance: Center of rotation offset—±1 mm.

Slice Thickness at the Center of the Field of View

The aim is to test the thickness of the tomographic slice at center of the FOV and ensure that spatial resolution in z-axis is within limits. A small point source of ^{99m}Tc is required. QA frequency is acceptance testing and half yearly.

Carry out the procedure as stated in test of tomographic resolution air. Only the data is analyzed differently. To analyze, the slice in which point source is most clearly seen is located. Pixel of maximum number of counts is also located. The x and y co-ordinates of the pixel and the maximum values are noted. Find the number of counts for the same x and y pixel position on all other adjacent slices. Include the slices containing more than 5% of the maximum counts. A profile is created along the z-axis by using the above values. FWHM of the profile is calculated and converted into mm by using pixel size.

Tolerance: Center of rotation offset—±10% of reference.

Variations of Uniformity of Sensitivity with Angle

The aim is to test the variations of systems sensitivity for different angular position of the detector. Requirement is a flood source of 200 MBq of ^{99m}Tc which is attached to the collimator face. A ^{57}Co source can also be used if field uniformity per angle is not required. It is done during acceptance testing.

After attaching the flood source firmly to the collimator, tomographic acquisition is made to have 10^6 counts per angle, for normal matrix size. Rotating time is recorded. Repeat the acquisition for slow (4 min) and fast (30 min) rotation. Repeat the same for other head, if any.

Total number of counts for each angle is obtained. Correction for radionuclide decay is performed, if acquisition time is longer. The mean, standard deviation, and maximum deviation are estimated. Same calculation is done for central ROI also. Data is analyzed by using vendor's software or IAEA human series 6, 2009. Integral uniformity per angular position is found on pixel-by-pixel basis. In continuous rotation system, analysis is done for both slow and fast rotation speed. Speed of rotation is also recorded.

Tolerance: Center of rotation offset—±10% of reference.

Alignment (Registration Calibration SPECT/CT)

The aim is to test spatial registration of FOV between reconstructed SPECT and CT images. SPECT image quality phantom or vendors' registration test phantom, and 70 kg lead weights are required. To test table deflection, lead weights are uniformly distributed over the table along with phantom. QA frequency is acceptance testing and annual.

To evaluate spatial registration, series of SPECT emission images and CT transmission images are acquired by using SPECT phantom. Reconstructed images of SPECT phantom are inspected with image fusion software. Location of objects in the SPECT phantom should be seen clearly in the CT images. It should also spatially align with objects in the SPECT phantom images. Hot spots of point sources should be centered within corresponding CT objects. Cold spots within the SPECT phantom should align within corresponding spheres seen in CT images.

If there is mismatch in the location of each source between CT and SPECT images, fusion software is used to move CT images to align them with SPECT images. The absolute value of offset in each direction is recorded as Δx, Δy, and Δz in terms of pixel shift or mm for all sources. Calculate the mean deviation between SPECT and CT images along the x, y, and z direction.

Tolerance for alignment (registration): ≤1.05 of reference.

Box 9.2: Recommended QA tests for PET and PET/CT.

Parameter

- PET spatial resolution
- PET and CT registration evaluation
- PET sensitivity evaluation
- PET count rate performance and accuracy of corrections evaluation
- PET energy resolution
- PET image contrast and scatter/attenuation correction evaluation
- Coincidence timing resolution for TOF positron emission tomography
- PET image uniformity
- Normalization

Note: QA part of CT component same as diagnostic CT, refer Chapter 6, Quality assurance in Diagnostic Radiology. Additional test includes alignment of table to gantry, accuracy of gantry tilt, and table indexing accuracy.

(CT: computed tomography; QA: quality assurance; PET: positron emission tomography; TOF: time-of-flight)

QUALITY ASSURANCE FOR PET AND PET/CT

Quality assurance of PET or PET/CT consists of the following tests. All the tests are carried out as per IAEA human health series 1, 2009 and AAPM task group 126, 2019 recommendations **(Box 9.2)**.

PET Spatial Resolution

Aim

The aim is to measure the tomographic spatial resolution of the system in air and to ensure that spatial resolution is not degraded by acquisition and reconstruction process. Spatial resolution refers to system's ability to distinguish two close point sources as distinct reconstructed images. It is defined as FWHM of a point spread function. It is calculated from the line profile of the reconstructed image of a point source of radioactivity in air (AAPM TG-126). QA frequency is acceptance testing and annual.

Materials

Using syringes, a solution of water and ^{18}F with a concentration of 185–370 MBq/mL is prepared and mixed with 3–5 drops of contrast solution. About 1 mm droplets are spread on a plastic sheet and sucked by the capillary tubes. Thus, three glass capillary sources of length of 1 mm are prepared. Radioactivity of the solution is such that when all the sources are inside the FOV, the percentage of dead time losses and random must be <5% of the local event rate.

Using a source holder, the three glass capillaries containing the point sources are positioned in the transverse plane at: (1) x = 0 cm, y = 1 cm; (2) x = 0 cm, y = 10 cm; (3) x = 10 cm, y = 0 cm. The sources are suspended in air with ±2 m accuracy. Spatial resolution is obtained at: (1) center of the axial FOV, (2) 1/4 of the axial FOV from the center of FOV, and (3) 3/8 of the FOV from the center of FOV.

Acquisition

The PET and CT acquisition is made with 5–10 million counts for 3–4 minutes to make two sets of data, namely: (1) point sources at the isocenter and (2) point sources at 1/4 of the FOV or 3/8 of the FOV (totally six source positions). Data is reconstructed with all corrections except attenuation and scattering. Reconstruction parameters used should match the clinical parameters. For example, smallest pixel size and FOV to cover the three sources, and largest matrix size may be optimal to sample PSF. The reconstructed image pixel size should not be >1/4 of the expected FWHM in all three dimensions.

Analysis

Calculate the FWHM from the line profile of the point source. Obtain the maximum value of the line profile and divide by two to get half maximum. Identify the position of half maximum values on each side of the maximum value. Distance between the two half maximum value positions is measured.

Acquisition has been made in axial positions with three-point sources so that there are three-point sources per axial position. Find the slice containing largest count in the point source of ROI. Line profiles are drawn across the point source in perpendicular, radial and tangential directions by using interpolation. Axial line profiles are also drawn in sagittal and coronal reformations of the reconstructed image by using interpolation. FWHM of the axial, radial, and tangential of each point source at each axial position (0, 0, 0, 10, and 10, 0) is obtained. Totally nine FWHM values are reported. It should be within 5% of the baseline value or vendors' reference value.

Tolerance of spatial resolution: $FWHM_{observed} \leq 1.05\ FWHM_{of\ reference}$

PET and CT Registration Evaluation

Aim

Aim is to assess qualitatively the accuracy of registration of CT and PET images. Since it involves fusion, different parts of FOV should be perfectly registered over a range of patient weights. Proper coregistration of PET and CT images must be maintained to ensure proper attenuation correction and localization. It is much important in radiotherapy application of PET/CT. QA frequency is acceptance testing (AAPM TG-126).

Material

This test can be done as extension of spatial resolution test as stated under the hedaing PET spatial resolution, in two steps: (1) contrast media is added to radioactivity concentration and (2) analysis of PET and CT images for misregistration.

Analysis

After acquisition, PET and CT point source images are fused to axial, sagittal, and coronal images. It ensures that both are adequately registered, spatially within one voxel. The edges of the phantom seen in the PET scan should correctly match with that of CT scan. Measure the distance between the center of point sources in PET and CT images respectively for three-point sources, at three pre-axial position. Centers of all point sources are visually inspected or distance between corresponding PET and CT centroid is measured. This should be kept as baseline data for future comparison. Limit for coregistration is ±1 mm.

Tolerance of image registration is ±1 pixel or ±1 mm, whichever is smaller.

PET Sensitivity Evaluation

Aim

Sensitivity refers to measure of number of counts per second per unit radioactivity in the FOV.

The aim of the test is to determine the rate of detected true coincidence events per unit radioactivity concentration for a standard source in a circular phantom. QA frequency is acceptance testing and annual (IAEA Human Health series 1).

Material

Required materials are: (1) NEMA PET sensitivity phantom with innermost sleeves of 700 mm length, 3.9 mm inside diameter (ID), and 6.4 mm outside diameter (OD), (2) fillable plastic tubes of 1 mm ID, 3 mm OD and length 700 mm, (3) 5.5–7 MBq (0.15–0.2 mCi) of ^{18}F, and (4) 2.5 mL syringes, and (5) 20–23-gauge needles **(Fig. 9.2)**.

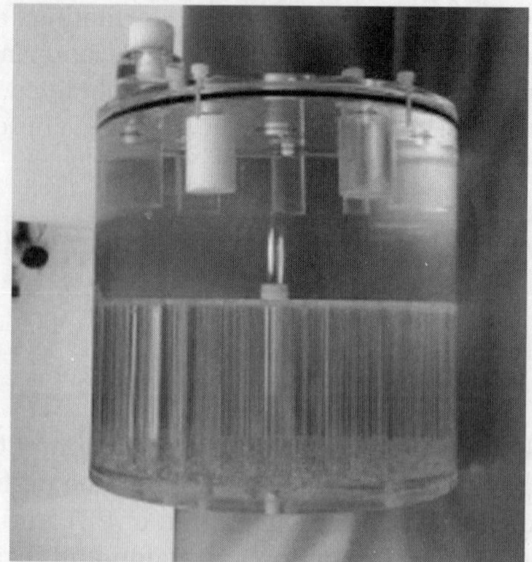

FIG. 9.2: NEMA PET sensitivity phantom.

Courtesy: Nuclear supplies.

Each syringe is drawn 5.5–7 MBq of activity of ^{18}F. The dose in the syringe and time of measurement is recorded. Activity is transferred to the plastic tubes without air gap and its end is sealed with Critoseal. Residual activity in the syringe is measured with time. Thread the line sources through the thinnest aluminum sleeves or equivalent. Mark the center of the thinnest aluminum sleeve and place it at the end of the table by positioning device. The center of source should be at the isocenter of PET and parallel to the table. It is also centered in all directions in the FOV.

Acquisition

The time and activity of assay information are recorded into the console computer. Start with a smallest sleeve containing the line source at the isocenter; three numbers of 1-minute PET scans are acquired. The line source is moved to 10 cm lateral and three additional PET scans of 1-minute duration are performed. Images are reconstructed using clinical protocols and analyzed. Record the scan start time, scan duration, and total prompt and random counts. The random counts are subtracted from the prompt counts to get total counts. Divide the total counts by acquisition duration to get counts per second. Phantom activity is corrected (kBq) for decay up to start of PET scan time. The sensitivity is obtained by dividing the total counts by corrected phantom activity (cps/kBq). Calculate the average sensitivity for three scans at the isocenter and at 10 cm lateral.

Analysis

Single slice rebinning should be used to assign counts in oblique lines of response (LORs) to the image slice whose LORs cross the scanner axis. Let T_j is the time of measurement and T_{acq} is the time duration, including detector movement time. Thus, the number of counts are collected. The counts per second ($R_{j,i}$) are determined for each of the five sleeves (j = 1, 2, 3, 4, 5), and for each slice (i = 1, 2.) by dividing the number of counts collected in the sinogram of the slice by the duration (T_{acq}).

Correspondingly, count rate for radioactive decay is corrected ($R_{CORR\ j,i}$) for all five sleeves, for each slice:

$$R_{CORR,j,i} = R_{j,i}\exp\left[\frac{(T_j - T_{cal})}{T_{1/2}}\right]$$

where T_j is the time of jth acquisition and T_{cal} is the time of calibration of phantom radioactivity. The cumulative count rate for each accumulated sleeve thickness is given by:

$$R_{CORR,j} = \sum_i R_{CORR,j,i}$$

The data is fitted to the following equation:

$$R_{CORR,j} = R_{CORR,0}\exp(-2\mu_M X_j)$$

where, $R_{CORR,0}$ refers to unattenuated count rate, μ_M is the linear attenuation coefficient of the sleeves material that allowed to vary to compensate scattered radiation, and X_j is accumulated sleeve wall thickness. From the curve fitting, the values of $R_{CORR,0\ and}$ μ_M are determined. The system sensitivity (S_{tot}) is finally obtained as follows:

$$S_{tot} = \frac{R_{CORR,0}}{A_{cal}}$$

where A_{cal} is total radioactivity. The same procedure is repeated when phantom and line source are offset at 10 cm from the central axis. The axial sensitivity profile is calculated using the data from the acquisition with the smallest sleeve, for the phantom at 0 cm offset. Using corrected count rates ($R_{CORR\ 1,i}$) for the slices, and the total count rate ($R_{CORR,1}$), the axial sensitivity for slice i is obtained as follows:

$$S_i = \frac{(R_{CORR,1,i})}{(R_{CORR,1})} \times S_{tot}$$

A sensitivity profile is plotted, S_i against slice number and the maximum and minimum values are recorded. The system sensitivity for 2D and 3D modes should be > vendors' specification.

$$\text{Tolerance: } S_{tot} > 0.95 S_{tot,expected}$$

PET Count Rate Performance and Accuracy of Corrections Evaluations

Aim

The aim is to measure count rate and scatter fraction and evaluate the count losses of the scanner under various radioactivity present in the FOV. Count rate performance refers to ability of the system to accurately measure high and low radioactivity sources. In clinical setting, count losses due to dead time are not negligible and rate of random coincidence increases with total single event count rate (AAPM TG-126). QA frequency is acceptance testing and annual.

Scatter fraction is the ratio of scatter coincidence to the sum of the scattered and true coincidences, while random coincidence is negligible. It varies with energy resolution, 2D verses 3D mode and CTW length. Scattering, count losses, and random count rates affects image quality and quantification accuracy. Hence, smaller scatter fraction is preferable.

Noise equivalent count rate (NECR) refers to tomography count rate performance as a function of radioactivity concentration:

$$R_{NEC} = \frac{R_T^{\ 2}}{R_T + R_S + (k + f + R_T)}$$

where, R_T, R_S and R_R are the true, scatter, and random count rates (kcps), f is the area of FOV subtended by the phantom and k = 1. R_{NEC} calculation requires knowledge of scatter fraction R_S which is not readility available. Hence, pseudo noise equivalent count rate (R_{PNEC}) term is used, which depends on prompt (total) and delayed (random) coincidence count rates:

$$R_{PNEC} = \frac{(R_P - R_D)^2}{R_P + \left[\left(\frac{k}{2} - 1\right) \times R_D\right]}$$

where, R_P and R_D are the prompt and delayed counts, and k = 1.

Material

A circular cylindrical phantom (20 cm diameter × 19 cm length), 700–750 MBq (20 mCi) of ^{18}F-FDG source, syringes, and gauge needles (20–23) are required.

Phantom is filled with water and 60 mL water is removed and kept for reuse. This is to create large air bubbles to air radioactivity mixing. Syringes of 3–5 cc are loaded with dose, and the time and activity is noted. The syringe dose is added to water in the phantom and mixed enough. Residual dose of the syringe is measured with time and activity. Previously removed 60 mL water is added now to the phantom to minimize air bubbles. Total volume of the phantom is estimated to calculate activity concentration.

Position the phantom on the table axially and centered in tarnsaxial and axial FOV. As baseline scan data, acquire multiple scans over 6–7 half lives; 15-minute scan, 15-minute delay, followed by 15 scan and so on. Images are reconstructed with all corrections. As follow-up scan data, acquire two 15-minute scans as did earlier. First scan should have activity concentration 1/2–1/3 of baseline scan activity. Second scan activity should be mimic clinical activity (≈0.5 mCi). Images are reconstructed with all corrections and each scan time is recorded.

Analysis

Obtain scan time, scan duration (t_s), total prompt counts (C_p), and total delayed counts (C_D) for each acquisition. Calculate the kBq/cc, corrected for decay to scan time. The prompt count and delayed count rate are calculated as follows:

$$R_P = \frac{C_P}{t_S}, R_D = \frac{C_D}{t_S}$$

From the above values, the R_{PNEC} is calculated using the relation stated earlier.

To simplify the method, water-filled phantom with large range of activity concentration is used initially to get baseline value. As periodic QA, two-activity concentration can be scanned to compare with baseline values. To address the accuracy of corrections, standard uptake value (SUV) is calculated from the reconstructed images as a function of range of activity concentration. In follow-up, SUV is calculated for two-activity concentration and compared with baseline data. SUV of water-filled phantom is unity.

Tolerance: >0.95 of reference

PET Energy Resolution

Aim

The aim is to assess photomultiplier calibration and ensures that the efficiency of light collection is within specification. This test is possible in equipment that uses signals-based attenuation correction and calibration. QA frequency is acceptance testing and change of detector response (IAEA Human Health Series No. 1).

Material

A point source in a capillary tube of ID <1 mm and OD <2 mm is prepared. The extent of the source both in axial and transaxial directions is <1 mm. Radioactivity quantity is chosen so that the percentage of dead time and random loss are <5%. Hence, radioactivity concentration of 1000 MBq /mL of ^{18}F is used and is placed at the center of the FOV. Source used in the spatial resolution test can also be used. The source is suspended in air to avoid scatter and at the center of FOV.

Acquisition and Analysis

Energy testing or energy spectra collection display is done as per vendors' specification. At least 10,000 counts in the peak energy distribution are obtained. The percentage of energy resolution of the system is obtained as per vendor's procedure. Alternatively, energy spectra are analyzed and FWHM of the peak distribution is obtained. FWHM is converted into units of energy (keV) by using energy calibration factor. The energy calibration factor is obtained by calculating the peak position using a parabolic fit to the top of the peak. Energy resolution (R_E) is given by:

$$R_E = \frac{1{,}000\ \text{FWHM}}{500}$$

Tolerance is $R_{E\ \text{measured}} < 1.05\ R_{E\ \text{Reference}}$

PET Image Contrast, Scatter/Attenuation Corrections Evaluation

Aim

The aim is to evaluate PET image quality based under the conditions of clinical imaging. It is desirable to compare the image quality of different imaging systems for a standardized imaging situation. QA frequency is acceptance testing and quarterly. (AAPM TG-126).

Material and Preparation

Requirements are: (1) PET ACR phantom, (2) 185 MBq activity of ^{18}F-FDG, (3) 1,000-mL bag or water bottle, (4) two 5-cc and one 60-cc syringes, and (5) gauge needles (16 gauge). The ACR phantom consists of seven cylinders of variable diameter of which six are fillable cylinders and seventh one is Teflon made **(Fig. 9.3)**.

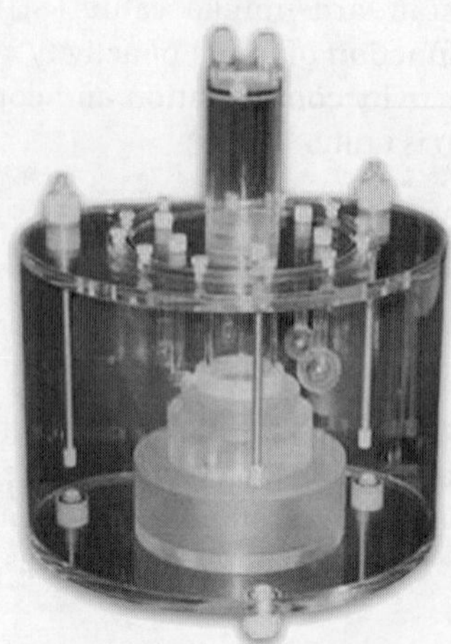

FIG. 9.3: ACR phantom for PET quality assurance.
Courtesy: AAPM TG 126.

The AAPM-TG 126 has given the ACR patient dose chart, which gives the dose of hot cylinders and background, equivalent to patient dose. First dose per ACR patient chart is diluted in 1,000 mL bag and mixed thoroughly and filled in 5-cc syringe. The syringe activity and time of measurement are noted. Syringe dose is transferred to four cylinders of 8 mm, 12 mm, 16 mm, and 25 mm diameters, referred as hot cylinders. Amount of air is minimized in each cylinder. Residual activity of the syringe and time of measurement are recorded. Remaining fillable two cylinders of 25-mm diameter are filled with air and cold water.

Second dose for background activity is prepared by filling the phantom with water. Remove about 60 mL of background water to create sufficient air bubbles. This is to help in mixing radioactivity thoroughly. Prepare dose as per ACR patient chart for background in 5-cc syringe. The syringe activity and time of measurement are noted. Syringe dose is transferred to the phantom. Remaining 60 mL of water is added to the phantom, to minimize bubbles.

Acquisition

Phantom is positioned in the isocenter and aligned in the three axes of the scanner with the help of lasers. Enter the patient weight as 70 kg and first dose activity as selected earlier. Acquisition is made as per whole body clinical scan protocol. Time between time of assay and the start of scan is recorded. Images are reconstructed as 1-mm slices.

Select the image containing four hot cylinders and draw 6–7 cm diameter background ROI in the center of the image. Also, draw second ROI just inside 25 mm hot cylinder and copy the same to remaining six cylinders. Record the mean SUV of the background, Teflon, air and water cylinders and minimum SUV of Teflon, air, and water cylinders. Maximum SUV of four hot cylinders is also recorded. Calculate the ratio between maximum SUV of hot cylinders and mean SUV of background. Also, calculate the ratio between maximum SUV hot cylinder and maximum SUV of 25 mm hot cylinder.

Limits for background mean SUV is 0.85–1.15, for 25 mm hot maximum SUV is 1.8–2.8, and ratio of 25 mm and 16 mm hot maximum SUV is >0.7.

Tolerance is ±5% of reference.

Coincidence Timing Resolution for TOF Positron Emission Tomography

Aim

The aim is to determine the capability of the PET to estimate the difference in time arrival of two coincidence photons. It is helpful to obtain likely location of annihilation LOR. This test is applicable only PET scanners with time-of-flight (TOF) mode. QA frequency is acceptance testing and daily basis (IAEA Human Health Series No. 1).

Material

A point source ^{22}Na (half-life = 2.6 years) or equivalent is kept in a scattering medium (steel or brass) and positioned at the center of the PET scanner.

Acquisition

The coincidence with time of arrival is acquired; difference in time of arrival histogram is made based on vendor's protocol.

Analysis

From the measurement, time of FWHM is estimated that gives the timing resolution of PET.

Tolerance of timing resolution (R_T): <1.05 of reference value.

PET Image Uniformity Assessment

Aim

The aim of this test is to measure deviation in activity concentration within slice and across the slices of uniform phantom. It is performed with cylindrical phantom used in count rate performance and accuracy of corrections evaluations as stated previously under the heading, PET Sensitivity Evaluation (AAPM TG-126). Frequency is as specified by the vendor.

Analysis

Images are reconstructed by using clinical protocols. Images are evaluated at two levels of activity concentration, namely: (1) 0.5 mCi and (2) 1/2–1/3 activity of peak, $R_{NEPC.}$ The images are visually inspected. Activity concentration is recorded in the phantom at the time of scanning. Five circular ROIs of 30-mm diameter are drawn on the central slice; one at the center and four at the cardinal locations (say 12′, 3′, 6′, and 9 ′o clock positions) and 10 mm from the phantom edge. The activity concentration on five ROIs is estimated. Mean activity concentration of slice i($ROI_{i,j}$) of five transverse locations (j) is also estimated. Similarly, draw five ROIs on other slices and find out activity concentration and mean activity concentration in all ROIs in all slices. The integral uniformity within a slice (IU_i) for all slices and integral uniformity between axial slices (IU_{axial}) for each of ROI locations are calculated by using suitable equations. The integral uniformity within slice $i = N$ is:

$$U_{I,N} = \frac{\overline{ROI_{N.max}} - \overline{ROI_{N,min}}}{\overline{ROI_{N,max}} + \overline{ROI_{N,min}}}$$

$\overline{ROI_{(N\ max)}}$ and $\overline{ROI_{(N\ min)}}$ are the maximum and minimum of five $\overline{ROI_{(N,\ J)}}$ values measured in slice N, where $i = N$ is the slice in which maximum and minimum activity concentrations are measured in five ROIs. The integral axial uniformity for a single transverse location is calculated using:

$$IU_{axil,M} = \frac{\overline{ROI_{max,M}} - \overline{ROI_{min,M}}}{\overline{ROI_{max,M}} + \overline{ROI_{min,M}}}$$

where, M is the transverse location in which maximum and minimum activity concentrations are measured in all slices. The limits for integral uniformity within a slice and across slices are 5%.

Tolerance is ≤1.05 of reference value.

Positron Emission Tomography Normalization

Aim

The aim is to acquire crystal efficiency data for correcting sinogram for detector nonuniformity in PET. The requirements are: (1) a rotating ^{68}Ge line source, (2) uniform cylindrical ^{68}Ge phantom, and (3) rotating ^{137}Cs point source. QA frequency is as specified by the vendor (IAEA Human Health Series No. 1).

Acquisition

The phantom is centered horizontally and vertically in the FOV of PET scan. Normalization data is acquired as per vendor's protocol. Backup copy of the previous normalization file is made before starting the acquisition. Normalization sonograms are visually inspected. If it is normal, new normalization data is stored in the file, as per vendors' flowchart.

Tolerance is only visual observation.

QUALITY CONTROL FOR RADIOPHARMACEUTICALS

All radiopharmaceuticals administered to patients must have safety, quality, and efficacy required for their intended use. The use of short-lived radionuclides in radiopharmaceuticals poses problems in QC testing since it is not possible to complete the necessary QC testing before the product's use-by date. This makes it imperative to employ a range of quick validation techniques to test the final product.

The objective of QC is to ensure whether the quality of radiopharmaceutical meet the predefined acceptance criteria. The criteria depends on the radionuclide and tracer, preparation, formation, and route of administration. QC involves number of steps, namely: (1) radionuclide identity, (2) radiochemical purity, (3) chemical purity, (4) pH, (5) osmolality, (6) filter integrity, and (7) sterility. More detail description is found in IAEA-TECDOC-1856.

Radionuclide Identity

It is necessary to ensure that the correct radionuclide with correct activity to be administered to the patient. First step is to identify the radionuclide by—(1) half-life, (2) gamma spectrometry, (3) radionuclide purity, (4) dose calibrator measurement, and (5) radiochemical identity.

Short-lived radionuclide half-life is determined by measuring the activity in a dose calibrator over time (ΔT):

$$\text{Half-life} = -0.693 \frac{\Delta T}{\ln\left(\frac{A_f}{A_o}\right)}$$

where, A_o is the standard activity and A_f is the activity measured at the end. The expected accuracy is within 10%. The dose calibrator must ensure its correct functioning and accuracy.

In the case of long-lived radionuclides, gamma spectrometry is used by identifying gamma peak. Radionuclide purity is meant for validation of batches not in every batch. Dose calibrator measurements are useful to determine impurities that have same emission pathways that of test radionuclide, cyclotron produced ^{99m}Tc, ^{99}Mo content in $^{99}Mo/^{99m}Tc$ generator, percentage of ^{68}Ge in ^{68}Ga labeled radiopharmaceutical in batches in $^{68}Ge/^{68}Ga$ generator, and the amount of radionuclide gamma-emitting impurities. Radiochemical identity mainly uses thin and instant layer liquid chromatography to identify radiolabeled molecule by comparing its retention factor to that of standard value.

Accurate measurement must take place during the preparation of radiopharmaceuticals and the dispensing of individual doses. It is always advisable to measure the vial before and after dispensing the radiopharmaceutical into the syringe. The difference between the readings gives a more reliable indication of the dispensed activity.

Radiochemical Purity

Radiochemical purity is defined as percent of total radioactivity present in the desired chemical form in a radiopharmaceutical. For many radiopharmaceuticals, the radiochemical purity will be expected to be >95%, but this is not universally so. Manufacturers will normally declare the radiochemical purity, for which further testing is not necessary. For materials prepared in house, either totally from original materials or purchased kits, radiochemical purity determinations are useful to establish the suitability of the final product.

Low-radiochemical purities may lead to an unintended biodistribution of the radiopharmaceutical. For diagnostic agents, this may lead to confusion in the diagnosis and for therapeutic radiopharmaceuticals; it can produce significant dosimetric problems. A range of techniques is available for such determinations, but the techniques must be reliable and simple, and preferably rapid, to perform such that, in an ideal situation, the radiochemical purity of materials containing short-lived radionuclides can be established prior to their administration.

Suggested method includes: (1) chromatography and (2) enantiomeric purity. Chromatography methods include thin and instant layer chromatography, solid phase extraction (SPE), high performance liquid chromatography (HPLC), paper electrophoresis, and size exclusion HPLC. All the methods determine radiochemical purity except size exclusion HPLC, which gives information about radiolabeled macromolecules protein integrity. Enantiomeric purity is performed by chiral HPLC, whereas filtration is used to know the amount of activity in albumin aggregate, especially in ^{99m}Tc.

It is expected that radioactive area corresponding to the radiopharmaceutical should represent at least 95% of total peak areas detectable on the radiochromatogram.

Chemical Purity

Chemical purity refers to an element that contains single substance without any other elements that tarnish its existence. Measurements usually determine amounts of impurities in the chemical sample. First step is to ensure the correct chemical purity of starting materials for radiopharmaceuticals. In addition, there are certain situations where the chemical purity of the final material can be affected by the process used in the preparation. The most likely situation to be met in radiopharmacies is the presence of Al ions in ^{99m}Tc radiopharmaceuticals. These can arise from alumina being washed off the columns used in ^{99m}Tc generators. Very high levels of Al can be toxic to patients, but it is unlikely that such problems will arise from administration of a radiopharmaceutical. Methods of ensuring chemical purity include: (1) chromatography and (2) specific activity.

In chromatography, HPLC and calorimetric assays—ultraviolet (UV) or visible spectrophotometer (VIS) methods—are used to determine chemical purity of radiopharmaceutical. Concentration of trace metal ions in radiolabeling solution can be done by using inductively coupled plasma atomic emission spectrophotometer (ICP-ACS) and inductively coupled plasma mass spectrometer (ICP-MS). Polarography can be used to quantify $SnCl_2$ in radiopharmaceutical cold kits, which is an accurate method.

In specific activity, HPLC is used to determine specific radioactivity of the radiopharmaceutical, UV/VIS method is used to determine radiolabeled antibody concentration, and immunoreactivity test is used to determine immunoreactive fraction in a radiolabeled antibody drug.

It is expected that the area corresponding to the radiopharmaceutical should cover at least 90% of the total peak area detected by chromatography. The limits for trace metal ions (Cu, Fe, and Zn) should be <0.1 PPM/GBq on the date of production. In radiolabeling solutions, it depends on the specific radionuclide or radiopharmaceutical.

pH

To ensure stability and integrity, all pharmaceuticals should have pH value equal to blood. However, range of pH is acceptable due to blood's higher buffer capacity. Hence, control of pH is essential to ensure that they retain their original specification. For example, ^{111}In chloride must be maintained at a pH of 1.5. If the pH rises, the material becomes colloidal and unsuitable for labeling reactions. With ^{99m}Tc compounds, the chemical composition and, hence, biodistribution of dimercaptosuccinic acid (DMSA) complexes are affected by the final pH of the solution. Normal renal imaging agent must be maintained at a pH <3.5.

Easiest method of determining pH is to use pH paper, since only small samples are needed. Generally, pH paper is exposed to the solution, its color changes to a certain pH value, and the color change is compared with the reference chart. It gives information about acidity or alkalinity of the solution. Papers are readily available from a variety of sources. Assessment of pH is subjective and such papers are normally only accurate to about 0.5 of a pH unit.

Alternate method is to use pH meter, which determines the pH of the solution by using a glass electrode. It is more accurate than pH paper test. Though pH has a range of 3.5–8.5, the ideal value for radiopharmaceutical is 7.4. It depends on the route of administration, injection volume, and rate.

Osmolality

Radiopharmaceutical is divided as labeled compounds and radiopharmaceutical kit. It is injected through intravenous injection that demands certain criteria. Osmolality is one such criterion which refers to the concentration of dissolved particles of chemicals and mineral in the solution. For human administration, radiopharmaceutical must possess certain ionic strength, isotonicity, and osmolality. Proper dilute is used to dilute radiopharmaceutical so that it has pH and isotonic strength to provide stability. Various methods to determine osmolality are—(1) freezing point depression osmolality measurement, (2) sodium chloride equivalent, (3) visual inspection, (4) radioactive concentration, and (5) endotoxin content. The specification for isotonic solution is 290 mOsm/kq and the deviation depends on the volume of administration, injection rate, and route of injection.

Filter Integrity

Radiopharmaceuticals are administered as sterile parenteral solutions. Sterilization can be done in two ways, namely: (1) autoclave and (2) using membrane filters. Though autoclaving is highly effective, it is not routinely used due to risk of chemical integrity of the labeled molecule and decay of activity during sterilization (≈15 minutes). Membrane filter method is often used even though it is not safe as autoclave. Membrane filter has limited bacterial load capability and may be damaged. This may allow microorganisms to enter the final product. Hence, filter integrity should be checked often by using—(1) diffusion rate and (2) pressure hold bubble point test. The later test is used most often with wet membrane.

Membrane bore diameter of 0.22 µm of different materials is generally used to suit different solutions. Filter integrity can be checked either before or after use, but later is most common. Radiopharmaceutical's final formulism is made with saline physiological solution with or without ethanol, ascorbic buffer, etc. Manufacturer's specification is valid only if certain media is passed through the membrane. Acceptance criteria may vary based on the solution composition. Test method should be validated for a specific radiopharmaceutical formulism.

Sterility

Radiopharmaceuticals administered parenterally need to be sterile and apyrogenic. It is achieved by using a suitable sterilization technique during preparation of the radiopharmaceutical. Control of the environment in which such manipulations take place is also important.

Direct inoculation method is used for sterility. Small sample volume of the radiopharmaceutical inoculated directly into a suitable culture media preferably fluid thioglycollate and soybean-casein digest medium, followed by an incubation period of 32.5 ± 2.5°C and 22.5 ± 2.5°C for 14 days. Sample volume should represent the batch and is within 10% of total volume of culture media. The media is inspected for microscopic evidence of microbial growth during the interval and end of the incubation. If no microbial growth is found, the sample complies with the test of sterility.

BIBLIOGRAPHY

1. American Association of Physicists in Medicine. PET/CT acceptance testing and quality assurance. AAPM-Task Group 128. Virginia, United States: AAPM; 2019.
2. Halama J, Graham G, Harkness BA, Kappadath SC, Madsen MT, Massoth RJ, et al. Acceptance testing and annual physics survey recommendations for Gamma camera, SPECT, and SPECT/CT systems. AAPM-Task Group 177.2019 [online] Available from https://www.aapm.org/pubs/reports/detail.asp?docid=184. [Last accessed October, 2022].
3. International Atomic Energy Agency. Quality control in the production of radiopharmaceuticals, IAEA, TECDOC-1856. Vienna, Austria: IAEA; 2018.
4. International Atomic Energy Agency. IAEA Health Human Series No. 6: Quality assurance for SPECT systems. Vienna, Austria: IAEA; 2009.
5. International Atomic Energy Agency. IAEA health human series No. 1: Quality assurance for PET and PET/CT systems, Vienna, Austria, 2009. [online] Available from https://www-pub.iaea.org/MTCD/Publications/PDF/Pub1393_web.pdf. [Last accessed November, 2022]
6. National Electrical Manufacturers Association. NEMA standards publication NU 1-2007: performance measurements of Gamma camera, USA, 2007. Virginia, United States: NEMA; 2007.
7. National Electrical Manufacturers Association. NEMA standards publication NU 2-2007: performance measurements of positron emission tomographs, USA, 2007. [online] Available from https://psec.uchicago.edu/library/applications/PET/chien_min_NEMA_NU2_2007.pdf. [Last accessed December, 2022]
8. National Electrical Manufacturers Association. NEMA standards publication NU 1-2001: performance measurements of Gamma camera, USA, 2001. Virginia, United States: NEMA; 2001.
9. National Electrical Manufacturers Association. NEMA standards publication NU 2-2001: performance measurements of positron emission tomographs, USA, 2001. Virginia, United States: NEMA; 2001.

CHAPTER 10

Radiation Protection and Safety in Nuclear Medicine

INTRODUCTION

Diagnostic nuclear medicine uses radiopharmaceuticals/tracer to image or quantify organ function. The tracer is given to the patient by intravenous injection or orally. The activity used for patient depends on body weight, metabolic characteristics, clinical conditions, type of equipment, and type of study and duration. The uptake or excretion and turnover is studied by an imaging system, either by γ camera or positron emission tomography (PET) scan. Higher activity may give high-quality images with higher risk to the patient. Lower activity may give inadequate information with lesser risk. Hence, optimal activity should be used to get the required diagnostic information. Hence, balance is required between image quality and radiation risk. Absorbed dose or organ dose can be calculated by *Medical Internal Radiation Dosimetry (MIRD) or biokinetic models* of International Commission on Radiological Protection (ICRP). Nuclear medicine is safe based on the activity used for the study.

In therapeutic nuclear medicine, ^{131}I as sodium or potassium iodide of 6 GBq is used in liquid/gelatin capsule form for thyroid cancer. It is used to treat hyperthyroidism and thyroid cancer. It can also be used to treat benign thyroid diseases such as thyrotoxicosis, Grave's disease, and toxic goiter. Iodine-131 or ^{90}Y-labeled monoclonal antibodies of 3 GBq is used as antibody therapy, especially in non-Hodgkin's lymphomas. Potassium-32 as sodium phosphate therapy is used for polycythemia vera and leukemias, and pain palliation in metastases in bone. Rhenium-188, strontium-89 chloride, and samarium-153 lexidronam are used to treat intractable pain from metastatic bone diseases. Primary radiation safety for the above therapy is contamination control.

PROTECTIVE DEVICES

Time, distance and shielding is the basic principle of reducing radiation dose. Fixing intravenous (IV) line to the patient is done before dispensing radioisotope to reduce time. Long forceps/tongs and bottle openers are used to keep distance from the radioisotopes **(Fig. 10.1)**. Protective devices with suitable shielding material should be used for personnel protection. Usually, tungsten, lead, leaded glass, and lead acrylic shields are used as shielding materials to reduce radiation exposure from vials and syringes in nuclear medicine. These materials are used to design the following protective devices:

- Syringe shield (Exposure ↓ 100-fold)
- Leaded glass (radiopharmaceutical preparation areas)

- Lead pigs (dispensing system)
- L-bench
- Transport container
- Waste storage: Lead dustbin

Syringe Shields

Syringe shields are useful to reduce radiation exposure during preparation and administration of radiopharmaceuticals by a factor of 100. Syringe-shielding is made up of 3 mm thick lead to reduce finger and body doses by about 200 times from syringe activities. The dose rate from an unshielded vial containing 100 mCi (4 GBq) of ^{99m}Tc would be 800 μSv/h at 30 cm. The required minimum thickness of shielding is 1.5 mm Pb to keep the surface dose level within regulatory limits which will reduce the dose by 94% **(Fig. 10.2)**.

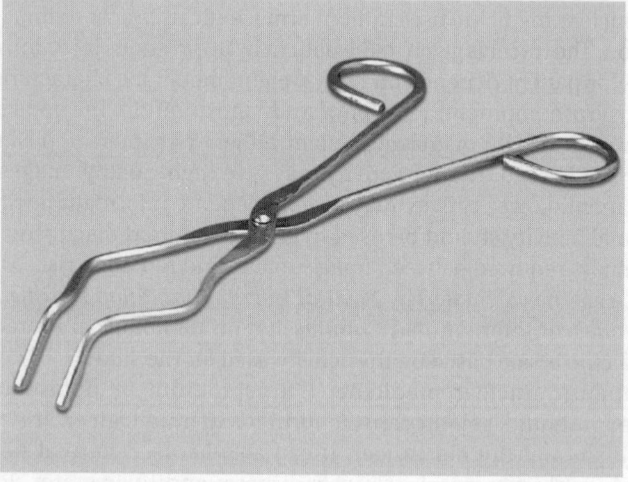

FIG. 10.1: Long crucible tongs.

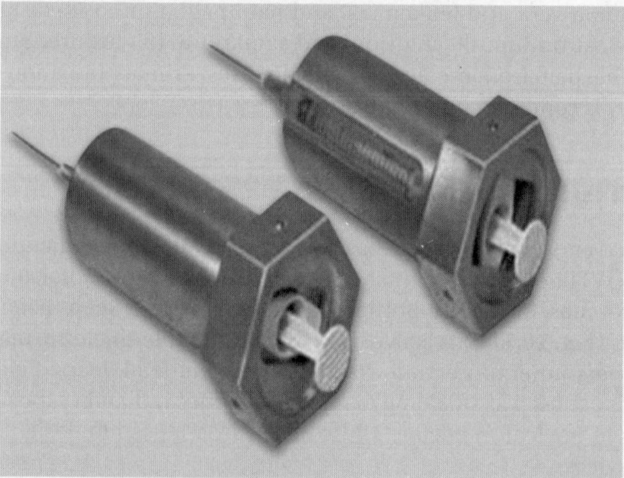

FIG. 10.2: Syringe shield.

TABLE 10.1 **Few radionuclide's dose rate constant and tenth value layer for lead.**

Radionuclide	*Γ (μSvh⁻¹MBq⁻¹)*	*TVL (mm lead)*
^{18}F	0,1851	13.5
^{51}Cr	0,0063	6.0
^{58}Co	0.0409	0.57
^{67}Ga	0,0300	4.8
^{75}Se	0,2323	2.5
^{99}Mo	0,0305	19.7
^{99m}Tc	0,0332	0.83
^{111}In	0,1356	2.23
^{123}I	0,0748	1.19
^{125}I	0,0743	0.06
^{131}I	0,0764	9.5
^{153}Sm	0,0244	0.32
^{201}Tl	0,0236	0.88

Courtesy: ICRP-106 ANNEX E.

The half-value layer (HVL) and tenth-value layer (TVL) of lead ($\rho = 11.35$ g/cm^2) for ^{99m}Tc of energy 140 keV is 0.25 mm and 0.83 mm, respectively. PET-CT uses fluorine-18 of energy of 511 keV which is higher energy than technetium. The HVL and TVL of lead for ^{18}F is 4 mm and 13.5 mm, respectively, it requires thicker syringe-shield than that of technetium. One HVL of lead attenuates 50% of ^{99m}Tc γ rays, whereas its effective attenuation is only 5% for ^{18}F. Hence, tungsten (ρ = 18 g/cm^2) syringe-shields are preferred in PET-CT. The TVL of tungsten is 0.59 mm and 9.62 mm for technetium 99m and fluorine-18, respectively. The required TVL of fluorine-18 should be 16 times that of technetium-99m. Tungsten syringe-shields for PET-CT energy are available in 8.64 mm and 14 mm with tungsten shielding. They will reduce the finger dose by 88% and 97%, respectively. Few radionuclide's dose rate constant and tenth value layer for lead is given in **Table 10.1**.

Lead Glass, L-bench, Pigs, and Transport Container

Leaded glass or acrylic shields is used along with solid lead in radiopharmaceutical preparation rooms. Lead pigs are used to dispense activity to various patients. Radiopharmaceutical containing vials are kept in lead pigs inside the L-bench **(Fig. 10.3)**. Required activity can be taken through syringe for each patient. The pig has tilting provision so that entire activity can be taken out easily. Generally, mirror is mounted in the back walls of the L-bench. This will easy the retrieval and manipulation of sources without direct exposures to head and neck area of the worker.

Transport container is used to move syringe with activity or activity from one location to another. It finds greater role today in transporting fluorodeoxyglucose (FDG) from cyclotron center to various hospitals by road and air. It can transport 2,500 mCi safely from cyclotron to PET-CT centers **(Fig. 10.4)**.

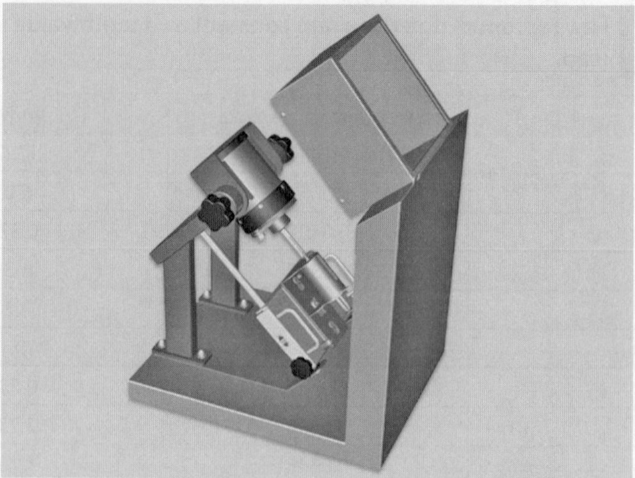

FIG. 10.3: Dose drawing system with lead pig in a L-bench.

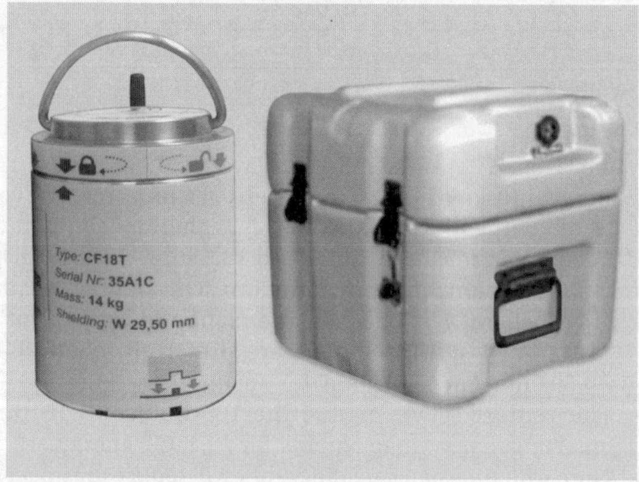

FIG. 10.4: Transport container (PET-CT).
Source: GE health care.

Generator Shielding

The radiation levels from a medium size unshielded technetium generator having 500 mCi (18.5 GBq) would be 6 mSv/h at 0.5 m **(Fig. 10.5)**. A typical shielding used is 9.5 cm of lead, that includes the core shielding of 5.0 cm lead + additional shielding of 4.5 cm. This shielding is higher than the minimum required shielding. For example, 6.3 cm lead shielding (9 HVL) is the minimum required to keep the radiation level at 15.0 μSv/h in the case of Mo (HVL = 7 mm lead).

Beta Shielding

Low atomic number shields such as plastic or glass or led glass are used to shield β radiation effectively. It not only attenuates but also reduces bremsstrahlung

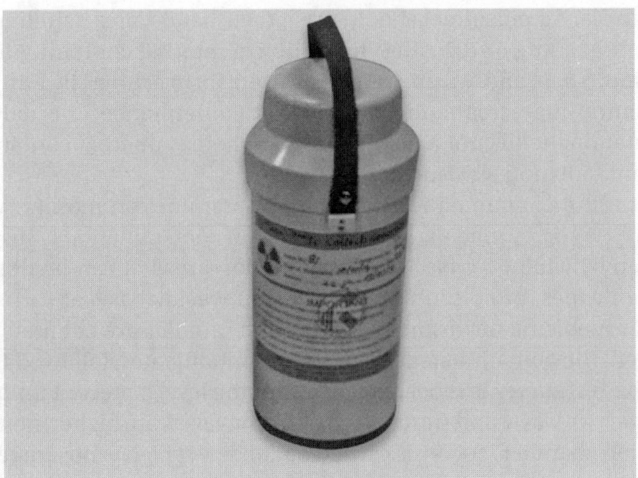

FIG. 10.5: Molebedinun-99 Technitium 99m generator.
Source: Board of Radiation and Isotope Technology(BRIT).

production. In the case of high energy β (^{32}P), the isotope is first kept in glass vial and then placed in lead container to prevent bremsstrahlung X-rays.

Personnel Wear

Personnel should wear laboratory coat, disposable gloves, finger ring thermo-luminescent dosimeter (TLD), body dosimeters, and lead apron. Lead apron has limited value in nuclear medicine as it does not attenuate enough medium energy photons (140 keV) as in diagnostic X-rays. Detail description is given in the later paragraphs.

CONTAMINATION CONTROL AND SURVEY

Contamination refers to uncontained radioactive material which is unwanted. Areas that are greater than twice the background level are said to be contaminated. Contamination control is carried out to prevent radioactive material that contact with personnel and prevent its spread to other work surfaces. Protective clothing such as disposable plastic gloves, laboratory coats, closed toe shoes, and handling precautions are the basic methods of contamination control. The personnel and work surfaces are periodically surveyed for contamination and areas should be classified as radioactive and nonradioactive areas. Nonradioactive areas such as patient examination room should be labeled as clean area and radioactive material is prohibited. Work surfaces where unsealed radioactive material is handled should be covered with plastic backed absorbent paper. If it is contaminated or worn, it should be changed. Volatile radionuclides (e.g., ^{131}I, ^{133}Xe gas) should be stored in a 100% exhaust fume hood to prevent airborne contamination and subsequent inhalation.

Collimators of scintillation cameras should be covered with plastic to avoid contamination. Personnel should discard gloves in the radioactive waste dustbin after work and monitor their hands, shoes, and clothing for contamination at periodic intervals. All personnel should wash their hands after handling radioactive material (before eating or drinking) to minimize internal contamination. For skin contamination, soap and warm water are used for washing and any aggressive decontamination may create aberrations that can enhance internal absorption. External contamination is not a health hazard, whereas internal contamination can give significant radiation exposures.

To monitor the contamination control, a contamination monitor with Geiger-Müller (GM) type survey meter is made available. If contamination is suspected, wipe tests are taken by wiping surface of contamination areas. It can be done with filter paper, alcohol wipes, or cotton tipped swabs on weekly basis at various locations of the nuclear medicine department. These wipe samples are counted in a NaI (Tl) γ-well counter. The contaminated areas are decontaminated followed by additional wipe tests. The GM survey is repeated to confirm the level of decontamination. In the areas of radioactive waste and storage, the radiation levels are higher, hence, exposure rate meters (ion chamber) survey is carried out to detect high exposure rates.

RADIOACTIVE MATERIAL SPILLS

Radioactive spills do happen in nuclear medicine. Though it is not a life-threatening hazard, but to be handled with special acre. When radioactive spills occur, area and personnel decontamination is required. Various steps involved in spills are: (i) to inform, (ii) to contain, and (iii) to decontaminate.

Individuals are alerted to stay in their workplace until they are monitored by GM survey meter. No workers to be moved in or out of the spilled area. Disposable shoe covers and plastic gloves are made available for decontamination. The vial that caused fill should be made upright and absorbent pads are put over the spill. Door should be closed to avoid escape airborne activity. Contaminated personnel should not leave the area until they are decontaminated. Personnel decontamination should follow area decontamination.

Persons doing decontamination should wear protective clothing. Skin contamination should be washed with water. Attention should be paid to wounds, eyes, nose, and mouth. Contaminated clothes should be removed and kept in a plastic bag. A shower path may be advised to the contaminated workers.

Area decontamination starts from outer area to center area to limit spread of contamination. It should be done under the supervision of radiation safety officer (RSO). Absorbing material is used initially to absorb the spill followed by detergent and water. Collected spills are contained and area is isolated and posted with warning signs. If complete decontamination is not possible, the surface area should be covered or rarely need replacement. After the decontamination, person doing the decontamination should subject their protective clothing for survey. It will ensure whether the clothing is contaminated or not. If the spill is a volatile radionuclide, there is a possibility of internal contamination, then bioassay should be performed.

MISADMINISTRATION

Misadministration refers to administration of radiopharmaceutical to a wrong patient, giving wrong pharma or wrong activity to a patient, or wrong route of administration or unjustified examinations of pregnant or lactating female patient. Generally, any variation of ±25% from the planned activity is unacceptable.

Misadministration of radioisotopes to patients have been reported in literature. A patient meant for whole body bone scan has been mistakenly given 370 MBq of ^{131}I, instead of 740 MBq of ^{99m}Tc. It resulted a thyroidal dose of 100 Gy with 20% uptake and the reason is verbal communication. Another case of administration of therapeutic ^{131}I therapy dose to a breast-feeding mother, without telling her to discontinue breast-feeding. Dose of 300 Gy was resulted to infant's thyroid.

The causes of misadministration are communication, busy environment, distraction, ignorance of regulatory rules, lack of training in emergency, not defining responsibilities, and lack of quality assurance. As a remedial measure, every effort should be taken to minimize adverse effects. The physician and patients should be informed, and dose due to misadministration is calculated. Corrective measures are planned and implemented. Report of the same should be made for submission to the management and the regulatory body. All the staff members are briefed about the report details to avoid such incidents in future.

PERSONNEL PROTECTION

Occupational Dose from Patients

Nuclear medicine involves low exposure rates of longer duration. Patients with injected activity contribute significant radiation exposure to staffs. For example, a patient with 750 MBq of ^{99m}Tc activity for bone scan emits an exposure of 10 μSv/h at 1 m. Due to radioactive decay and urinary excretion it will be reduced to 5 μSv/h after 2 hours. Exposure rates may range from 1,000 mSv to natural background values. Hence, knowledge of exposure rate and how it changes over a time is very important in reducing personnel dose. Wearing a lead apron of 0.25 mm Pb may reduce the exposure to certain extent in γ camera but not in PET-CT.

Hence, reasonable distance should be kept by the staff. Typical radiation dose from the patients injected with activity are given in **Table 10.2**. Patient who has received radionuclide injection should be kept in a separate area or isolation in the department. Suitable precautions are required to reduce staff's radiation dose. Patients should be given instruction leaflets detailing contact with other people and appropriate action if clothing becomes contaminated.

When using radionuclides for patient studies, the following points will reduce dose to the staffs:

- Good counting statistics in laboratory tests
- Diagnostic image within a reasonable time

TABLE 10.2 **Occupational staff exposure from patients.**

Radionuclide	*Investigation*	*Half life*	*Activity (MBq)*	*Exposure (μSv/h at 1 m)*
^{201}Tl chloride	Myocardial perfusion	73 h	111	0.87
^{99m}Tc RBC	Cardiac-gated study	6.0 h	740	7.90
^{99m}Tc MDP	Bone scan	6.0 h	925	10.5
^{18}F-FDG	Tumor imaging	110 m	370	43.7
^{131}I (NaI)	Thyroid therapy	8.0 d	7,400	306

(FDG: fluorodeoxyglucose; MDP: methylene diphosphonate; RBC: red blood cell)

Courtesy: Bushberg JT et al, 2012.

- Acceptable radiation dose to the patient from the target organ and excretion pathway
- Cost of expensive isotopes (e.g., ^{123}I, ^{111}I)

However, patient radiation doses in nuclear medicine studies are much lower than the radiology investigations using X-rays. For example, an urography study using iodine contrast may yield an ovarian dose of 30 mSv, bladder wall dose of 43 mSv, and whole-body dose of 30 mSv, respectively. Dose administration is the major contributor of radiation dose to the staffs. Hence, technologist duties are rotated often so that radiation dose is evenly distributed all.

Protection of Patient in Imaging

Nuclear medicine physician shall endeavor to ensure the use of methods for blocking the uptake of radionuclides in organs not under study and for accelerated excretion whenever applicable to protect the normal tissues. Container of radioactive material is labeled as, *Caution-radioactive material,* along with radionuclide name, calibration date, activity, and chemical form details. Each syringe or vial containing radiopharmaceuticals should also be labeled so that it is visible. Patient's name and activity should be written on the syringe. Patient's identity is verified by two means, e.g., name and date of birth.

Administration of radionuclides to pregnant women and children must be carried out only if there is a strong clinical indication. Adult female or pregnant women or breast-feeding women must be ascertained before administering activity **(Table 10.3)**. In ^{131}I therapy procedure, if activity >30 μCi, pregnancy should be ruled out by pregnancy test within 72 hours before the procedure. Written consent must be obtained from the patient before administrating such activity. It should contain details of patient's name, radiopharmaceutical, activity, and the route of administration. For some patients, counseling may be required to discontinue

TABLE 10.3 **Cessation of breast-feeding after administration of radiopharmaceutical to nursing mothers.**

Activity	*Administered activity (MBq)*	*Cessation of breast-feeding*
^{99m}Tc DTPA, MDP, PYP, and RBC	740	None
^{99m}Tc sulfur colloid	444	None
^{99m}Tc sestamibi or terofosmin	1,110	None
^{99m}Tc disofenin	300	None
^{99m}Tc sodium pertechnetate	185	4 h
^{18}F FDG	740	12 h
^{123}I NaI	14.8	24 h
^{99m}Tc WBC	185	48 h
^{201}Tl chloride	111	96 h
^{67}Ga citrate	185	Discontinue
^{131}I	1	Discontinue

(DTPA: diethylene-triamine-pentaacetate; FDG: fluorodeoxyglucose; MDP: methylene diphosphonate; PYP: pyrophosphate; RBC: red blood cells)

Courtesy: Stabin and Breitz, 2000.

breast-feeding until the radioactivity in the breast milk is reduced to safe level. Infant doses have been calculated in many such patients. As per the data, no interruption in breast-feeding is needed to keep the infant dose within 1 mSv.

Diagnostic reference level (DRL) is set in terms of dose quantity to monitor nuclear medicine practices. DRL quantity is the *activity administered or administered activity per kg of body mass,* which is easily measurable. It helps to develop examination specific protocol, optimal to age, or site and clinical indication. It also ensures the patient dose is as low as reasonably achievable for the examinations.

Pediatric Patient Exposure in Imaging

The injected activity depends upon the weight and age of the pediatric patient. Guidelines are given for a standard man on the radiopharmaceutical package. Several multiplication factors are used for obtaining children doses from the adult dose as follows:

- Body surface area (BSA) ÷ 1.73
- Child's age +1, divided by age +7
- Child's weight ÷ 70 kg
- Child's height ÷ 174 cm

For static imaging studies, first three steps are used and for dynamic study last step is used. Most radionuclides used in nuclear medicine investigations are concentrated in breast milk. A neonate thyroid gland can receive a high radiation dose from these nuclides in mother's milk. Hence, either nuclear medicine investigations should be avoided, or the mother is instructed to bottle feed after the investigation for a suitable period. Over 90% of the ^{99m}Tc activity appears in the breast milk over 24 hours and breastfeeding can continue after this term. The trauma imposed on the child and mother restricting contact should be weighed against the radiation risk.

Iodine-131 Therapy

After ^{131}I therapy, patients are either discharged or kept in isolation based on the administered activity. About 2% of the activity is taken by the organ as uptake and the remaining activity goes via excretion. The half-life of ^{131}I is 8 days and it is excreted through urine, saliva, feces, sweat, lacrimal fluid, and breast milk. Mostly 50–60% of activity is excreted in the first 24 hours and about 85% excretes over 4–5 days, resulting chance of contamination.

Main route of excretion is through kidney and patients are advised to take plenty of water to minimize the dose to kidney, bladder, and gonads. Second route of excretion is via saliva which will contaminate eating and drinking utensils and pillow covers. Hence, before administration, plastic-backed absorbent paper is used to cover floor, bed, mattress, light switches, toilet, and telephone. Patient's meals are served by disposable meal trays. Waste containers are placed in patient's room to dispose meal trays and contaminated linens.

Third route of excretion is via breast-feeding. Breast milk contain sufficient activity and requires control measures. This represents a potential radiation hazard to the newborn child. The principal risk to the child will be induction of cancer and is a factor of two to three times higher than for the average population. Therapy radionuclides are designed to damage the target tissue, and often have particulate emissions (usually β particles) and a longer half-life. Proximity of the child to the mother gives external radiation exposure to the child. Administration of therapeutic radiopharmaceutical orally, intravenously, or arterially is potentially hazardous to the child, and breastfeeding must cease.

Radiation survey is made around the bedside, doorway and the neighboring room, and the levels are posted for information along with instructions to nurses and visitors. The nursing staff should wear dosimeters, disposable shoecovers, and gloves. The visitors are instructed to wear disposable shoecovers and the visiting times are limited. Visitor's dose should never exceed 5 mSv or 1 mSv in children.

Patient with ^{131}I therapy may be discharged once the activity is <1.2 GBq or 33 mCi or dose rate at 1 m is <0.07 mSv/h (NRC regulation). Generally, once activity is administered (A) the exposure rate at 1 m from the patient is measured (X_A). Expected exposure rate at the time of discharge (X_D) can be calculated as follows:

$$(X_D) = \frac{1.2\ \text{GBq} \times \text{Measured exposure rate}\ (X_A)}{\text{Administered activity}(A)}$$

After discharge, the room is completely surveyed and decontaminated. It must be confirmed by swipe tests and GM meter radiation survey. If the total dose equivalent is >1 mSv, the patient may be discharged with instructions. This is to minimize radiation exposure and contamination to other individuals. The radiation safety instructions may be given to the patients to adhere at home.

Safe Work Practices by the Personnel

- Wear personnel monitoring TLD badge all times where radioactive materials are used. Wear extremity dosimeter, if required.
- Personnel should wear laboratory coats and disposable gloves when handling radioactive sources. Gloves should be handled such a way to avoid contamination of their inside surfaces. Laboratory coats, aprons, and other protective clothing should not be taken home.
- Radioactive materials should be stored in shielded containers in the storage room (hot laboratory) when they are not in use, to avoid exposure to people. Other materials should not be stored in that area.
- Package receipt survey is performed to ensure that source shielding has not been damaged during transport, or the package is not leaking or contaminated.
- Activity of the isotopes to be administered should be checked and confirmed using the isotope calibrator.
- Dispose radioactive waste in the radioactive waste dustbin which is labeled and properly shielded. Radioactive waste disposal should follow the steps:
    - Dilute and disperse
    - Store and decay
    - Concentrate and bury
- Ensure that ^{133}Xe ventilation studies are performed in a room with negative pressure with respect to hallway (if the exhaust rate is higher than the supply rate, then air will flow from hallway to room). The ^{133}Xe exhaled by patients during ventilation studies must be exhausted into a Xe trap.
- Syringe shields should be used to disperse radiopharmaceuticals, administration to patients.
- Taps in the sink should be operated by elbow, and foot-operated dustbins must be used.
- Persons with an open wound should not work with radioisotope.
- Spills or accidents should be reported to the radiological safety officer (RSO).

Reduction of Radiation Doses from Internal Sources

- All efforts should be to avoid spillage and misadministration of radionuclides.
- Hazards should be minimized by adopting time, distance, and shielding.
- Do not pipette radioactive materials by mouth. Pipette and stirring rods should be placed in nonporous trays or pans.
- Personnel should wash their hands after working with radioactive sources or before leaving the area, and their hand and clothing should be checked for contamination in a low background area by a survey monitor.
- Work should be carried out on absorbent pads to catch spills and prevent spattering of liquids.
- Work with radioactive gases or other volatile materials should be performed in a ventilated fume hood. These materials also should be stored in a hood.
- Work areas should be kept tidy. Radioactive trash, contaminated pads, and so forth should be disposed of promptly.
- No eating, drinking, smoking, or applying of cosmetics should occur in areas where open sources may be present.
- Handbags, handkerchiefs, keychains, etc., should not be brought inside the laboratory.
- No foodstuffs or drinks should be stored where radioactive sources are kept, such as laboratory refrigerators.
- Unnecessary contamination of light switches, doorknobs, and other items that could result in unsuspected contamination to personnel should be avoided.
- Disposable polythene and absorbent sheets are used wherever necessary.
- Containers with sharp or broken edges should not be used for radioactive materials.

PET-CT AND SAFETY

Nowadays, PET-CT is used as hybrid imaging with ^{18}F-FDG as radiotracer. It is a positron emitter isotope of half-life of 110 m. It causes internal radiation exposure to the patient and low-level external exposure to others. Hence, protection of occupational workers and patient is much important. Patient may consist of children and pregnant women. Specific instructions are followed to adhere safety. A prudent medical justification must be made with every PET-CT referral to avoid repeated exposure or overexposure of the patient.

Occupational Worker

Technologists receive higher dose in PET-CT, it may be 3–14 μSv per study with a mean dose is of 10 μSv per ^{18}F-FDG scan. About 50–60% of dose arises from dose administration. Hence, rotation of duty is mandatory in PET-CT. I-V line must be fixed before injecting FDG. Dedicated syringe shields are used for PET-CT dose administration. About 50% technologists may be females, they should voluntarily declare to her employer that she is pregnant. It is employer's/RSO responsibility to protect the conceptus of the worker. Equivalent dose limit is applied to the surface of the women's abdomen (lower trunk) of 2 mSv for the remainder of pregnancy. They may be advised to abstain from work if exposure >2 mSv. Nursing and ancillary staff will not receive significant risk by nursing PET patients. No nurse is likely to receive dose more than the regulatory limits. However, their training on radiation safety is much important. Lead apron is not useful in PET-CT as its transmission is 91%.

Patients

Computed tomography (CT) scan radiates only the patient and the effective whole-body radiation dose may be of the order of 7–30 mSv. High-resolution CT may increase the whole-body effective radiation dose. PET activity irradiates both patients and others (staffs and patient relatives). Radiation dose from PET imaging is about 8 mSv for adults while using an activity of 400 MBq. Other investigations like ultrasound and MRI can be taken in the same day, if required. It will not interfere with investigations. Activity injected patients are isolated, restricting from family members and friends. Proper shielding of FDG is provided in such waiting rooms. Patients should not be transported through hospitals.

After 2 hours of PET scan, patient can leave the center and can travel on public transport. Remaining activity is only 20–30% after scanning, unlikely to cause 1 mSv to public. However, radiation sensitive detector is kept in airport like public areas as alarm. Therefore, patient should get a document from the physician stating that he is a PET-imaged patient. Patient can carry out all his activities following PET scan without restriction. It is better to limit contact with pregnant women and children for 24 hours.

Children and Pregnant Women

Children are more sensitive to radiation than adults. The effective dose from PET-CT may be 5–18 mSv. If the procedure is justified, it can be carried out with optimization of dose. Children should never accompany a patient to PET-CT center or hospital.

Pregnant women should not accompany a patient to PET-CT center. This will keep the dose to the fetus to low. If a pregnant mother accompanies a child to a PET-CT center, specific precautions are followed. Contact time should be as short as possible. ^{18}F-FDG excretes in small quantities in breast milk. The scan is delayed until breast-feeding is stopped. It is advisable to collect milk from lactating mother before the scan to provide feed, after the scan. Third party should bottle feed the infant to avoid infant exposure. After the scan, the milk should be collected and discarded for 2 hours. Normal feeding can be resumed afterward.

PREGNANCY AND NUCLEAR MEDICINE

Discretion is required to ascertain the possibility of pregnancy in an adolescent. To minimize the frequency of unintentional radiation exposures of the embryo or fetus, advisory notices should be posted at several places within the nuclear medicine department, and particularly at its reception area.

Many patients incorrectly assume that irradiation from a nuclear medicine examination begins when the γ camera begins imaging, and they may not mention a potential pregnancy until after the radiopharmaceutical has been administered. Therefore, before administering radiopharmaceuticals, it is necessary to consider as pregnant any woman of reproductive age presenting herself for a nuclear medicine examination at a time.

Many laboratories also ask all females to indicate if they are breastfeeding, since many radiopharmaceuticals can be transferred to a baby via breast milk. Cessation of breastfeeding for at least some period is recommended for the most nuclear medicine studies. Breast-feeding is usually stopped for 3 weeks after all ^{131}I and ^{125}I radiopharmaceuticals except labeled Hippurate, and after ^{22}Na, ^{67}Ga, and ^{201}Tl administration. It is stopped for 12 hours after iodine labeled Hippurates and all ^{99m}Tc compounds except labeled red blood cells, -phosphonates, and ± DTPA, and for at least 4 hours after the latter compounds.

Occasionally, questions arise about the advisability of becoming pregnant after a nuclear medicine examination or treatment. This is not usually a consideration except for radioiodine therapy or radiopharmaceuticals.

Radioisotopes used in nuclear medicine are mostly short lived and does cause large doses to the fetus. Some radionuclides do not cross the placenta, and dose to the fetus is calculated from the maternal tissues. Radionuclide that crosses the placenta concentrate in a specific organ of fetus and poses significant dose. The risk and control measures are considered as: (i) before irradiation, (ii) during irradiation, and (iii) after irradiation.

Before Irradiation

Before conducting the examination, it is to be ascertained whether the investigation is indicated for the medical condition of the patient. In the case of diagnostic study, the risk to the mother of not performing the study should be greater than the risk to the fetus. Attempts should be made to reduce the administered activity. In women of childbearing age, possibility of pregnancy and justification of examinations should be considered with precautions. The methods of minimizing the fetus dose are as follows (ICRP-84):

- The patient must be carefully interviewed to assess the likelihood of pregnancy in an adult.
- An advisory notice must be posted as follows:
  "If it is possible that you might be pregnant, notify the physician or technician before receiving any radioactive material".
- Menstrual period overdue or missed should be considered for women of reproductive age, considering the nuclear medicine examinations. If the menstrual cycle is irregular, pregnancy test may be indicated before administering activity.
- Patients should be asked whether they are breast-feeding since activity may be transferred to the fetus via breast milk.
- Cessation of breast-feeding for some period may be recommended in such cases.
- General recommendation is that women should be not pregnant until the fetus dose from the remaining radionuclides is <1 mGy. However, this need not be strictly adhered to all isotopes of short half-life in diagnostic imaging. Pregnancy may be avoided for 6–12 months while using long-lived radionuclides labeled with ^{59}Fe (for metabolism studies) or ^{75}Se (for adrenal imaging), respectively.

During Irradiation

The fetus receives dose from (i) placental transfer which is distributed in the fetus, and (ii) external radiation from mother's tissue or organ. Physical, chemical, and biological properties of the radionuclides are critical in deciding the dose. Radioisotopes that do not cross placenta offer only external irradiation to the fetus. Radioiodine-131 crosses the placenta freely and accumulates in fetal tissues and irradiates.

Smaller activity and longer imaging time can reduce the fetus dose. Sequence of examinations can also reduce dose. For example, if a patient is prescribed ventilation perfusion study to exclude pulmonary embolus, perfusion scan can be done first. If the result is normal, ventilation scan is not needed at all, which is advantages.

The choice of radiopharmaceutical for ventilation portion of lung scan can also affect the fetal dose. Use of ^{133}Xe gas offers very little fetal dose, whereas ^{99m}Tc-DTPA aerosol contributes higher doses. This will be absorbed and excreted via kidneys, and while in the bladder it will contribute to fetal dose.

If the patient has pregnant family members at home, no significant risk occurs to them. Fetal dose at 0.5 m and 1.0 m are 0.02–0.25 mGy and 0.05–0.10 mGy, respectively which add no risk to them.

Maternal Hydration

Those radionuclides that are rapidly eliminated by maternal kidneys, the urinary bladder acts as a major source of fetal irradiation. In such patients, maternal dehydration and frequent vomiting are encouraged. Administration of laxatives is rarely helpful in patients having gastrointestinal excretion. For those radiopharmaceuticals that have gastrointestinal excretion, however, administration of laxatives is only rarely helpful in reducing fetal dose.

After Irradiation

Estimation of fetus dose is not necessary in diagnostic studies involving ^{99m}Tc. However, explanation may be given to the patient/relatives regarding the administration of activity and the related radiation risks.

The fetus dose depends on the activity rather than the imaging equipment as in radiology. Typical fetus doses are given in **Table 10.4**.

TABLE 10.4 Fetal whole body dose from common nuclear medicine examinations in early pregnancy and at term (dose includes maternal and fetal self-dose contributions).

Radio-pharmaceutical	*Procedure*	*Administered activity (MBq)*	*Early pregnancy (mGy)*	*9 months (mGy)*
^{99m}Tc	Bone scan (phosphate)	750	4.6–4.7	1.8
^{99m}Tc	Lung perfusion (MAA)	200	0.4–0.6	0.8
^{99m}Tc	Lung ventilation (aerosol)	40	0.1–0.3	0.1
^{99m}Tc	Thyroid scan (pertechnetate)	400	3.2–4.4	3.7
^{99m}Tc	Red blood cell	930	3.6–6.0	2.5
^{99m}Tc	Liver colloid	300	0.5–0.6	1.1
^{99m}Tc	Renal DTPA	750	5.9–9.0	3.5
^{67}Ga	Abscess/Tumor	190	14–18	25
^{123}I	Thyroid uptake*	30	0.4–0.6	0.3
^{131}I	Thyroid uptake*	0.55	0.03–0.04	0.15
^{131}I	Metastases imaging*	40	2–2.9	11

*Fetal thyroid doses are much higher than fetal whole-body dose, viz., 5–15 mGy/MBq for ^{123}I and 0.5–1.1 Gy/MBq for ^{131}I.

Source: Russell, Stabin, Sparks, et al., International Commission on Radiological Protection (ICRP) 84.

If the patient is found pregnant shortly after therapy, maternal hydration and frequent vomiting are encouraged. This is to reduce maternal radioactivity and reduce radioiodine storage at the bladder so that fetus external dose is reduced.

If pregnancy is found several hours of administration of activity, thyroid blacking agent (KI) may be given. If pregnancy is found later, placental transfer of iodine might have happened, resulting high dose of fetal thyroid. Since the fetal dose is <100 mGy, no need of termination of pregnancy. Mothers may be given useful levels of replacement thyroid hormone.

Actions and Precautions to Reduce Radiation Exposure to the Fetus

Pregnancy need not be considered as contraindication for nuclear medicine procedures, especially diagnostic examinations involving short-lived radionuclides, provided there are strong clinical justifications. However, efforts should be made to explore alternatives involving nonionizing radiation.

Since radionuclides in maternal tissues contribute to fetal dose, maternal hydration and frequent voiding can reduce the fetal dose after the administration of a number of radiopharmaceuticals.

Irradiation of the fetus results from placental transfer and distribution of radiopharmaceuticals in the fetal tissues, as well as from external irradiation from radioactivity in the mother's organs and tissues. The physical, chemical, and biological properties of the radiopharmaceuticals are the critical factors in possible placental transfer.

Using smaller administered activities and longer imaging times can reduce the absorbed dose to the fetus. This is feasible if the patient is not too sick and is able to remain still. Occasionally, the sequence of the examinations and choice of radiopharmaceutical can be adjusted to reduce radiation dose.

Treatment of Pregnant Patients with Radionuclides

As a rule, a pregnant woman should not be treated with a radioactive substance unless the radionuclide therapy is required to save her life: in that extremely rare event, the potential absorbed dose and risk to the fetus should be estimated and conveyed to the patient and the referring physician. Considerations may include terminating the pregnancy.

In general, if any therapy is to be performed during pregnancy, it will be surgery during the second or third trimester. In therapeutic doses, radionuclides cross the placenta and pose greater risk to the fetus, e.g., ^{131}I, ^{32}P.

Radioiodine Therapy for Hyperthyroidism and Thyroid Carcinoma

In women, thyroid carcinoma comprises over 80% of head and neck cancer between ages of 15–45 years. Thyroid cancers are relatively nonaggressive compared to other cancers. As a result, both surgical and radioiodine treatment are often delayed until after pregnancy. In general, if any therapy is to be performed during pregnancy, it will be surgery during the second or third trimester.

Radioiodine therapy is essentially contraindicated in patients who are known to be pregnant. ^{131}I easily crosses placenta and the fetal thyroid accumulates iodine at about 10 weeks of gestational age. If radioiodine treatment of thyroid carcinoma is to be performed, it should be delayed until after delivery. If this is done, the physician should also be aware that radioiodine is excreted in breast milk and breastfeeding should be stopped completely after a therapeutic dose. If this is not done the infant may become permanently hypothyroid or be at high risk for subsequent thyroid cancer.

Maternal hypothyroidism can happen during pregnancy. Serum hormone studies can be used instead of radioiodine uptake study in such patients. Iodine therapy may be delayed until after pregnancy.

Patients Become Pregnant after Administration of Radioiodine Therapy

Patients have been often treated with ^{131}I, who not thought of pregnant, and are found pregnant after iodine therapy for thyroid carcinoma. Hence, menstrual history alone not enough, pregnancy test is a must before therapy or high dose ^{131}I scan for women of childbearing age unless there is a clear history of prior tubal ligation or hysterectomy precluding pregnancy. However, still pregnant patients are getting treated due to false history or early-stage pregnancy test is not yet positive.

If the pregnancy is early, and the major problem is fetal whole-body dose due to γ emissions from radioiodine in the maternal bladder. The effective dose to the conceptus is about 50–100 μGy/MBq of administered activity. This dose can be reduced by hydrating the patient and by encouraging frequent voiding.

If the conceptus is >8 weeks postconception (and the fetal thyroid may accumulate iodine) and the pregnancy is discovered within 12 hours of iodine administration, giving the mother 60–130 mg of stable potassium iodide (KI) will partially block the fetal thyroid and reduce thyroid dose. 12 hours after radioiodine administration, this intervention is not very effective.

Avoid of Pregnancy after Radionuclide Therapy

Most female patients are advised not to become pregnant for at least 6 months after radioiodine therapy. This is to ensure that (i) hypothyroidism or cancer is controlled, (ii) another treatment with iodine is not needed during pregnancy. It will also ensure that unborn child will not get 1 mGy dose as recommended per ICRP. There are occasional circumstances in which ^{32}P, ^{89}Sr, or ^{131}I meta-iodobenzylguanidine are used for therapy. To keep the dose to the fetus below 1 mGy, pregnancy should be avoided for 3, 24 and 3 months respectively based on the radionuclide therapy **(Table 10.5)**.

Risk to a Pregnant Woman, When a Family Member is Treated with Radioiodine

Patients treated with radioiodine can be a significant radiation source to pregnant family members. The dose to a family member staying at a distance of 0.5 meters from a patient until the radioactivity totally decays (about 10 weeks) is about 1.3 mGy from a hyperthyroid patient and 6.8 mGy from a thyroid cancer patient. Also, these patients must be careful not to transfer radioiodine contamination to family members by direct or indirect means.

TABLE 10.5 **Avoid of pregnancy in months after radionuclide therapy for various isotopes and maximum activity.**

Radionuclide	*Therapy*	*Activity, up to MBq*	*Avoid pregnancy, months*
^{131}I iodide	Hyperthyroidism	800	4
^{131}I iodide	Thyroid cancer	6,000	4
^{131}I MIBG	Neuroendocrine tumors	7,500	3
P-32 phosphate	Myeloproliferative	200	3
Sr-89 chloride	Bone metastases	150	24
Y-90 colloid	Radiation synovectomy	400	0
Y-90 colloid	Malignancy	4,000	1
Au gold	Malignancies	10,000	2
ER-169	Synovectomy	400	0

(IAEA: International Atomic Energy Agency; MIBG: metaiodobenzylguanidine)

Courtesy: IAEA, 2009.

Patients with Iodine-131 Therapy without Hospitalization

Some patients are discharged after administration of low activity. They may have vomiting symptoms in 4–6 hours. Patient is advised to vomit in a container or into the toilet and may be fleshed clean. The nuclear medicine physician should be informed about the same. Cross contaminations are minimized by exchange of fluids, kiss or sextual intercourse must be avoided at least for 2 days. A condom should be used for the first week after therapy. The condom will reduce the risk of contamination but will not shield from the ^{131}I gamma radiation.

Patient Preparation for Iodine-131 Therapy with Hospitalization

Before admission, patients are counseled and history such as pregnancy, breast-feeding, incontinence, nausea, type of work, use of public transport, and living conditions are collected. Pretherapy patient instruction card is given to the patient to get prepared well in advance. Before 1 month, patient should stop all iodine-related compounds, cough syrups, and vitamins. They should not undergo any iodine contrast studies in CT and X-rays. They should stop thyroid medicine for at least 6 weeks prior to therapy. Certain blood tests may be needed on the day of admission. Instruction also includes the following:

"If you are, or could be, pregnant or are breastfeeding, please notify staff before proceeding with the therapy dose. You must also not become pregnant for at least 6 months after the ^{131}I therapy dose".

Administration of ^{131}I activity, isolation, and daily monitoring of external radiation are informed to the patient. Precautions to be followed for 7 days, after discharge is given to the patient in advance:

- *Pretherapy instructions*:
  - Avoid contact with children and pregnant women. Stay one arm's length away from people.
  - Avoid unnecessary trips in public transport for 5–7 days.

  - Toilet is flushed twice after use, and wash hands frequently.
  - Do not attend work if this involves prolonged contact with people.
  - If convenient, sleep in a single bed if partner is <50 years of age.
  - Wash hands before preparing food. Sharing food or eating utensils should be avoided.
  - Avoid activities like kissing with family members.
  - If hospitalized within 4 days for any illness, nuclear medicine physician should be informed.
- *Post-therapy instructions during discharge*:
  - Avoid all close contact with children or pregnant women until (date).
  - Avoid extended periods of close contact with children or pregnant women until (date).
  - Avoid prolonged personal contact with adults at home until (date).
  - Avoid prolonged close personal contact with adults away from home until (date).
  - You may return to work on (date).
  - Do not sleep with an adult in the same bed until (date).
  - Male patients are advised to sit and urinate
  - Daily showering will remove sweat.
  - Clothing should be separately laundered.
  - Breastfeeding must be ceased before iodine therapy and not be resumed under any circumstances.

Pregnant Staff and Continuation of Work

For most diagnostic procedures, there would be no need for pregnant staff to take any additional precautions other than limiting their direct contact to as short as necessary. Because the exposure from patients who have been administered radiopharmaceuticals is quite low, there is no radiological reason not to continue imaging procedures. Moreover, the *International Basic Safety Standards* require that "notification of pregnancy shall not be considered a reason to exclude a female worker from work". If the institution administers therapeutic activities of ^{131}I for thyroid cancer, it should be considered refraining from this part of the practice. Not only that there are higher exposures associated with the administration of ^{131}I, but also iodide is volatile, increasing the potential for internal uptake.

Some radiopharmaceuticals cross the placenta freely, e.g., radioactive iodides, and are taken up in fetal tissues, where they irradiate the tissues. Some analogs of natural metabolites (e.g., radiostrontium for calcium and radiocesium for potassium) are less readily transferred. Radiopharmaceuticals that are retained by the mother, and do not cross the placenta (e.g., radiocolloids), only act as external sources of irradiation to the fetus. In nuclear medicine departments, a pregnant technician can be restricted from spending a lot of time in the radiopharmacy or working with radioiodine solutions.

PROTECTIVE CLOTHING REQUIREMENTS

The protective clothing requirements in a contaminated area depend on the nature and amount of the contamination. For low levels of surface contamination, an ordinary laboratory coat with overshoes and gloves may be sufficient. When there are substantial levels of airborne contamination it is usually necessary to have a fully-enclosed dry suit and a filter mask or a mark fitted with an air supply. Again, when the contamination is in liquid form, it is often necessary to wear a fully enclosed PVC suit with a filter mask or fresh air supply.

Whatever the standard of protective clothing, the change and barrier arrangements must be efficient and should have the following facilities:

- Wash hand basin (and possibly a shower) and monitoring instruments (for example, a hand and clothing monitor).
- Suitable stowage on the nonactive side of the barrier for the workers' personal clothing.
- Conveniently-placed protective clothing ready for use.
- Containers for used clothing and radioactive waste.
- Noticeboards at the barrier, stating "no unauthorized entry", the hazards in the area, the clothing to be worn and any other precautions to be taken.
- *Emergency instructions*: Detailing actions in the event of possible incidents such as criticality, fire, and serious personal contamination should be posted in the area. Consideration must also be given to suitable emergency exists.

Special arrangements are made for laundering clothing worn in contaminated areas and the effluent from laundry facilities is treated as liquid radioactive waste.

Laboratory Coat

Conventional white cotton drill or nylon coat of proper size which should extend below the knees are suitable for clean areas.

Overalls (Boiler Suit)

These are one-piece cotton drill garments so designed as to cover the body completely except for the head and neck, wrists and hands, and feet and ankle. The fastenings for these garments are usually at the front. They are extremely useful as they protect all the clothing worn below.

Aprons

In areas in which the processes involve work at benches with liquids, an apron of suitable impervious material such as PVC, polyethylene or neoprene will be found useful in preventing the clothing below from becoming contaminated by corrosive liquids or dust.

Rubber Gloves

For general laboratory work, surgical gloves are adequate for most operations. Where it is necessary to handle β-active material directly with the hands, rubber gloves of a heavier type or leather gloves may be used to reduce the β-radiation dose to the hands.

Footwear

These should be preferably rubber-soled to prevent the uptake of contamination and to facilitate cleaning. It is recommended that the pattern of the rubber sole should not be too deeply indented. The upper part of the shoes should be well waxed to resist the absorption of contaminated solutions.

Overshoes

These are worn over the normal walking shoe and are suitable for use by visitors to active areas or for general use in laboratories. The conventional rubber overshoes are suitable, but the soles should not be too deeply indented. A cheaper form of overshoe made of rubber, plastic, or canvas is also available.

Rubber Boots

These are particularly useful for wear in areas in which the processes involve contaminated solutions or wet conditions, such as in areas being decontaminated. The half-length rubber boot is usually adequate for this purpose. The soles of these boots should not be too deeply indented.

Breathing Apparatus

For work in areas of low or medium level of airborne activity, a full-face respirator with an efficient filter provides adequate protection. The filter used must be reliable; suggested types are the resin wool and charcoal or the highly efficient paper filters which are commercially available. Care must be taken to ensure that these respirators fit properly and do not allow air to be taken in from the sides of the face-piece. For work in areas of very low activity a half-face respirator may be used.

RADIOACTIVE WASTE DISPOSAL AND RADIATION MONITORING

Disposal of Radioactive Waste

Radioactive waste can be disposed by the following methods: (i) dilute and disperse, (ii) store and decay, and (iii) concentrate and bury. Radioactive liquid through sink or radioactive gases through ventilation may be released to the environment by the first method. However, its concentration should not exceed the recommended limits.

Short half-lives (less than few weeks) may be stored for decay and then disposed. After a decay period of 10 half-lives or 0.1% of the initial activity they are categorized as wastes with half-lives <3 days and wastes with half-lives >3 days. This will reduce the volume of accumulated waste. Now it can be disposed as per regulatory norms.

Disposal of waste with long half-lives >1 month is not suitable by store and decay method. It should be disposed by concentrate and bury method.

Radiation Monitoring

Portable and battery operated GM type meters are used for radiation survey. They are more sensitive and display count rates in counts per minute (CPM). It is also provided with thin mica or aluminum entrance for β measurements. It is useful for detecting small quantities of radioactivity like spills.

Ionization chamber type survey meter is also available with a range of 0–300 mR/h. It gives accurate measurements within ±10%. If chamber is not sealed, ambient temperature and pressure correction is required. Its accuracy must be checked periodically by using a sealed radioactive source.

Zone or area monitors are fixed on the wall and operated continuously. They are mostly GM type and gives audible sound when radiation is detected along with display of count rate. This type of meter is required in radiopharmacy like area, to warn the presence of high-level radiation. It can be used to monitor hands also for check contamination.

All workers are provided with TLD personnel monitoring badges. They are evaluated for dose once in 3 months. It will give the dose received by the personnel. Pocket dosimeter can also be used additionally for measuring over short period or on the spot assessment.

Wipe test is done to detect small amounts of radioactive contamination on work bench or package surface and radioactive leakage. Alcohol-soaked gauze or cotton-swab is wiped over the suspected surface or leaky source. Then it is tested under a liquid scintillation detector for contamination. Any contamination less than KBq limits can be tested by wipe test method.

BIBLIOGRAPHY

1. Bushberg JT, Seibert JA, Leidholdt EM, Boone JM. The Essential Physics of Medical Imaging, 3rd edition. Philadelphia: Wolters Kluwer/Lippincott Williams and Wilkins; 2012.
2. International Atomic Energy Agency. (2009). Release of patient after radionuclide therapy. IAEA Safety Report Series No. 63, Vienna 2009. [online] Available from https://www.iaea.org/publications/8179/release-of-patients-after-radionuclide-therapy [Last accessed September, 2022].
3. International commission on Radiological Protection. Pregnancy and Medical Radiation, ICRP Publication 84. Oxford: Pergamon Press; 2000.
4. Russell JR, Stabin MG, Sparks RB. Radiation absorbed dose to the embryo/fetus from radiopharmaceuticals. Health Phys. 1997;73:756-69.
5. International commission on Radiological Protection (ICRP). How to protect your hands in Nuclear Medicine work -ICRP Publication 106 Annex E. Oxford: Pergamon Press; 2008.

CHAPTER 11

Planning a Radiation Therapy Facility

INTRODUCTION

Radiological installation requires specific rooms to house an individual equipment. It involves proper layout, location, and room design, etc. These rooms consist of primary and secondary barriers based on beam direction. The primary barriers are thicker than the secondary barriers. The extent of primary barrier will depend on the divergence of primary beam. The radiation beam energy, workload, type of occupancy around the installation, and use of beam direction toward a particular wall will decide the thickness of the barrier. Construction material and density are crucial in making such wall thickness. Teletherapy and brachytherapy rooms requirements are different. The overall objective of radiotherapy planning is to protect the occupational workers and public, so that the radiation exposure is within prescribed limits.

GENERAL PLANNING REQUIREMENTS

Location

Radiotherapy departments are usually located on the periphery of the hospital complex to avoid radiation protection problems since therapy rooms being adjacent to high occupancy areas. Operational efficiency, initial cost, as well as provision for future expansion and/or increased workload, should be considered when locating a therapy installation. Proximity to adjunct facilities, ready access for in-patients and outpatients, and consolidation of all therapeutic radiological services are important than construction cost. For rooms below ground level, the reduction in shielding costs for floors and outside walls should be weighed against the expense of excavation, watertight sealing and of providing access. Rooms above the ground floor requires shielding in outside walls.

Additional structural support is needed for heavy equipment. Shielding re-equipment depends on type of occupancy of surrounding areas and occupancy levels decide the shielding thickness. Mostly lower occupancy is advised around the treatment room. Either restricted entry or prohibition of unauthorized entry is imposed in such location. All the facilities at the vicinity of 20 m from the external walls of the radiotherapy room should be shown in the layout plan. The installation should have approval from the competent authority.

Access

Access to the room for the delivery and replacement of the treatment unit and patients must be considered. It shall permit transport of equipment, source transfer flask, and patients on wheelchairs or trolleys or beds. Entrance to the room may be through a shielded door or via a maze. It is necessary to include in the room design an open access conduit for dosimetry equipment cables. This dosimetry duct should always be through a secondary barrier so that the primary beam can never strike it. Ideally, it should run at an angle through the barrier to the treatment control area.

Also, for security purposes, access by members of the public to the rooms where sources are used and stored is restricted. Further, the proximity of source storage facilities to personnel that may respond in the event of a security breach should also be considered.

Room Size

The room should be large enough to allow full extension of the couch in any direction, with room for an operator to walk around it. The desirable size depends upon the type of treatments; for example, a total body irradiation (TBI) procedure will require a larger treatment distance to one wall. Intraoperative procedures (IORT) require extensive support staff and equipment; the room may need to be larger. The accessory equipment such as electron applicators, breast positioning boards, etc., are usually stored within the room, and should be located to minimize the walking distance for each patient set-up. Rooms comprising the facility should be integrated suitably, so that it will be able to function efficiently. It will also help to perform source loading, commissioning, patient treatment, maintenance and decommissioning within the area with ease and safety.

The supporting facility of the radiotherapy department such as simulator room, treatment planning system room, mold room, patient waiting areas, change room, UPS room, chiller room, air handling room (AHS), medical physicist room, radiation oncologist room, examination room, nurse's room, and record room, etc., should be incorporated in the layout as shown in **Figure 11.1**. Rooms located at near the plot boundary should maintain a distance 2–3 m between the external walls of the room and plot boundary for any contingency in future.

Shielding

Adequate structural shielding shall be provided for the walls, ceiling, floor of the treatment room, so that radiation doses outside the room shall not exceed the regulatory limits. The shielding is calculated based on workload, use factor of the radiation beam and occupancy around. The entry of the room shall be of indirect type to minimize shielding requirements at the entrance door (IAEA SRS No.47).

Maze

To reduce the radiation dose near the entrance, a restricted access passageway (Maze) leading to the room may be incorporated in the design. Maze should be long in length and small in width. The minimum width may be determined by the dimensions of the treatment unit to be delivered by this route or by access for a hospital bed. The maze ensures the exit of the photon radiation after sufficient scattering. A maze reduces the need for a heavy shielding door. If the length of the maze is sufficient, or if there are enough bends, there may be no need for a radiation protection door at the maze

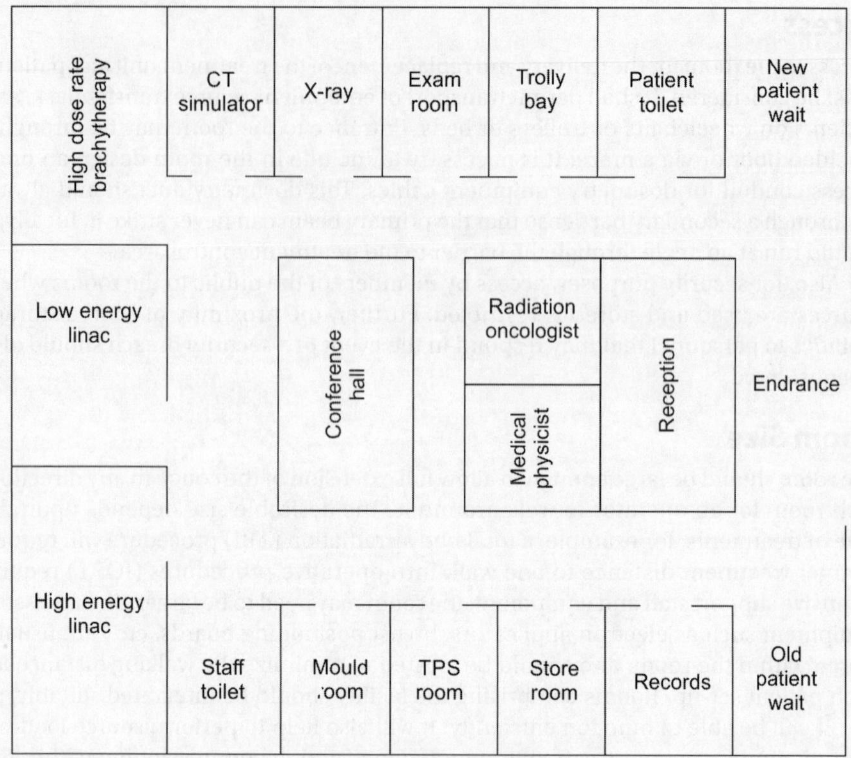

FIG. 11.1: A model layout of radiotherapy department.

entrance. However, it is recommended that a physical barrier such as a normal door(s) or gate be installed to discourage entry to the maze during patient treatment. Linear accelerators usually require a gate to prohibit entry during treatment times and/or motion detectors to detect unauthorized entry if a shielded door is not required to reduce dose rates. Another advantage of a maze is a route for ventilation ducts and electrical conduits without compromising the shielding.

Doors and Interlocks

The treatment room is a controlled area and a barrier should be installed at the entrance to the maze or treatment room to restrict access during exposures. If a shielded barrier is required to reduce dose rates, a motorized door may be necessary. A motorized door must have a manual means of opening the door in the event of a power or mechanical failure. There should also be an emergency means by which the motion of the door is stopped. Additionally, any motorized door that is too heavy to be stopped manually should have sensors that stop the motion of the door to prevent injury to personnel and patients.

All doors, gates, photoelectric beams, and motion detectors must be interlocked to the treatment unit to prevent an exposure if a door is open. The interlock must also ensure that when the door is opened the irradiation will be terminated. The radiation output of the device should not be resumed automatically after the door is closed again. The interlock should be fail-safe so that safety is not jeopardized in the event of failure of any one component of the system.

In certain centers, it is advised that a door-reset switch be situated near the exit from the treatment room at the position where the person leaving the room has a clear view of the room. Only after activation of the reset switch, can the radiation be turned "on". If there is a maze, this switch should have a delayed action to allow the person time to leave the room and maze after resetting the switch. This switch should be connected in series with a second switch just outside the door. The same person should operate both switches. In cases where the door is clearly visible from the control panel, closing the door may activate the second switch. Only after activation of both switches can the radiation be turned "on" (IPEM Report 75).

In facilities using radioactive sources, a barrier that restricts access to the treatment room outside normal working hours may also meet certain specifications. An unauthorized access to the source can be detected in a timely fashion. To achieve this, a video camera that provides continuous remote surveillance of the device, a photoelectric beam or motion detector system installed in the maze and/or treatment room, or a door interlock can be incorporated. If these devices indicate the potential presence of an unauthorized person, an alarm should indicate this locally and remotely so that personnel can respond in a timely fashion. These technical measures will be independent of any interlocks that terminate the radiation beam during normal operation because they will not be operational when the treatment unit is powered "off" outside operational times.

Treatment Control Area

The operators control the machine from the treatment control area. This area should be close to the entrance to the treatment room with interlocked doors. The doors are under direct supervision from the control console without barrier in between the interlocked door and control console. The control area should be sufficiently large to accommodate the treatment unit control console and associated equipment. There may be computer terminals for record and verification, electronic portal imaging, hospital information system and dosimetry equipment, as well as closed circuit TV (CCTV) monitors for patient observation. There should be clear access to any dosimetry ducts.

Patient Observation and Communication

Control rooms of teletherapy and nurse's rooms of remote after loading brachytherapy are outside the treatment room. The operator/nurse should be able to visually monitor the patient during treatment with closed CCTV. Two cameras are recommended with a fixed and movable camera. These should be situated 15° off and above the gantry rotation axis for optimum observation of the patient on the treatment couch. The cameras should be located far away from the radiation source, consistent with tele-zoom capabilities, to minimize degradation of the image receptor by scatter radiation. There should also be provision for two-way audio communication between the treatment control area and the room. A patient activated alarm may be required for patients unable to give an audible call.

Ducts and Shielding

Ducts and conduits between the treatment room and the outside must be adequately shielded. This includes ducts for cables necessary to control the treatment unit, heating and ventilation ducts, ducts for physics equipment, and other service ducts.

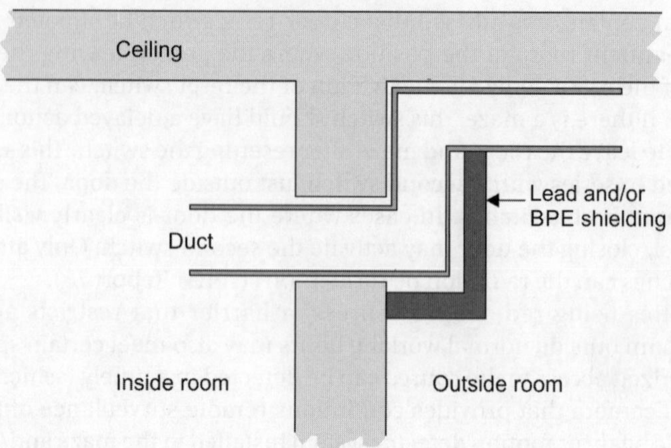

FIG. 11.2: A bend in duck to avoid radiation streaming.

It is recommended that ducts should only penetrate the treatment room through secondary barriers. No duct with a diameter >30 mm should penetrate the primary shielding.

The ducts should be placed in such a way that radiation passing through them will require the least amount of compensation for the barrier material it displaces. No duct should run orthogonally through a radiation barrier. It could either run at an angle through the barrier or have one or more bends in it so that the total length of the duct is greater than the thickness of the radiation barrier. If required, lead or steel plates are suitable materials to compensate for the displaced shielding. To shield the scattered radiation that passes along the duct, it is better to place the additional shielding outside the treatment room, where the radiation has a lower average energy and therefore, less shielding material is needed as shown in **Figure 11.2**.

Treatment machine cables are usually run below the floor level under the primary or secondary barriers, before bending up to reach the treatment control area. Provided there are no rooms below, additional shielding is not usually required unless the treatment control area is directly behind a primary barrier, and the cable passes beneath the same primary barrier.

Water pipes and narrow electrical conduits are usually placed in groups inside a larger duct. It is recommended that they also should not penetrate through barriers but follow the maze to exit the treatment room as described above or follow a route beneath the shielding barrier.

Heating and ventilation ducts should not penetrate through primary barriers because of their large cross-sectional area, which makes it costly to compensate for the shielding material they displace. If the ducts must pass through a secondary barrier, the cross-section of the duct should have a high aspect ratio to decrease the radiation passing through the duct because of multiple scattering interactions with the duct/shielding walls. The axis of the duct and the longer side of the duct cross-section should be as orthogonal as possible to the direction of the leakage radiation from the target toward the duct.

The amount of additional shielding required to shield penetrations in shielding walls depends on the energy of the radiation beam, room layout, and the route of the duct(s). The shielding must be evaluated carefully if the ducts must penetrate the primary barrier. The recommended placement of these ducts is above a false ceiling along the path of the maze, to exit the maze at or near the external maze door where the photon and/or neutron fluence are lowest. For accelerators of energies up to 10 MV, usually no additional shielding around the duct is required. For higher energies, an additional shielding is required. If it is necessary for the ducts to pass through the secondary barrier, they should be placed as high as possible to minimize the scattered radiation to personnel outside the room.

Conduit

Conduits are required for dosimetry cables, beam data acquisition system control cables, quality assurance (QA) equipment cables, and in vivo dosimetry equipment cables. The conduits are usually PVC pipes of 80–100 mm diameter included in the concrete formwork. They should be inclined at an angle (20–45°, in the vertical and horizontal planes), and penetrate through the secondary barrier but not through the primary barrier. If the openings are at least 300 mm above floor level, they are more convenient to use. Ideally, the opening in the treatment control area should be at the countertop level and the opening in the treatment room side should be at a different level but within easy reach.

Atomic Energy Regulatory Board (AERB) recommends a conduit of 5 cm diameter, at angle between 20 and 40° to the horizontal and lower end located at a height of 15–20 cm from the finished floor level (FFL) in the treatment room. It will enable cables of radiation measuring instruments to pass through from the control room to the treatment room. Conduit are described above usually do not need additional shielding unless the barrier is constructed of material with a much higher density than 2,350 kg/m^3.

Shielding requirements of ducts depend on photon energy and maze length. An 18 MV accelerator with 5 m length maze requires no shielding for the duct. If the maze length is 3 m, shielding is necessary. **McGinley** suggests a 1.2-m long duct shielding wrapped with 10-mm thick lead and 25-mm thick polyethylene for a 3.6-m long maze. The lead should be wrapped around outside first, followed by polyethylene layer. This will offer a reduction of one-fourth for neutrons and half for photons. Rooms having more than one bend need not have duct shielding.

Warning Signs and Lights

It is recommended that an illuminated warning sign should be displayed at the entrance to the maze or treatment bunker. It should be possible to see a warning sign from any position within the treatment bunker. These signs should be mounted at eye level (1,650 mm above FFL) and interlocked with the treatment unit control. The illuminated signs may have two or three stages. For a two-stage sign, the first stage will be illuminated when there is power to the treatment unit, and the second stage will illuminate when the beam is turned “on”. For a three-stage sign, stage one will be illuminated when there is power to the treatment unit, stage two will light when the treatment unit is programmed to deliver a radiation beam and stage three will illuminate when the beam is turned “on”. The color of the warning light will be green when the beam is “off” position, red in the “on” position and yellow in the transit position. A warning sign should indicate the nature of the hazard. If there are controlled areas with restricted access outside the treatment bunker it should be labeled appropriately.

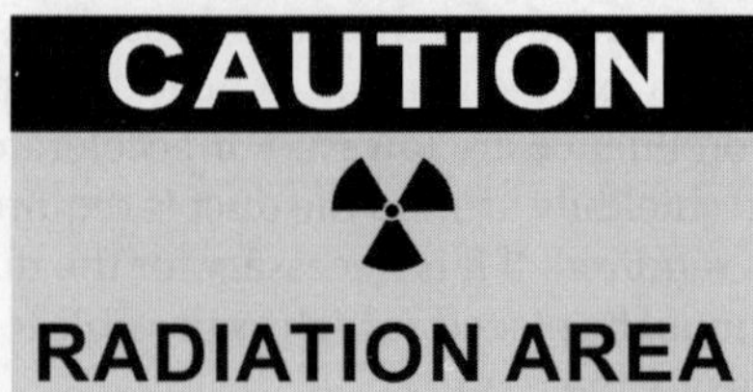

FIG. 11.3: Radiation warning placard. ***(For color version, see Plate 1)***

A suitable warning sign such as the red light must be provided at a conspicuous place outside the room and kept "on" when the unit is in use, to prevent entry of persons not connected with the examination or treatment. An appropriate warning placard must also be posted outside the room entrance or door. AERB recommends a radiation symbol, specified under rule 14 of Atomic Energy (Radiation Protection) Rules, 2004 **(Fig. 11.3)**. It will be pasted conspicuously and prominently at the treatment room entrance and at the entrance of the controlled and supervised areas. A legend in Hindi/local language and in English indicating radiation hazards and restricted entry shall be pasted near the radiation symbol.

Treatment rooms of teletherapy and remote after loading brachytherapy shall have suitable door interlock and warning light at the entrance door which will warn against inadvertent entry of persons during irradiation.

Room Lighting and Lasers

To set up a patient for radiotherapy treatment, the room lights should be dimmable so that the field light of the treatment unit and the alignment lasers can be seen easily. It is useful to be able to control the room lights and lasers from the treatment unit control pendant in the treatment bunker. When the field light is switched "on", the room lights should dim to a preset (but variable) level, and the alignment lasers should also be switched "on". Since fluorescent lights do not dim very satisfactorily, it is recommended that incandescent lights be used for the dim level. The main room lighting can be fluorescent lights that extinguish when the field light is turned "on" and the incandescent room lights are used for the dim level. When the field light is switched "off", the main room lighting is switched "on" and the lasers are switched "off". The dimmable lights may remain "on", at all times.

If junction boxes or alignment of lasers are to be in set in walls, then the voids should be backed with 40 mm thick steel plate with a 30 mm margin all around **(Karzmark et al.)**. Based on the occupancy of the adjacent area, reduction of shielding over a small area, especially in secondary barrier may be accepted.

Four alignment lasers are recommended; two lasers are aligned with the gantry positions of 90° and 270°, third laser should project a sagittal line along the gantry axis. This laser is usually mounted on an angled bracket on the wall opposite the gantry. Fourth laser is mounted in the ceiling directly above the isocenter. The laser switching should be controlled from the hand pendant, but it is also useful to be able to switch them off independently for QA tests.

Air-conditioning

The treatment room as well as the control room should be air-conditioned. If it is a central air-conditioning, the ducts should be taken along the wall of the entrance

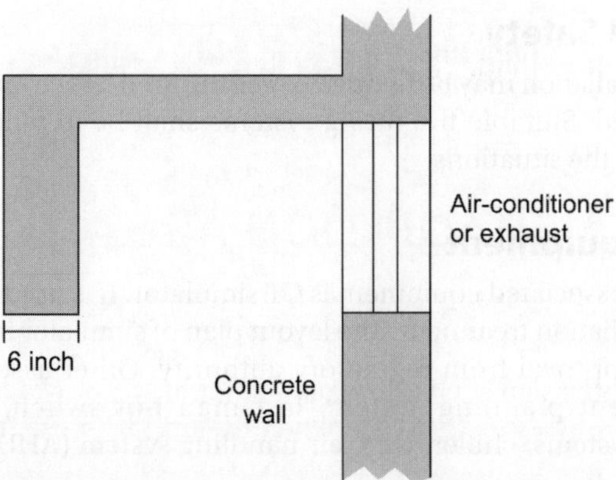

FIG. 11.4: Baffle design for air-conditioner or exhaust.

door and left at the desired location without making any opening on any wall. In case of split air-conditioners, the conduit of minimum diameter consistent with requirements and making an angle of 20–45° with the horizontal should be provided. The opening of the conduits in the treatment room should be at height of above 1.5 m from the floor of treatment room. The details may be finalized in consultation with AC engineers. In the case of accelerator installation, special ventilation arrangements are required. Air-conditioners of the control room may be located anywhere in its brick walls as per convenience.

The opening for the air-conditioners should be provided in the specified outer wall of the treatment room in the case of cobalt teletherapy room. The lower end of the openings should be located at a minimum height of 2.5 m from the floor level outside and further be covered with a baffle arrangement **(Fig. 11.4)**. The width of the baffle and the length of its vertical portion should be such that 30 cm wide overlap is available all around the openings. If split type air-conditioners are planned, the baffle arrangements are not necessary. However, conduit for passing the AC duct is to be provided in the specified wall at an angle to avoid direct scattered radiation passing through it.

Zone Monitor

A radiation zone monitor shall be provided at a location near the entrance to the treatment room of telecobalt and brachytherapy facilities to monitor radiation continuously. It is not necessary for a linear accelerator facility.

Ramp

Telecobalt installations require a ramp which may be provided in near proximity to the teletherapy room to facilitate easy movement of the crates carrying the unit to the site. It is also useful in future source loading operation. This usually happens at 5–7 years and a new source container of weight 2–3 tons may arrive the site. This container needs to be unloaded from the truck and to be moved to the teletherapy room. The height and slope of the ramp is so adjusted so that the transport container will be unloaded with ease from the truck into the teletherapy room on a suitable trolly.

Conventional Safety

Radiotherapy installation may be flooded or getting fired hence, preventive measures should be adhered. Suitable fire fitting systems shall be in place with manpower training to handle the situations.

Associated Equipment

One of the major associated equipment is CT simulator. It is used to simulate patient before starting radiation treatment. The layout plan of simulator installation requires site and layout approval from regulatory authority. Other associated equipment includes treatment planning system, last man out switch, beam modifiers, immobilization systems, chiller, UPS, air handling system (AHU), dosimeters, and QA devices.

Waiting Area

To avoid crowding of patients and relatives near the entrance door, a waiting area must be provided outside and adjacent to the treatment room. It should have sufficient area to match the patient workload with toilet facility.

Regulatory Clearance

For obtaining requisite regulatory clearance, the user needs to submit relevant application through AERB's e-Licensing of Radiation Applications (e-LORA). Prior to this, institution get registered with AERB and obtain USERNAME and PASSWORD.

The site and layout plan of radiotherapy installation is prepared in 1:200 scale and submitted through e-LORA by the user and get approved from AERB. Plan should indicate various rooms along with their dimensions, positions of doors, windows, type of occupancy around, etc. Cross-sectional views in XX, YY, and ZZ directions may be required. Further details can be obtained from www.aerb.gov.in.

MODEL LAYOUT PLANS FOR TELETHERAPY FACILITY

Model Layout Specification for Telecobalt Therapy Installation

Telecobalt machine uses Cobalt-60 radioactive source as source of radiation. Its isocenter is 80 cm with maximum field size of 35 × 35 cm and mean energy 1.25 MeV gamma rays. Symmetric and asymmetric collimators are used. Machines with add on multi leaf collimator with 100 SSD is available now. Leakage radiation is always present even in source "off" position. Since large amount of primary and secondary radiation incident on the floors, walls, and ceilings, it requires special consideration. A typical model plan is shown in **Figure 11.5**.

- *Land area*: About 10 × 10 = 100 m^2 (not to scale)
- *Internal area*: About 5 × 6 m^2
- *Ceiling height*: 3 m
- *Isocenter from floor*: 1.3 m
- *Primary barrier thickness*: 1.3 m
- *Ceiling thickness*: 1.3 m
- *Conduit*: 100 mm diameter, 150 mm above FFL at an angle 45°

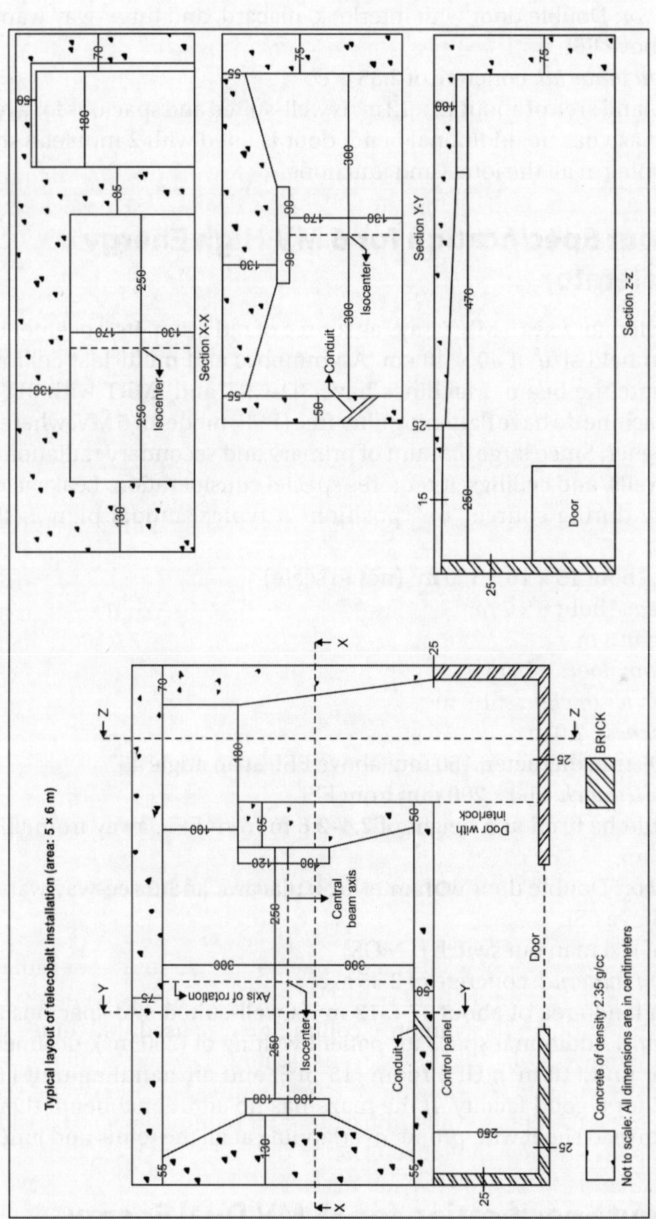

FIG. 11.5: Model layout for telecobalt installation.
Courtesy: AERB. https://www.aerb.gov.in

- *Core conduit/trench*: 200 × 200 mm from FFL
- Lasers should be fixed at a height of 2.4–2.6 m from FFL away from the path of the primary beam.
- Zone monitor at 2 m from floor
- Provision of last man out switch (LMOS)
- *Entrance door*: Double door with interlock, placard, and three-way warning sign at 1.65 m above FFL.
- *Construction material*: concrete of 2.35 g/cc

However, a land area of about 12 × 12 m^2 is well-suited and spacious for a telecobalt facility. If the maze has no additional bend, door is lined with 2 mm lead sheet with proper overlapping at all the joints and junctions.

Model Layout Specification for 6 MV High Energy Linear Accelerator

This linear accelerator uses 6 MV X-rays as source of radiation. Its isocenter is 100 cm with maximum field size of 40 × 40 cm. Asymmetric and multi-leaf collimator are used to collimate the beam. Machines have 3D-CRT and IMRT with 3D-imaging capabilities. Machine do have flattening filter free (FFF) mode for 6 MV, where the dose rate may be higher. Since large amount of primary and secondary radiation incident on the floors, walls, and ceilings, it requires special consideration. Leakage radiation is present only during source "on" position. A typical model plan is shown in **Figure 11.6**.

- *Land area*: About 15 × 10 = 150 m^2 (not to scale)
- *Internal area*: About 6 × 7 m^2
- *Ceiling height*: 3 m
- *Isocenter from floor*: 1.25 m
- *Primary barrier thickness*: 1.9 m
- *Ceiling thickness*: 2.0 m
- *Conduit*: 100 mm diameter, 150 mm above FFL at an angle 45°
- *Core conduit/trench*: 200 × 200 mm from FFL
- Lasers should be fixed at a height of 2.4–2.6 m from FFL, away from the path of primary beam.
- *Entrance door*: Double door with interlock, placard, and three-way warning sign at 1.65 m above FFL
- Provision of last man out switch (LMOS)
- *Construction material*: concrete of 2.35 g/cc

However, a land area of about 17 × 12 m^2 is well-suited and spacious for 6 MV linear accelerator. Additional space for patient waiting of (250 m^2), dosimetry room (15 m^2), chiller unit (10 m^2), UPS room (15 m^2), and air handling unit (15 m^2) is recommended for a good facility. If the maze has no additional bend, then door is lined with 4 mm lead sheet with proper overlapping at all the joints and junctions.

Model Layout Specification for 15 MV Dual Energy Linear Accelerator

This linear accelerator uses 6, 10, 15 MV X-rays as source of radiation. If it is a dual-energy accelerator it may have 6, 8, 9, 12, and 15 MeV electrons or different combination. Its isocenter is 100 cm with maximum field size of 40 × 40 cm.

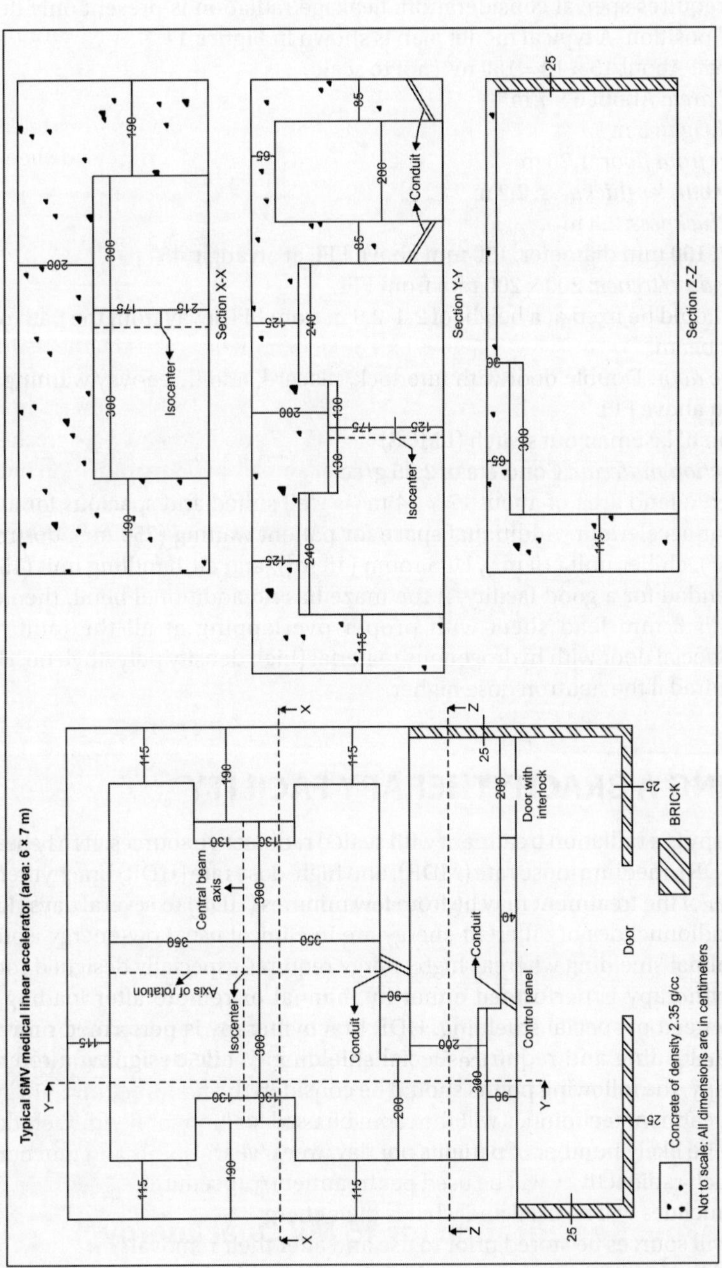

FIG. 11.6: Model layout for 6 MV linear accelerator installation.
Courtesy: AERB. https://www.aerb.gov.in.

Asymmetric and multi-leaf collimators are used to collimate the beam. Machines have 3D-CRT, IMRT with 3D imaging, VMAT, and SRS/SRT treatment capabilities. Machine do have FFF mode in 6 and 10 MV, where the dose rate may be higher. Since large amount of primary and secondary radiation incident on the floors, walls, and ceilings, it requires special consideration. Leakage radiation is present only during source "on" position. A typical model plan is shown in **Figure 11.7**.

- *Land area*: About 15 × 12 = 180 m^2 (not to scale)
- *Internal area*: About 6 × 7 m^2
- *Ceiling height*: 3 m
- *Isocenter from floor*: 1.25 m
- *Primary barrier thickness*: 2.2 m
- *Ceiling thickness*: 2.3 m
- *Conduit*: 100 mm diameter, 150 mm above FFL at an angle 45°
- *Core conduit/trench*: 200 × 200 mm from FFL
- Lasers should be fixed at a height of 2.4–2.6 m from FFL away from the path of the primary beam.
- *Entrance door*: Double door with interlock, placard, and three-way warning sign at 1.65 m above FFL
- Provision of last man out switch (LMOS)
- *Construction material*: Concrete of 2.35 g/cc

However, a land area of about 17 × 14 m^2 is well suited and spacious for a dual energy linear accelerator. Additional space for patient waiting (250 m^2), dosimetry room (15 m^2), chiller unit (10 m^2), UPS room (15 m^2), and air handling unit (15 m^2) is recommended for a good facility. If the maze has no additional bend, then door is lined with 6 mm lead sheet with proper overlapping at all the joints and junctions. Special door with hydrogenous material (high density polyethylene, HPE), may be required if the neutron dose higher.

PLANNING A BRACHYTHERAPY FACILITY

Brachytherapy is a radiation treatment with sealed radioactive sources. It may be low-dose rate (LDR), medium-dose rate (MDR), and high-dose rate (HDR) brachytherapy. The duration of the treatment may be from few minutes (HDR) to several days (LDR). Variety of radionuclides of different energy are in clinical use. Low-energy isotopes require minimal shielding whereas high energy requires especially designed rooms. LDR brachytherapy is performed either by manual or remote after loading and requires no need of special shielding. HDR brachytherapy is performed only with remote after-loading and requires special shielding. While designing a room for brachytherapy, the following points should be considered:

- Which treatment techniques will the room be used for?
- What is the likely number of patients per day/week/year?
- How much radioactivity will be used per treatment/procedure?
- Which nuclides will be used and what is their energy?
- Where will sources be stored prior to use and after their removal?
- How will the security performance objectives for brachytherapy be achieved?

In brachytherapy, the protection must be sufficient to reduce the primary and scattered radiation to the design limit in all directions since the sources are unshielded in all directions. The dose rate within the room will be much higher and the room will be designated as controlled area. The dose rate outside the brachytherapy room

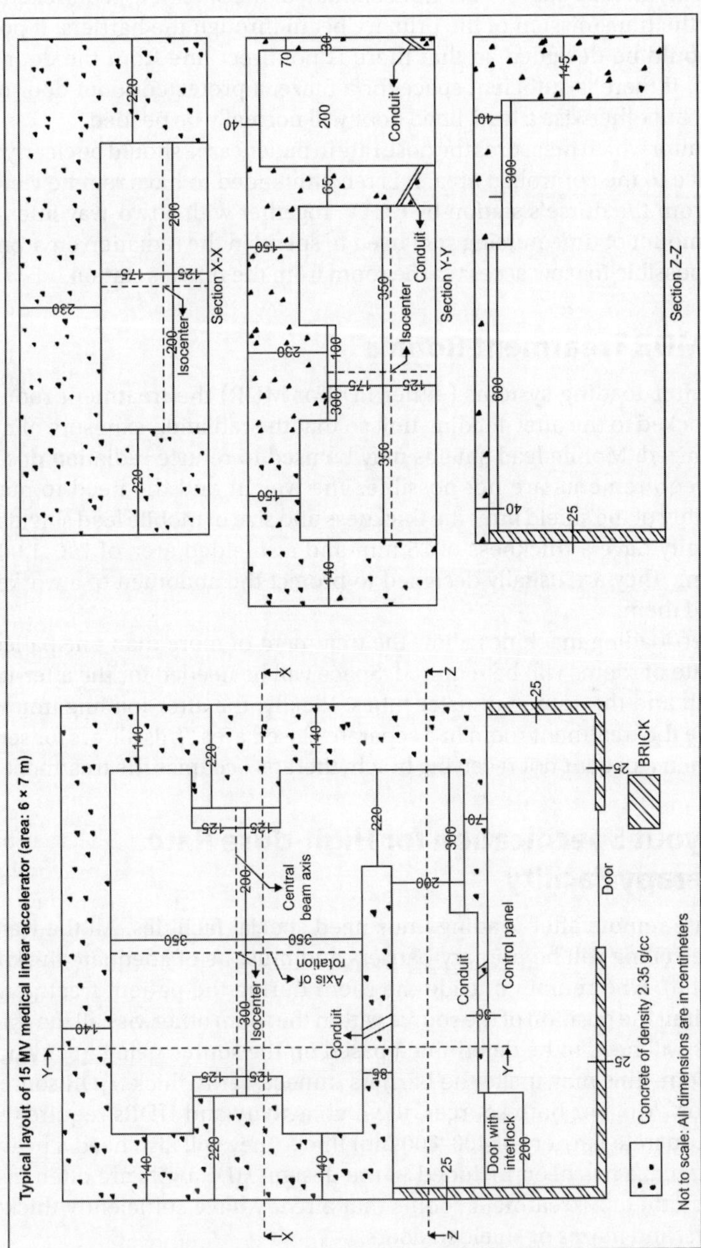

FIG. 11.7. Model layout for 15 MV dual energy linear accelerator installation.
Courtesy: AERB. https://www.aerb.gov.in.

should be reduced to <1 mSv/year that depends on occupancy. The patient receiving brachytherapy will attenuate the radiation. The extent of the attenuation will depend on the energy of the nuclide in use, the size of the patient, and the location of the source(s) within the patient.

Since brachytherapy sources are not collimated, the shielding requirements will be based on the transmission of the primary beam through the barriers. If possible, the room should be designed so that there is no direct line from the door to the patient's bed. If there is sufficient space for a maze, a protected room door may be unnecessary, but otherwise a lead-lined door will normally be needed.

Zone monitor which measures the dose rate in patient area should be clearly visible at the entrance to the controlled area. It is recommended to have remote viewing of the patient from the nurse's station by CCTV, together with a two-way intercom to reduce the amount of time nursing staff need to spend in the radiation environment. It should be possible to view access to the room from the nurse's station.

LDR and MDR Treatment Rooms

For remote after-loading systems (either LDR or MDR) the treatment room door will be interlocked to the after-loading unit so that the radiation exposure of nursing staff is minimized. Mobile lead shields may be used to reduce radiation dose rates when ideal requirements are not possible. The weight and the need to maintain maneuverability of the shield limit the thickness and size of mobile lead shields. Lead shields typically have a thickness of 25 mm and a shielded area of 700–1,000 mm × 500–600 mm. They are usually designed to protect the abdomen of a worker who stands behind them.

Some after-loading machines allow the treatment of more than one patient at a time so as suite of rooms will be required. Space will be needed for the after-loading machine itself and the source transfer tubes. Ideally, the after-loading unit will be stored outside the treatment room in a separate closed area. This allows for servicing of the unit when a patient not receiving brachytherapy occupies the treatment room.

Model Layout Specification for High-dose Rate Brachytherapy Facility

High-dose rate remote after-loading units need special facilities. All the walls, the floor, and the ceiling will be primary barriers and must be of adequate thickness to protect the staff, who remain outside the room during the patient treatment. It is advisable to limit the position of the source within the room otherwise all the shielding requirements will need to be determined based on the source being in any position within the room. This may make the barriers unnecessarily thick. HDR sources are usually ^{192}Ir or ^{60}Co. For both sources, the high activity and HDRs require that the rooms have concrete barriers of 400–800 mm thick. They will also need a heavy lead door unless a maze has been included in the design. HDR units are often installed in former radiotherapy treatment rooms that already have sufficiently thick walls, ceilings, floors, and mazes or shielded doors.

In HDR brachytherapy the patients are often treated directly after the appliances have been positioned. Ideally, there will also be an X-ray (C-arm) facility within the room so that the correct placement of the applicators can be confirmed immediately prior to the treatment being delivered. A waiting area for the patient and a trolley may be required where the patient may be nursed while the treatment planning calculations are completed. An HDR facility should have an interlocked room door so that the source is returned to the safe position whenever the door is opened, and there should be a radiation warning sign at the room entrance indicating the "ON-OFF" status of the source. A model layout of the HDR room is shown in **Figure 11.8**.

- *Land area*: about 7 × 9 = 63 m^2 (not to scale)
- *Internal area*: about 4 × 5 = 20 m^2
- *Ceiling height*: 3 m
- *Barrier thickness*: 0.45 m
- *Ceiling thickness*: 0.45 m
- *Conduit*: 100 mm diameter, 150 mm above FFL at an angle 45°
- Zone monitor at 2 m from floor
- *Entrance door*: Double door with interlock, placard, and three-way warning sign at 1.65 m above FFL. Doors are lined with 2 mm lead sheet with proper overlapping at all the joints and junctions.
- *Construction material*: Concrete of 2.35 g/cc

However, wall thickness of 60 cm concrete is required for ^{60}Co HDR source. If the maze has additional bend, there is no need for lead lined doors, only aluminum with glass partition is sufficient.

CLASSIFICATION OF AREAS

Controlled Area and Supervised Area

International basic safety standard (BSS)-series No. 115 classifies controlled and supervised areas. Controlled area is one in which specific protection and safety are provided for (i) controlling normal exposures or preventing the spread of contamination during normal working conditions, and (ii) preventing or limiting the extent of potential exposures. Controlled areas include (i) external radiotherapy treatment room, (ii) remote after loading brachytherapy treatment room, (iii) operation theater doing brachytherapy with real sources, (iv) brachytherapy patient ward with sources, and (v) radioactive source storage and handling area. Generally provided with physical boundaries and radiation signs with restricted access.

Supervised area is an area for which occupational exposure conditions are kept under review even though specific protective measures and safety provisions are not normally needed. Areas adjacent to treatment room where the dose levels are sufficiently low is referred as supervised area. However, it is beneficial to classify the area based on dose rate at the boundary.

Controlled Area and Uncontrolled Area

NCRP-151 classifies radiotherapy areas as controlled and uncontrolled areas. Controlled area is limited access area in which occupational exposure of personnel to radiation or radioactive material is under the supervision of an individual or RSO. Its access, occupancy, and working conditions are controlled for radiation protection purposes. Areas such as treatment room and control console comes under this category. Workers of the controlled area are specially trained to use ionizing radiation and are individually monitored.

All other areas in the hospital are uncontrolled areas. Rest rooms and examination rooms near controlled areas fall under this category.

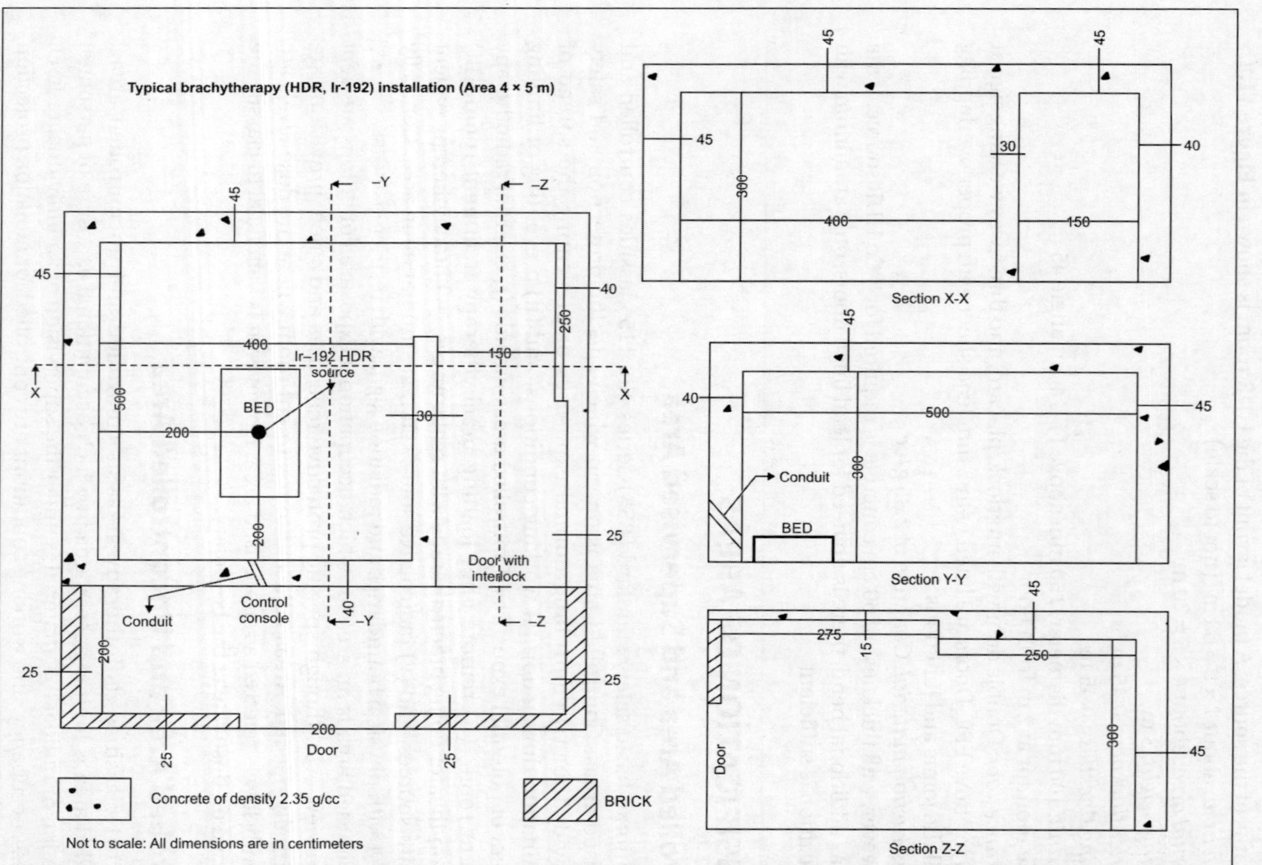

FIG. 11.8: Model layout of high dose rate brachytherapy with Iridium-192 installation. In case of ^{60}Co HDR source, the wall thickness should be 60 cm instead of 45 cm.

Courtesy: AERB. https://www.aerb.gov.in.

Effective Dose Limits for Design

Occupational exposure effective dose limit is 20 mSv/year, averaged over 5 consecutive years, and 30 mSv in any single year. The public dose limit is 1 mSv in a year (ICRP-90). It corresponds to an effective dose limit of 0.4 mSv/week for controlled area (restricted entry) and 0.02 mSv/week for uncontrolled area (Assuming 8 h/day and 50 week/year for shielding design).

However, IAEA has given lesser effective dose limits for shielding calculations for the occupational areas adjacent to radiation therapy treatment rooms **(Table 11.1)**. NCRP-151 recommends a weekly dose limit of 0.1 mSv/week (5 mSv/year) for controlled areas, and 0.02 mSv/week (1 mSv/year) for uncontrolled areas.

The effective dose limit is expressed as "P" in shielding calculation. It is the exposure in mR/week at a given location in an adjacent area. It is a function of treatment technique, workload, primary, scattered and leakage level, and corresponding distance to the point of interest.

WORKLOAD, USE FACTOR AND OCCUPANCY FACTOR

Workload

Workload (W) indicates the radiation output per week of an external beam X-ray or gamma-ray source. It is a measure of an expected exposure levels obtained from patient load and machine "on" time. It is expressed in mA-min/week (equal to mAs/60) in diagnostic radiology. In radiotherapy, the workload is number of patients treated per week multiplied by average dose (MU) per patient at the isocenter, expressed in Gy/week.

For example, if a linear accelerator treats 50 patients per day with dose of 3.5 Gy for each patient at 1 m, then the clinical workload:

$$W_{clin} = (3.5\ \text{Gy/patient}) \times (50\ \text{patient/day}) \times (5\ \text{days/week}) = 875\ \text{Gy/week}$$

Physics workload: In addition to patient treatment, medical physicists use the accelerator for calibration, QA, radiation survey, patient dosimetry, and service and maintenance. It involves considerable workload referred as physics workload (W_{Phys}), amounts to about 7,100 Gy/year or 142 Gy/week, as per IAEA. Hence, total workload is the sum of the clinical and physics workload:

$$W_{tot} = W_{clin} + W_{phys}$$

The total workload comes around 10^3 Gy/week or 5×10^4 Gy/year. It includes conventional, TBI, IMRT, and physics workloads. NCRP recommends a workload of 500 Gy/week for high-energy accelerators and 1,000 Gy/week for low-energy accelerators (NCRP-151).

TABLE 11.1 **Effective dose limits (P) in design for occupational areas adjacent to radiation therapy treatment room.**

Personnel	*Annual effective dose (mSv/year)*	*Weekly effective dose (mSv/week)*
Occupational worker	10	0.2
Public	0.5	0.01

Courtesy: IAEA, 2006.

Intensity modulated radiation therapy (IMRT), SRS, and SRT are much complex. It uses much smaller field sizes with large number of beamlets to get highly conformal dose distribution. More MU will be delivered per Gy which impact the head leakage workload (W_L).

$$W_L = W_{con} + W_{IMRT}$$

where, W_{con} is the conventional workload. The IMRT factor (C_I) is the ratio of MU with IMRT to the MU with conventional treatment delivering same dose, and ranges from 2 to 10:

$$C_I = \frac{MU_{IMRT}/Gy}{MU_{Con}/Gy}$$

This only influences leakage workload but not that of primary and scatter. Helical Tommotherapy has C_I value > 10 whereas, it is 15 for cyber knife.

$$W_{IMRT} = W \times C_I$$

However, TBI has higher workload due to extended distance of treatment. It is the product of TBI patient dose per week and square of the TBI treatment distance. Though the leakage workload is higher, but that of patient and wall scatter is less.

Use Factor

Use factor (U) is the fraction of operating time during which the radiation is directed towards a particular barrier (wall) per week. In other words, it is the fraction of primary beam workload that is directed towards a primary barrier. It describes different orientations used for treatment when calculating the required barrier thickness for each beam orientation. It depends on particular use of the facility and the energy used.

For example, a facility performing large number of TBI may have a use factor >0.25 for one wall, and lower for other walls. IMRT may also change values assigned to the use factor. NCRP-49 has suggested a use factor of 1 for floor, 0.25 for ceiling, and 0.25 for lateral walls. However, NCRP-151 suggested use factor distribution in terms of gantry angles **(Table 11.2)**.

TABLE 11.2 Use factor distribution for 90° and 45° gantry intervals in dual X-ray mode radiotherapy.

Barrier type	*Use factor % (U)*
90° interval	
0° down	31
90° and 270°	21.3 each
180° up	26.3
45° interval	
0° down	25.6
45° and 315°	5.8 (each)
90° and 270°	15.9 each
135° and 225°	4.0 each
180° up	23

Courtesy: NCRP-151.

Occupancy Factor

The occupancy factor (T) refers to the amount of time rooms adjacent to the treatment room is occupied. It is the fraction of the operating time spent by a single person who is there the longest. The target is nonradiation workers of the hospital. Area below ground would have no occupancy at all, and therefore "T" would equal zero. Areas that are intermittently occupied, such as corridors would have a slightly greater occupancy. Occupancy factor is best defined as the fraction of 8 h/day or 2,000 h/year for a single individual to occupy a particular area. Occupancy factors are based on local regulations and specific conditions at the facility. Nature of occupancy may be full, partial, and occasional occupancy **(Table 11.3)**.

CONSTRUCTION MATERIALS

Concrete, lead, steel, and bricks are generally used as construction material while designing radiation facility **(Table 11.4)**. However, concrete is the preferred choice which is least expensive. Concrete density varies widely; however, its density of 2,350 kg/m^3 is accepted as standard. If the radiation energy >1 MV, Compton interaction dominates, and the shielding material will absorb the radiation that varies with density of the material. Concrete is normally specified by strength, and density being of secondary importance. By adding more cement in the aggregate, the strength of concrete may be increased, in turn the density. Increase of water in the aggregate will reduce overall density along with air pockets. Hence, the barrier should be formed in one pour to avoid seams, and the mix is vibrated enough while pouring. The density of preformed concrete is only 2,000 kg/m^3.

Wherever space is a limitation, higher density building material such as baryte, steel, and lead may be recommended. Different materials such as magnetite, baryte, iron scrap, and hematite may be mixed with concrete to have high density of about

TABLE 11.3 **Occupancy factors for different occupancy in radiotherapy.**

Type of occupancy	*Occupancy factor (T)*
Administrative/clerical office, treatment planning areas, treatment control rooms, nurse stations, reception areas, attended waiting rooms and occupied space in nearby building	1 Full occupancy
Adjacent treatment room, patient examination room adjacent to vault	0.5 or 1/2
Corridors, employee lounges, staff rest rooms	0.2 or 1/5
Treatment vault doors	0.125 or 1/8
Public toilets, unattended vending rooms, storage areas, outdoor areas with seating, unattended waiting rooms, patient-holding areas, attics, and Janitor's closets	0.05 or 1/20
Outdoor areas with only transient pedestrian or vehicular traffic, unattended parking lots, vehicular drop off areas, stairways, and unattended elevators	0.025 or 1/40

Courtesy: NCRP-151.

TABLE 11.4 Barrier design materials and density.

Barrier material	***Density, kg/m³***	***Atomic number (Z)***	***Remarks***
Iron ore with ferrosilicon	4,000–5,000	26	Density depends on ore mixture to sand
Ledite	3,844 and 4,613	–	Premolded high-density interlocking bricks
Barytes concreate	3,400–3,500	26	Dense concrete but expensive
Lead (Solid)	11,340	82	Used as shield in an existing treatment room
Steel	7,900	26	Used as supplementary shield
Concrete	2,350	11	Vary with mineral content
Clay bricks	1,100–1,400	–	Used up to 500 kV_p with supplementary to lead or steel
Breeze bricks	1,600	–	
Earth fill	1,600	–	Used in bunker below the ground

Courtesy: IAEA, Safety report series 47.

3,000 kg/m³. When high-density bricks are used, it is important to use heavy mortars to avoid shine paths between the bricks. Ordinary sand mortar has only density of 2,000 kg/m³. Rooms which are upgraded mostly use steel plate of 10 mm thickness which is fixed one layer at a time to the existing wall, taking care that the fixings do not overlie each other.

Influence of Neutron

Machines >10 MeV may produce photoneutrons and protection against neutron is necessary. Generally, concrete contains relatively high hydrogen, its designed thickness is sufficient to shield against fast neutrons. The TVL for primary X-ray beam is approximately double the photoneutron produced by medical linear accelerators, so any shield designed as primary barrier against X-rays will be more than adequate against photoneutrons. However, fast neutrons interact with hydrogen through elastic scattering in concrete and goes with reduced energy. After number of collisions, they become slow neutrons which undergo capture reaction with materials and produce capture gamma rays. The capture gamma ray spectrum in concrete extends to >8.0 MeV and the average energy is 3.6 MeV. The capture of slow neutrons by hydrogen in concrete results in a pronounced peak in the photon spectrum at 2.21 MeV.

Boron and cadmium are suitable as shield to capture slow neutrons. Generally, boron is incorporated in polyethylene to have high hydrogen content and become an effective neutron shield. However, slow neutron capture in boron will produce low energy gamma of 0.473 MeV. This can be shielded best by 5% composition by weight of boron in polyethylene (high density polyethylene, HPE), especially in treatment room door design.

BIBLIOGRAPHY

1. AERB Safety Code No. AERB/RF-MED/SC-1 (Rev. 1): Radiation Therapy Sources, Equipment, and Installations, 2011.
2. IAEA safety report series 47: Radiation protection in the design of Radiotherapy facilities, IAEA, Vienna, 2006.
3. Structural shielding design and evaluation for Megavoltage X- and Gamma-ray Radiotherapy facilities. NCRP Report No. 151 Bethesda, MD, 2005.
4. NCRP report 49. Structural shielding design and evaluation for medical use of X-rays and Gamma the rays of energies up to 10 MeV, 1976.
5. Varian medical systems: Linear accelerator planning data, 2000.
6. Patrick Horton and David Eaton: Design and shielding of radiotherapy facilities, IPEM report 2nd edition., 2017.
7. Atomic Energy Regulatory Board (AERB), Website: https://www.aerb.gov.in

CHAPTER 12

Design and Shielding Requirements for Radiotherapy

INTRODUCTION

Radiotherapy uses much higher energy of ionizing radiations. It is used as external beam radiation therapy, brachytherapy, and X-ray simulator. External beam radiation therapy includes telecobalt units and linear accelerators including tommotherapy, and cyber knife. They require special design and shielding requirements to keep the radiation dose the public and workers within regulatory limits. The primary and secondary barriers are much thicker for these machines, compared to diagnostic X-ray units. Hence, the workload and shielding calculation is different from diagnostic X-rays.

SHIELDING CALCULATION METHODS

Any radiological facility has six barriers/walls that includes four walls, floor, and ceiling. Radiotherapy facility consists of seven barriers including maze, floor, and ceiling **(Fig. 12.1)**. If the installation is in ground floor or bunker, no floor calculation is necessary. If it is on the first floor, floor calculation for shielding is mandatory. The calculation is performed by *weekly dose rate method* for seven barriers individually.

Primary Barrier

General approach is to calculate the fraction of transmission based on the dose constraint. This dose constraint is either occupational worker dose limit or public dose limit per week. Number of TVL required is calculated to control the radiation within the limits. In the case of primary barrier, the transmission factor (B) is given by the relation:

$$B = \frac{P(d + SAD)^2}{WUT} \tag{12.1}$$

where, P is the allowed dose per week outside the barrier,
d is the distance between isocenter and the point of interest outside the barrier, in meter
SAD is the source to axis distance,
W is the workload,
U is the use factor, and
T is the occupancy factor.

NCRP-51 has given beam attenuation graphs for different energies and barrier materials, under broad beam geometry for concrete density of 2.35 g/cc **(Fig. 12.2)**. The thickness of the concrete is determined from the attenuation graphs.

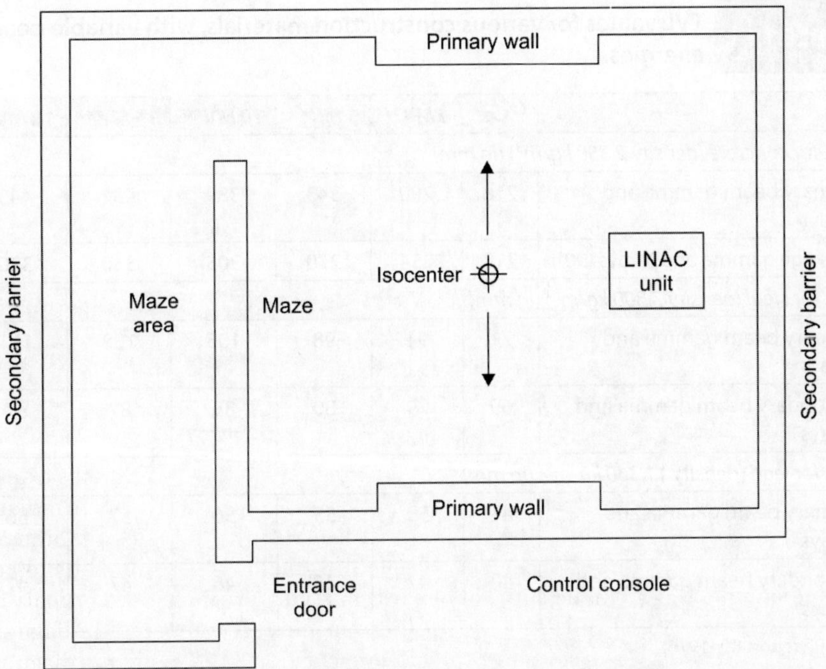

FIG. 12.1: Model layout plan of linear accelerator for radiation therapy (not to scale).

Note: Gantry rotation axis is perpendicular to maze axis.

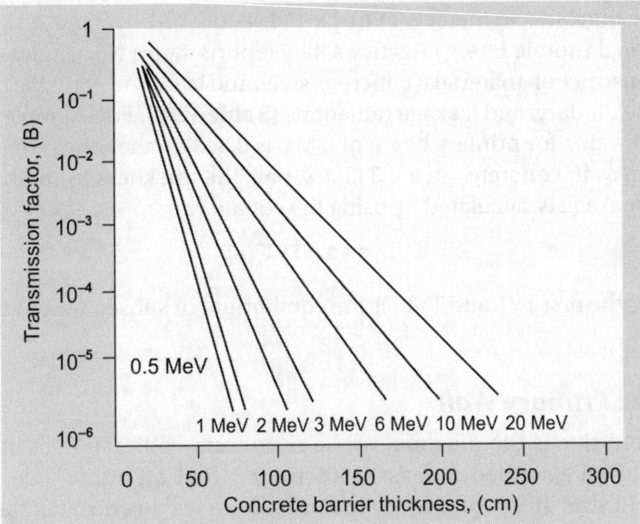

FIG. 12.2: Transmission curves of a thick target X-rays for different photon beam energies under broad beam geometry, for concrete with density 2.35 g/cc as barrier material (NCRP1977).

Alternatively, thickness of concrete can also be determined by *tenth value layer (TVL)* concept by calculation. From the transmission factor, the number of TVL required, TVL(n) to produce required attenuation is:

$$\text{TVL(n)} = \log_{10} \times (1/B) \tag{12.2}$$

TABLE 12.1 TVL values for various construction materials, with variable beam energies.

	^{60}Co*	4 MV**	6 MV**	10 MV**	15 MV**	18 MV**
TVL for concrete (density 2,350 kg/m^3) (in mm)						
Primary beam gamma and X-rays	218	290	343	389	432	445
Leakage gamma and X-rays (90°)	218	254	279	305	330	330
TVL for steal (density 7,800 kg/m^3) (in mm)						
Primary beam gamma and X-rays	71	91	98	105	108	111
Secondary beam gamma and X-rays	69	79	80	85	87	87
TVL for lead (density 11,360 kg/m^3) (in mm)						
Primary beam gamma and X-rays	41	53	55	56	57	56
Secondary beam gamma and X-rays	40	47	45	46	47	47

*NCRP report 49 (1976),

**Varian Associates, Nelson and LaRiviere (1984).

Courtesy: IAEA safety series 47.

Actual barrier thickness in meter = TVl(n) × TVL value

International Atomic Energy Agency safety reports series No. 47 gives TVL values for various construction materials (concrete, steel, and lead) with variable beam energy for primary, secondary, and leakage radiations **(Table 12.1)**. For example, if TVL(n) is 6 and the TVL value for primary beam of 6 MV is 0.343 m, then the required primary barrier thickness in concrete = 6 × 0.343 = 2.0 m. The thickness (S) of the barrier for primary and leakage is calculated by using the equation:

$$S = TVL_1 + (n - 1)\, TVL_e \tag{12.3}$$

where, TVL_1 is the first TVL and TVL_e is the equilibrium or subsequent TVL of concrete **(Table 12.2)**.

Width of the Primary Wall

Maximum field size is the diagonal of the maximum collimator settings. Primary barrier should be extended at least 0.305 m or 1 foot on either side beyond the maximum field size. This is to prevent radiation from leaking through the secondary barrier that abuts the primary. Most of the linear accelerator has 40 × 40 cm as maximum field size at 1 m from the target. When the collimator is rotated to 45°, the above dimension become equal to its diagonal (56.6 cm or 0.566 m). The horizontal barrier width (W) required is given by the relation:

$$W = 0.566\, d + (0.305 \times 2)$$

$$W = 0.566\, d + 0.61 \tag{12.4}$$

where, d is the distance from the source to the barrier,

TABLE 12.2 **Tenth value layers (TVL) for primary barriers, for concrete (2.35 g/cm³), steel (7.87 g/cm³), and lead (11.35 g/cm³) versus beam energies.**

Endpoint energy (MV)	*Shielding material*	*TVL_1 (cm)*	*TVL_e (cm)*
6	Concrete	37	33
	Steel	10	10
	Lead	5.7	5.7
10	Concrete	41	37
	Steel	11	11
	Lead	5.7	5.7
15	Concrete	44	41
	Steel	11	11
	Lead	5.7	5.7
18	Concrete	44	41
	Steel	11	11
	Lead	5.7	5.7
^{60}Co	Concrete	21	21
	Steel	7	7
	Lead	4	4

Courtesy: NCRP-151, 2005.

Ceiling

The roof section that struck directly by the radiation beam is a primary barrier. Method of calculation is same as discussed above. The design dose limit for the roof will depend on the location of the bunker. If it is a single-story building, then the only consideration may be the limitation of access to the roof space. However, the effect of *sky shine* must be considered. It refers to radiation scattered off the atmosphere back to the ground or surrounding buildings. It becomes an issue in vault's ceiling which are lightly shielded.

If there is a nuclear medicine department nearby, then it should be noted that gamma camera and possibly other imaging equipment are particularly sensitive to low levels of radiation that can affect certain patient investigations.

If the building has further floors above the bunker, then consideration should be given to locate a storage room or chiller plant and UPS room immediately above the bunker. It will have limited occupancy and restricted access, thus allowing a greater design dose limit than if an office was placed directly above the bunker. Generally, point of calculation is taken as 0.5 m above the ceiling.

Ground shine: It refers to radiation scattered off the ground below the vault back to the surface outside the vault. It may become an issue in vault designs that use earth as floor shielding.

Secondary Barriers

Secondary barriers are not facing the primary beam, but it is necessary to shield the leakage radiation from the machine head, and scattered radiation from the patient and room walls.

For a linear accelerator, national and international protocols state that the leakage from the treatment head must not exceed 0.5% of the primary beam, outside the useful beam at 1 m from the path of the electrons between the gun and target window and averaged over 100 cm^2. In the plane of the patient, the leakage must not exceed an average of 0.1% and a maximum of 0.2% over a 2-m radius measured from the beam central axis. In general, manufacturers have protected their machines to better than 0.1%, and it would be reasonable to assume this value when determining the required secondary barrier thickness.

Leakage Radiation

The barrier transmission factor (B_L) required to reduce the leakage radiation within permissible dose per week (P) is given by the relation:

$$B_L = \frac{P}{0.1\%\text{ of primary} \times WT} \times d^2 = \frac{1{,}000 \times P}{WT} \times d_s^2 \tag{12.5}$$

where, P is the design dose limit,
d_s is the distance from the isocenter and the point of interest in meter since the average position of the treatment head is taken at the isocenter,
W is the workload, and
T is the occupancy factor.

The leakage radiation is present whenever the machine is switched ON hence, the use factor (U) is unity. It is assumed that the treatment head reduces the leakage radiation to 0.1% or 1/1,000 of the useful beam. The energy of the leakage radiation is lower than the primary beam due to scattering inside the treatment head. It is also suggested to have distance measured from the waveguide gun to the barrier behind the accelerator, for accelerator with horizontal waveguide.

Barrier thickness for leakage radiation is always greater than the scattered radiation since leakage radiation is more penetrating in nature. In the case of low energy, the difference in barrier thickness is very small. An optimally designed primary barrier will ensure adequate protection against scattered and leakage radiation.

Scattered Radiation

Let us consider a situation as shown in **Figure 12.3**. If B_P is the transmission factor required to reduce the scattered radiation dose within permissible dose per week (P) in area of interest:

$$B_P = \frac{P}{aWT} \times \frac{400}{F} \times d_{Sca}^2 \times d_{sec}^2 \tag{12.6}$$

where, a is the scatter fraction defined at d_{sca}
W is the workload,
T is the occupancy factor,
U = 1 since scattered radiation is always present,
F is the field area incident on the patient, in cm^2,
d_{sca} is the distance from the radiation source to the patient, in meter,
and d_{sec} is the distance between the patient and the point of interest, in meter.

Scatter fraction of dose (a), at 1 m are available for 20 × 20 cm = 400 cm^2 incident beam. It is the ratio of the scattered dose to incident dose, which varies with scattering angle and beam quality **(Table 12.3)**.

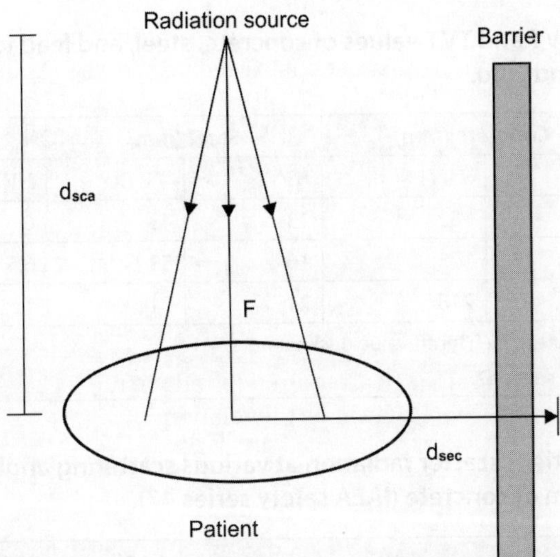

FIG. 12.3: Patient scatter at the point of interest transmitted through the barrier.

TABLE 12.3 **The maximum values of scatter fraction of dose (*a*) at 1 m, 400 cm² incident beam, for different scattering angles-^{60}Co and linear accelerator beams (IAEA safety series 47).**

Scattering angle, degree	*^{60}Co (10^{-3})*	*4 MV (10^{-3})*	*6 MV (10^{-3})*	*10 MV (10^{-3})*	*18 MV (10^{-3})*
10	11	2.7 (NCRP-34)	16.8	16.9	24.3
20	80		11.5	10.3	11.7
30	6.0		5.36	6.73	7.13
45	3.7		2.97	3.25	3.05
60	2.2		1.74	1.84	1.42
90	0.91		0.727	0.714	0.375
135	0.54		0.488	0.370	0.259
150	0.15		0.328	0.316	0.226

The scattered radiation from the patient is <0.1% of the incident radiation per 0.1 m² area irradiated. For large scatter angles, the energy of the scattered radiation is degraded, and the protection designed for leakage radiation is enough to protect against scattered radiation from the patient. However, it should not be ignored for small angle scatter, say 10° since scatter fraction is high (24.3×10^{-3} for 18 MV), and energy of the scattered photons may be closer to that of incident beam.

When a primary beam strikes the wall, the barrier transmission needed to shield against scattered radiation is given the relation:

$$B_W = \frac{P \times d_w^2 \times d_r^2}{\alpha \times A \times W \times U \times T} \quad (12.7)$$

TABLE 12.4 HVT and TVT values of concrete, steel, and lead for ^{192}Ir, ^{137}Cs, and ^{60}Co.

	Concrete (mm)		*Steel (mm)*		*Lead (mm)*	
Source	***HVT***	***TVT***	***HVT***	***TVT***	***HVT***	***TVT***
^{192}IR	43	152	13	43	6	16
^{137}CS	48	175	16	53	6.5	22
^{60}Co	62	218	21	71	12	41

(HVT: half value thickness; TVT: tenth-value thickness)

Courtesy: IAEA Safety series 47.

TABLE 12.5 Patient scatter radiation at various scattering angles-first TVL in mm of concrete (IAEA safety series 47).

Scatter angle	*^{60}Co*	*4 MV*	*6 MV*	*10 MV*	*15 MV*	*18 MV*
15	223	320	367	410	436	449
30	213	248	261	275	285	288
45	197	223	229	233	237	238
60	189	201	205	209	211	211
90	151	169	171	173	174	174
135	128	143	144	144	145	145

where, d_w is the distance from the radiation source to the scattering surface/wall, in meter
d_r is the distance from the scattering surface to the point of interest, in meter
α is the wall reflection coefficient, which depends on the wall material, scattering angle, and beam energy (Refer Tables 6 and 7, IAEA safety report series 47),
and A is the field area projected on the scattering wall in m^2, W, U and T are the workload, use factor and occupancy factor, respectively.

Two Source Rule

The patient scatter and leakage components of the secondary radiation is treated as two distinct sources. The photons scattered from the wall and the patient will have same energy. If the patient scattered and leakage transmission factor are equal, shielding thickness may be taken as the larger of the two-barrier thickness plus one HVL. If the thickness of leakage and scatter protection differs by 1 TVL or more, the larger barrier thickness may be used. It may be applied to different beam energies.

Half value thickness and TVT values of concrete, steel, and lead for ^{192}Ir, ^{137}Cs, and ^{60}Co are given in **Table 12.4**. TVL values of concrete for various beam energies with function of scattering angle are given in **Table 12.5**.

Dose at the Maze Entrance

While designing the maze, the scattering characteristics of X-rays by the patient, and room walls are much important. The maze entrance dose (door level) arises from (i) patient scatter (D_p), (ii) primary beam scatter (D_W), (iii) head leakage scatter (D_L), and (iv) head leakage transmission (D_T).

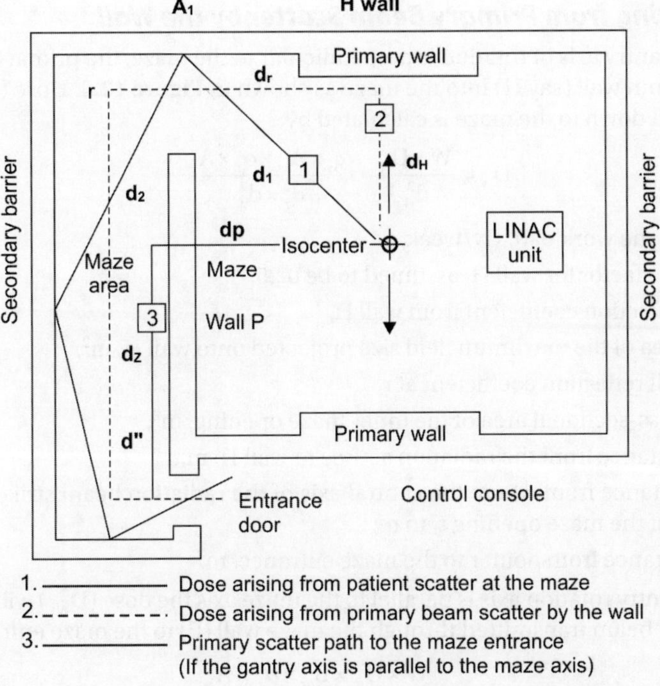

FIG. 12.4: Dose at the maze entrance due to: (i) patient scatter path from the patient and (ii) scatter path for the primary radiation beam to the maze entrance, (iii) primary beam scattered by the wall (Gantry rotation axis is perpendicular to the maze axis).

Dose Arising from Patient Scatter at the Maze Entrance

Let us consider a layout in which the gantry is rotating with its axis perpendicular to the maze axis **(Fig. 12.4)**. Dose (D_p) at the maze entrance due to patient scatter is calculated by the relation:

$$D_p = \frac{W \times U_0 \times a \times (F/400) \times (\alpha_1 A_1)......(\alpha_{n-1} A_{n-1})}{(d_{Sca} \times d_1......d_n)^2} \tag{12.8}$$

where, W is the workload, Gy/week

U_0 is the use factor, generally = 0.25,

a is the scatter primary ratio at the patient,

$\alpha_1 ... \alpha_n$ are wall reflection coefficients for 0.5 MeV for scattered X-rays (Assuming this energy is constant),

F is the field area incident on the patient, cm^2,

$A_1 ... A_n$ are the areas of wall that scattered radiation can strike and be reflected down the maze and subsequent areas are taken to be the cross-sectional area of the maze,

d_{sca} is the distance of the radiation source from the patient in meter,

$d_1 ... d_n$ are the distances of next scattering surface, and subsequently the length of each leg of the maze, in meter.

Dose Arising from Primary Beam Scatter by the Wall

When the gantry axis of rotation is perpendicular to the maze, the primary beam gets scattered from wall (say H) into the maze as shown in **Figure 12.4**. Dose (D_w) arising by such wall down to the maze is calculated by:

$$D_W = \frac{W \times U_H}{d_H^2} \times \frac{\alpha_H \times A_H \times \alpha_r \times A_r}{d_r^2 \times d_z^2} \tag{12.9}$$

where, W is the workload, Gy/week,

U_H is the use factor for wall H, assumed to be 0.25,

α_H is the reflection coefficient from wall H,

A_H is the area of the maximum field size projected onto wall H, m^2,

α_r is the wall reflection coefficient at r,

A_r is the cross-sectional area of the inner maze opening, m^2,

d_H is the distance from the radiation source to wall H, m,

d_r is the distance from where the central axis of the radiation beam strikes wall H to the center of the maze opening r, in m,

d_z is the distance from point r to the maze entrance, m.

If the gantry rotation axis is parallel to the maze axis the dose (D_{WT}) will arise from the primary beam transmitted through the maze wall (P) to the maze entrance:

$$D_{WT} = \frac{W \times U_m \times B_{pr} \times \alpha_p \times A_p}{(d_p \times d'')^2} \tag{12.10}$$

where, W is the workload, Gy/week,

U_m is the use factor for the beam directed at the maze wall, assumed to be 0.25,

B_{pr} is the transmission of the primary through the maze wall,

d_p is the distance from the source to the center of wall p,

d″ is the distance from the center of wall P to the maze entrance,

α_p is the wall reflection coefficient at p,

A_p is the area of maximum field size projected to wall p, in m^2.

Dose Arising from Head Leakage Scatter

Let us consider a layout in which the gantry is rotating with its axis perpendicular to the maze axis **(Fig. 12.5)**. The dose (D_L) at the maze entrance (door) due to from head leakage scatter can calculated by the relation:

$$D_L = \frac{L_0 \times W \times \alpha_1 \times A_1}{(d_i \times d_m)^2} \tag{12.11}$$

where, L_0 is the fraction of dose due to head leakage at 1.0 m from the radiation source relative to the dose on the beam axis at 1 m,

W is the workload, Gy/week,

α_1 is the wall reflection coefficient,

A_1 is the area of wall that can be seen from the maze entrance,

d_i is the distance from the radiation source to the maze centerline, in meter

d_m is the centerline distance along the maze, in meter

The fraction of dose due to head leakage is assumed as 0.1%, and the leakage radiation energy is taken as 1.4 MeV for 6 MV and 1.5 MeV for 10 MV X-rays.

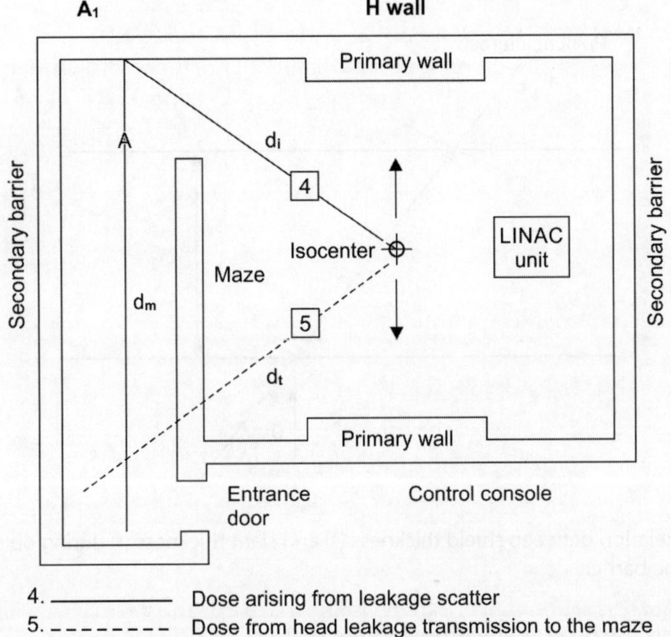

FIG. 12.5: Dose at the maze entrance due to (i) leakage scatter and (ii) head leakage transmission (Gantry rotation axis is perpendicular to the maze axis).

Dose from Head Leakage Transmission to the Maze

The radiation dose (D_T) at the maze entrance (door) due to leakage transmitted through the maze can be calculated by using the relation **(Fig. 12.5)**:

$$D_T = \frac{L_0 \times W \times B}{(d_t)^2} \tag{12.12}$$

where, d_t is the distance from the radiation source to the maze wall, in meter
B is the transmission through the maze wall.
The above equation depends on gantry axis rotation, whether it is perpendicular or parallel to the maze. In later case, the maze happens to be the primary barrier, and the head leakage transmission is negligible.
Note: The above transmission involves oblique transmission and involves obliquity factor **(Fig. 12.6)**. Slant thickness (t) is higher than the shielding thickness (S):

$$t = \frac{S}{\cos\theta}$$

where, θ is the slant angle. As a rule of thumb, if the angle is >45° and B is <0.001, 2 HVL is added for low energy photons whereas 1 HVL is added for high-energy photons.

Total Dose at the Maze Entrance

Total dose (D_d) at the maze entrance is the sum of patient scatter, primary beam scatter, head leakage scatter, and head leakage transmission (H refers to wall):

$$D_d = 2.64 \times (D_{pH} + f \times D_{WH} + D_{LH} + D_{TH}) \tag{12.13}$$

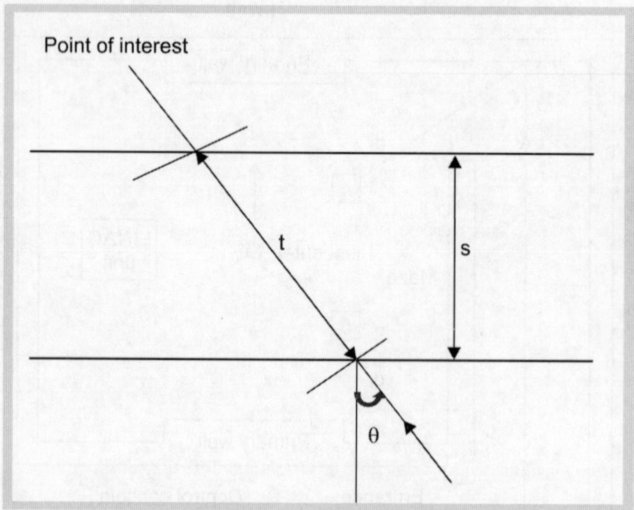

FIG. 12.6: Relation between shield thickness (s) and slant thickness (t) during oblique transmission in the barrier.

where, D_{PH} is the dose arising from patient scatter,

D_{WH} is the primary beam scattered by the wall

f is the patient transmission factor,

D_{LH} is the head leakage scatter to the maze entrance

and D_{TH} is the leakage transmission to the maze entrance

Capture Gamma Dose at the Maze Entrance

When photon interact with collimator, target, flattening filter, and other materials photoneutrons are produced. The head shield is made up of lead, tungsten, and other high Z materials which shield only photons but not the neutrons. They may lower the neutron energy by (n, p), (n, 2n), and inelastic scattering. The neutron fluence at any point in the room is made up of (i) direct neutrons (φ_d), (ii) scattered neutrons (φ_{sc}), and (iii) thermal neutrons (φ_{th}):

$$\varphi = \varphi_d + \varphi_{sc} + \varphi_{th} \tag{12.14}$$

The capture gamma dose at the maze depends on maze length and the total neutron fluence at the inner maze point A **(Fig. 12.7)**. The inner maze point A is the point of intersection of the centerline of the maze, and the line joining the isocenter and the end of the maze wall, at 1 m above floor level. The total neutron fluence (φ_A) at the inner maze point A per X-ray. Gy at 1 m is expressed in neutrons (n) m^2:

$$\varphi A = \frac{Q_N}{4\pi d_1^2} + \frac{5.4\,Q_N}{2\pi S} + \frac{1.26 Q_N}{2\pi S} \tag{12.15}$$

where, Q_N is the neutron source strength (obtained from literature or Table 9, safety report series No. 47, IAEA),

d_1 is the distance from the isocenter to the inner maze point A in meter, and

S is the surface area of the treatment room, in m^2.

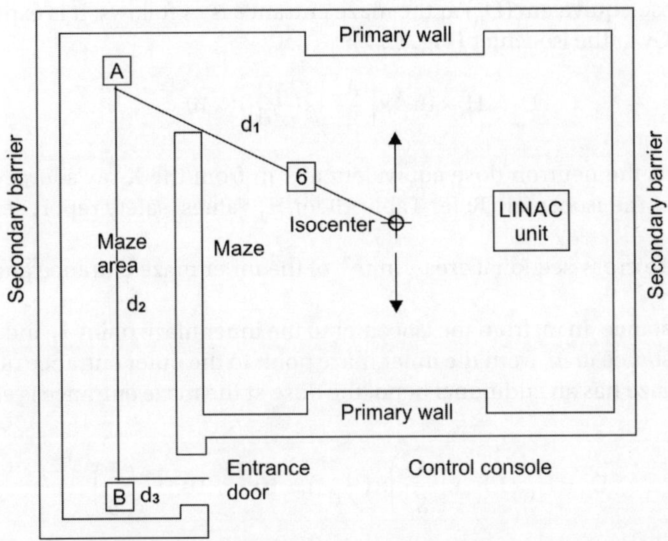

FIG.12.7: Dose at the maze entrance due to (i) capture gamma dose at the maze entrance and (ii) neutrons for high energy accelerators.

Knowing the total neutron fluence at the inner maze point, the capture gamma dose (D_φ) is expressed in Gy per isocenter photon × Gy, for a given maze length for a maze length d_2. It is determined by the relation:

$$D_\varphi = 5.7 \times 10^{-16} \times \varphi_A \times 10^{\frac{-d_2}{6.2}} \quad (12.16)$$

The weekly dose equivalent (D_C) due to capture gamma in Sv per week is the product of workload and capture gamma dose:

$$D_C = W \times D_\varphi \quad (12.17)$$

where, W is the workload, in Gy.m^2.
Total weekly dose due to photons is $D_d + D_C$ mSv/week.

Neutrons in High-energy Linear Accelerators

Neutron dose estimation is much important for accelerators of >10 MeV. It decreases along the maze with a TVL of 5–7.5 m. A maze with small cross-sectional area permits more interactions between neutron and wall, resulting reduction of dose at the maze entrance. The neutron dose is higher for a gantry angle when the LINAC head is closest to the inner maze entrance. The dose is lower for a gantry angle when the head is farthest away. A neutron dose may differ by factor of two between two gantry angles. When the beam is pointing downward, the dose is slightly higher than the average of the two gantry angles. Smaller field size results in higher neutron dose at any point down the maze. A difference of about 10–20% found between largest and smallest field sizes. Hence, calculation of neutron dose is done with beam pointing downwards with fully closed collimators. **Kersey's** empirical method of calculating neutron dose equivalent (D_n) at the maze entrance is as follows. It is expressed in Sv per X-ray. Gy at the isocenter **(Fig. 12.7)**:

$$D_n = H_1 \times 10^{-3} \times \left(\frac{A_r}{S_1}\right) \times \left(\frac{1}{d_1}\right)^2 \times 10^{\frac{-d_2}{5}} \qquad (12.18)$$

where, H_1 is the neutron dose equivalent at 1 m from the X-ray source in mSv per X-ray. Gy at the isocenter (Refer Table 10 for H_1 values, safety report series No. 47, IAEA),

A_r and S_1 are cross-sectional areas, in m^2, of the inner maze entrance and the maze, respectively,

d_1 is the distance, in m, from the isocenter to the inner maze point A, and

d_2 is the distance in m, from the inner maze point to the outer entrance of the maze.

If the maze has an additional bend, the dose at the maze entrance is estimated as follows:

$$D_n = H_1 \times 10^{-3} \times \left(\frac{A_r}{S_1}\right) \times \left(\frac{1}{d_2}\right)^2 \times 10^{\frac{-d_2}{5}} \times 10^{\frac{-d_3}{5}} \times \left(\frac{1}{3}\right)$$

where, d_2 is the distance in m from inner maze point to outer maze point B before bend, and

d_3 is the distance in m from outer maze point to maze entrance at the end of bend. Addition of bend reduces the neutron dose by a factor of 1/3.

The weekly neutron dose (D_E) is the product of weekly workload (W) and the neutron dose equivalent (D_n) and expressed in Sv per week:

$$D_E = W \times D_n \qquad (12.19)$$

The dose at the maze entrance is made up of: (i) scatter and leakage photon dose (D_d), (ii) capture gamma dose (D_c), and (iii) neutron dose (D_E). Total weekly dose at the maze entrance due to photons and neutrons is given by:

$$D_W = D_d + D_c + D_E \qquad (12.20)$$

DESIGN AND SHIELDING CALCULATIONS FOR LINEAR ACCELERATOR INSTALLATION

Leakage Limit for Linear Accelerator

The leakage radiation outside the beam limiting device in a plane of circular surface radius centered on and perpendicular to the radiation beam axis at normal treatment distance (NTD) shall not exceed a maximum of 0.2% and an average of 0.1% of the maximum absorbed dose measured at the center of the plane in a 10 × 10 cm radiation field size. The leakage radiation outside the patient plane shall not exceed 0.5% of the maximum absorbed dose measured on the radiation beam axis in a 10 × 10 cm radiation field at NTD. The stray X-radiation during electron irradiation shall not exceed 4% for electron energies up to 6 MeV, 5% between 6 and 15 MeV and 10% beyond 15 MV up to 30 MeV.

The neutron leakage in the patient plane, outside the beam limiting device at electron energy >10 MeV shall not exceed a maximum of 0.05% and an average of 0.02% of the maximum absorbed dose in a 10 × 10 cm radiation field at the point of intersection with the radiation beam axis. Neutron leakage outside the patient plane shall not exceed 0.05% of the maximum absorbed dose due to electron or X-radiations (AERB safety code 2011).

Worked Example 12.1

It is proposed to design a 15-MV linear accelerator facility for a workload of 750 Gy/week at the isocenter. The location of a particular primary wall is at 5.5 m from the isocenter. Assume the use factor = 0.25, occupancy factor = 1, and SAD = 1 m. Calculate the primary wall thickness to yield an effective weekly dose of 0.4 mSv/week (Occupational limit)?

SAD = 1 m, d = 5.5 m, W = 750 Gy/week, U = 0.25, and T = 1, using equation 12.1.

$$B = \frac{P(d+SAD)^2}{WUT}$$

$$B = \frac{0.4\times10^{-3}(5.5+1)^2}{750\times0.25\times1} = \frac{0.4\times42.25\times10^{-3}}{187.5} = 9.0\times10^{-5}$$

$$TVL(n) = \log_{10}\times(1/B), \text{ by using equation 12.2,}$$

$$TVL(n) = \log_{10}\times(1/9.0\times10^{-5}) = 4.04$$

From **Table 12.1**, the TVL for 15 MV X-rays in concrete is 432 mm, then thickness required = 4.04 × 432 = 1,745 mm or ≈1,750 mm.

Note: If the occupational limit of 0.02 mSv/week (public limit) is used, the number of TVL is 5.34 and required primary barrier is 2,306.8 mm ≈ 2,310 mm.

As per NCRP the actual concrete primary thickness required for both primary and leakage radiation is:

$$S = T_1 + (n-1)T_e, \text{ by equation 12.3,}$$

$$= 44 + (5.04 - 1)41, \text{ (from **Table 12.2**)}$$

$$= 209.6 \text{ cm}$$

$$= 2.09 \text{ m}$$

Worked Example 12.2

It is proposed to design a 15-MV linear accelerator facility for a workload of 750 Gy/week at the isocenter. The location of a particular secondary wall is at 5.5 m from the isocenter. Assume the occupancy factor = 0.1, and SAD = 1 m. Calculate the leakage, scattered radiation, and the secondary wall thickness to yield an effective weekly dose of 0.02 mSv/week (public)?

Leakage Radiation

SAD = 1 m, d_s = 5.5 m, W = 750 Gy/week, P = 0.02 mSv/week (public limit), T = 0.1, (occupancy factor for secondary wall at the control console area is 1, for other walls it is 0.1), using equation 12.5,

$$B_L = \frac{1{,}000\times P}{WT}\times d_s^2$$

$$= \frac{1{,}000\times0.02\times10^{-3}}{750\times0.1}\times5.5^2 = 8.0\times10^{-3}$$

$$\text{TVL(n)} = \log_{10} \times (1/\text{B}),$$
$$\text{TVL(n)} = \log_{10} \times (1/8.0 \times 10^{-3}) = 2.09$$

From the **Table 12.1**, the TVL in concrete for 15 MeV leakage radiation is 330 mm. Secondary barrier required against the leakage radiation is:
= 2.09 × 330 = 689.70 mm, it is rounded to the nearest 10 mm, 690 mm.

Scattered Radiation

In this case, SAD = d_{sca} = 1 m, d_{sec} = 5.5 m, W = 750 Gy/week, F = 20 × 20 cm = 400 cm², P = 0.02 mSv/week, for scatter fraction *a* for 90° scatter from 15 MV X-rays is 5.02 × 10^{-4} per 400 cm² of irradiated area (Table 5, IAEA safety report series 47, this value is extrapolated from 10 and 18 MeV energy for its maximum, from **Table 12.3**), T = 0.1, using equation 12.6:

$$B_P = \frac{P}{aWT} \times \frac{400}{F} \times d_{sca}^2 \times d_{sec}^2$$
$$= \frac{0.02 \times 10^{-3}}{5.02 \times 10^{-4} \times 750 \times 0.1} \times \frac{400}{400} \times 1 \times 5.5^2$$
$$= 5.31 \times 10^{-4} \times 30.25 = 1.60 \times 10^{-2}$$

(Value *a* is interpolated from the Table 5, safety report series No. 47, IAEA for 15 MeV for concrete).

$$\text{TVL(n)} = \log_{10} \times (1/\text{B}),$$
$$= \log_{10} \times (1/1.60 \times 10^{-2}) = 1.79$$

The barrier requires 2.09 TVLs against leakage radiation and 1.79 TVLs against scattered radiation. These two values are within one TVL of each other, so the required barrier secondary wall thickness in concrete:

= TVL + 1 HVL

= (2.09 × 330) + 99.39 = 789.09 mm, rounded to 790 mm

(1 HVL of concrete = 99.39 mm, for 15 MV X-rays)

Worked Example 12.3

Find the width of a primary barrier, which is 3.6 m away from a 6-MV linear accelerator. By using equation 12.4:

$$W = 0.566\,d + 0.61,$$
$$= (0.566 \times 3.6) + 0.61$$
$$= 2.03 + 0.61$$
$$= 2.64\text{ m}$$

Maze and Door Design

The door design depends on the annual dose limit in force. AERB recommended public dose limit is 1 mSv/year. This will be 0.02 mSv/week taking 50 weeks for 1 year. Ratio of the dose limit and the calculated value of dose at the maze entrance will give the attenuation of door. Either protected door or physical barrier can be used depends on the attenuation. The doors should be lockable, especially in telecobalt therapy.

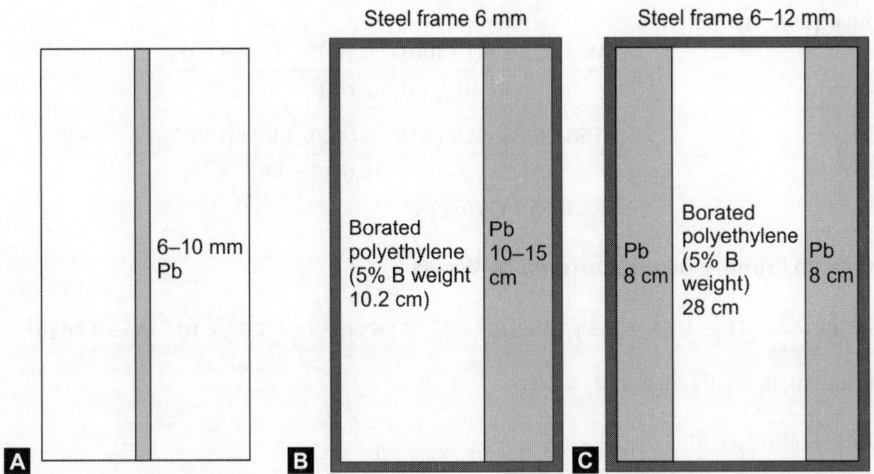

FIGS. 12.8A TO C: Door designs: (A) low energy LINAC with maze, (B) high energy LINAC more than 10 MV with maze, and (C) High energy LINAC more than 10 MV with no maze.

Generally, the scatter and leakage component are low compared with capture gamma and neutrons. Mean energy of capture gamma is 3.6 MeV for short mazes up to 10 MeV. Rooms with long mazes like >5 m, the gamma energy much lower, and require about 6 mm lead. Average neutron energy at the maze entrance may be 100 keV and require either polyethylene (TVL = 45 mm) or borated polyethylene (5% Wt.). Borated polyethylene (PBE) is more effective in thermal neutrons compared to fast neutrons or bare polyethylene **(Figs. 12.8A to C)**. Its TVL is 38 mm, and 12 mm for 2 MeV neutrons and thermal neutrons, respectively. Generally, doors with 6–12 mm lead and 20–40 mm PBE is recommended for accelerator facility. The BPE should be sandwiched between the layers of lead in such design. Lead at the radiation side (inner) reduce neutron energy by inelastic scattering and makes the BPE more effective in shielding. The outer lead will attenuate the capture gamma of energy 0.473 MeV, arising from BPE.

Rooms with short maze length requires much thicker shielding. The capture gamma from concrete may be 7.2 MeV with TVL of 61 mm. Neutrons at the entrance are less thermalized and require three times higher BPE for such door shielding. Door weight mostly depends on neutron shielding. Generally, rooms with long maze, less area of inner maze opening, and addition of bend to the maze is preferred.

Worked Example 12.4

A 15 MV linear accelerator has a workload of 750 Gy/week and the gantry axis is rotating perpendicular to the maze, with following specifications. Calculate the (i) dose from patient scatter to the maze entrance, (ii) dose from primary beam scattered by wall, (iii) dose from leakage radiation scattered down the maze, (iv) dose from leakage radiation transmitted through the maze, and the (v) total dose at the entrance door (refer **Figs. 12.4 and 12.5**)?

Dose from Patient Scatter to the Maze Entrance

$W = 750\,\frac{\text{Gy}}{\text{week}}$, $U = 0.25$, $a = 2.03 \times 10^{-2}$, $F = 20 \times 20\ \text{cm} = 400\ \text{cm}^2$, $\alpha_1 = 1.207 \times 10^{-3}$,

$A_1 = 9.225\ \text{m}^2$, $d_{sca} = 1\ \text{m}$, $d_1 = 6.56\ \text{m}$, $d_2 = 9.9\ \text{m}$.

Using equation 12.8:

$$D_{pH} = \frac{W \times U_0 \times a \times (F/400) \times (\alpha_1 A_1)......(\alpha_{n-1} A_{n-1})}{(d_{sca} \times d_1......d_n)^2}$$

$$= \frac{750 \times 0.25 \times 2.03 \times 10^{-2} \times (400/400) \times (1.207 \times 10^{-3} \times 9.225)}{(1 \times 6.56 \times 9.9)^2}$$

$$= 1.0 \times 10^{-5} \text{ Gy/week}$$

Dose from Primary Beam Scattered by Wall H

$W = 750 \dfrac{\text{Gy}}{\text{week}}$, $U_H = 0.25$, $\alpha_H = 1.75 \times 10^{-3}$, $A_H = 3.063 \text{ m}^2$, $\alpha_r = 7.54 \times 10^{-3}$, $A_r = 9.56 \text{ m}^2$, $d_H = 4.37$ m, $d_r = 5.02$ m, and $d_z = 9.0$ m

Using equation 12.9:

$$D_{wH} = \frac{W \times U_H}{d_H^2} \times \frac{\alpha_H \times A_H \times \alpha_r \times A_r}{d_r^2 \times d_z^2}$$

$$= \frac{750 \times 0.25}{4.37^2} \times \frac{1.75 \times 10^{-3} \times 3.063 \times 7.54 \times 10^{-3} \times 9.56}{5.02^2 \times 9.0^2} = 1.85 \times 10^{-6}$$

Dose from Leakage Radiation Scattered Down the Maze

$L_o = 1 \times 10^{-3}$, $W = 2 \times 750 \dfrac{\text{Gy}}{\text{week}}$, $\alpha_1 = 4.34 \times 10^{-3}$, $A_1 = 9.225 \text{ m}^2$, $d_i = 7.28$, and $d_m = 9.90$ m

Using equation 12.11:

$$D_{LH} = \frac{L_0 \times W \times \alpha_1 \times A_1}{(d_i \times d_m)^2}$$

$$= \frac{1 \times 10^{-3} \times 2 \times 750 \times 4.34 \times 10^{-3} \times 9.225}{(7.28 \times 9.90)^2} = 1.15 \times 10^{-5} \text{ Gy/week}$$

Note: Since the LINAC is having IMRT provision, an IMRT factor of two is used to multiply the regular workload.

Dose from Leakage Radiation Transmitted Through the Maze

$L_o = 1 \times 10^{-3}$, $W = 2 \times 750 \dfrac{\text{Gy}}{\text{week}}$, $B = 4.89 \times 10^{-6}$, and $d_t = 8.48$ m, and $d_m = 9.90$ m,

Using equation 12.12:

$$D_{TH} = \frac{L_0 \times W \times B}{d_t^2}$$

$$= \frac{1 \times 10^{-3} \times 2 \times 750 \times 4.89 \times 10^{-6}}{8.48^2} = 1.02 \times 10^{-7} \text{ Gy/week}$$

Note: Since the LINAC is having IMRT provision, an IMRT factor of two is used to multiply the workload. B is obtained from $10^{-1754.9}/330 = 4.89 \times 10^{-6}$. The oblique thickness of the maze wall t is 1754.9 mm concrete and the TVL in concrete for leakage radiation is 330 mm **(Table 12.1)**.

Total Dose at the Entrance Door

Using equation 12.13:

$$D_d = 2.64 \times (D_{pH} + f \times D_{wH} + D_{LH} + D_{TH})$$

$$= 2.64 \times [1.0 \times 10^{-5} + (0.34 \times 1.85 \times 10^{-6}) + 1.15 \times 10^{-5} + 1.02 \times 10^{-7}]$$

$$= 5.87 \times 10^{-5}\,\frac{\text{Gy}}{\text{week}} = 0.0587\ \text{mGy/week}$$

Worked Example 12.5

Calculate the capture gamma dose for a 15 MV linear accelerator facility having the following specifications?

$Q_N = 3.2 \times 10^{11}$ neutrons per photons, $S = 234.91\ m^2$, $d_1 = 6.07$ m, $d_2 = 9.04$ m, $W = 2 \times 750$ photon Gy/week.

Using equation 12.15 the total neutron fluence at a point in maze per photon Gy at 1 m is:

$$\phi_A = \frac{Q_N}{4\pi d_1^2} + \frac{5.4\,Q_N}{2\pi S} + \frac{1.26Q_N}{2\pi S}$$

$$= \frac{3.2\times10^{11}}{4\pi\times6.07^2} + \frac{5.4\times3.2\times10^{11}}{2\pi\times234.91} + \frac{1.26\times3.2\times10^{11}}{2\pi\times234.91}$$

$$= \frac{3.2\times10^{11}}{462.77} + \frac{17.28\times10^{11}}{1{,}475.23} + \frac{4.03\times10^{11}}{1{,}475.23}$$

$$= (6.91 \times 10^8) + (11.7 \times 10^8) + (2.73 \times 10^8)$$

$$= 21.34 \times 10^8\ \text{n.m}^2$$

The capture gamma dose per photon Gy at the isocenter is estimated by using equation 12.16.

$$D_\phi = 5.7 \times 10^{-16} \times \phi_A \times 10^{-\frac{d_2}{6.2}}$$

$$= 5.7 \times 10^{-16} \times 21.34 \times 10^8 \times 10^{-\frac{9.04}{6.2}}$$

$$= 5.7 \times 10^{-16} \times 21.34 \times 10^8 \times 10^{-1.45}$$

$$= 4.25 \times 10^{-8}\ \text{Gy/photon Gy}$$

The weekly dose equivalent due to capture gamma is obtained by multiplying with IMRT workload (W):

$$D_c = W \times D_\phi\ (\text{Gy/Photon Gy}) \times (\text{photon Gy/week})$$

$$= 2 \times 750 \times 4.25 \times 10^{-8}$$

$$= 6.37 \times 10^{-5} = 0.063\ \text{mGy/week}$$

Total weekly photon dose at the maze entrance is the sum of the photon dose (D_d) and capture gamma dose (D_c) at the maze entrance:

Total photon dose = 0.0587 + 0.063 = 0.121 mGy/week

Note: Photon dose is taken from worked example 12.4, calculated for maze entrance dose.

Worked Example 12.6

Calculate the weekly equivalent neutron dose at the maze entrance for a 15 MV linear accelerator facility having the following specifications?

$H_1 = 7.0 \times 10^{-4}$ Sv per Gy photons, $A_r = 9.56\ m^2$, $S_1 = 9.12\ m^2$, $d_1 = 6.07$ m, $d_2 = 9.04$ m, $W = 2 \times 750$ Gy/week

Using the equation 12.18:

$$D_n = H_1 \times 10^{-3} \times \left(\frac{A_r}{S_1}\right) \times (1/d_1)^2 \times 10^{\frac{-d_2}{5}}$$

$$= 7.0 \times 10^{-4} \times 10^{-3} \times \left(\frac{9.56}{9.12}\right) \times (1/6.07)^2 \times 10^{-\frac{9.04}{5}}$$

$$= 7.0 \times 10^{-7} \times 1.04 \times 0.027 \times 0.015$$

$$= 2.94 \times 10^{-10}\ \text{Sv/Gy}$$

Weekly neutron equivalent dose (D_E) is obtained by multiplying the neutron dose (D_n) with IMRT workload (W) of the accelerator:

$$D_E = W \times D_n$$

$$= 2 \times 750 \times 2.94 \times 10^{-10}$$

$$= 4.41 \times 10^{-7}\ \text{Sv/week or } 4.41 \times 10^{-4}\ \text{mSv/week}$$

DESIGN AND SHIELDING CALCULATIONS FOR TELECOBALT INSTALLATION

Leakage Limits for Telecobalt Therapy

OFF condition leakage limit: The radiation in the beam OFF condition at distance of 1 meter from the source shall not exceed 0.02 mGy/h or 2 mR/h. The stray radiation measured at any accessible position 5 cm from the surface of the protective shielding shall not exceed 0.20 mGy/h or 20 mR/h (AERB safety code, 2011).

ON condition leakage limit: The leakage radiation outside the maximum radiation beam in a plane circular surface radius 2 m centered on and perpendicular to the radiation beam axes at NTD shall not exceed a maximum radiation measured at distance of 1 m from the source shall not a maximum of 0.2% and an average of 0.1% of the maximum absorbed dose measured at the point of intersection of radiation beam axis and the plane of surface for a 10 × 10 cm radiation field size. The absorbed dose rate due to leakage radiation measured at the distance of 1 m from the radiation source shall not exceed 0.5% of the maximum absorbed dose rate on the radiation beam axis measured at a distance 1 m from the radiation source (AERB safety code, 2011).

Worked Example 12.7

It is proposed to design a telecobalt-60 facility for a workload of 1,000 Gy/week at the isocenter. The location of a particular primary wall is at 4 m from the isocenter. Assume the use factor = 0.25, occupancy factor = 1, and SAD = 0.8 m. Calculate the primary wall thickness to yield an effective weekly dose of 0.02 mSv/week (Public limit)?

SAD = 0.8 m, d = 4 m, W =1,000 Gy/week, U = 0.25, and T = 1, using equation 12.1.

$$B = \frac{0.02 \times 10^{-3}(4+0.8)^2}{1{,}000 \times 0.25 \times 1} = \frac{0.02 \times 23.04 \times 10^{-3}}{250} = 1.84 \times 10^{-6}$$

By using equation 12.2:

$$TVL(n) = \log_{10} \times (1/1.84 \times 10^{-6}),$$

$$= \log_{10} \times (1/1.84 \times 10^{-6}) = 5.73$$

From the **Table 12.1**, the TVL in concrete for telecobalt-60 primary radiation is 218 mm. The required primary barrier is:

= 5.73 × 218 = 1,249.14 mm, it is rounded to the nearest 10 mm, that is 1,250 mm.

Note: If the occupational limit of 0.4 mSv/week is used, the number of TVL is 4.43 and required primary barrier is 965.7 mm ≈ 970 mm.

Worked Example 12.8

It is proposed to design a telecobalt-60 facility for a workload of 1,000 Gy/week at the isocenter. The location of a secondary wall is at 3 m from the isocenter. Assume the occupancy factor = 1, and SAD = 0.8 m. Calculate the primary wall thickness to yield an effective weekly dose of 0.02 mSv/week (Public limit)?

Leakage Radiation

Manufacturer usually states two leakage limits, the maximum limit is always <0.1% (1/1,000) of the primary radiation. By using equation 12.5:

$$B_L = \frac{1{,}000 \times P}{WT} \times d_s^2$$

$$= \frac{1{,}000 \times 0.02 \times 10^{-3}}{1{,}000 \times 1} \times 3^2 = 0.18 \times 10^{-3}$$

$$TVL(n) = \log_{10} \times (1/0.18 \times 10^{-3}) = 3.74$$

From the **Table 12.1**, the TVL in concrete for telecobalt leakage radiation is 218 mm. Secondary barrier required against leakage radiation is:

= 3.74 × 218 = 815.3 mm, it is rounded to the nearest 10 mm, 820 mm.

Scattered Radiation

In this case, SAD = d_{sca} = 0.8 m, d_{sec} = 3 m, W = 1,000 Gy/week, F = 20 × 20 cm = 400 cm^2, P = 0.02 × 10^{-3} mSv/week, for scatter fraction *a* for 90° scatter from telecobalt gamma rays is 9.1 × 10^{-4} per 400 cm^2 of irradiated area **(Table 12.3)**, T = 1, using equation 12.6:

$$B_P = \frac{P}{aWT} \times \frac{400}{F} \times d_{sca}^2 \times d_{sec}^2$$

$$= \frac{0.02 \times 10^{-3}}{9.1 \times 10^{-4} \times 1{,}000 \times 1} \times \frac{400}{400} \times 1 \times 3^2 = 2.19 \times 10^{-5} \times 9 = 1.97 \times 10^{-4}$$

$$TVL(n) = \log_{10} \times (1/1.97 \times 10^{-4}) = 3.70$$

The secondary barrier requires a thickness of 3.70 × 151 mm = 558.7 ≈ 560 mm (for 90° scatter, from **Table 12.5**). The TVL for both leakage and scatter are <1 TVL (almost same), one HVL may be added to the highest thickness. It comes around 820 + 45 = 865 mm (1 HVL of concrete = 45 mm).

DESIGN AND SHIELDING CALCULATIONS FOR HDR BRACHYTHERAPY INSTALLATION

Brachytherapy treatment is carried out with low-dose rate (LDR), medium-dose rate (MDR) and high-dose rate (HDR), and HDR brachytherapy is most common. It is used either with ^{192}Ir or ^{60}Co stepping source. The source with treatment unit can be placed anywhere in the treatment room. The radiation is isotropic in nature and not collimated. Hence, all barriers are considered as primary barriers and patient attenuation is excluded. Workload is expressed in air kerma per year in air. Knowledge of radioactive source, its maximum activity, number of patients treated per day, maximum treatment time, number of days per week, and air kerma rate (AKR) of the source are important to carry out shielding calculation. Brachytherapy workload (W) is calculated as follows:

$$W = RAKR \times A \times t \times n \qquad (12.21)$$

where, RAKR is the reference air kerma rate for a source of unit activity,
A is the maximum activity or total activity (activity per source × number of sources),
t is the average duration of treatment in hours,
n is the number of treatments per week.

RAKR values of different brachytherapy sources are given in **Table 12.6**. The workload can also be written by using AAPM report 21 specifications as follows:

$$W = S_k \times t \times n \qquad (12.22)$$

where, S_k is the air kerma strength of the source in units of U or $\mu Gy{\cdot}m^2/h = RAKR \times A$. It is also possible to relate the dose rate (D_0) as follows:

$$D_0 = RAKR \times A = S_k \qquad (12.23)$$

For brachytherapy the sources are not collimated so the use factor U will always 1. The transmission (B) of the barrier is calculated as follows:

$$B = \frac{P \times d^2}{RAKR \times A \times t \times n \times T} \text{ or } \frac{P \times d^2}{S_k \times t \times n \times T} \qquad (12.24)$$

where, P is the design limit,
d is the distance, in meter, from the exposed source position to the point of interest outside the barrier, and
T is the occupancy of the area outside the barrier.

TABLE 12.6 **Physical data of brachytherapy radionuclides.**

Nuclide	*Mean photon energy (MeV)*	*Half-life*	*RAKR (μGy m²/MBq/h)*
^{60}Co	1.25	5.27 years	0.308
^{125}I	0.028	60.1 days	0.034
^{137}Cs	0.662	30.0 years	0.077
^{192}Ir	0.37	74.0 days	0.111
^{198}Au	0.42	64.7 hours	0.056
^{226}Ra	0.78	1,600 years	0.195

Courtesy: IAEA Safety reports series No. 47, 2006.

Leakage Limits for High-dose Rate Brachytherapy

The brachytherapy source storages (LDR/HDR equipment), emergency storages, and in-house transport containers must meet the following limits for leakage radiation. In the case of remote after loading system, the leakage radiation dose rate at 5 cm from the source storage and at 1 m from the source shall not exceed 10 μGy/h and 1 μGy/h, respectively, for unrestricted access, whereas it shall not exceed 100 and 10 μGy/h, respectively, for restricted access. In the case of manual after loading system/emergency storage container/in-house transport container the above levels shall not exceed 500 μGy/h and 20 μGy/h, respectively for portable, whereas it shall not exceed 1,000 μGy/h and 50 μGy/h for mobile systems (AERB safety code, 2011).

Worked Example 12.9

An HDR brachytherapy machine has 10 Ci (370 GBq) activity of ^{192}Ir source of RAKR of 0.111 μGy·m^2/MBq/h. The intended workload is 30 treatments per week and the average treatment duration of 12 minutes (0.2 h) for each patient. Calculate the barrier thickness at 3.5 m?

P = 0.02 mSv = 20 μSv, d = 3.5 m, t = 0.2 h, n = 30, RAKR = 0.111 μGy·m^2/MBq/h, A = 370 GBq = 370 × 10^3 MBq

Weekly workload is obtained from equation 12.21:

$$W = RAKR \times A \times t \times n$$

$$= 0.111 \times 370 \times 10^3 \times 0.2 \times 30$$

$$= 24.64 \times 10^4 \ \mu Gy.m^2$$

The design limit is 0.02 mSv/week for a public area of occupancy, T = 1 at 3.5 m from the treatment position of the sources. The required transmission through the barrier by equation 12.24 is:

$$B = \frac{P \times d^2}{RAKR \times A \times t \times n \times T}$$

$$= \frac{20 \times 3.5^2}{24.64 \times 10^4 \times 1} = 9.94 \times 10^{-4}$$

$$TVL(n) = \log_{10} \times (1/9.94 \times 10^{-4}) = 3.0$$

The TVL for ^{192}Ir for concrete is 152 mm (from **Table 12.4**) and the total thickness of concrete required is 3.0 × 152 mm = 456 mm ≈ 460 mm (from **Table 12.4**).

Note: Similarly, if the design limit is taken as 0.4 mSv/week, the barrier thickness changes relatively. Individuals are advised to use their specific values for barrier calculation.

Worked Example 12.10

A HDR brachytherapy machine has 2 Ci (74 GBq) activity of ^{60}Co source of RAKR of 0.308 μGy·m^2/MBq/h. The intended workload is 30 treatments per week with an average treatment duration of 12 minutes (0.2 h) for each patient. Calculate the barrier thickness at 3.5 m?

P = 0.02 mSv = 20 μSv, d = 3.5 m, t = 0.2 h, n = 30, RAKR = 0.308 μGy·m^2/MBq/h, A = 74 GBq = 74 × 10^3 MBq

Weekly workload is obtained from equation 12.21:

$$W = RAKR \times A \times t \times n$$
$$= 0.308 \times 74 \times 10^3 \times 0.2 \times 30$$
$$= 13.67 \times 10^4\ \mu Gy.m^2$$

The design limit is 0.02 mSv/week for a public area with occupancy, T = 1 at 3.5 m from the treatment position of the sources. The required transmission through the barrier is by equation 12.24:

$$B = \frac{P \times d^2}{RAKR \times A \times t \times n \times T}$$

$$= \frac{20 \times 3.5^2}{13.67 \times 10^4 \times 1} = 1.79 \times 10^{-3}$$

$$TVL(n) = \log_{10} \times (1/1.79 \times 10^{-3}) = 2.74$$

The TVL for ^{60}Co for concrete is 218 mm and the total thickness of concrete required is 2.74 × 218 mm = 597.3 mm ≈ 600 mm (from **Table 12.4**).
Note: Similarly, if the design limit is taken as 0.4 mSv/week, the barrier thickness changes relatively.

Worked Example 12.11

The Cesium manual after loader has five sources of each 100 mCi (3.7 GBq) to be used for gynecological treatments. The reference air kerma rate (RAKR) for ^{137}Cs is 0.077 $\mu Gy \cdot m^2/MBq/h$. The intended workload is five treatments per week. The shielding design will be based on the use of five sources per patient with a total activity of 18.5 GBq (0.5 Ci). The average treatment duration is 30 hours to deliver an absorbed dose of 30 Gy to the prescription point. The weekly workload is obtained from equation 12.21:

$$W = 0.077 \times 18.5 \times 10^3 \times 30 \times 5 = 2.13 \times 10^5\ \mu Gy.m^2$$

The design limit is 20 μSv/week for a public area (T = 1) at 3.5 m from the treatment position of the sources. The required transmission through the barrier is determined from equation 12.24 is:

$$B = \frac{P \times d^2}{RAKR \times A \times t \times n \times T}$$

$$= \frac{20 \times 3.5^2}{2.13 \times 10^5 \times 1} = 1.15 \times 10^{-3}$$

$$TVL(n) = \log_{10} \times (1/1.15 \times 10^{-3}) = 2.93$$

The TVL for ^{137}Cs for concrete is 175 mm and the total thickness of concrete required is 2.93 × 175 mm = 512.75, rounded to 520 mm (from **Table 12.4**).

DESIGN AND SHIELDING CALCULATIONS FOR CT SIMULATOR INSTALLATION

Simulator can be either fluoroscopic or CT simulator and the latter is most common. It is housed in such a way that it will not direct the primary beam toward doors and windows. Patient attenuates the primary beam >1,000 times and the primary scattered by the walls is negligible. Patient scatter can be evaluated as did earlier (Equation 12.6):

$$B_P = \frac{P}{SW_{DAP}T} \times d^2{}_{sca} \times d^2{}_{sec}$$

where P, $d^2{}_{sca}$, $d^2{}_{sec}$, and T are a same as discussed earlier, s is a scatter kerma at 1 m from the scatterer per dose area product (DAP) at the location of the scatterer. Scatter factor, s is related to the scatter fraction, a:

$$S = \frac{a}{400}$$

Scatter fraction values are given in the form of table for various kV as a function of scatter angle (IAEA safety report series No. 47, Table 12). W_{DAP} is the average dose-area product per week which may be measured by a DAP meter, expressed in Gy/cm^2. If measurement is not possible a weekly workload of 1 Gy at 1 m or W_{DAP} = 400 Gy/cm^2 may be assumed. This is enough to carry on 25 simulations in a week. A use factor of 0.25 is used for walls and ceiling and one for the floor. The use factor for leakage radiation is always one. Once transmission is calculated the required barrier thickness is obtained from standard table. Thickness of lead, concrete, and steel for 100 kV both primary and secondary shielding are available in IAEA safety report series No. 47, Table 15, 16 and 17.

Worked Example 12.12

Primary calculation

P = 0.02 mSv, d = 3 m, W = 2,000 mSv/week, U = 0.25, T = 1/16 = 0.0625

$$B = \frac{0.02 \times (3+1)^2}{2,000 \times 0.25 \times 0.0625} = 1.02 \times 10^{-2}$$

$$n = \log_{10}\left(\frac{1}{1.02 \times 10^{-2}}\right) = 1.99 \text{ TVL}$$

Referring the safety report series No. 47, Table 15, the lead thickness for the transmission of 1.02×10^{-2} is found to be 0.9 mm. Similarly, the leakage and scattered radiation transmission is found out as follows:

Leakage Calculation

P = 0.02 mSv, d_s = 3 m, W = 2,000 mSv/week, T = 1/16 = 0.0625

$$B_L = \frac{1,000 \times 0.02 \times 3^2}{2,000 \times 0.0625} = 1.44 \approx 0 \text{ TVL}$$

Since the primary transmission is lower than the leakage in several order of magnitude, primary barrier thickness is sufficient for leakage radiation.

Scatter Calculation

P = 0.02 mSv, d_{sca} = 1 m, d_{sec} = 3 m, F = 400 cm^2, W = 2000 mSv/week, T = 1/16 = 0.0625

a = 0.0021 is the scatter fraction for 125 kV

$$B_P = \frac{0.02 \times 1 \times 3^2}{0.0021 \times 2,000 \times (400/400) \times 0.0625} = 0.68 \approx 0 \text{ TVL}$$

In the case of scatter calculation, there is more than 1 TVL difference from the primary (1.99 TVL), no additional primary barrier thickness is required.

BIBLIOGRAPHY

1. Thayalan K. Basic Radiological Physics, 2nd edition. New Delhi: Jaypee Brothers Medical publishers (P) Ltd.; 2017.
2. National Council on Radiation Protection and Measurement. Structural shielding design and evaluation for Megavoltage X- and Gamma-ray Radiotherapy facilities. NCRP report No. 151 Bethesda, MD, 2015. [online] Available from https://ncrponline.org/publications/reports/ncrp-reports-151/ [Last accessed December, 2022].
3. IAEA. Radiation protection in the design of radiotherapy facilities, Safety reports series No. 47, IAEA, Vienna, 2006. [online] Available from https://www.iaea.org/publications/7197/radiation-protection-in-the-design-of-radiotherapy-facilities. [Last accessed December, 2022].
4. Podgorsak FB. Radiation oncology physics: A handbook for teachers and students. Vienna: IAEA; 2005.
5. IAEA. (1996). International basic safety standards for protection against ionizing radiation and for the safety of radiation sources-BSS-115. [online] Available from https://www.ilo.org/wcmsp5/groups/public/---ed_protect/---protrav/---safework/documents/publication/wcms_171036.pdf [Last accessed December, 2022].
6. NCRP. Radiation protection design guidelines for 0.1-100 MeV particle accelerators facilities. Report No. 51. Washington DC: National Council on Radiation Protection and Measurements, 1977.
7. Structural shielding design and evaluation for medical use of X-rays and Gamma: The energies up to 10 MeV. NCRP report No. 49, Bethesda, MD, 1976.
8. McGinley PH. Shielding Techniques for radiation oncology facilities, 2nd edition. Madison WI: Medical physics publishing. 2002.
9. Atomic Energy Regulatory Board. (2011). AERB safety code No. AERB/RF-MED/SC-1 (Rev.1): Radiation therapy sources, equipment, and installations, 2011. [online] Available from https://www.aerb.gov.in/images/PDF/CodesGuides/RadiationFacility/MedicalApplicationsInvolvingRadiation/4.pdf [Last accessed December, 2022].
10. NCRP, Medical x-ray, electron beam and gamma-ray protection for energies up to 50 MeV. Report No. 102. Bethesda, MD: National Council on Radiation Protection and Measurements, 1989.
11. American Association of Physicists in Medicine (AAPM) report 21: Specification of brachytherapy source strength, Report of AAPM TG-32,1987.

CHAPTER 13

Quality Assurance in Radiotherapy

INTRODUCTION

Quality assurance (QA) is a set of procedures carried out in an equipment to verify manufacturer's specifications. In medical use of radiation, QA policies are helpful to maintain the quality of patient care. It is designed specific to an equipment to meet international standards. Every equipment is subjected to exhaustive performance testing to meet the technical specification and clinical intent. Professional organizations like American Association of Physicists in Medicine (AAPM) have recommended QA programs for radiological practice. International Atomic Energy Agency (IAEA) and Atomic Energy Regulatory Board (AERB) have recommended a set of QA procedure for radiotherapy equipment.

Quality control (QC) is a regulatory task by which the quality performance is measured, compared with existing standards. It also gives corrective measures to meet the standards. It is one part of QA, and its aim is: (i) to check whether the quality requirement is correct, and (ii) if not, to adjust and correct performance.

The intent of QA in radiation therapy is to ensure consistency of clinical dose prescription to the target volume and its satisfactory execution. It also ensures minimal dose to normal tissue, minimal exposure to staffs, and patient monitoring. QA reduces uncertainty and errors in dosimetry, treatment planning and delivery. It also reduces accidents, provides high degree of accuracy for complex gadgets, and permits intercomparison of patient outcome.

Usually, QA tests are performed at the time of installation, known as acceptance testing and commissioning. In this process, the supplier demonstrates the baseline parameters performance to the satisfaction of the customer. Commissioning is the process of accessing full character performance of the equipment for clinical use, for all possible treatments. QC tests or periodic QA are established and initiated for the entire life of the machine. Periodic QA will ensure the integrity of its basic physical and functional specification through time. Additional QC tests are required after any major repairs or replacement of parts. This will also ensure that the fundamental parameters have not changed since last measured. A planned preventive maintenance program is also required from the vendors.

Some of the basic QA parameters and procedures of: (i) CT simulator, (ii) linear accelerator, (iii) HDR brachytherapy unit, and (iv) Telecobalt machine is given below. However, individual hospital must devise their own QA methodology and periodicity to suit their machine and model.

Quality assurance parameters and tolerance values of specific modality are obtained from: (i) AERB QA format, and (ii) American Association of Physicists in Medicine Task Group reports: AAPM TG-40, 142, 198, and 218.

QUALITY ASSURANCE FOR CT SIMULATOR

Mechanical Tests

Alignment of Table Gantry

Congruence between gantry midline and table midline is checked using plumb line. The tolerance should be within ±5 mm.

Gantry Tilt

A non-screen cassette loaded with film is used for this study. A particular kV_p and mAs are selected in the scanner. The gantry is tilted for a set value and the corresponding tilt is measured. The difference between the set and measured gantry tilt is found. The tolerance should be within ±1°.

Scan Localization Light Accuracy

A non-screen cassette loaded with film is used for this study. The kV_p, mAs, and slice thickness are suitably selected. Alignment of the internal laser light and the external laser light is checked. The tolerance should be within ±2 mm.

Table Position/Increment

A non-screen cassette loaded with film is used for this study. An initial table position is chosen (arbitrary) and a given load is put on the couch. The kV_p, mAs, and the slice thickness are selected. The table is set with different increments from the reference position; say 1, 2, 3, 4, and 5 cm, respectively. At the same time the couch increments are measured correspondingly. The difference between the set couch position and the measured is found. The tolerance should be within ±2 mm.

Collimator Test

Radiation Profile Width/Slice Thickness

A non-screen cassette is used for this study. A given kV_p (100) and mAs (100) are selected. For a given slice thickness of 1 mm, density profile is recorded on the film. This is repeated for 2 and 3 mm slice thicknesses. From the density profile, profile width, i.e., full wave half maximum (FWHM) is found for each slice thickness **(Table 13.1).**

X-ray Generator Tests

Measurement of Operation Potential

Operating potential is measured by using a kV_p meter or diagnostic sensor. A given mA station is selected and a kV_p is set on the scanner, say 80 kV_p. After exposing the meter, measured kV_p is noted. Later, the mA station is changed, and the measurement is repeated for same 80 kV_p. In the same way, kV_p readings are taken for one

TABLE 13.1 **Density profile width for different slice thickness.**

Applied slice thickness (mm)	*Measured density profile width (FWHM) (mm)*	*Tolerance*
1		0.5 mm for <1 mm slice
2		±5 mm for 1–2 mm slice
3		±1 mm for >2 mm slice

TABLE 13.2 **Operation potential.**

Set kV_p	*mA station 1*	*mA station 2*	*mA station 3*	*Average kV_p*
80				
100				
120				

TABLE 13.3 **Timer accuracy.**

Set time (second)	*Observed time (second)*	$\% \text{ error} = \left(\dfrac{\text{oberved time - set time}}{\text{Set time}}\right) \times 100$
1.0		
1.5		
2.0		

more mA station. Average of three kV_p reading are estimated and recorded. The whole exercise is repeated for 100 kV_p and 120 kV_p, respectively **(Table 13.2)**. Finally, the difference between the measured and set kV_p is obtained. The tolerance should be within ±2 kV_p.

Timer Accuracy

Position all in one diagnostic sensor in the couch and set time 1 second in the scanner. The observed scan time is noted. This is repeated for 1.5 second and 2 second, respectively **(Table 13.3)**. The percentage of difference between set time and observed time is found, which should be within ±10%.

Measurement of mA linearity

The diagnostic sensor is positioned with 100 kV_p and 10 mm slice thickness settings. The meter reading is noted for 100 mA range. Readings are repeated to get three measurements and their average is found. From the average value mGy/mA is calculated X. The whole procedure is repeated for 200 and 300 mA range, respectively and each time the value of X is calculated **(Table 13.4)**.

The coefficient of linearity (COL) is estimated by using the relation:

$$\text{COL} = \frac{X_{max} - X_{min}}{X_{max} - X_{min}} \tag{13.1}$$

The tolerance value of COL is ± 0.1.

TABLE 13.4 **mA linearity.**

	Output (mGy)				
mA range	***1***	***2***	***3***	***Average***	***(X), mGy/mA***
100					
200					
300					

TABLE 13.5 **Output consistency.**

		Output (mGy)				
kV_p	***mA range***	***1***	***2***	***3***	***4***	***Average, X***
80	100					
100	100					
120	100					

Output Consistency

The pocket dosimeter or remote-control exposure meter is positioned with 100 mAs and 10 mm slice thickness settings. The meter reading is noted for 80 kV_p range. Readings are repeated to get four measurements and an average is obtained. Similarly, the procedure is repeated for 100 and 120 kV_p, keeping mAs constant **(Table 13.5)**. The coefficient of variation (CoV) is calculated by using the relation:

$$\text{CoV} = \frac{1}{X} \times \sqrt{\frac{\sum (X_i - X)^2}{(n-1)}} \tag{13.2}$$

where, X is the average value:
CoV for 80 kV_p =
CoV for 100 kV_p =
CoV for 120 kV_p =
Tolerance of CoV is ±0.05

Total Filtration

Total filtration of the X-ray tube is evaluated by determining the half-value thickness (HVT) of the beam, by using a pocket dosimeter. The HVT is measured for maximum operating potential of the tube.

The pocket dosimeter is kept at the center of radiation field area on the table. For a given kV_p and mAs the dosimeter is exposed, and reading is noted. The measurement is repeated, and average value is obtained. An aluminum filter of 0.5 mm is interposed (at the collimator level) and the measurements are repeated. Similar measurements are repeated for aluminum filters of known thickness 1, 1.5, 2, 3, 4, and 5 mm. Transmission curve of the X-ray beam can be plotted on a graph between absorber thickness (X-axis) and measured dosimeter readings (Y-axis). The absorber thickness for 50% transmission will be the HVT of the X-ray beam.

Alternatively, a diagnostic sensor is positioned, and operating parameters are set as kV_p = 120, mAs = 100, and mA = 100. The filtration directly obtained is expressed in mm Al.

Tolerance is 2.5 mm Al for kV_p >100.

Resolution

Low-contrast Resolution

A low-contrast resolution test phantom is used for this study. A given kV_p, mAs, and slice thickness and window width are set on the scanner. For example, operating parameters are kV_p = 110, mAs = 100, slice thickness = 10 mm and widow width = 400. Test phantom is exposed, and resolution is measured from the phantom in millimeter and the percentage of contrast difference is calculated, say 3 mm at 1.0% contrast difference (minimum).

The tolerance is 5.0 mm at 1% contrast difference (minimum) and the expected is 2.5 mm at 0.5% contrast difference (maximum).

High-contrast Resolution

A high-contrast resolution test phantom is used for this study. A given kV_p, mAs, and slice thickness and window width are set on the scanner. For example, operating parameters are kV_p = 110, mAs = 100, slice thickness = 10 mm and widow width = 400. The phantom is exposed using a high-resolution algorithm. The size of the smallest resolvable bar/hole pattern is found in lp/cm and the percentage of contrast difference is calculated.

Tolerance: At 10% contrast difference the size of the bar/hole pattern to be resolvable should be 1.6 mm (~3.12 lp/cm). The expected high-contrast resolution is 0.8 mm (~6.25 lp/cm).

Radiation Dose Tests

Measurement of Computed Tomography Dose Index

A pencil type ionization chamber with suitable electrometer is used in conjunction with a head/body CT phantom. The phantom is positioned in the couch and the chamber is inserted in it. The kV_p is set as 80 for 100 mAs and slice thickness of 10 mm. The axial dose and peripheral dose are measured in mGy, then mGy/mAs is calculated. The measurements are repeated for different kV_p, i.e., 100, 140, and same mAs and slice thickness settings. This procedure is carried out for both for head and body phantoms **(Table 13.6)**. The mean of the peripheral dose is found for both head and body phantoms. Then the axial Computed Tomography Dose Index (CTDI) and the mean peripheral CTDI is found. From the above, the weighted CTDI is calculated both for head and body.

$$\text{Weighted CTDI } (CTDI_w) = \frac{1}{3}\, CTDI_c + \frac{2}{3}\, CTDI_p \tag{13.3}$$

Tolerance: ±20% of the quoted value (expected),
± 40% of the quoted value (maximum)

Radiation Leakage from X-ray Tube

Radiation leakage measurement is carried with an ionization radiation survey meter. For checking the leakage radiation, collimator of the tube housing is fully closed,

TABLE 13.6 CT dose index measurements.

Chamber position	*Head (mGy/mAs)*	*Body (mGy/mAs)*
Axial/Center ($CTDI_C$)		
Peripheral-1		
Peripheral-2		
Peripheral-3		
Peripheral-3		
Peripheral average ($CTDI_P$)		

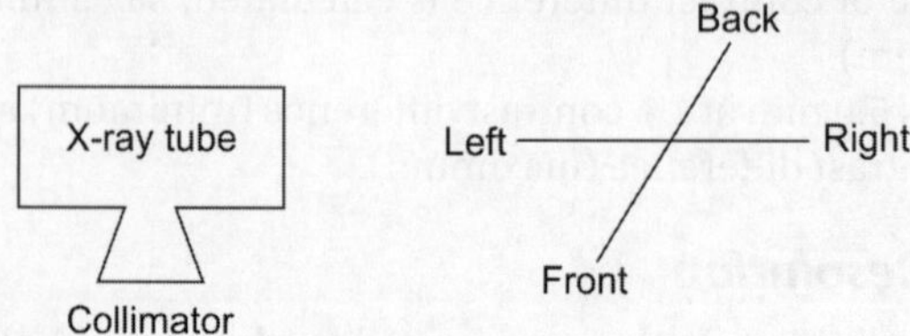

FIG. 13.1: Measurement of leakage radiation.

TABLE 13.7 Leakage radiation levels.

Radiation leakage level (mR/h)			
Front (Cathode)	*Back (Anode)*	*Left*	*Right*

and the tube is energized at maximum rated tube potential and current at that kV_p. The operating time should be greater than the time constant of the survey meter. Radiation leakage levels from the X-ray tube housing at 1 m is measured at front, back, left, and right side of the housing **(Fig. 13.1 and Table 13.7)**. Operating parameters are kV_p = 100, mA = 100, and exposure time = 1 second. Maximum leakage level of the X-ray tube in 1 hour:

$$= \frac{500 \text{ mA-min in 1 h} \times \text{maximum leakage measured, mR/h}}{60 \times 100 \text{ mA used for measurement}} \quad (13.4)$$

The maximum leakage level is obtained from the measured readings in the **Table 13.7**.

Tolerance: The maximum leakage radiation level at 1 m from the focus should be ≤115 mR in 1 hour.

Radiation Protection Survey

Radiation protection survey of CT installation is done with a pressurized ionchamber survey meter and a head phantom in position. The operation settings are: kV_p = 100, mA = 100, exposure time = 1 second and workload = 25,000 mA-min/week. The measurements are done at various locations namely, control console, outside patient entrance door, behind widows (if applicable), patient weighting areas, and control console door **(Table 13.8)**.

TABLE 13.8 **Radiation protection survey.**

Location	*Maximum radiation level (mR/h)*
Control console (operator position)	
Outside patient entrance door	
Behind windows (if applicable)	
Patient waiting areas	
Control console door	

$$\text{Maximum radiation level, mR/week} = \frac{25{,}000 \times \dfrac{\text{mA-min}}{\text{week}} \times \text{Maximum radiation level measured, mR/h}}{60 \times 100 \text{ mA used for measurement}} \quad (13.5)$$

The maximum radiation level is obtained from the measured readings in the **Table 13.8.**
Tolerance: 20 mSv in a year or 40 mR/week for radiation worker, and 1 mSv in a year or 2 mR/week for location of members of public.
(*Note*: Survey meter should have valid calibration certificate).

QUALITY ASSURANCE FOR LINEAR ACCELERATOR

Radiation Survey

After the installation, radiation protection survey of the installation should be carried out. The survey will ensure that the exposure levels outside the room will not exceed the permissible limits, considering the dose rate, machine on time, use factors, and occupancy factors for the adjacent areas. A good survey program includes checking the equipment specification, calibration of the machine, measurement of head leakage, area survey, testing of interlocks, warning lights, and emergency switches. The survey should duplicate the conditions that are expected during the patient treatment in terms of workload, use factor, and occupancy factor.

The radiation survey requirements are: (i) pressurized ionchamber survey meter, (ii) GM type contamination monitor, (iii) neutron survey meter (BF3), (iv) radiographic or radiochromic film, and (v) water phantom or slab phantom.

Source ON Position Leakage

The gantry of the linear accelerator unit is placed at 180°. Choose 20 measurement points located on the surface of a sphere of radius 2 m from the source. Consider two points on the poles of the sphere, four equally spaced points on its equator and distribute the remaining points uniformly on the surface of the sphere. Now the collimator is closed completely, and it is covered with two TVL of lead shielding **(Fig. 13.2)**. The ionchamber is positioned at any one of the location points at 2 m from the source. The CCTV camera is positioned to cover the ionchamber location. This will enable us to read the ionchamber through the TV monitor. The machine is switched ON and the ionchamber reading is noted. The ionchamber position is changed to different location points around the head at the same 2 m distance from

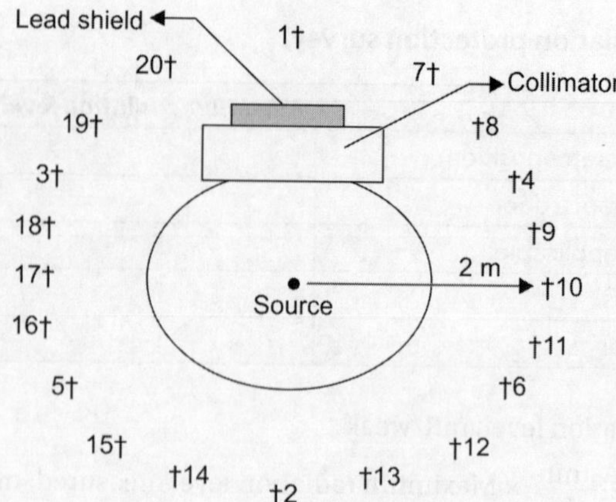

FIG. 13.2: Linear accelerator, radiation survey leakage measurements in μSv/h at 2 m, for source ON condition.

the source. The readings in exposure rates (μSv/h) are noted for all the 20 locations individually.

The leakage radiation outside the beam limiting device, in a plane of circular surface radius centered on and perpendicular to the radiation beam axis at normal treatment distance (NTD) shall not exceed: (i) a maximum of 0.2% and (ii) an average of 0.1% of the maximum absorbed dose measured at the center of the plane in a 10 × 10 cm radiation field size. The leakage radiation outside the patient plane shall not exceed 0.5% of the maximum absorbed dose measured on the radiation beam axis in a 10 × 10 cm radiation field at NTD. The stray X-radiation during electron irradiation shall not exceed 4% for electron energies up to 6 MeV, 5% between 6 and 15 MeV, and 10% beyond 15 MV up to 30 MeV.

The neutron leakage in the patient plane outside the beam limiting device at electron energy >10 MeV shall not exceed a maximum of 0.05% and an average of 0.02% of the maximum absorbed dose in a 10 × 10 cm radiation field at the point of intersection with the radiation beam axis. Neutron leakage outside the patient plane shall not exceed 0.05% of the maximum absorbed dose due to electron or X-radiations.

Area Survey

The sketch of the linear accelerator installation is drawn on a paper. The occupancy around the installations, controlled area, and uncontrolled areas are marked in the drawing, preferably multiple locations. Mark number of locations in the drawing, in which the exposure rate is to be measured. These locations may include primary wall (1), primary wall (2), primary wall ceiling (3), secondary wall (4, couch side), secondary wall (5, gantry side), control console (6) and doors (7). The LINAC machine is set at 100 cm (SSD) with maximum field size (40 × 40 cm). The gantry is kept at 0° position for the maximum photon energy available, e.g., 15 MV without phantom. Now the unit is switched ON and the exposure rate is measured in each location by a wide range pressurized ionchamber survey meter. It is repeated to complete the measurements in all the locations. Similarly, the exposure rate measurements are repeated for different gantry positions of 90°, 180°, and 270°. The maximum values of measured readings are tabulated **(Table 13.9)**.

TABLE 13.9 Linear accelerator radiation survey: Measured exposure rates in µSv/h at different locations.

	Radiation levels in µSv/h for different gantry angles			
Locations	***0°***	***90°***	***180°***	***270°***
Primary wall (1)				
Primary wall (2)				
Primary wall ceiling (3)				
Secondary wall (4, couch side)				
Secondary wall (5, gantry side)				
Control console (6)				
Doors (7)				

A water phantom (30 × 30 × 30 cm) is kept on the couch to create maximum scatter condition and the above procedure is repeated. The same is repeated for different photon energies, say 10 and 6 MV. If the machine is provided with FFF facility, radiation survey is repeated for 6 and 10 FFF beams also. Thus, radiation survey is done without and with phantom for all energies, including both FF and FFF beams.

Neutron radiation survey needs to be done for all the photon energies >10 MV without phantom for largest (40 × 40 cm^2) field size and the jaws completely closed, by using a suitable neutron survey meter at various locations for different gantry angles. The procedure is repeated with phantom also for the above two energies. It is repeated for the smallest possible field size, say 0.3 × 0.3 cm also for various gantry angles without and with phantom.

Jaw Symmetry

To study jaw symmetry, a machinist's dial indicator is used. First the gantry is set at horizontal, and jaws open to a large field size. The feeler of the dial indicator is made to touch the face of one of the jaws and the indicator reading is noted. Now the collimator is rotated to 180° and the feeler is touching the opposite jaw and the dial reading is again noted. The difference between the two readings is noted. The symmetry error is half of the difference in readings. The procedure is repeated for the second jaw. Spirit level is used to check the collimator angle. The tolerance for jaw symmetry is ±1 mm.

Coincidence

Collimator Axis, Light Beam Axis, and Crosshairs Coincidence

Crosshairs are used as visual aid to show the beam central axis entry position. It is projected onto the patient through mylar sheet with crosshairs are engraved. Cross hair projection should rotate about the isocenter with <1 mm. If the cross hairs drifts but not the front pointer, this may be due to decal or light/mirror assembly is out of alignment.

Gantry is set at vertical, and the SSD is set at 100 cm. A graph sheet is fixed on the couch or at the surface of a phantom and the field size is kept as 10 × 10 cm. Switch ON the light field and mark the edges of the light field, intersection of diagonals and the position of the crosshair images. Rotate the collimator through 180° and mark the above parameters in the graph sheet. Check the coincidence of light field edges, intersection of diagonals and position of cross hair images. If there is a misalignment, it should be adjusted to bring down to coincidence.

Optical and Radiation Beam Congruence

A therapy verification film or a radiochromic film is placed on the couch with SSD of 100 cm. A field size of 10 × 10 cm is set, and collimator angle is set to 0°. The light beam is made ON and the light field edges and the center is marked with lead wires or radio-opaque markers. Alternatively, perforating the film by a pin can also be done. Marking cross hair position and film with a perforation will give reference position if asymmetry is found. A plastic (2–5 mm) sheet or phantom slab is placed over the film to give electronic build-up and eliminate electron contamination. The film is exposed so that an optical density of around one is achieved. The procedure is repeated for a collimator angle 90°, 180°, and 270°. The coincidence of the optical and radiation beam is checked visually or by cross beam optical density profiles **(Fig. 13.3)**. The tolerance is ±2 mm.

Mechanical Isocenter

Mechanical isocenter is a point about which the gantry rotates at a fixed distance, say 100 cm. It is also the point from which the axis of collimator and the axis of couch rotates.

Collimator Rotation

A graph sheet is fixed on the couch and front pointer is put on the accessory mount with a gantry angle of 0°. With the pointer extended, the SAD is set to 100 cm. Now the pointer tip position is marked on the graph sheet. The collimator is rotated to 90°, 180°, and 270° and each time the pointer tip position is noted. A sharp edge or wiggler may be attached to the end of the pointer rod to have effective observation. The tolerance of the isocenter is ≤2 mm diameter.

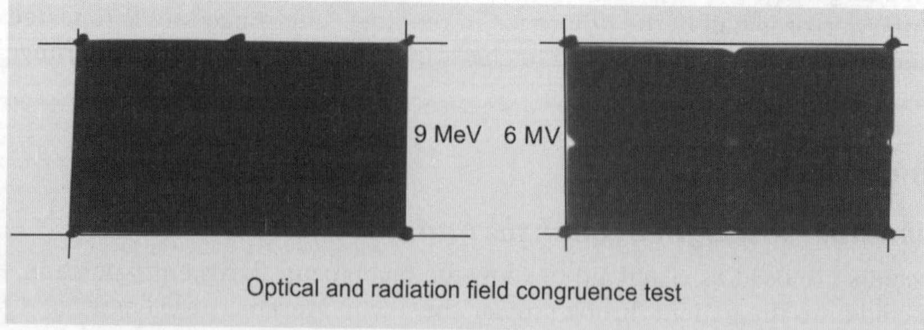

FIG. 13.3: Optical and radiation field congruence: 9 MeV electron and 6 MV photon beam.

Gantry Rotation

In the above procedure, another horizontal rod with fine pointer is positioned by means of a stand. The stand should be kept away to avoid gantry collision. The horizontal rod tip and the front pointer tip are made to coincidence at 100 cm SAD with gantry position of 0°. The gantry is rotated to 90°, 180°, and 270° and the displacement between front pointer tip and the horizontal rod tip is observed. If the isocenter drifts with gantry rotation, it points the gantry bearing assembly. The tolerance of the isocenter shift is ≤2 mm diameter.

Couch Rotation

In the case of couch, mechanical isocenter is checked for both radial and vertical couch axis. The front point is placed at 100 cm SSD with a graph sheet pasted on the couch. When the couch is rotated, the front pointer describes a smaller semicircle on the graph sheet, which gives isocenter. To check the vertical axis, a sharp pointer is mounted on the couch, so that it is protruding from the couch and its pointer is set at the isocenter. The front pointer is made to describe small arc around the isocenter. If the isocenter drifts when the table is rotated, it means that the LINAC is not physically located correctly with relative to table. The radius of the arc should be within 1 mm.

Radiation Isocenter

Radiation isocenter is defined as the smallest sphere through which the axis of radiation beam pass through in all situations. Mechanical and radiation isocenter should coincidence within 1 mm. Radiation isocenter is much more important since it falls on the clinical target. This can be checked with spoke shots as described below.

Gantry

A ready pack film is sandwiched between two plastic sheets, and it is kept on the couch vertically in the gantry rotation plane. This means that the plane of the film should be perpendicular to the plane of the couch top. A slit beam is created by closing one set of collimator jaws optimally, parallel to the gantry axis. The film is exposed for different gantry angles (12 number × 30°) and the final star pattern is obtained **(Fig. 13.4A)**. The spokes of film blackening should coincide. If the spokes are too wide, diagonals can be drawn from entry to exit position to get exact position of the isocenter. The lines should intersect within 2 mm diameter circle.

Collimator

The gantry is set to vertical, 0° with a SAD of 100 cm. A ready pack film is kept flat on the couch. The upper jaws are fully opened, and the lower jaws are closed to have a narrow slit of beam. A build-up sheet is placed over the film, and it is exposed to create a density of unity (=1). Collimator is rotated to different angles (4–8) and each time the film is exposed. The procedure is repeated for upper jaws of narrow slit, while the lower jaws are wide open. The developed film will show the star pattern with dark center region **(Fig. 13.4B)**. Using a film marker, the lines are drawn through the middle of the slit images, which will show clearly the intersection point. The lines should intersect within ≤2 mm diameter circle. This test ensures that the electron beam, the target, and the jaws are aligned properly.

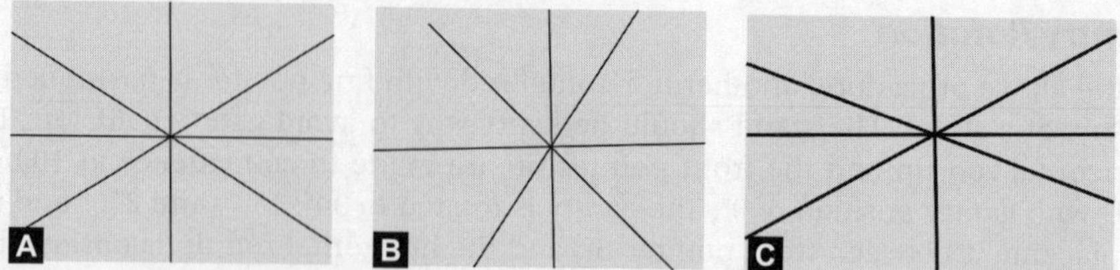

FIGS. 13.4A TO C: Mechanical isocenter verification: (A) Gantry rotation (B) Collimator rotation, and (C) Couch rotation.

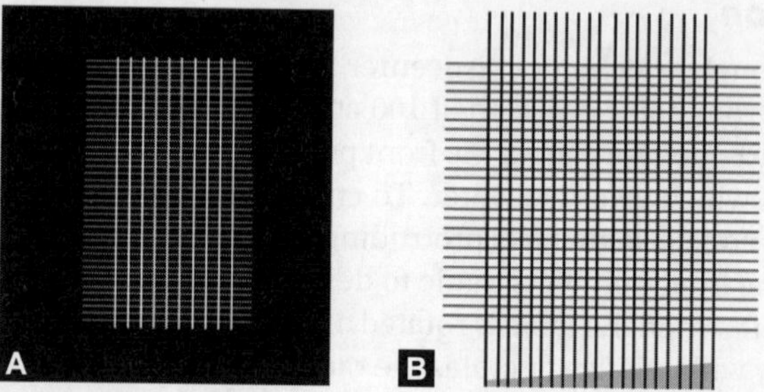

FIGS. 13.5A AND B: Multi leaf collimator leaf positional accuracy: (A) Picket fence test (Static), (B) Garden fence test pattern.

Table

The film is placed flat on the couch and a narrow slit of beam is created as stated above. The gantry and the collimator are in fixed position. The table is rotated (4–8) to different angles and each time the film is exposed. A final star pattern is obtained, and it is examined **(Fig. 13.4C)**. The lines should intersect within ≤2 mm diameter circle.

Multiple Beam Alignment Check

When more than one beam is used misalignment may occur. This may be due to: (i) focal spot displacement, (ii) asymmetry of collimator jaws, and (iii) displacement in the collimator rotation axis or the gantry rotation axis **(Lutz et al. 1981)**. To check the beam misalignment a split field test is recommended. A ready pack film is sandwiched between build-up sheet and is exposed twice. First the one-half (region 1) of the field is exposed by blocking the other half (region 2). The gantry is rotated through 180° and exposed again by blocking region 1. Relative shift of the two images is the indicator of the misalignment.

Multi-leaf Collimator

Garden Fence and Picket Fence Test

The garden and picket fence tests are performed to check the stability of the MLC movement in IMRT delivery and the reproducibility of gap between the leaves **(Figs. 13.5A and B)**. The aim of this test is to verify leaf position accuracy and interleaf leakage transmission. Leaf gap width in dynamic MLC can also be accessed with the test with slight change in the picket fence test. A well-calibrated MLC will create a pattern at the location of the abutting fields. Leaves out of alignment with the neighbor may break the pattern at the location of field junction, any displacement >1 mm can be detectable. For a given leaf pair, leaf position difference between the opposed leaves may create low or higher dose at the location of the field junction. Any error of >1 mm is easily detectable, and the tolerance is ±2 mm, to be performed on weekly basis.

The beam used to generate picket fence pattern should have all MLC leaves and cover the entire leaf travel range. The picket fence pattern is formed by radiation fields measured on an Electronic Portal Imaging Device (EPID) when all leaves are moved across the field of view at the same speed with several stops at measured intervals. There are two versions of the test, namely static and rapid arc. The static test is done while gantry is stationary, whereas rapid arc is done with moving gantry. The two-dimensional (2D) dose distribution produced by the picket fence pattern should be analyzed by visual inspection or can be measured with a radiochromic/radiographic film of suitable dimension. An equal number of MUs should be used for each beam of picket fence pattern. For example, 8 fields of 5 × 40 cm^2, spaced in every 5 cm can be used for the test. In the case of dynamic MLC, 1 mm irradiation strip with every 2 cm can be used to verify dynamic gap width consistency. Impact of gravity on MLC position accuracy can be checked by having different cardinal gantry angle for each week, so that all four angles can be covered in a month.

Daily Quality Assurance Tests

Daily QA tests are performed to find any significant change in LINAC functionality that will influence patient treatment. Generally, these tests are simple and can be completed before starting the patient treatment. These tests are dived into dosimetry, mechanical, safety, and imaging. Dosimetry tests are designed to find out any change in output >3%. Mechanical tests include laser, optical distance indicator accuracy, and acceptable collimator position. Safety checks are intended so that patient can be seen, heard, function of the radiation monitors and the working of interlocks. Imaging tests check the collision interlock function and imaging and treatment isocenters are within 2 mm. An outline of daily QA check of basic LINAC is given below.

Photon and Electron Output Constancy

This test is done to verify whether the patient dose is constant during that day of treatment and nominally accurate to the expected prescribed dose. It confirms that the output has not changed within a reasonable tolerance. To perform the test a phantom embedded with multiple ionization chamber or diodes with an electrometer is used. Alternatively, QUCKCHECK (PTW) or Daily QA (Sun-nuclear corporation), or StarTrack (IBA) phantom can be used. It can support both output and profile constancy of photon and electron beams. One can measure the output, beam flatness, in plane and cross plane symmetry and beam quality within 3% from the baseline value.

Laser Localization

There are three or four lasers in the treatment room for initial patient setup of patients before treatment or acquiring images. They have electronic control systems that can drift with time. Hence, it is important that the positional errors are as small as possible. It will help to deliver clinical plan accurately to the desired target and sparing critical targets. Commercially available cube with markings on the sides is positioned at the isocenter. Using crosshairs and the light field as reference point, accuracy of the coincidence of laser at the isocenter is determined. The tolerance is ±2 mm for non-IMRT, ±1.5 mm for IMRT and ±1 mm for SRS/SBRT.

Optical Distance Indicator

Optical distance indicator (ODI) is used for setting up SSD for patient treatment and phantom dosimetry. ODI is redundancy to the coronal laser and is the only setup reference when the surface is located away from the machine isocenter. To carry out the test, the ODI is set coinciding with crosshairs on a surface at the machine isocenter. It is checked then the coronal lasers graze the surface illuminated by the ODI field light. The tolerance is ±2 mm.

Collimator Size Indicator

Collimator is used to define treatment field edges. Its positions are set by hand pendant or console. The objective is to verify that the collimator indicators are consistent with desired setting. A graph paper and template with predetermined rectangular shape is used to carry out the test. The paper surface is illuminated by the light field for visual inspection against collimator setting. The light field serve as surrogate of the radiation field. The tolerance is ±2 mm per jaw for non-IMRT and IMRT, whereas it is ±15 mm for SRS/SBRT.

Door Interlock

This is to verify the safety of the personnel so that it ensures that the beam is turned OFF when the door is opened. To carry out the test the door is opened while the beam is ON. The beam must be turned OFF as the door gets opened. Alternatively, the machine can be made ON, while the door is opened. It is expected the beam should be in OFF condition. It is also known as beam ON indicator test. The tolerance is functional.

Door Closing Safety

Treatment room doors are heavy in some installations, it may cause injury to the personnel while closing. If the door has emergency stop switch it will stop closing if personnel are accidently caught in the path. When the door is in open position, close the door by standing away in a safe position. When the door is halfway closed, activate emergency switch. The door should stop closing, ensuring proper function. The tolerance is functional.

Audio-visual Monitor

Audio-visual monitor (two-way) ensures safe patient treatments. To check this, switch ON the music system and place a sound producing device on the couch. Observe from the control console whether the sound device is observable on the monitor and the sound is heard. Next enable the two-way communication system at the console and talk into the microphone, record the communication by a smartphone. Instead, one can listen the communication sound, near the open treatment room door. The tolerance is functional.

Stereotactic Interlocks

This is to check the devices used are interlocked and correct dose rate is delivered under specific treatment mode. The stereotactic device is attached to the LINAC and a non-stereobeam is programmed. The LINAC should indicate interlock and prevent beam delivery. Then program a stereotactic beam delivery for a given dose.

Now remove the stereotactic device from the LINAC and try to deliver the same dose. The LINAC should not deliver the dose. This test is performed only on days of stereotactic treatment of patients. The tolerance is functional.

Radiation Area Monitor

This is to verify that the area monitor is functional and prevent personnel to the enter the treatment room while beam is ON. The radiation area monitor is connected to a remote device or CCD camera, to be observed from the console. When the door is closed, observe the monitor display; no radiation, while the beam is OFF. When the beam is ON, the monitor should indicate radiation inside the treatment room. The tolerance is functional.

Beam ON Indicator

The beam ON indicator is provided at the door level needs to be checked for their proper functioning. Usually it is green, yellow, and red indicators, green indicates beam OFF, red indicates beam ON, and yellow is for transition mode. When the door is closed, observe visually that the indicator is ON, while beam is ON. Similarly, the indicator should be OFF when the beam is OFF. The tolerance is only functional.

Imaging Test

A dedicated imaging phantom such as *QUASAR PentaGuide* or equivalent can be used for imaging tests. Tests include collision interlocks (functional test), positioning and repositioning and imaging treatment coordinate coincidence (single gantry angle) for planar kV and MV (EPID) imaging system. The image is taken and compared with DRR or CT image to access the coincidence of isocenter and the tolerance should be ≤2 mm. In the case of cone-beam CT (kV and MV) the above tests are applicable but positioning and repositioning tolerance should be ≤1 mm, especially for SRS/SBRT facilities.

QUALITY ASSURANCE FOR HIGH DOSE RATE BRACHYTHERAPY

Commissioning Tests

During commissioning, wipe tests, autoradiography, and uniformity tests for activity checks, and source calibration must be carried out. It should be followed by regular QA tests.

Once the source consignment reaches the hospital, the package is subjected to wipe test. The radiation level at 5 cm and at 1 m from the package is measured to access the physical damage or any excessive exposures. This should be done at the time of arrival and then once in 6 months intervals for long half-life sources.

Autoradiography and radiography can be done by using film with single exposure. It can be helpful to check the uniform distribution of radioactive material within the source capsule. Later, the film is scanned by a densitometer to get iso-density and isodose profiles. This method is much useful to check the uniformity of activity and presence of any cold material (nonradioactive), especially in seeds and ribbons.

Source must be calibrated to achieve traceability with national standards. Well type or re-entrant ionchamber is most suited for calibration of either low or high activity sources. However, these chambers need to be calibrated at the standard laboratories for different quality of radiations. The chamber calibration factor is obtained by interpolation or extrapolation method. Generally, calibration factor for ^{192}Ir is obtained from the calibration factors of 250 kV X-rays and ^{60}Co gamma rays. The measured activity is compared with vendors stated source strength.

After the source is loaded into the HDR machine radiation protection survey is carried out.

Radiation Survey

The high-dose rate brachytherapy equipment requires radiation protection survey measurements for both sources OFF and ON condition. When the source is in OFF condition, the leakage radiation levels in μSv/h is measured both at 5 cm from the surface of the treatment head and at 1 m from the center of the treatment head at various positions **(Fig. 13.6)**. A wide range survey meter of ionchamber type can be used to perform the measurements. The measured readings are tabulated as shown in **Tables 13.10 and 13.11**. Radiation survey measurements are also carried out when the source is in ON condition. Various locations are selected in and around the HDR installation and radiation levels are measured by using the above survey meter, by simulating the HDR treatment without patient.

Leakage Limits HDR Brachytherapy

In the case of remote after loading system, the leakage radiation dose rate at 5 cm from the source storage and at 1 m from the source shall not exceed 10 and 1 μGy/h, respectively, for unrestricted access, whereas it shall not exceed 100 and 10 μGy/h, respectively, for restricted access. In the case of manual after loading system/emergency storage container/in-house transport container, the above levels shall not exceed 500 and 20 μGy/h, respectively for portable, whereas it shall not exceed 1,000 and 50 μGy/h for mobile systems (AERB safety code, 2011).

Electrical and Mechanical Tests

After the installation of the HDR unit, the electrical and mechanical tests should be carried out. In the electrical tests, the interlocks in the treatment room doors,

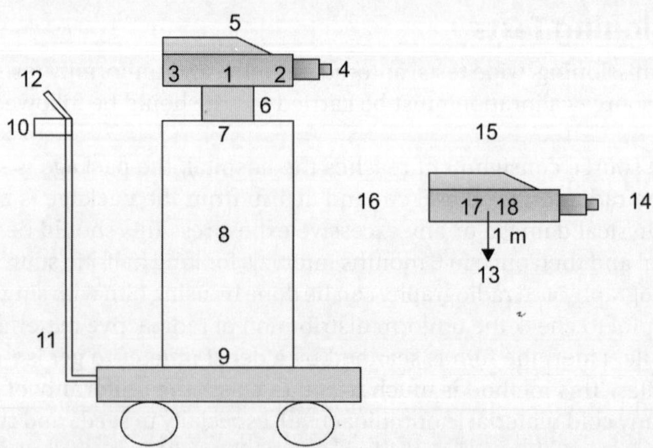

FIG. 13.6: HDR brachytherapy system: OFF position leakage measurements.

TABLE 13.10 **Radiation survey HDR brachytherapy: Radiation levels at 5 cm and 1 m during source OFF condition.**

Survey meter: Date:
Make: Activity:
Model:

Position	*5 cm from the source housing (µSv/h)*	*Position*	*1 m from the center of the source housing (µSv/h)*
1		13	
2		14	
3		15	
4		16	
5		17	
6		18	
7			
8			
9			
10			
11			
12			

TABLE 13.11 **Radiation survey HDR brachytherapy: Radiation levels during source ON condition.**

Survey meter: Date:
Make: Activity:
Model:

Position	*Radiation levels (µSv/h)*
1	
2	
3	
4	
5	
6	
7	
8	
9	
10	

guide tube and treatment unit, applicator and guide tubes, emergency stop button to interrupt the irradiation are to be tested. Source safe display and treatment ON/OFF indicator are also be tested. Control console display and control console functions should also be tested for electrical safety. The mechanical tests included are functioning of sensors such as pressure, torque, optical, and coupling between (i) guide tube and unit, (ii) guide tube and applicator, and (iii) drive cable and source, etc. Time taken to drive the source to ON/OFF position and integrity of applicators are also very important.

Positional Accuracy

Applicator Integrity

The positional accuracy is tested by combining autoradiography and radiography. A graph sheet is pasted on the therapy verification film. Over the graph sheet, the tandem of the standard gynecology applicator (IU3) is fixed. A small lead wire is kept at the end of the tandem in a transverse direction **(Fig. 13.7A)**. The film is exposed with suitable factors with an X-ray machine. This will confirm the mechanical integrity of the applicator. Now the applicator is moved laterally and fixed in a different position in the film. Using a graph sheet, the tip of the applicator must be maintained in the same level as before. Then the applicator is connected to the HDR unit in channel 3. Programs are made to create dwell positions at 1,500, 1,450, 1,400, and 1,350 (50 mm gap). Autoradiography was performed in HDR for a period of 0.3 second or less at each dwell position. Later, the whole test package is taken to X-ray machine and again exposed. When the film exposed, the remaining part of the film was shielded with lead partition. This is repeated for various other applicators.

Pin Prick Method

A graph sheet is pasted on a therapy verification film. The gynecology tandem applicator or a flexible implant tube is pasted on the graph sheet. A pin is used to mark several cardinal treatment lengths 1,500, 1,480, 1,460, 1,440, 1,420, and 1,400 mm parallel to the applicator. The distance between the applicator and the pin prick is 50 mm on both sides. The applicator is connected to the transfer tube, and the HDR source is used to expose the film. The film was developed and checked for the positioning accuracy and uniformity. The criterion for positional accuracy is ±1 mm.

Staggered Autoradiography

Staggered autoradiography is used to confirm the correct delivery of each unique sequence of dwell positions to the programmed channel, the correct spacing of adjacent dwell positions, and the accurate relative positioning of the most dwell position. Autoradiography is performed for 1–5/6 channels, with dwell spacing of 15 mm, consisting of 8 dwell positions. The dwell time for each dwell is selected optimally to create an optical density of around one. The first position in each catheter was offset from the previous one by 2.5 mm, resulting in a pattern of descending dots in which errors are readily discernible. In the same way all the 10/18/24 channels need to be tested **(Fig. 13.7B)**.

Temporal Accuracy

Verification of temporal accuracy consists of identically measuring the length of time the HDR source remains at the specific dwell position and comparing it with the set time. In this study, the timer error, timer linearity, and end error were determined.

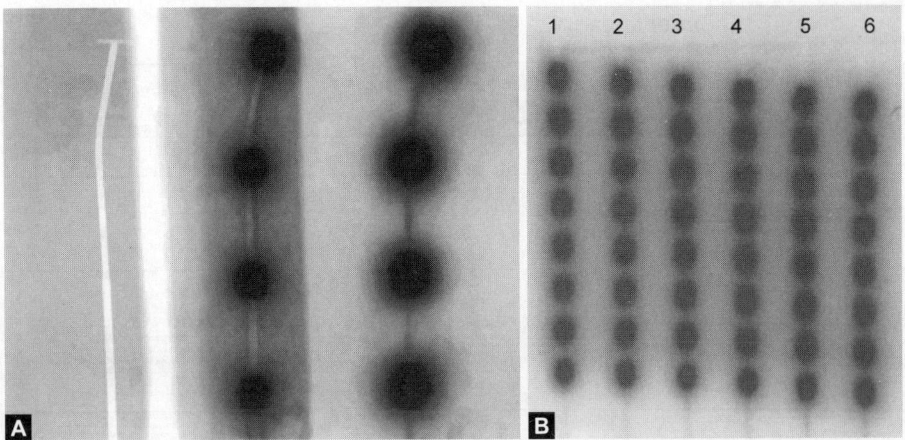

FIGS. 13.7A AND B: (A) Radiography and autoradiography; (B) Staggered autoradiography.

TABLE 13.12 Timer error.

Reading	*Charge 1, nC*	*Charge 2, nC*	*Charge 3, nC*	*Charge 4, nC*	*Charge 5, nC*	*Charge Average, nC*
R_1						
R_2						
Timer error = $(R_2 - R_1)\,t/(2R_1 - R_2)$						

Timer Error

The HDR system is programmed for 60 seconds in maximum response position of a well-type ionization chamber with respect to the catheter used. The charge for 60 seconds is noted as R_1. Again, the system is programmed for 60 seconds, and the machine is made ON. At 30 seconds an interruption is made, and the system is restarted again. The accumulated charge taking the additional transit time into consideration is noted as R_2. Five sets of reading are taken as follows and the average R_1 and R_2 were found **(Table 13.12)**.

Timer Linearity

The HDR system is programmed for about 320 seconds in maximum response position of a well type ionization chamber and the charge (Q) for 300 seconds (T) is collected by using an independent timer. Five sets of readings are taken and the average charge of five sets of reading (Q_{ave}) is taken and corrected current (I_{cor}) is calculated **(Table 13.13A)**:

$$I_{cor} = \frac{Q_{ave}}{T} \tag{13.6}$$

Now the system is programmed for 60 seconds, taken as T_{set} and the charge for 60 seconds is collected by operating the machine timer. Five sets of reading are

TABLE 13.13A Timer linearity.

Reading	***Charge 1 nC***	***Charge 2 nC***	***Charge 3 nC***	***Charge 4 nC***	***Charge 5 nC***	***Average charge, (Q_{ave}), nC***
R_1						

TABLE 13.13B Timer linearity.

T_{set} (second)	***Charge 1, nC***	***Charge 2 nC***	***Charge 3 nC***	***Charge 4, nC***	***Charge 5, nC***	***Average charge (Q_{ave}) nC***	***T_{meas} = Q_{ave}/I_{cor}***
60							
120							
180							
240							
300							

taken, and the average charge is found. Then the value of T_{meas} is calculated using the formula:

$$T_{meas} = \frac{Q_{ave}}{I_{cor}} \tag{13.7}$$

Similarly, the readings were taken for 120, 180, 240, and 300 seconds and tabulated **(Table 13.13B)**. A graph has been plotted with T_{set} in X-axis and T_{meas} in Y-axis. From the graph the slope is found using the most deviated readings on both sides:

$$\text{Linearity error} = 1 - [T_{meas}\ \text{Max}\ (T_1) - T_{meas}\ \text{Min}\ (T_2)] \times 100\% \tag{13.8}$$

The T_{set} corresponds to T_1–T_{set} leads to T_2. End error is the intercept at Y-axis. Alternatively, the intercept can also be calculated by using an excel sheet.

Leakage and Contamination

The HDR machine is connected to a flexible implant tube and made ready for dummy treatment. Trial treatment is performed with the ^{192}Ir source for about 5 times. The flexible implant tube is now cut longitudinally, and the wipe test is performed using gauze. The gauze is tested for contamination using a contamination monitor and the reading is recorded as—Counts per minute (CPM) and converted into activity units. The source is said to be leaky if the measured contamination is >200 Bq or 5 nCi.

Source Strength Verification

The HDR system is to be calibrated with re-entrant type ionchamber (well chamber). As a first step the axial response of the chamber is obtained, by programming all dwell positions (say 1–48). Secondary standard dosimeter is used to measure the current in nA. Repeated readings are taken for at least two times for a given dwell position and tabulated **(Table 13.14A)**. A plot is made between dwell position and relative meter readings. The dwell position (Dwell_{max}) corresponding to the maximum response is found.

TABLE 13.14A Source strength verification.

Dwell position	Meter reading (nA) (i)	Meter reading (nA) (ii)

TABLE 13.14B Source strength verification.

Dwell position	Meter reading (nA) (i)	Meter reading (nA) (ii)	Meter reading (nA) (iii)	Average meter reading (nA) (M)
$Dwell_{max}$				

Now the machine is set for the dwell position of $Dwell_{max}$ and the measurements are repeated for three times. The readings are tabulated, and the average of the readings is also found **(Table 13.14B)**. The temperature (T) and pressure (P) parameters are also noted:

$$\text{Air - kerma strength } (S_K) = I \times N_e \times k_{tp} \times N_{SK} \times A_{ion} \times P_{ion} \quad (13.9)$$

where, I is the measured ionization current,
N_e is the electrometer calibration coefficient,
k_{tp} is the temperature and pressure correction factor,
N_{SK} is the air-kerma strength calibration coefficient,
A_{ion} is correction for recombination at the time of calibration,
and P_{ion} is the correction for recombination at the time of measurement.
The temperature and pressure correction factor are estimated as follows:

$$k_{tp} = \frac{273.15 + T}{273.15 + 22} \times \frac{1{,}013}{P} \quad (13.10)$$

where, 1,013 mbar and 22°C are the pressure and temperature during the calibration of well type ionization chamber at the secondary standard dosimetry laboratory (SSDL). The % of variation of the measured activity with that of the stated activity (vendor) is calculated as follows and the tolerance is within ±3%:

$$\% \text{ of variation} = \frac{\text{Stated activity} - \text{Measured activity}}{\text{Stated activity}} \times 100 \quad (13.11)$$

Quality Assurance for Treatment Planning System

Quality assurance of treatment planning system (TPS) is an essential and indispensable part before commissioning any TPS. After installation, the TPS is tested for its accuracy of: (i) checking the reconstruction procedure, (ii) consistency tests between quantities and units, (iii) test the computer dose with manual dose for a single source, and (iv) verify the decay correction.

Checking the Reconstruction Procedure

Accuracy of digitizer and plotter should be routinely checked. Simple test cases with a small number of sources placed in a known geometry, as seen on two orthogonal radiographs, should be run to check the accuracy of source reconstruction. A 5, 10, and 12 cm catheter length are drawn in a graph sheet and its AP and lateral images are fed into the system through the digitizer. A printout is obtained, and its dimensions are compared with input data. Similarly, input is made through keyboard and the hard copy is compared. This can be repeated for different catheter lengths and orientation with marking points. The verification test should include translation from film to Cartesian coordinates, rotations, and corrections for magnification. Tolerance limit for data transfer is ±1 mm.

Consistency Tests between Quantities and Units

Incorrect quantities and units lead to dose distribution errors in calculation. One must verify the correct labeling of the input and output quantities and units. The strength of the sources (activity) may be specified in one unit out of several alternative units. The user should carefully use correct unit of source strength as input in the TPS. An inconsistent use of units for this parameter could lead to serious errors in patient treatment.

Test the Computer Dose with Manual Dose for a Single Source

The computer calculated dose distribution around a linear source should be compared with literature dose rate values for a similar source or to the Sievert integral. When comparing with the Sievert integral, scatter and attenuation corrections should not be included. A single pellet is programmed in a gynecology application, so that it can deliver a dose of 10 Gy at 10 mm distance. The isodose print out is made and checked. Additional tests should include:

- Inverse square law for point sources
- Summing of the dose for multiple sources
- Scaling of the dose rate with source strength
- Scaling of the dose with time

Verify the Decay Correction

Computer calculations of dose rates at specific times within the duration of the implant should be verified with manual calculations. Similarly, the computer calculated dose to total decay for permanent implants should be verified. A proper choice of units should be made for these calculations.

The treatment time can be verified either by: (i) *Mante carlo* data or (ii) *Meisberger polynomial.* The tolerance limits is ±3% for dose.

Regular Quality Assurance Checks

Dosimeter Constancy Checks

Calibrated dosimeter must be checked periodically for its constancy. A cesium-137 check source with a special holder is required. The holder helps in positioning the source in a reproducible manner in well-type chamber. This test will strengthen the entire QA process.

Source and Applicator Checks

Mechanical integrity of the source must be checked at regular intervals by visual inspection, leak test, and activity measurements. Applicators may undergo changes due to handling, cleaning, and sterilization. Visual inspection and radiographic evaluation of applicators is required at regular intervals. In the case of gynecology applicators, its assembly, function of screws, clamps, and seating of colpostats must be checked.

Source Strength

Source strength of long-lived sources must be checked at periodic intervals. The measured activity should be compared with decay corrected activity. Short-lived isotopes are used either as temporary or permanent implants. Their activity is verified at the time of arrival and compared with manufacturer's values.

Wipe Tests

All sources that are in storage should be subjected to wipe tests for leakage radiation. The frequency of such tests is once in 6 months.

Source Positioning Checks

Source position can be checked with autoradiography with millimeter precision. Treatment catheters are loaded with predetermined source position. Use of radiographic markers or combination of radiography and autoradiography image are the suitable methods for source position checks.

Four flexible catheters are taped on a sheet and placed on the ready radiographic pack film at 2 cm apart. Dummies were inserted in each catheter, making sure that the stop collar on the dummies abuts the coupler on each catheter **(Fig. 13.8)**. After radiographing the dummies, the HDR machine is programmed to dwell 0.1 second at each dwell position. At each catheter, dwell positions are 1, 5, 9, 13, 17, 21, 25, 29,

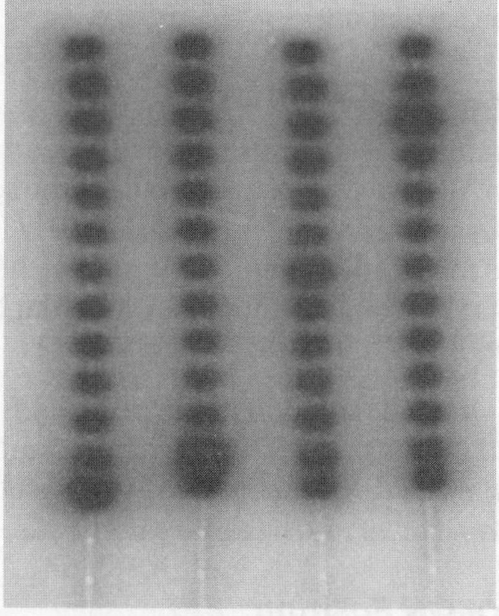

FIG. 13.8: Periodic quality assurance test.

33, 37, 41, 45, and 48. After the exposure, the HDR machine is again programmed as follows:

Catheter 1	Dwell 5	Length 1,490
Catheter 2	Dwell 5	Length 1,450
Catheter 3	Dwell 5	Length 1,400
Catheter 4	Dwell 5	Length 1,390

After HDR autoradiography, the film is developed and the maximum deviation from the dummy position is checked, and the tolerance is 2 mm.

Radiation Survey

After implantation, radiation survey must be done within and around the patient room. Radiation levels should be measured and recorded. The radiation levels in adjoining rooms should be low and any individual should not receive >0.2 mSv in 1 hour. All implant patients must be surveyed before their discharge from hospital. In temporary implants, survey must be done after the removal of the source to confirm the removal of all sources from the patients. In permanent implant, patients may be discharged from the hospital, provided the radiation levels at 1 m is <0.5 mSv/h.

QUALITY ASSURANCE FOR TELECOBALT THERAPY

The acceptance testing and commissioning and periodic QA is similar to that of linear accelerator with lesser accuracy. Hence, those details are not repeated here due to lesser number telecobalt units are in clinical today. The radiation survey procedure is only outlined in the following paragraphs. Readers are advised to refer relevant documents for more information.

Radiation Survey

In the case of Cobalt-teletherapy machine radiation survey, the head leakage for both source OFF and source ON conditions and area survey of the installation are the essential procedures to be carried out.

Head Leakage-source OFF Condition

The gantry of the teletherapy unit is placed at 90° or 270° and the machine is switched OFF. Exposure rate (mSv/h) at 5 cm from the surface of the source head is measured, at eight different positions around the gantry **(Fig. 13.9)**. A wide range ionchamber survey meter may be used for the measurement. Similarly, the exposure rates (mSv/h) are measured at 1 m distance from the source for different locations (8) around the source.

OFF condition leakage limit: The radiation in the beam OFF condition at distance of 1 m from the source shall not exceed 0.02 mGy/h or 2 mR/h. The stray radiation measured at any accessible position 5 cm from the surface of the protective shielding shall not exceed 0.20 mGy /h or 20 mR/h (AERB safety code, 2011).

Head Leakage Source ON Position

The gantry of the machine is positioned at 180° and the collimator is closed completely, and it is covered with two TVL of lead shielding **(Fig.13.10)**. The ionchamber is

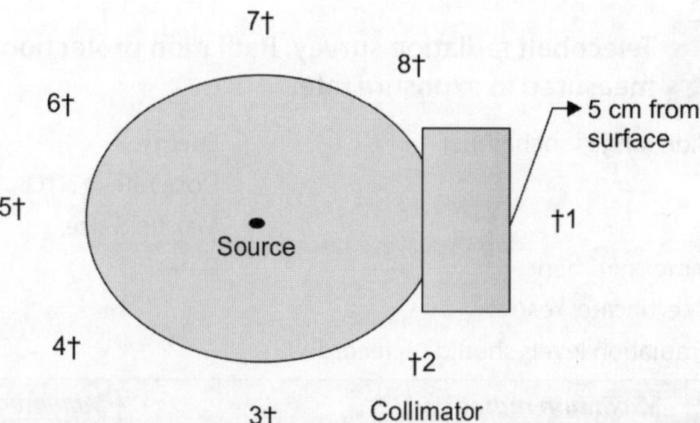

FIG. 13.9: Teletherapy Cobalt-60 machine. Radiation survey, leakage exposure measurements in mSv/h, for source OFF condition.

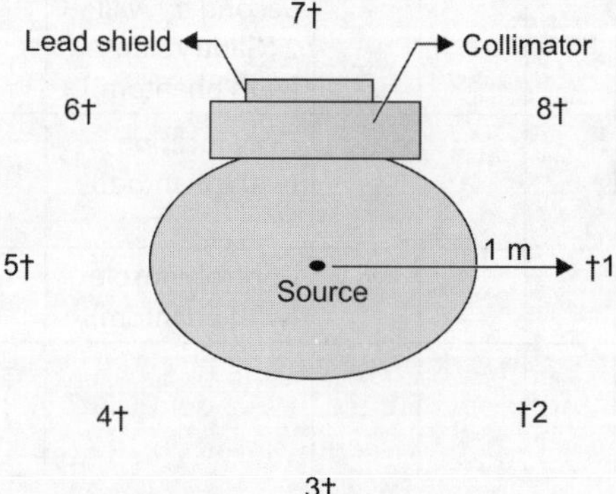

FIG. 13.10: Teletherapy Cobalt-60 machine. Radiation survey: Exposure rate measured in mSv/h for source ON position.

positioned at 1 m from the source around the head. The CCTV camera is positioned to cover the ionchamber location. This will enable us to read the ionchamber through the TV monitor. The machine is switched ON and the ionchamber reading is noted. The ionchamber position is changed to different locations around the head at the same 1 m distance from the source. The readings in exposure rates (mR/h) are noted for at least eight locations around the head.

ON condition leakage limit: The leakage radiation outside the maximum radiation beam in a plane circular surface radius 2 m centered on and perpendicular to the radiation beam axis at NTD shall not exceed a maximum radiation measured at distance of 1 m from the source shall not (i) a maximum of 0.2% and (ii) an average of 0.1% of the maximum absorbed dose measured at the point of intersection of radiation beam axis and the plane of surface for a 10 × 10 cm radiation field size. The absorbed dose rate due to leakage radiation measured at the distance of 1 m from the radiation source shall not exceed 0.5% of the maximum absorbed dose rate on the radiation beam axis measured at a distance 1 m from the radiation source (AERB safety code, 2011).

Area Survey

The sketch of the teletherapy installation is drawn on a paper. The occupancy around the installations, controlled area, and uncontrolled areas are marked in the drawing.

TABLE 13.15 Telecobalt radiation survey: Radiation protection survey, measured in exposure rate.

Survey meter: Wide range ionchamber | Energy:
Make: | Dose rate @ NTD:
Model: | Max field size:
Unit of radiation measurement: | Date:
Valid calibration certificate: Yes/No

Note: Maximum radiation levels should be recorded

Location	***Maximum radiation level (mSv/h) each cardinal gantry angle***				***Location***	***Maximum radiation level (mSv/h) each cardinal gantry angle***			
	0°	***90°***	***180°***	***270°***		***0°***	***90°***	***180°***	***270°***
Primary wall 1 (without phantom)					Secondary wall 2 [Gantry side (with phantom)]				
Primary wall 2 (without phantom)					Door location (with phantom)				
Ceiling (without phantom)					Control console (with phantom)				
Secondary wall 1 (Gantry side (with phantom)									

Locations in the drawing in which the exposure rate is to be measured are marked. These locations may include control panel, door, all four sides, above ceiling, below the floor if occupancy any and patient-weighting area, etc. The teletherapy machine is set at 80 cm (SSD) with maximum field size. The gantry is kept at 0° position. A water phantom (30 × 30 × 30 cm) is kept in the couch to create maximum scatter condition. Now the unit is switched ON and the exposure rate is measured by using a wide range ionchamber survey meter. It is repeated to complete the measurements in all the locations. Similarly, the exposure rate measurements are repeated for different gantry positions of 90°, 180°, and 270°. The readings are tabulated as shown in the case of linear accelerator **(Table 13.15)**.

Primary Barrier Adequacy

This survey will reveal and ensure the shielding adequacy of the primary barriers. The collimator is set for larger field size (35 × 35 cm) and the gantry is kept at 90°. Now the beam is focused on the primary wall 1. Exposure rate behind the barrier is measured by using the pressurized ionchamber survey meter. Then the gantry is set at 270° and the exposure rate is measured behind the primary wall 2. Similarly, measurements are made by focusing beam on the ceiling and basement with occupancy, if any.

BIBLIOGRAPHY

1. American Association of Physicists in Medicine Task Group-198 report: An implementation guide for TG 142 quality assurance of medical accelerators. Med Physics. 2021;48(10): e830-85.
2. Moyed Miften, Arthur Olch, Dimitris Mihailidis, Jean Moran, Todd Pawlicki, Andrea Molineu et al. Tolerance limits and methodologies for IMRT measurement-based verification QA: Recommendations of AAPM Task Group no.218. Med Phys. 2018;45(4): e53-83.
3. Khan FM, Gibbons JP. Khan's The Physics of Radiation therapy, 5th edition. Philadelphia: Wolters Kluwer; 2014.
4. Radiation therapy sources, equipment, and installations: AERB safety code No. AERB/RF-MED/SC-1 (Rev.1), 2011.
5. American Association of Physicists in Medicine Task Group-142. Quality Assurance of Medical Accelerators 2009.
6. Podgorsak FB. Radiation oncology physics: A handbook for teachers and students, IAEA, Vienna 2005.
7. Comprehensive QA for radiation oncology: Report of AAPM radiation therapy committee Task Group 40. Med Phys. 1994;21(4):581-618.
8. Nag S. High Dose Rate Brachytherapy: A Textbook, Futura publishing 1994. [online] Available from www.aerb@org.in.
9. American Association of Physicists in Medicine Task Group-198 report: An implementation guide for TG 142 quality assurance of medical accelerators. Medical physics. 2021; 00:1-56.

CHAPTER 14

Radiation Protection and Safety in Radiotherapy

INTRODUCTION

Radiation therapy uses ionizing radiations to treat cancer. It is in the form of external beam radiation therapy (EBRT) and brachytherapy. Linear accelerator and telecobalt machines are used in EBRT. Brachytherapy uses single encapsulated source to deliver radiation directly into or near the volume of interest. Though low-dose rate (LDR) sources have been used, nowadays high-dose rate (HDR) remote after loaders are common. Appropriate equipment and accessories must be made available for performing dosimetry, treatment planning, simulation, and radiation safety. All these equipment are calibrated periodically with suitable gadgets for treatment use. Relevant quality assurance tests are conducted during installation and over a period.

PROTECTION IN BRACHYTHERAPY

Security of Brachytherapy Sources

Brachytherapy sources should be stored in a secure room with adequate shielding. Safety of radioactive sources requires controlling exposures from the sources during normal operating conditions and during incidents. It includes compromises to the security of sources. Licensee responsibility includes security measures to prevent loss, theft, or unauthorized access to radioactive sources. Since the safety and security of sources are intimately linked, any measures which address one aspect, will also address the other. For example, doors and walls interlocks which limit the radiation exposures will also contribute to the security of sources.

A logbook should be maintained, indicating details such as, number of sources of each radionuclide, date of receipt, batch ID, activity quoted and measured with time and date, leak test report, identification mark, and exact place of storage. The logbook should clearly illustrate the TO and FROM movements of the sources(s), from the storage. Carriers used for the transporting the sources to insertion room and back to the storage room should have adequate shielding and good mobility.

The maximum radiation level outside the storage and transport containers should be within the maximum allowable limit of 200 μSv/h at 5 cm from the surface of the container and 10 μSv/h at 1 m from the center of the container. A radiation monitoring instrument should be readily available at the entrance of the room.

Security of Low-dose Brachytherapy Sources

Low-dose rate brachytherapy sources come under security Group C (BSS). The security measures should address unauthorized access and checking the presence of sources at regular intervals. Sources should be stored in a locked and fixed container and in a room with access control. It should also ensure that authorized person uses the source only in an area that has controlled access.

Security of Medium-dose Rate and High-dose Rate Brachytherapy Sources

Medium-dose rate (MDR) and HDR brachytherapy sources come under security Group B. Security measures should deter unauthorized access, detect unauthorized access, and permits acquisition of sources in a timely manner. Sources in storage should be (i) in locked and fixed container, (ii) kept in a locked room to separate the container from unauthorized access, (iii) have access control to the room, and (iv) capability to detect unauthorized access or removal of the source. Sources that are in use should be (i) in a locked area or controlled area, (ii) have continuous surveillance of the source, and (iii) access control to the room.

Low-dose Rate Brachytherapy

Preloading Brachytherapy

In preloading brachytherapy, the sources are loaded in the applicator first and then inserted into the patient. Radiation hazards are much higher and complete safety is required in every stage of preloaded brachytherapy as follows:

- Receipt of sources, verification, and quality-control checks
- Preparation of applicators for use in the patients
- Insertion of the applicators into the patient at the operation theater
- Radiographic localization of implants
- Treatment time duration
- Removal of applicators
- Sterilization of applicators
- Keeping inventory of sources

After Loading Brachytherapy

After loading techniques were introduced to overcome the limitations of preloading and achieve radiation safety. In this, the applicator is inserted first into the patient and the sources are loaded later. After loaders can be either manual or remote. Both preloading and after loading involves LDR sources, consists of ^{192}Ir, ^{137}Cs, ^{60}Co and ^{125}I or ^{103}Pd radioisotopes. ^{125}I and ^{103}Pd are used as seeds for prostate and ophthalmic brachytherapy. Their half-life is 60 days and 17 days, respectively hence used as permanent implants.

Safe Operations of Brachytherapy: General Aspects

- Source strength of each source is calibrated.
- Unit of activity used in calibration is same as used in the TPS.
- Source movements should be documented.
- Assign an in-charge person for accountability of source.
- Source inventory with location and current activity

- No source will be left on the preparation site.
- In HDR units, wipe test for after loading drive assembly and transport containers.
- Periodic area survey
- Identification of responsible person for emergency handling
- Storage facility should be under lock and key.
- Patient survey after every treatment

Safe Operations Specific to Manual Iridium-192 Wires/Ribbons

In the case of manual ^{192}Ir wire, the following precautions are adhered: (i) forceps, cutting devices, magnifying lens, and good illumination of work area, (ii) container to hold full length of cut wires, (iii) collection of radioactive waste and storage, (iv) decontamination of surface and tools. Brachytherapy treatment should have informations like:

- Identification of patient
- Sources used
- Date and time of insertion and removal
- Nursing required
- Time allowance for nurses and visitors
- Instructions for unplanned source and applicator removal in emergency

After removal of therapy implant sources, the patient is monitored with survey meter to ensure that no source is within the patient. Linen, dressings, and clothing shall be kept within the room, until the sources are accounted. Rubbish bins, soiled dressing bins, and laundry baskets from the brachytherapy ward needs monitoring.

Safe Operations Specific to Manual Brachytherapy

- Sources should be inspected visually after each treatment.
- Chart showing the location of source within the safe is displayed.
- Source is transported in shield containers with shortest route.
- Sterilization of source must be done with great care to prevent damage.
- Drainage system should have filter in the sink to prevent loss of sources.

Patient Care

Low-dose rate brachytherapy patients should have separate treatment ward with adequate shielding on all sides and at the entrance, approved by the regulatory authority. Positioning of two patients and the distance between them should be such that the dose contribution from one patient to another is negligible. A mobile lead shield may be provided near each patient to minimize the dose to attending staffs. A warning sign of radiation hazard should be posted on the door, accordance with the regulatory requirement. Entry by family members should be restricted. A radiation monitor with audio system (zone monitor) should be kept always near the entrance door to ensure inadvertent movement of sources from the treatment room. The patient chart kept near the bed should have details, such as type of radionuclide, activity used, date and time of insertion and removal, total dose delivered to reference patient, etc.

High-dose Rate Remote after Loading Brachytherapy

High-dose rate brachytherapy delivers high dose of radiation to the tumor with a sharp fall-off dose outside the tumor. It is a remote after loading technique in which the applicator is inserted first, and sources loaded later by remote mechanism.

Single stepping source is used to contain the radioactive material within the sealed capsule and filter the unwanted radiation. Source size is small due to higher specific activity. Miniature source gives greater flexibility to use smaller diameter applicators, with increasing patient comfort. Effective photon energy is 340 keV for ^{192}Ir and 1.25 MeV for ^{60}Co source. ^{192}Ir source needs replacement in every 3–4 months due its half-life of 74 days, whereas it is 5–10 years for ^{60}Co. Maximum activity of 10 Ci (^{192}Ir) or 2 Ci (^{60}Co) is generally loaded in the remote after-loader HDR unit. It is carried out in the form of intracavitary, interstitial implant, surface mold, and intraluminal procedures.

Optimization

Protection in brachytherapy includes (i) treatment optimization and (ii) protection of accidental exposure. Remote after loading HDR systems has advantages over manual after loading systems. It reduces radiation exposures to staffs since the source is not manually handled. Treatment can be better optimized with enhanced reproducibility. It gives sufficient absorbed dose at a distance from the source to create homogeneous dose to the target.

Accidental Exposure

Accident exposure can be prevented by using proper unit for source strength which is specified in air kerma strength, and reference air kerma rate (RAKR). Literature reveals that (i) wrong unit of source strength entry in the TPS, whereas TPS requirement is different, and (ii) source activity ordered in one unit and the supplied activity in another unit. To minimize this error both end user and the manufacturer should use same unit of source strength.

After radiation treatment, the patient should be surveyed with portable survey meter. This will identify the failure of welding between transfer wire and source capsule and patient is free from radiation. Area monitor indications were ignored on many occasions in the past stating that it is monitor malfunction. Hence, area monitor and post-treatment survey should be brought under the safety system. The selection of dwell position and dwell time are programmed in such way that the target coverage and avoidance of organ at risk are optimized. Accidents are reported due to dwell step position in the program of incorrect length causing undesired dose distribution. Hospital should use a constant dwell step position, namely 5 mm or 10 mm to avoid such errors. Sufficient training and knowledge about the equipment and optimization in protection of treatment is required.

High-dose Rate Brachytherapy Accidents

A patient underwent HDR brachytherapy treatment with 5 catheters. After pretreatment checks, four catheters were treated. The fifth catheter showed error even after several attempts and its treatment was abandoned. The staff went inside the room and disconnected the HDR unit from the patient. Patient was shifted to the nursing home. Area monitor indicated high-radiation levels, but it was ignored. Survey meter was available but not used.

Staff believed that the area monitor is malfunctioning as it did earlier. The HDR console displayed that the source is in the safe.

The HDR source has broken from the transfer wire and remained inside the catheter. The source fell out from the patient after 4 days and it is put into the medical biohazard trash bag. A detector identified the source from the trash tailer and the source was retrieved. The patient died immediately after the source fell out due to overexposure.

Safe Operation of Remote after Loaders

- Quality control is done before each treatment day
- Transfer tubes and couplings require checking before each treatment
- Zone monitor's function to be checked
- Location of emergency container
- Aware of emergency procedures, before it arises

Radiation Safety: Remote after Loaders

As the sources do not contact with body fluids, sterilization of sources is not required. Probability of loss is also minimized, as there is reduced handling of sources. Radiation exposure during preparation of applicators has been eliminated. The radiation exposure during insertion and removal of sources has also been almost eliminated. As radiographic/CT localization of implant is done with dummy sources, exposure during the procedure has also been eliminated. Thus, remote after-loading techniques eliminate the radiation hazards associated with all stages of treatment procedure.

PROTECTION IN EXTERNAL BEAM RADIATION THERAPY

External beam radiation therapy is performed from outside to inside the patient's body. The prescribed absorbed dose should be delivered to the PTV and minimizing dose to organs at risk (OAR). A 1% change in dose may decrease 0.5–5% probability of tumor control, corresponding to 2–3% normal tissue complications. Hence, a high level of accuracy of dose delivery is required for clinical practice.

Treatment with curative intent should safely optimize the volume of treatment. Optimization should ensure that (i) the tissue target volume has a probability being included within the volume receiving high absorbed dose every day, (ii) accounts geometric variations like organ motion and setup variations in the target region, and (iii) accounts organs surrounding the targets. It can be achieved by planning target volume (PTV) and planning organ volume at risk (PRV) and drawing optimal margins around the target volume. Conformal radiation therapy reduces geometric variations to a desired level. Finally, quality control is carried out in all the steps of treatment chain to improve the quality of patient treatment as per national, and international standards.

Radiation equipment should be calibrated to achieve national traceability through secondary standard dosimetry laboratories (SSDL). It will ensure that 1 Gy at one hospital will be close to 1 Gy at another hospital. The calibration frequency is based on regulatory recommendations.

Security of Teletherapy Radioactive Sources

Radioactive sources used in teletherapy comes under security group A (BSS). Security aim is to deter unauthorized access and to detect unauthorized access and acquisition of the source in a timely manner. Security measures should delay the acquisition until a response is possible. To satisfy security objectives, provisions are implemented while (1) sources in storage and (2) sources in use.

Sources in storage should have:

- A locked and fixed source storage container like source head or transport container
- A locked storage room separating the container from unauthorized personnel
- Access control to the storage room
- Detection of unauthorized access or removal of sources
- Ability to respond in a timely manner to such detection

Sources in use should have the following:

- A locked teletherapy head in an area to which access can be controlled
- Access control to that area
- Continuous monitoring for unauthorized intrusion attempts, either by personnel surveillance or electronic equipment
- Security guards capable of providing a timely response

The above may be achieved by incorporating proper technical design in the radiotherapy facility. It includes locking the teletherapy head, locking the treatment/storage room and adding an intrusion alarm that notifies compromise of security.

Safe Operation of External Beam Radiotherapy

External beam machine's safe operation procedure requires the following:

- Wipe tests
- Area survey
- Interlock checks
- Emergency off switch check
- Last man out switch check
- Emergency during source struct in the ON position, either fully or partially

Necessary radiation survey meters are made available: (i) GM type survey meter, (ii) Ionization type survey meter, (iii) Wipe test devices—well counter and multichannel analyzer (MCA), and (iv) Personnel alarm dosimeter during emergency.

Accidents due to Equipment Malfunction

Patient undergoing radiation treatment getting benefit compared to radiation risk. However, patient may have chance to being exposed to radiation in future, and the probability of harm should be low. If harm occurs, it may be serious for the patient which will create a risk to the individual. Equipment's malfunction due to (1) software, (2) incorrect repair, and (3) interlock failure have been reported. Several lessons have been learned from such accidents and investigations.

Software Accident

An accelerator delivered overdose due to wrong carousel setting (USA, Canada, 1980) in six events. The technologists wrongly selected X-ray mode instead of low-energy electron mode for the patient. Operator realizing the mistake promptly corrected for the mode using edit-key facility. The computer displayed the electron beam mode and the "beam ON" command was given to start the treatment. The treatment was abruptly terminated after 1 second with the patient writhing in pain calling for help from inside treatment room. Physicist later simulated the malfunction "Malfunction-52" and measured the dose in water phantom as 250 Gy/s. Vendor subsequently informed all users to suspend the use of the accelerator.

Incorrect Repair of Accelerator

During treatment, a linear accelerator broke down (Spain, 1990). A technologist working nearby in a Cobalt unit was called for repair. After the repair the control panel displayed 36 MeV, irrespective of 7, 10, and 13 MeV electron selection. Treatment was resumed for 10 days on 27 patients using electrons, and 17 died due to overexposures over 1 year. Technologists came to know the difference between the energy selection and the console display only later.

A transistor gets short circuited and full current was flown to the magnet system. This made the selection of maximum electron energy and displayed as 36 MeV. The accelerator is designed such a way that homogeneous electron field is achieved by scanning the electron beams by deflection magnets. Current to the scanning magnet should match the selected electron energy. Since the electron energy is maximum, the current to the deflection magnet is too low. This made the field to be centered at the center resulting increased energy fluence and dose.

Accelerator Interlock Failure

During treatment an accelerator was shut down automatically due to power failure *(Poland, 2001)*. When power resumed, restarted again and few tests were conducted. Low-dose rate was indicated, and the staff increased the filament current to high level. Remaining treatment was completed, and two patients reported burning sensation during treatment. Physicist measured the dose which was extremely high. Five patients had local injuries of varying severity.

Investigations revealed two faults namely: (i) failure of fuse of power supply to beam monitoring system which leads to high-dose rate, though lower value is displaced, (ii) diode was broken in the safety interlock chain which normally indicates dosimetry faults. Due the above, nothing was indicated, though the dose was very high than planned.

Accidents due to Equipment Calibration and Errors

Accidents due to equipment calibration and errors includes: (1) Incorrect decay data and (2) Errors in treatment planning which are discussed below.

Incorrect Decay Data

A tele-Cobalt unit in *Ohia* was not calibrated between 1974 and 1976. Physicist failed to do calibration of the machine and obtained dose rate from source decay data to calculate treatment time. He plotted the dose rate on a semi-log graph sheet and extrapolated the decaying dose rate over time. He plotted the page with linear scales on both axes. Y-axis did not correspond to the original log Y-axis, leads to incorrect output. X-axis did not correspond to the original calendar axis, and leads to incorrect date values. The dose rate being underestimated is about 10–55% that passed on to the patients. About 462 patients received high doses and reported symptoms of overexposure. Physicist showed falsified calibration documents attempting to prove correct output of the machine. In fact, the machine was due for calibration for more than 22 months.

Errors in Treatment Planning

A treatment planning system (TPS) was purchased (*UK, 1982*) and the hospital started using it for isocentric (Non-SSD) calculations. Technologists applied distance correction factor for all non-SSD treatment calculations. TPS has already corrected the plans for distance which was ignored. As a result, every patient was given corrections twice for distance in all isocentric plans, resulting lower dose to the patients. Since 1991, about 6% of patients have been given isocentric treatments, over 9-year period. It includes 1,045 patients whose received lower doses, out of which 492 developed local recurrences. The underdose varied between 5 and 35%.

CONTROL OF OCCUPATIONAL, MEDICAL, AND PATIENT EXPOSURES

Radiation areas are classified as controlled area and supervised areas or controlled and uncontrolled areas as described earlier. Controlled area is one in which specific protection and safety provisions are required to prevent normal and potential exposures. Supervised areas do not require specific protection and safety policies.

Occupational Exposure

Workers are provided with personnel monitoring devices [thermoluminescent dosimeter (TLD)] to access the radiation doses. These workers include radiation oncologists, medical physicists, radiation safety officer, radiotherapy technologist, nursing personnel, and maintenance staffs. Health surveillance program should be organized to all workers. If workers are exposed to high-level radiation, biological dosimetry, and other medical investigation may be required. Counseling is made available to pregnant workers, over exposures, and those worried about potential or acute radiation exposures. Workers shall have access to dose-monitoring records. These records must have details about nature of work involving occupational exposure, dose and dose-assessment data, number of employees exposed, date of employment, and doses due to emergency handling or accidents.

Medical Exposure

Medical exposure involves only justification and optimization but not dose limits. Medical exposures are justified by weighing the diagnostic or therapeutic benefits. It should be accounted based on risk versus benefits.

Exposure of normal tissues should be kept as low by ALARA principle and organ shielding is provided. Exposure of the abdomen or pelvis of women who are likely to be pregnant is avoided. Any therapeutic dose to pregnant women should be with minimum dose. Fetal dose <100 mGy should not be considered as reason for pregnancy termination.

Calibration of radiation sources and machines with international protocols is necessary to prevent mistakes. Quality assurance for medical exposures with internal and external audit may be advisable.

Comforters and visitors who help knowingly to the patient should not exceed a dose of 5 mSv during that procedure. The dose to the children who visit the patients having radioactive sources should be <1 mSv. Accidental exposure of patients may be investigated to arrive the following data:

- Estimate the dose received within the patient
- Corrective measures to prevent recurrence of such events
- Reporting such events to the regulatory authority
- Sharing information with patient and his doctor

Public Exposure

Public exposure is controlled by the following:

- Physical shielding design
- Keeping the sources under secure and shielding
- Ensuring the function of interlocks
- Secure the control area to have restricted access

Exposure to public from brachytherapy sources could arise during transportation of patients/sources in hospital premises, during treatment in case of manual after loading, and loss of accidental mishandling. Some of the reported radiation incidents includes loss of sources with hospital wastes, inadvertent discharge of patient/cremation of dead body with source within, spread of contamination by cutting applicator with source struck in, leakage due to uncontrolled sterilization and rough handling, etc. To minimize hazards associated with brachytherapy application, it is necessary to ensure safe work practices at all the levels.

Hence, radioactive waste and unused sources should be disposed as per regulatory norms. Shielding material like depleted uranium should be disposed as radioactive waste. Decontamination of telecobalt-60 or HDR brachytherapy source shall be notified to the competent authority.

Visitors to the radiotherapy facility should be controlled. They must be provided information and instruction before they enter the control area. Public must be accompanied by a radiation oncology staff during such entry. Public exposures during their visit require monitoring.

Possibility of Potential Exposures and Emergency Plans

Common types of emergencies arise from:

- Lost source
- Struct source
- Contamination
- Off-site accidents
- Patient accidental exposure

In the case of lost source, the identity, type, and activity of the source, where the lost source was last seen and by whom is important. The area is closed, and entry is restricted until radiation survey is carried out.

In struct sources, emergency procedures should be carried out, it should be short, concise, and unambiguous. If the source struct is in the external beam unit, the first step is to return the source driving mechanism to the shielded position. If it is not successful, the patient is removed from the table and the room is closed. All effort should be made to avoid primary beam exposure to the staffs. If the source struct is in HDR brachytherapy unit, the emergency container should be placed closer to the patient and the applicator along with source is removed from the patient and transferred to the container. Long-handled forceps are useful to handle applicator and transfer tubes. Brachytherapy supplier suggested emergency procedures are carried out as follows:

- Observation of error message at the console
- Pressing emergency off button
- Enter the room with portable survey meter and wearing TLD badge
- Monitor the radiation levels in the room
- Recovery from the after-loading unit
- Manual retraction of the source by hand crank

- Survey of patient in HDR unit to conform source position
- Removal of applicator and placement in the emergency container
- Survey of patient and emergency container

Contamination generally arises from Radium-226 which is in powder form. Nowadays, it is replaced by ^{137}Cs sources and contamination is unlikely. If contamination arises, the area should be closed, and further entry is restricted. All the personnel in the area should remain there until it is surveyed and decontaminated. Off-site accidents arise due to loss of security of unused tele-therapy sources which may warrant regulatory intervention. It may cause high-level contamination or external exposure.

Patient Accidental Exposure

Overall, accidental exposures are much rare in radiation therapy. Past experiences indicate that attention, alertness or awareness, procedures and checks, qualified and trained manpower and co-ordination are the key factors to reduce accidents, if any. Over exposures may be without symptoms in patients. Incidents have greater probability to occur than accidents. Hence, incidents may create much more harm or risk to the patients. One can learn from the incidents took place elsewhere, and every incidence varies with magnitude.

In the case of telecobalt unit's source struck in beam ON position is the major issue. It can be overcome as follows:

- Terminate the radiation using emergency button
- Enter the treatment room and wear TLD badge
- Other person should be in the console and make note of the time taken for the task to complete.
- Collimator is closed to minimal field size
- Gantry is rotated so that beam is directed on the opposite primary wall.
- Couch is lowered down, and patient is removed safely and quickly from the couch
- If the source does not return, push it back to the safe position by using an emergency T-rod
- RSO should be informed about source struct incident
- Room door is closed with a warning sign pasted on the door.

RESPONSIBILITIES OF HEALTHCARE PROFESSIONALS

Responsibility of Radiation Oncologist

- Ensure that the exposure of normal tissue is kept as low as reasonably achievable while required dose is delivered to the planning target volume.
- Establish optimized protocols for therapeutic procedures in consultation with the medical physicist.
- Ensure radiotherapeutic procedures of women who are pregnant or likely to be pregnant be avoided unless there are strong clinical indications.
- Evaluate any radiation accident or incident from a medical point of view.

Responsibility of Medical Physicist

- Ensure the correct calibration of treatment units both during commissioning and on a regular basis.

- Ensure the correctness and accuracy in patient dose calculations, both computerized and manual.
- Design, implementing, and supervising quality assurance procedures
- Participate in the continuing review of the radiotherapy practice's resources (including budget, equipment, and staffing), operations, policies, and procedures.
- Plan, in conjunction with the radiotherapy physician and the RSO, the facilities for radiotherapy practice.
- Prepare performance specifications for equipment about radiation protection.
- Ensure the establishment and maintenance of a radiation protection program for the safety of staff and the public.
- Test equipment for acceptance, commission of equipment for clinical use and supervise equipment maintenance.
- Participate in the investigation and evaluation of incidents and accidents.
- Contribute to the radiation protection training program.

Responsibility of Radiotherapy Technologist

- Identify the patient prior to treatment occasion.
- Administer the radiotherapy to the patient, including the correct set up and delivery.
- Inform the physician and seek advice if the female patient is pregnant or likely to be pregnant.
- Inform the physician in case you are concerned about an unusual reaction of patient.
- Inform the physicist in case you are concerned about an unusual event related to a treatment unit or treatment parameters.
- Contribute to the preparation of specifications for new equipment.
- Contribute to the quality control of radiological equipment.

Safe Work Practice in Radiotherapy

- Daily quality assurance checks should be performed before starting the patient treatment.
- Electric power, room temperature, humidity, AC function, door interlock, and radiation warning light display should be checked daily.
- Technologist should wear the TLD badge at the chest level.
- Patient should be briefed about the treatment procedure in their own language.
- As far as possible the patient should be treated in supine position with isocenter setup.
- For head and neck treatment, proper head rest must be used along with suitable patient positioning boards. Flexible headrests such as pillows should be avoided. Shoulder retraction device is used whenever required.
- Proper immobilization methods: Thermoplastic mask/vacuum cushions are used for patient positioning to suit the location of treatment.
- Correct patient positioning board should be used for each patient unless it is an all-in-one board. In the case of breast board proper angulation is to be set.
- The patient must be positioned with great care for a given SAD/SSD, field size, photon, or electron energy, etc.
- The beam-directing devices and wedge filter must be used whenever is needed.
- Proper time or MU is set in the control console with correct energy.

- The door must be closed properly before the machine is switched ON.
- During irradiation, the patient must be observed through the CCTV.
- Treatment details must be entered in the patients register.
- Any interruption in treatment must also be recorded in a separate logbook.
- Make use of the last man out switch (LMOS) and its alarm after the treatment.
- In brachytherapy, the patient should be surveyed before leaving the treatment room, for radioactive source, if any.

PREGNANCY AND RADIOTHERAPY

Cancers that are remote from the pelvis can be treated in radiotherapy with careful planning. However, cancer of the pelvis cannot be treated adequately without severe or lethal consequences for the fetus.

Cancer in pregnancy is uncommon, it is 0.1% of the total pregnancies. About 4,000 women are treated with radiotherapy in the USA during pregnancy. Surgery, chemotherapy, and radiotherapy combinedly may pose risks to the unborn child. The patient-mother get the benefit, whereas the fetus gets the risk. It is not only an ethical but also a risk versus benefit issue.

Most common neoplasms that occur during pregnancy are breast, cervix, leukemia, lymphoma, melanoma, thyroid, ovary, nasopharynx, esophagus, and brain cancers. Each cancer site requires different management strategy. For example, fetus receives scattered radiation from the chest area is likely to get childhood cancer with IQ reduction. If the fetus is close to the pelvic region, the effect on the fetus is much severe. Considerations should be given in terms of (1) before radiotherapy, (2) during radiotherapy, and (3) after radiotherapy. Special cares are required while planning radiotherapy for patients during pregnancy.

Before Radiotherapy

It is important to ascertain whether the female patient is pregnant prior to radiotherapy. It should be based on history, age, and prior surgery or pregnant test, etc. Even if the patient is not pregnant, she should be counseled to avoid pregnancy until the radiotherapy is over and the tumor is cured completely. If she is found pregnant, the husband or relative should be informed about the course of treatment and its outcome. There are no hard and fast rules, but the patient, family members, treating oncologist, and other team members should carefully discuss the decisions made. ICRP-84 has suggested few important points for consideration as follows:

- Stage and aggressiveness of the tumor
- Potential hormonal effects of pregnancy on the tumor
- Various therapies and their length, efficacy, and complications
- Impact of delaying therapy
- Expected effects of maternal ill-health on the fetus
- Stage of pregnancy
- Fetal assessment and monitoring
- How and when the baby could be safely delivered.
- Whether the pregnancy should be terminated.
- Legal, ethical, and moral issues

Chemotherapy drugs may exhibit major malformation in 10% of fetus during the first trimester. After the first trimester the risk decreases, it is also reported that in-utero exposure to chemotherapy may cause increased risk of pancytopenia at birth, and possibility of neoplasms in the offsprings.

Surgery and anesthesia also pose problems such as hypotension, hypoxia, and infection. Many patients are reported fever or infection due to tumor or immunosuppression. The hyperthermia is related to teratogenic effects like neural tube defects and microphthalmia. The maternal issue is malnutrition of fetus.

During Radiotherapy

Nonpelvic Pregnant Patients

Nonpelvic radiotherapy can be done but with estimation of fetal dose that may require additional shielding. Nonpelvic cancers are breast, lymphoma, etc. Breast cancer occurs 1 out of 3,000 pregnancies. It is quite away from the fetus and can be treated in different ways. If a breast cancer patient is pregnant, most radiation oncologists advise their patients not to become pregnant for 1–2 years after completion of therapy. This is not primarily related to concerns about potential radiation effects, but rather to considerations about the risk of relapse of the tumor that would require more radiation, surgery, or chemotherapy.

Lymphomas can be treated with chemotherapy/radiotherapy or delayed until late pregnancy or until after pregnancy.

The first step is that the treatment can be postponed until the fetus is at a later gestation age. If radiotherapy is decided, it is important to calculate the dose to the fetus before the treatment is given. When external radiotherapy is used for treatment of tumors at some distance from the fetus, important parameter is fetus distance from the edge of the radiation field. The fetus dose decreases exponentially with distance. Fetus dose may be 30 mGy for photon radiotherapy in brain cancers. In the case of Hodgkin's disease, it may be 400–500 mGy for unshielded fetus.

For ^{60}Co with 10 × 10 cm^2 field, the estimate of off-axis dose is available in literature. The dose is reduced by a factor of 2–5 for photon accelerators. Phantom and in-vivo dosimetry measurements can be done to avoid dose uncertainty. The *American Association of Physicists in Medicine (AAPM)* recommends that the following points:

- Complete all planning as though the patients were not pregnant. If the fetus is near the treatment beam, do not take portal localization films with open collimation and blocks removed.
- Consider modifications to the treatment plan that would reduce the radiation dose to the fetus by changing field size, angle, radiation energy and field trimmers on the edge nearest to the fetus. If possible, use photon energies of <25 MV.
- Estimate dose without shielding to the fetus by using phantom measurements at symphysis pubis, fundus, and midpoint.
- If the fetus dose is 50–100 mGy shield may be constructed with 4–5 half-value layers of lead. Fetus dose again measured in phantom with shield in place.
- Document the treatment plan and discuss it with the staff involved in patient set-up. Document the shielding (perhaps with a photograph).
- Check the weight and load-bearing specifications of the treatment couch or other aspects of shielding support.
- Be present during initial treatment to assure that shielding is correctly placed.
- Fetal size and growth throughout the course of treatment should be monitored and reassess fetal dose if necessary.

- After treatment, total dose including the range of dose to the fetus during therapy should be documented.
- If equipment and personnel are not available for reducing and estimating the fetal dose, refer the patient to another institution.

Pelvic Pregnant Patients

Carcinoma of the cervix is the most common with pregnancy and the incidence is one out of 1,250 to 2,200 that varies with country. It is often treated by surgery or radiotherapy (including brachytherapy). Absorbed dose of both forms of radiotherapy will causc termination of pregnancy. If the tumor is infiltrative and is diagnosed late in pregnancy, an alternative is to delay treatment until the baby is delivered. Radiotherapy in pelvic region during pregnancy results in severe consequences including fetal death. The ovarian cancer is very rare, it is one out of 10,000 pregnancies. It may be treated with surgery and chemotherapy, whereas radiotherapy is rarely used.

Brachytherapy patient is treated as outpatient or hospitalized until sources are removed. They occasionally become the source of radiation. The fetal dose of a visiting pregnant woman relative is much low. Iodine-131 seed prostate implant patients discharged from hospital, pose no damage to pregnant family members.

Fetal Shielding

Radiotherapy during pregnancy may harm the developing fetus. Fetal dose depends on the gestational period and cancer treatment site. A fetal dose of 5.6–58.7 cGy has been reported during the treatment of Hodgkin's lymphoma. Radiation effects like mental retardation and organ malformation may arise if the threshold dose is >0.1–0.2 Gy. This dose is unlikely if the tumor is located away from the fetus. However, additional shielding can reduce the dose by 50–60% and prevents the risk of childhood cancer and leukemia. Such shielding is found useful in brain, breast, lung, nasopharynx, and Hodgkin's lymphoma and can limit the fetus dose within 10 cGy.

Seonghee Kang et al. (2021) designed a fetal shielding device for treating brain tumor in pregnant patients. It is aimed to reduce scatter leakage radiation at various gantry angles during IMRT and VMAT by 6 MV X-rays. A fetal dose reduction of 50% is achieved at 50 cm from the field edge. **Mohammed K Islam** et al. (2001) used 5-cm thick lead bricks and heavy mental steel cart, and designed a 50 cm × 50 cm portable shield. It reduced the fetal dose from collimator scatter and head leakage, while the gantry is positioned at 90°/270° position to treat nasopharyngeal cancer by 6 MV and 9 MV X-rays.

AAPM-TG-36 (1995) has suggested suitable shields to protect the fetus during radiotherapy. It includes (i) bridge over patient, (ii) table over treatment couch, and (iii) mobile shields. In the first method about 4–5 HVL of lead (5–7 cm of lead or 6-8.5 cm of Cerrobend) is kept over the abdomen as bridge format. Second type consists of a single unit that rests on the treatment couch. It protects the fetus from anterior, posterior, and lateral treatment fields. Third type consists of single mobile shield for anterior-posterior treatment, but independent of treatment couch. It is vertically adjustable from 80 to 125 cm SSD with a motor assistance. All types of shields can reduce the fetal dose by 50%.

After Radiation Therapy

Records of the radiotherapy techniques, total dose estimation should be maintained. Proper counseling is recommended. Pregnancy usually found before or during radiotherapy. It is rare to be pregnant after radiotherapy since treatment take several weeks. Hence, prior counseling and shielding are required during treatment.

Fetal dose estimate is calculated and documented. Trained medical physicist must do such exercise and the associated risk is conveyed to the mother. Records should be kept as per local regulations.

Illustration 1

A patient just finished 4 weeks of radiation treatment to the neck area for *non-Hodgkin's lymphoma.* After 1 month, she got pregnant. What are the possible effects on the fetus?

There is no likely effect. Radiation exposure occurred before conception, so any effect on the offspring would be classified as genetic effect. No data from humans show any statistically significant genetic effect in any population, even the *Japanese Atomic bomb survivors.* All estimates of genetic radiation risk come from studies of rodents, which show that males are far more sensitive than females. However, it is not easy to extrapolate this data to humans. There is very low risk of any effect on the unborn child. The *World Health Organization* estimates that the worldwide incidence of inherited disease (ranging from severe to as trivial as an inconspicuous birthmark) is about 10%. In the unfortunate event that the child is born with any genetic abnormality, it is extremely unlikely that it would be related to the earlier radiation exposure.

Illustration 2

What is the risk to a fetus if a man who has had a radiation pellet/seed inserted into his prostate for cancer treatment comes into proximity with a pregnant woman?

There is no danger involved. Prostate brachytherapy can be performed with permanent implantation of radioactive ^{103}Pd or ^{125}I seeds, and the patient is discharged from hospital with sources in place. The short range of the emissions from these radionuclides is the reason that the patient can be discharged and patients pose no danger to pregnant family members. Other brachytherapy patients are kept in the hospital until the sources are removed. While these patients can occasionally be a source of radiation to a pregnant family member, the potential dose to the fetus is very low, irrespective of the type of brachytherapy.

Pregnant Staffs and Continuation of Work

A pregnant worker can continue to work in radiotherapy department if there is reasonable assurance that the fetal dose can be kept <1 mGy during pregnancy. It is important to ensure that pregnant women are not subjected to unnecessary discrimination. There are responsibilities for both the worker and the employer. The pregnant radiation worker should inform the pregnancy to the employer and RSO. Suitable remedial measures can be taken to reduce the fetal dose. They may be posted in equipment which are remotely operational. In radiotherapy with sealed sources, pregnant technicians or nurses might not participate in manual brachytherapy.

RADIATION SAFETY DURING SOURCE TRANSFER OPERATIONS OF TELETHERAPY AND HDR BRACHYTHERAPY

Owing to the decay of the radiation sources in radiotherapy units, replacement of the decayed sources with fresh sources of higher activity is necessary and the frequency of replacement depends upon the half-life of radioactive source used (e.g., 5 years for ^{60}Co, 3–4 months for ^{192}Ir). Sometimes the repair work of the unit's head also demands source transfer operation. The activity of these sources depends on the make and model of the therapy unit. The activity of a teletherapy source is much higher than in a remotely controlled after loading brachytherapy unit. Therefore, more attention is needed during the source transfer of the teletherapy units. Ignoring any of the recommended procedures and steps may result in a serious radiation accident and elaborate and expensive management of the situation.

Make and Models

Different make and models of teletherapy and brachytherapy units have been installed and under service by various manufacturers, all over India. **Table 14.1** gives details about some of the teletherapy units available in the country and the type of source drawer of each mode, which is replaced during the source transfer operation. **Table 14.2** gives the details about the remotely controlled brachytherapy units available in India and abroad.

The new sources loaded in drawers or capsules are transported in special source flasks designed for a specific make and model of the therapy unit **(Fig. 14.1)**. The source flask is used to carry out the source transfer operation. The decayed source is first removed from the unit and loaded into source flask. New source is then loaded into the unit. During repair works (involving head of the unit) also, the source flask is used for removing the source from the unit and for reloading it into the therapy unit on completion of the repair work.

TABLE 14.1 Teletherapy units and manufacturers.

Model	*Type of source drawer*	*Manufacturer*
Equinox 80/100	Cylindrical	M/s TeamBest Theratronics Asia Pvt Ltd
Bhabhatron-II	Cylindrical	M/s Panacea Medical Technologies Pvt Ltd

TABLE 14.2 Brachytherapy sources and manufacturers.

Model	*Type of source*	*Manufacturer*
Flexitron	^{192}Ir, ^{60}Co	M/s Elekta
GammaMedplus iX Bravos	^{192}Ir	M/s Varian Medical Systems
SagiNova	^{60}Co ^{192}Ir	M/s Eckert and Ziegler BEBIG

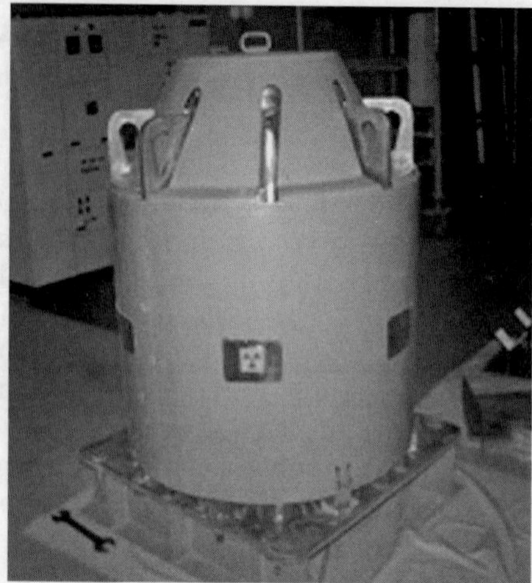

FIG. 14.1: Telecobalt 60, source transportation flask.

Courtesy: Board of Radiation and Isotope Technology (BRIT), India.

General Precautions

- It is the responsibility of serving company to ensure safe transport of the source flask loaded with new source either supplied by *Board of Radiation and Isotope Technology (BRIT), Mumbai* or imported, and the return of the decayed source back to the supplier. All the regulations for safe transport should be strictly followed.
- All the gadgets required for the source transfer operation as per the checklist should be made available before undertaking the operation. Non-standard gadgets which may delay the source transfer operation and may lead to radiation accidents should not be used.
- Personnel monitoring badges, pocket dosimeters, and pocket alarm type radiation monitor should be used by all personnel involved in the operation.
- Proper procedure should be adopted for the alignment of the source flask with the unit head. Necessary coupling devices should be used to facilitate proper alignment.
- Proper arrester/s should be provided on the source flask after removing the lids so that source drawer does not slip down accidentally during the alignment process.
- After confirming the alignment between the source flask and unit head, the source flask should be immobilized. Also, all unnecessary materials around the flask should be removed.
- In case the source transfer operation is to be carried out in beam ON position (e.g., Theratron), proper locking device should be provided to prevent the movement of the system in case of power failure.
- Wherever dummy drawer is required in the source transfer operation (Theratron and Siemen's Model), source transfer operation without dummy drawer should not be carried out.
- After the transfer of the new source into the teletherapy unit, proper arrester or arresting plates should be employed to prevent the slipping of the source drawer in case the unit is moved accidentally.

- Proper functioning of the unit, after loading of new source, should be checked with shutter open to minimum size and beam pointing opposite to maze wall.
- Parking rod required for pushing the stuck source drawer or shutter should always be available in the control room.

Preparation During Source Transfer Operations

- Loading, unloading, and handling of radioactive sources shall be undertaken under close supervision of Radiological Safety Officer (RSO) under a well-defined radiation protection program.
- Source loading/unloading operations shall not be carried out if all the operating, control and safety systems are not functioning in the intended manner.
- Motive power for source and product movement shall be disabled during source loading/unloading operations.
- Mock runs shall be carried out with dummy sources prior to undertaking actual operations using proper tool for picking lifting of source pencils.
- The hoist to be used for lifting the source transport cask shall be tested periodically through the authorized testing agency and valid certificate of testing shall be submitted to regulatory body prior to source loading operations.
- Radiation safety assessment of the whole operation shall be made by RSO and protection and safety shall be optimized.

Guidelines for Source Loading/Unloading Operation

- Procedures described by the manufacturer/supplier and accepted by the Competent Authority shall be strictly adhered to.
- Radiation survey of the transport cask including external radiation survey and external removable contamination shall be performed prior to opening it.
- Proper under water lighting system in the water pool shall be provided to facilitate smooth source handling operation.
- It shall be ensured that water inside the pool remains clear for proper visibility for the operation.
- It shall be ensured that no inflammable or explosive material is present in the vicinity of area of sources loading/unloading operation.
- All sources loading/unloading operations shall be carried out by trained personnel of source supplier.
- The personnel involved in source loading/unloading operation shall use appropriate safety gears such as safety belts and helmet.
- The physical barrier shall be used during source loading/unloading operation to prevent accidental fall of any personnel inside the water pool.
- All personnel involved in the operation shall be monitored with personnel monitoring badges and pocket dosimeters and individual dose records shall be maintained.
- Good housekeeping practices shall be observed during and after source loading/unloading operations to prevent any abnormal situations/incidents.

Emergency

- The source supplier shall provide assistance to handle any emergency situations involving radiation source and ensuring safe disposal, if necessary.

- In case of any emergency or abnormal situation during the operation, the source shall be brought back to its fully shielded position either in the cask or shielded position in the radiation processing facility.

After Completion of Source Loading/Unloading

- The record of the position of each source unit in the source rack and its activity as on date shall be maintained.
- Following the source loading operations, source supplier shall carry out internal contamination survey of the empty transport cask by taking swipe samples from inside the cask cavity.
- After completion of source loading/rearrangement/redistribution operation, report on the above operation, radiation protection survey and product dosimetry report shall be submitted to Regulatory Body. The routine operation of the radiation processing facility shall be subject to obtaining prior license/permission from the Competent Authority.

PATIENT PROTECTION: AERB SAFETY CODE

Quality Assurance

Prior to commissioning of radiation therapy equipment including sources and accessories for patient treatment, the entire prescribed acceptance tests shall be performed. It shall be ensured that the results of the tests are within tolerance limits. Records of list of tests performed and their results shall be maintained by the medical physicist in a logbook. Quality assurance tests shall be repeated at specified intervals and records of the list of tests performed and their results maintained by the medical physicist in a logbook. The licensee shall inform the competent authority if the results of the tests show any unexpected deviation and corrective action taken.

Equipment and Accessories

Appropriate equipment and accessories, as required shall be made available for measuring source strength and for performing dosimetry, treatment planning, treatment simulation and quality assurance tests. These shall be maintained in good working condition.

Calibration of Dosimetry Instruments

The dosimetry instruments shall be calibrated at specified intervals and the dose measurements shall have accuracy within ±3%. These calibrations shall be traceable to national/international standard laboratories and as per internationally accepted dosimetry protocols.

Dose Delivery

- For both teletherapy and high-dose rate brachytherapy patients, the radiation therapy technologist shall keep a close watch to ensure that the treatment is terminated at the intended time.

- In the case of brachytherapy patients, the positions of the applicator/sources in/on the patient shall be verified with the help of appropriate imaging systems. It shall be ascertained that, as far as possible, the positions of the sources are retained in the same way throughout the treatment, unless planned otherwise.

Patient Treatment Chart

A patient treatment chart shall be maintained for each patient as per institution's requirement. The chart shall be signed by the members of the radiation oncology team. The modifications, if any, in the treatment schedule shall be recorded in the chart. The chart shall also be reviewed at regular intervals, at least once a week, by the radiation oncology team, signed and dated by the reviewers.

Misadministration

Misadministration of doses resulting in accidental medical exposures involving: (i) any treatment given to either the wrong patient or the wrong site, or using the wrong radioisotope, or wrong type of radiation, or with a dose or dose fractionation differing substantially from the values prescribed by the radiation oncologist or that may lead to undue acute secondary effects, and (ii) any equipment failure, accident, error, mishap, miscalculation or other unusual occurrence with the potential for causing a patient dose significantly different from that intended shall be promptly investigated by the employer/licensee.

A report of the investigation including: (i) calculation or estimation of the doses received and their distribution within the patient, (ii) corrective measures required to prevent recurrence of such an accident, and (iii) method to implement any corrective measures shall be promptly sent to the competent authority by employer/licensee.

Treatment Records

The licensee shall maintain treatment records of each patient for at least 15 years, including source configurations in case of brachytherapy, to facilitate unambiguous and correct post-treatment follow-up. In general, the following records are required:

- Patient case sheet
- Patient immobilization record
- Patient simulation record
- Patient treatment planning record
- Patient treatment chart and record
- Quality assurance (machine/patient) record
- Machine calibration record
- Radiation survey record
- Machine logbook

In brachytherapy also all the above records and logbooks are required. In addition, the following logbooks are maintained:

- Source inventory record
- Source movement record
- Source disposal record
- Source calibration record

In general, the number of logbook and type of entries vary with machine and type of treatment. Every machine should have separate logbook describing the entry and exit of the equipment. The logbook details include date of purchase, breakdown, remedial measures, name of service engineer, down time, remarks, and RSO signature.

BIBLIOGRAPHY

1. Radiation Protection and Safety of Radiation Sources: International Basic Safety Standards, IAEA safety standards, Vienna, 2014.
2. International Commission on Radiological Protection, Prevention of High-Dose-Rate Brachytherapy Accidents, ICRP Publication 97, Pergamon Press, Oxford, and New York, 2005.
3. Podgorsak FB. Radiation Oncology Physics: A Handbook for Teachers and Students, IAEA, Vienna, 2005.
4. International Atomic Energy Agency, Accidental Overexposure of Radiotherapy Patients in Białystok, STI/PUB/1180, IAEA, Vienna, 2004.
5. International Commission on Radiological Protection, Pregnancy and Medical Radiation, ICRP Publication 84, Pergamon Press, Oxford, and New York, 2000.
6. International Atomic Energy Agency, Lessons Learned from Accidental Exposures in Radiotherapy, IAEA Safety Reports Series No. 17, IAEA, Vienna, 2000.
7. International Atomic Energy Agency, Absorbed Dose Determination in External Beam Radiotherapy: An International Code of Practice for Dosimetry Based on Standards of Absorbed Dose to Water, IAEA Technical Reports Series No. 398, IAEA, Vienna, 2000.
8. Stovall M, Blackwell CR, Cundiff J, Novack DH, Palta JR, Wagner LK, et al. Fetal dose from radiotherapy with photon beams: Report of AAPM Radiation Therapy Committee Task Group No. 36. Med Phys. 1995;22(1):63-82.
9. Ash D, Bates T. Report on the clinical effects of inadvertent radiation underdosage in 1045 patients. Clin Oncol. 1994;6:214-25.
10. Levson NG, Turner CS. An investigation of the Therac-25 accidents, IEEE Computer. 1993;26:18-41.
11. Nuclear Regulatory Commission, Report to Congress on Abnormal Occurrences. 92-18. Loss of Iridium-192 Source and Medical Therapy Misadministration at Indiana Regional Cancer Center in Indiana, Pennsylvania, NUREG-0090, Volume 15, No. 4. USNRC, Washington DC (1992).
12. Williamson JF, Nath R. Clinical implementation of AAPM Task Group 32 recommendations on brachytherapy source strength specification. Med Phys. 1991;18:439-48.
13. Sociedad Espanola De Fisica Medica, The Accident of the Linear Accelerator in the "Hospital Clínico de Zaragoza", SEFM, Madrid (1991).

CHAPTER 15

Disposal of Radioactive Waste

INTRODUCTION

Every industry generates some amount of waste and nuclear industry is one among them. The waste generated in the nuclear industry is called radioactive waste. It is in the form of solid, liquid, or gaseous waste produced during the manufacture or use of radioactive substance. Hazards related to radioactive waste gives rise to certain amount of fear and unacceptability in the minds of public. The radioactive waste needs to be managed safely to ensure protection of man and environment, without imposing significant burden on future generations. If not handled carefully, ionizing radiations emitted by the radioactive waste can cause somatic and genetic effects in the living beings. Radioactive waste can be treated to some extent by physio-chemical methods, adopted to conventional pollutants. However, they undergo decay, and the radiation comes to the background level after a certain period. This period depends upon the half-life of the waste, which varies from seconds to thousands of years.

Hence, effective waste management methods are the need of the hour. It includes safe radioactive disposal methods and preventing pollution of the environment. Waste disposal refers to safe disposal of waste in which no number of the public will get a dose exceeding regulatory clearance limits.

RADIOACTIVE WASTE

Sources of Radioactive Waste

Mainly radioactive waste is generated from: (i) nuclear fuel, (ii) research and power generation reactors, and (iii) isotope applications. In nuclear fuel, it begins with mining, milling, refining of uranium and thorium from their ores, fuel fabrication and fuel reprocessing. The second type includes isotope production and electricity generation. The third, isotope application includes medicine, nuclear research, industry, and agriculture. The waste generated may be liquid, solid or gaseous with radioactive content varying from insignificant to extremely high levels.

A wide range of radionuclides is used in medicine for treatment, diagnosis, and research. The waste arises from the above applications is called medical radioactive waste, which requires a comprehensive management system. The types of radioactive waste that may arise in medicine are mainly from radiotherapy and nuclear medicine. The sources from which the wastes arise are source storage, preparation, source administration and injection needles, counting room, toilet-improper use (vomiting by patients), and decontamination. In radiation therapy, the waste arises from:

- Telecobalt-60 sources
- Enriched uranium components (shutter, collimator, etc.)
- Brachytherapy sources (^{60}Co, ^{137}Cs, ^{192}Ir, and ^{125}I)
- Leaking sources
- Contaminated cotton, etc.

In nuclear medicine, the radioactive waste arises from:

- Decayed sealed sources
- Spent radionuclide generators (^{99m}Tc, ^{81m}Kr, ^{185m}Au, etc.)
- Laboratory solutions of low activity
- Low-activity liquid washings from vials
- Liquid scintillant immiscible with water
- Biologically contaminated solid waste (e.g., syringes and vials)
- Radioactive gases

Classification of Waste

Radioactive waste cannot be discarded due to associated hazards to public and environment. It is classified as solid, liquid, and gaseous. The solid waste is categorized based on radiation dose on the waste package whereas liquid and gaseous wastes are based on amount of radioactivity. Wastes are categorized as follows for different types of processing:

- Liquid radioactive waste: Aqueous and nonaqueous.
- Solid radioactive waste: Combustible or noncombustible.
- Nonradioactive waste: Nonhazardous, biohazardous, glass, and sharps.

Solid Waste

Solid waste is generated at different stages in many different forms which include tissue papers, plastics, animal carcasses, contaminated materials, discarded radiopharmaceutical containers, bandages, protective wears, worn out metallic parts and contaminated equipment or organ and tissues, spend radiation sources, etc. Solid radioactive waste also consists of general biomedical waste that includes protective clothing, plastic sheets and bags, gloves, masks, filters, overshoes, paper wipes, towels, metal and glass, hand tools, and discarded equipment.

Liquid Waste

Liquid waste includes contaminated water and effluent, waste arising from chemical processing and decontamination solutions, solvents, blood, or body fluids, discharged liquid radiopharmaceuticals, wound and oral discharges, urine chemotherapy agents, small quantities of contaminated oil and scintillation fluids. Waste that includes both radioactivity and a hazardous chemical is referred as mixed waste. A safe disposal is one in which no member of the public should get more than the effective dose limits. The liquid discharge systems should be within 10^{-4} to 10^{-5} Ci/mL.

Gaseous Waste

Gaseous waste management is very important to take care of airborne radioactive particles and gases. The main contaminants of importance in nuclear facility are radioiodine (^{131}I and ^{125}I), tritium, fission products, noble gases, etc. ^{133}Xe and ^{81m}Kr are used in diagnostic imaging for assessment of regional lung ventilation.

Once the effluent is released in the air, the operator has no control and cannot escape the consequences arising out of air pollution. The emission of activity to the atmosphere may give rise to three possible types of hazards: (i) a direct irradiation hazard from the radioactive clout itself or from material, which is deposited on the ground, (ii) inhalation hazard to people breathing the cloud, and (iii) an ingestion hazard from material that finds its way into food chains. The type of hazard depends on the circumstances of a particular emission. For most isotopes, the hazard is usually caused either by first or third types.

International Atomic Energy Agency Classification of Waste

International Atomic Energy Agency (IAEA, 2011) classified the radioactive waste into six categories based on activity and half-life of radionuclides. They are (1) exempt waste (EW), (2) very short-lived waste (VSLW), (3) very low-level waste (VLLW), (4) low level waste (LLW), (5) intermediate level waste (ILW), and (6) high-level waste (HLW).

Very short-lived waste is stored for decay over a limited period and disposed. It includes primary radionuclides of short half-life used in medicine and research. VLLW contains radioactive material that is not harmful to the people and environment. It arises from demolished material from rehabilitation or dismantling of nuclear and industrial site. LLW refers to radioactive waste of 4 GBq per ton of alpha activity or 12 GBq per ton beta-gamma activity which does not require shielding during handling and transport. It arises from hospitals and industry and can be disposed by near surface facilities. It accounts 90% of volume and 1% of radioactivity of all radioactive waste.

Intermediate level waste waste activity is higher than LLW, but the heat generated is <2 kW/m^3 which requires some shielding. It arises from resins, chemical sludges, metal fuel cladding, and contaminated materials from reactor decommissioning. It accounts 7% of volume and 4% of radioactivity of all radioactive wastes.

High-level waste has higher activity and decay heat generated is >2 kW/m^3. It increases its temperature and its surroundings. Hence, shielding and cooling is required. It arises from burning uranium fuel in the nuclear reactor and contains fission products and transuranic elements. It accounts 3% of volume and 95% of radioactivity of all radioactive waste. HLW has both short lived and long-lived isotopes and is divided into two types:

1. Used fuel that has been designated as waste.
2. Separated waste from reprocessing of used fuel.

TREATMENT TECHNIQUES FOR SOLID, LIQUID, AND GASEOUS EFFLUENTS

Type of radioactive waste in practice include: (i) solid waste, (ii) liquid waste, (iii) gaseous waste, (iv) spent sealed sources, (v) decommissioning waste, and (vi) nonradiological hazards. Biomedical waste can be treated by (i) mechanical process, (ii) thermal treatment: incineration, steam autoclaving, microwave processing, and dry heat, and (iii) chemical treatment. However, the treatment is specific to either solid, or liquid, or gaseous waste.

Solid Waste

Solid waste contains low levels of radioactivity. It is produced for the application and use of radioactive materials in normal operation and maintenance. Solid waste is typically classified as combustible/noncombustible, and compactible/noncompactible waste. In general, noncompactible solids are treated by decontamination, cutting, and crushing whereas compactible waste is treated with compaction and incineration. Treatment of solid waste makes it suitable for handling, storage, and disposal.

Though above-said methods are useful, but incineration is the most preferred method. If the activity of the ash is within the clearance levels, it can be disposed as landfill. Alternatively, the waste may be chemically neutralized and fixed in concrete for disposal. Other treatment methods are maceration/pulverization, mummification, dissolution in acids, bases, or hydrogen peroxide.

Decontamination

Decontamination is the removal of contamination from areas or surfaces of facilities or equipment by washing, heating, chemical or electrochemical action, mechanical cleaning. Its aim is to reduce the volume of equipment and materials requiring storage and disposal, to remove contamination, and to reduce dose levels. Decontamination process is divided into chemical, electrochemical, and mechanical.

Compaction

Compaction is done to reduce the waste volume and concentrates the radionuclides. Plastics, paper, absorbent material, and cloth are compatible with conventional compactors. Metal pipe, values, conduit, and wood are compatible with super compactors. It is done through presses with a compaction force of few tons -1,000 tons. Achievable volume reduction factors are 3 and 10.

Cutting

Metal and plastics of large volume requires cutting and sawing so that it is reduced in size to suit the packing containers. Cutting is done either in dry state in cells, by using conventional tools, remote controls or underwater.

Liquid Waste

Low and intermediate active liquid waste from different sources is normally collected and transported to the treatment facility by means of permanent pipelines systems. In some cases, where volume involved is small, specially designed tankers are used for collection and transportation. Liquid residue after injection to the patients can be disposed after a delay period. Iodine-131 in thyroid treatment should be provided with delay tanks as described later.

Waste with long-lived isotopes may be collected and transported to the centralized waste management facility. If the quantity is small, it is conditioned in concrete or gypsum at the producer's facility. If the waste contains a lot of organic compounds, they are made to absorb in silicate material and fixed in concrete for further disposal.

A wide variety of treatment methods are available to meet the specific requirement of decontamination. Decontamination factor is defined as a ratio of radioactivity

TABLE 15.1 Decontamination factors for various processes.

Processes	*Decontamination factor*
Chemical precipitation	10–100
Ion exchange	10–10,000
Reverse osmosis	10–50
Evaporation	1,000–10,000

content of untreated and treated waste. Liquid wastes are divided into aqueous and organic wastes. In aqueous liquid waste, (i) chemical precipitation, (ii) ion exchange, (iii) evaporation, and (iv) solid/liquid separation treatments are used. In organic liquid waste (i) distillation, (ii) incineration, (iii) wet oxidation, (iv) acid digestion, and (v) electrochemical oxidation techniques are employed. A few commonly employed processes and the corresponding decontamination factors are given in **Table 15.1**.

Chemical Precipitation

Chemical precipitation is most common which is greatly versatile and economical. Radionuclides can be removed by precipitation, co-precipitation with a carrier or sorption on to particulates present in the waste. It can treat large volumes of liquid effluents containing relatively low concentrations of inactive salts. In some cases, oxidation of organic containments, decomposition of complexed species, pH adjustment, and change of valency state or adjustment of ionic species are applied as pretreatment before precipitation.

Ion Exchange

This is the technique used for removal of specific radionuclides from the bulk of wastes. An ion exchange or sorption method involves replacement of cations or anions between an insoluble solid matrix containing ionizable polar groups and a liquid solution. If the ionic group is negative, cations are exchanged, and if positive anions are exchanged. This process is selective, stoichiometric, and reversible.

Materials used for ion exchange are: (i) natural ion exchangers (clays, zeolites, cellulose, charcoals, and collagen), (ii) synthetic materials (zeolites, hydrous oxide gels of metals or organic resins, etc.). This process can be operated in batch or continuous mode. If the waste contains high concentrations of salts, suspended solids, and organic contaminants, it must be pretreated before ion-exchange process. It has wide application to remove radionuclides from liquid waste produced in nuclear fuel cycle operations, radioisotope production and research facilities. It is effective in converting large volume of radioactive liquid in small volume.

Evaporation

It is used for concentrating the liquid waste or removing salts, heavy metals, and hazardous materials from waste effluent, reducing large volume of liquid waste with high factor of decontaminations. Steam and natural evaporation methods are employed, depending upon the activity, volumes involved, and climatic conditions. This method is suitable for low, intermediate, and high-level effluents including treatment of small volumes of highly active effluents. Its limitations are unsuitable for waste effluents containing large concentration of inactive salts, and expensive. Involvement of large energy and presence of organic compound may cause explosions.

Reverse Osmosis

Reverse osmosis (RO) is the technique used for liquid radioactive waste. It will remove 99% of the radionuclides along with many other contaminants. It uses high pressure pumps to increase the pressure on the salt/waste side of the RO and the force of the liquid across the semi-permeable RO membrane. Likewise, it is a modern solution to liquid waste management. Special membranes remove the radioactive waste without chemicals, resins, or ion exchange.

Gaseous Waste

Gaseous waste is a minor concern in hospitals. ^{133}Xe and ^{81}Kr are noble gases, they are difficult to treat and are often released to the atmosphere through an exhaust system. It is essential to ensure that there is no possibility of re-entry of the released gases back into the building through open windows or ventilation system. Exhalation of ^{133}Xe during the diagnostic test is absorbed by the charcoal filter. Volatile radionuclides in fume hood release vapours which are usually trapped on a charcoal or HEPA filter. The filters need replacement, and stored for decay, before passed on to the incinerator for final disposal.

Therefore, the airborne activity in the working area should be kept within limits **(Table 15.2)**. The removal of particulate and gaseous contaminants from gaseous effluents is a complex and expensive one. It is advisable to design the plant and buildings so that the volume to be treated is as small as possible. This may be achieved by providing separate ducking systems for radioactive and nonradioactive effluents and filtration system for the radioactive fraction alone. In addition, negative pressure compared to atmosphere is maintained in the working areas to restrict the release of activity to the environment. The ventilation exhaust system is provided with suitable devices to contain airborne radionuclides. The exhaust gases are treated for removal of and retention of particulate activity by using high efficiency particulate air (HEPA) filters along with other cleaning techniques.

TABLE 15.2 **Airborne, water, and sewer concentrations that would result annual dose limits for public if continuously inhaled or ingested.**

Radionuclide	*Environmental concentrations (μCi/mL)*		*Sewage concentration (μCi/mL)*
	Air	*Water*	
^{18}F	1×10^{-7}	7×10^{-4}	7×10^{-3}
^{99m}Tc	2×10^{-7}	1×10^{-3}	1×10^{-2}
^{131}I	2×10^{-10}	1×10^{-6}	1×10^{-5}
^{14}C	3×10^{-9}	3×10^{-5}	3×10^{-4}
^{133}Xe	5×10^{-7}	—	—

Courtesy: Cherry SR et al, 2012.

Spent Sealed Sources

Sealed sources after their useful clinical life are referred as spent sealed sources. Sealed sources become surplus if it has sufficiently decayed, leaky, outdated, or clinical use is discontinued. These sources are in capsule form with high degree of containment and the activity ranges from few MBq to TMq. The sources are mostly gamma emitters and beta-calibration sources. It can be categorised as follows:

- Sources with half-life <100 days with high activity, e.g., ^{192}Ir
- Sources of low activity used for calibration
- Sources with a potential emanation and contamination hazard
- Sources with half-life >100 days, with low or high activity

These sources should be collected, segregated, and stored with physical protection. Small-sealed sources <4 MBq can be disposed, whereas >4 MBq activity is subjected to treatment and conditioning and disposed as low and intermediate waste. Sealed radioactive sources of long half-life are transferred to another licensed user or returned to the original manufacturer. Returning the source to the manufacturer will permit recycling of the source which is a part of original purchase agreement contract. If the manufacturer is not available, it can be returned to different vendor or centralized waste management facility (CWMF) of the country.

Decommissioning Waste

Linear accelerators and telecobalt machines are decommissioned after their clinical use. Activation of collimator-like accessories by neutron energy >10 MeV is a challenge. Depleted uranium has been used as shielding material which should be considered as radioactive waste during decommissioning. Activation product levels up to 1 kBq/g for cobalt and 26 kBq/g for wolfram have been measured at the end of the useful life of a 20 MeV accelerator after dismantling. However, the activation of concrete in the biological shield or base of a linear accelerator used for medical purposes is very low.

Cyclotrons pose more activation and waste during decommissioning than linear accelerators. Metal machine parts and infrastructures of beam lines and collimators are considered as radioactive waste during decommissioning. Activation in concrete has been measured up to 70 cm depth. The iron reinforcement bars in concrete may be activated with ^{60}Co to >10 kBq/kg. Hence, the use of iron and scrap metals in concrete shielding around cyclotrons is not preferred. Since cyclotron causes significant volume of metal and concreate wastes, usually decommissioning is delayed for decay until the accepted level arises.

Non-radiological Hazards

Biomedical waste creates non-radiological hazards like: (i) physical hazard, (ii) chemical hazard, (iii) biological/infectious hazard, and (iv) flammable/explosive hazards. Physical hazard arises from cuts and puncture injuries from needles, broken glass, scalpel blades or blood lancets (sharps). Chemical reactions or injuries arise from the presence of acids, alkalis, oxidizers or oxidizable organic matter. It involves liquid or vapors containing dangerous chemicals and mixing of incompatible wastes. Waste contaminated with human blood, other body fluids, or any potentially infectious material is referred as biohazardous. In such case universal precaution is adopted which includes hand washing, wearing of disposable gloves, use of protective gowns and use of face masks, protective eye glass, etc.

Flammable/explosive hazard arises when low flash point organic scintillant (<21°C) is stored. Radioactive store has spark-resistant lighting so that these wastes are securely stored in metal bins/cabinets. It should also adequate ventilation to let out fumes and located in the vicinity of other flammable hazards or highly combustible wastes.

PERMISSIBLE LIMITS FOR DISPOSAL

Authorized Limit

The activity limits for discharges or disposal of radioactive wastes may be derived from the dose constraint or it can be evolved from the design and/or operating experience of facilities or activities. In either of the cases, it can be correlated to the dose per unit release of a radionuclide for a particular site based on the following relation:

$$AL_i = \frac{AD_i}{CD_i}$$

where, AL_i is the authorized limit (Bq/y), AD_i is the assigned dose constraint for a particular radionuclide (μSv/y), and CD_i is the computed dose per unit release for that radionuclide for the site (μSv/Bq). There are regulatory activity limits for discharge of patients from hospital, administered with beta-emitting radionuclides **(Table 15.3)**.

Estimation of Exempt Activity for Discharge or Disposal

The exemption of certain category of the facilities and activities from waste discharge or disposal authorization requirements are based on the effective dose criteria of 10 μSv/y. The maximum exempt activity to be discharged or disposed from a facility can be evolved from the following relation. In case of more than one radionuclide, the rule of mixture should be followed so that the sum of the ratio of the total activity to the prescribed limit should be ≤1:

$$\sum\left(\frac{A_1}{A_i}\right) \leq 1$$

TABLE 15.3 **Activity limits for discharge of patients administered with beta emitting radionuclides from hospital.**

Radio-isotope	*Activity (MBq)*
Y-90	4,000
Sm-153	4,000
In-111	400
Sr-89	300
P-32	1,200
Re-188	4,000

Courtesy: AERB safety code, 2011.

where, A_1 is the actual activity (Bq/y) discharge of individual radionuclide, and A_i is the prescribed discharge limit (Bq/y) for individual radionuclide. However, in case of chemically toxic radionuclides, the concentration level prescribed by the relevant regulatory authority should be acceptable.

SAMPLING TECHNIQUES FOR AIR, WATER, AND SOLID: GEOLOGICAL, HYDROLOGICAL, METEOROLOGICAL AND ECOLOGICAL CONSIDERATIONS FOR WASTE DISPOSAL

Air sampling is of airborne radioactive material is done to evaluate the dose in each location or site. The sampling should be representative of actual working conditions. The objective of air sampling is:

- Evaluate exposures to the public and workers
- To control airborne concentration and to document
- Warn workers of unexpected releases
- Assist in materials balancing
- As part of a respiratory protection program
- Satisfy regulatory and license requirement
- Obtain data for use in potential litigation

Airborne radioactive material is in the form of (i) particulates, and (ii) gases and vapors. Particulate is a collective term that describes airborne solids and liquid droplets. They are categorized as:

- Aerosol: Refers to particulate that is stable or quasi stable suspension in air.
- Dusts: Larger than 1 micron (μm), disintegration of material due to grinding
- Fumes: 0.1–1 μm, particulate produced by chemical reactions like oxidation
- Smoke: 0.5 μm, small particle due to incomplete combustion
- Mist and fogs: Liquid droplets produced by condensation, 5–40 μm referred as fog, and particulate size of >40 μm is called mist.

Gases are defined as material exists in the gaseous state under normal conditions. Vapor is the gaseous phase of the substance that exists as liquid or solid at room temperature.

Air sample is collected over finite period and sent to laboratory for analysis, whereas monitoring refers to real-time analysis. Sampling systems that perform real-time analysis of airborne radioactive material is referred as *continuous air monitors (CAM)*. It will alert the workers if any unexpected release of radioactive material.

The concentration of airborne radioactive material may be determined for a specific radionuclide and as a gross alpha or beta concentration. Alternatively, representative samples are collected. In this, sample whose characteristics are identical to the atmosphere being analyzed. Characteristics of airborne material that affects dose are: (i) concentration, (ii) particle size, and (iii) clearance class. Air sampling is performed in three locations, namely (1) workplace, (2) stack (effluents), (3) sampling for iodine and (4) environment.

Workplace

Fixed air samplers (FAS) are used where the concentration in the location has the potential to frequently become excessive, e.g., glove boxes. Portable samples are used to obtain short-term samples in areas that do not require continuous sampling, areas where radioactive material is occasionally used. Sampling near the room air exhaust grill will give representative sampling so that average room calculation is calculated.

Breathing zone (BZ) samples are collected to calculate the concentration in air inhaled by the worker. It is usually higher than the room concentration value since the worker is close to the source. Meters used for the purpose are called *personnel air monitors (PAM)* which has filter holder attached to the collar with a pump and a flow meter attached to a belt. BZ meters are rarely used due to unacceptance of the worker, and mostly FAS is used to calculate concentration at the worker area. CAMs are used to alert the worker and not used to calculate the average concentration.

Stack/Effluent

Particle sampling is done in the stack both upstream and downstream of the cleaning equipment/filter. It is done continuously on daily or weekly basis. It is necessary to insert a baffle in the duct of stack to ensure distribution of the dust. A baffle which obstructs half of cross-sectional area of the stack, situated three diameter's upstream of the sampling point is recommended. Since the particle size distribution in the sample is same as that in the stack, the sampling is done *iso-kinetically*, that is the linear gas velocity in the entrance of the sampling device should be the same as the stack gas velocity at that point of sampling.

In subisokinetic sampling, the velocity entering the nozzle is lower which overestimates the activity associated with particulate, mostly in larger particulate. In superisokinetic sampling, the velocity entering the nozzle is faster than isokinetic, so that it underestimates the activity associated with particulate, mostly in larger particulate. Of late, probes with single-point extraction or multi-point extraction system are being used. They requires flat velocity profile at the sampling point and does not require isokinetic sampling.

The sampling device selected depends on the information required. If it is desired to determine the percentage of particulate activity which passes the gas-cleaning equipment, it will be sufficient to sample isokinetically through a suitable sampling nozzle on to a high-efficiency filter paper, which can then be counted for betas. On the other hand, information on the particle size of the dust which penetrates the gas-cleaning equipment is required, a high-efficiency cyclone followed by a fine-glass fiber filter is used.

Sampling for Iodine

Iodine-131 and iodine-125 are commonly used in nuclear medicine and have greater impact on the environment. Both are highly volatile Iodine hence, control of iodine contamination in air and around patients treated with iodine is much critical. Measurements can be done as aerosol measurements methods or scintillation counting methods and the later method is more specific.

Nowadays advance system like continuous monitoring system (CMS) is used for airborne concentration of radioiodine. Its filtration mechanism captures all forms of radioiodine and has automatic background compensation. It is provided with bremsstrahlung shield and temperature stabilization. Algorithm helps fast response to rising concentration. It can be installed at workplace, stacks, cells, and glove boxes.

Environment

Airborne concentration in the environment is low and requires long-sampling time and high-flow rate. There are two approaches, namely (i) gross alpha and or beta analysis after sampling for 1 week at 1–2 cubic feet meter (cfm) through a 47-mm filter, and (ii) nuclide specific analysis after sampling for 1 week at 40 cfm through an 8 × 10 inch filter. Problem may arise due to collection of large quantities of dust and other nonradioactive particulates, selection of sampling locations, and maintenance of equipment at remote sites.

Sampling Equipment

Basic sampling system consists of filter, flow meter, elapsed timer, and a pump. There are three types of filters, namely (i) membrane, (ii) glass fiber, and (iii) cellulose. Flow-rate meter is used to measure the volumetric flow rate of the sampler in cubic feet (cf) or liters (L) and milliliter (mL). Most common is the rotameter, dry gas meter, and mass flow meter. Elapsed timer is used in systems operating unattended for long periods. In resettable timer, the reading is set back to zero at the beginning of each sampling period. There are two types of pumps, namely (i) positive displacement pump, and (ii) centrifugal blower/fan. For low-volume sampling, <2 cfm positive displacement pump is used whereas centrifugal blower/fan is used where volume > 5 cubic feet per minute (cfm).

Release of Effluents from Chimney Stacks

Release of effluents has three effects, namely (1) geological effects, (2) topographical, and (3) meteorological parameters.

Geological Effects

Dilution of diffusion of radioactive gas or any other contaminant depends upon wind and temperature conditions. Since hills and mountains superimpose variations on the general wind and temperature conditions at a place, these must be considered before siting an installation. The variation of vertical temperature gradients is dependent on the location of the site, air mass and the time of the day. Again, this will depend upon the continent, i.e., whether it is in the temperature zone or the tropics.

Topographical Effects

The effects of terrain within a radius of 15–100 km from the source of release of the dilution and dispersion must be studied by actual field work, while some qualitative predictions can be made where topography is uniform, say a flat plain. It will be necessary to carry out a program of measurements in the case of irregular topography.

Meteorological Parameters

The location and the terrain are the important factors that decide the dilution efficiency of the atmosphere. In practice, space and time gradients of horizontal wind velocities and temperature are measured. At high wind velocities, dispersion of gas in the atmosphere gets enhanced, and the effect of obstructions, both natural such as hills and mountains and men-made buildings and other chimneys are also increased.

This will result not only in vertical motions of the air, but also in an increased lateral movement due to turbulent eddies.

In addition to the effect of mechanical turbulence caused by solely by wind speeds, thermal turbulence, as represented by the vertical temperature gradient, has at least an equal influence on the dispersed material in the air. The relationship of density and buoyancy of a gas can be interpreted in terms of the vertical temperature gradient, and the potential vertical motions of the air estimated.

The rate of decrease in the value of any meteorological element with elevation is usually referred to as *lapse rate*. With a normal lapse, the rate at which the temperature decreases with height is specified as 0.6°C/100 m. If the lapse rate is such that it shows no change of temperature with height is called an *inversion*. Of particular interest is the state which permits a volume of air to be displaced from one level to another so that the air always has the same density as the environment. Since the change of state of a gas is said to be adiabatic if it takes place without heat being supplied or withdrawn, the lapse rate referred to is known as the dry adiabatic lapse rate.

Stack Discharge

The main consideration in the release of radioactivity from the stacks is the concentration of the radioactivity at ground level. It depends upon the geographical and meteorological conditions that exist and on the method of release of the gas. As the distance from the stack increases, the ground level concentration starts from zero at the foot of the stack rises to a well-defined maximum value and then decreases slowly. The maximum concentration of the effluent at the ground level varies inversely as the square of the height of the orifice above the ground. Stack height is the distance from the ground level elevation at the base of the stack to the crown of the stack.

Plume refers to the path and extent of the gaseous effluents released in the atmosphere. From the appearance of effluent plums, it is found that the diffusion is largely regulated by vertical gradient of air density in the neighborhood of the stack. Plume behavior refers to dispersal pattern of gaseous pollutants in atmosphere depending upon wind conditions, atmospheric stability, and vertical temperature profile. There are seven types of plume behavior, namely (i) conning plume, (ii) fanning plume, (iii) looping plume, (iv) neutral plume, (v) lofting plume, (vi) fumigating plume, and (vii) trapping plume.

DECONTAMINATION PROCEDURES

Decontamination is the process of removal of radioactive contamination from skin or from surfaces such as wall or floor of working areas. Radioactive contamination may exist in loose or relatively fixed form due to physical and chemical factors. Whenever possible, contamination should be cleaned up as soon as it occurs which will prevent further spread.

Skin and Surface Contamination

In decontaminating the skin, it would be ideal to remove the entire contamination, but may not be possible always. Necessary measures that are taken in certain cases could result in skin damage, the radioactive material could enter the body and leads to internal hazards. In such cases, it should be satisfactory to reduce the levels of contamination to within permissible limits. Similar methodology may be used in the decontamination of surface (walls, floors, and table-tops), and for contaminated equipment. However, there may be situations in which experimental requirements render it essential that the decontamination be absolute. On the other hand, in dealing with contamination of certain articles and types of equipment, it might be economical to store the contaminated object temporarily, with a view of letting the activity die down naturally to within permissible level, or to dispose of it as waste.

The above considerations imply the setting up of maximum permissible levels of contamination for the skin and for surfaces in controlled and uncontrolled areas. The fundamental principles which are applicable to all decontamination procedure are:

- Wet decontamination method should always be used in preference to dry.
- Mild decontamination method should be tried before resorting to treatment which can damage the surfaces involved.
- Precautions must always be taken to prevent further spread of contamination during decontamination operations.
- Where possible, contamination involving short-lived activities should be isolated and segregated to allow natural decay to take its course.

Decontamination of Personnel

Once a radioisotope has become lodged in the body, very little can be done to increase the rate of elimination. This means that every effort must be made to prevent contamination entering the body. It is vital that all personnel should obey inhouse rules and always wear correct protective clothing. Even so, contamination incidents are bound to occur and so a knowledge of the current treatment is vital.

The first action when dealing with a contaminated person is to ascertain whether or not he is injured. If he has a serious injury, then he must be given first-aid treatment as quickly as possible. Following any necessary medical treatment, the next action is aimed at removing the contamination. Before decontamination can be started, a careful survey must be carried out over the entire body with a suitable contamination monitor to determine the location of contamination. In the case of partial contamination, it is only necessary to decontaminate the affected areas.

Soap and water are the first requirement for removing contamination from hands and other exposed areas of skin. The soap chosen should be mild so that it will not produce skin damage after frequent use.

For hands, soft-bristle nail brush should be used in conjunction with soap and water over the entire surface of the hands and the wrists. Particular attention should be given to the nails, to the ridges between the fingers, and to the edges of the hand. Frequent rinsing is essential during the entire operation.

For the face, copious amounts of water and soap should be used, the hands alone being used to create the lather. Isolated areas of high contamination should be carefully scrubbed. All personnel should be instructed to keep the eyes and mouth closed during treatment and to rinse the face frequently with copious amounts of water. While using towels or other materials suitable for drying, rubbing should be avoided. All cases of face contamination should be referred to the medical officer.

Contamination of hair should be washed several times with an efficient shampoo and copious amounts of water should be used for rinsing. The latter is particularly important to ensure that contamination removed from the hair does not remain in the ears or on the face.

In the event of contamination which persists even after the above-mentioned procedure has been followed a number of times, the individual concerned should be referred to the medical department where more effective decontamination can be carried out under medical supervision. It is essential that skin decontamination should not be taken to the point of damaging the skin.

In case of contaminated small open wounds, cuts, punctures, etc., the wound should be immediately washed, bleeding should be encouraged if necessary, and the medical officer should be consulted.

Whenever internal contamination occurs, it becomes a medical problem, parallel in some ways to the absorption of chemical toxins. All corrective measures should be carried out under medical supervision.

When contamination has been swallowed, substances designed to prevent or reduce absorption from the gastrointestinal tract, e.g., antacids or ion exchange resins, may be administered promptly after the intake. If radionuclides of high toxicity like *plutonium (Pu)* is absorbed through wound or inhaled as soluble form, certain chemical called *chelating agents* may be administered to promote excretion.

Unfortunately, these substances tend to be chemically toxic themselves. The absorption of certain radioisotopes can be blocked by prior ingestion of substantial amounts of a stable isotope of the same element. For example, the uptake of radioiodine to the thyroid can be greatly reduced by previous ingestion of a 200 mg tablet of *potassium iodate*. This has an important application in the event of a reactor accident.

Decontamination of Working Areas

A preliminary contamination survey will indicate those areas which require decontamination, and such areas should be clearly marked. The decontamination measures should be restricted to those areas and every endeavor should be made to prevent the spread of contamination. The decontamination measures depend on nature of the contamination, either (1) loose contamination or (2) reactively fixed contamination.

Removal of Loose Contamination

Special decontamination apparatus, such as vacuum cleaners fitted with special filters, may be used to remove loose contamination. No attempt should be made to brush or dust it off, if the floor is with slight contamination, a wet medium such as *dampened sawdust* sprinkled over the contaminated area before brushing is acceptable. For all other surfaces, wet methods such as webbing are essential. The removal of contamination should be done with minimum of rubbing and the swabs should be frequently discarded as radioactive waste. Decontamination solutions which contain complexing agents are particularly useful in such cases.

Where there is copious loose contamination, a suitable *strippable lacquer* may be carefully applied to the contaminated surfaces. This lacquer is allowed to dry and in so doing will take up the contamination. Afterward, the strippable lacquer can be removed together with the contamination. During this operation, care should be taken in using the spraying device to avoid disturbing the loose contamination and thus giving rise to an airborne hazard. As a precaution, personnel should be in fully protective clothing. After shipping, the affected areas should be washed as described above.

Removal of Relatively Fixed Contamination

In this case, only wet methods should be used. The first wash should be with suitable detergent solution which will remove loose contamination and all grease-held material. Only light rubbing should be used at this stage and the swabs should be discarded frequently as radioactive waste. Contamination remaining after this treatment should be removed by further washing with suitable decontaminating solutions. The decontaminating solutions to remain in contact with the contaminated surfaces as long as possible so that chemical reaction at the surface may assist the decontamination.

Contamination remaining after several attempts at removal with the above treatment will normally be confined to small areas (unless a major spill has occurred) and further proprietary abrasive cleaners are useful for general application in this spotting treatment. *Metal polish* can be used to advantage on metal surfaces, *abrasive creams* containing a complexing agent, may be rubbed into the affected areas, and left in contact for a period before being washed off. More stringent treatment would involve the use of *steel wool* or a similar *scouring agent.*

If contamination persists, it will be necessary to remove the surface on which the contamination is fixed, unless it is a place. In the latter case, precautions should be taken to seal in the contamination with concrete, paint, or other appropriate material. Such sealed in contamination must be recorded so that in any further modifications to the building, suitable precautions can be taken against dispersing the contamination and creating a hazard.

Decontamination of Equipment

It is difficult to summarize all decontamination process of individual equipment used in radiation work. However, such equipment may be classified based on the material of which they are made, and the decontamination:

- Removal of contamination without damage to the surface below.
- Removal of the surface of the equipment together with the adhering contamination.

In all cases, the first method should be used initially, and only if several attempts fail should the second method be tried, since damaged surfaces may be unsuitable for re-use because of their tendency to collect contamination easily.

Decontamination of equipment should be carried out as soon as possible after its removal from the active area. Contamination left in situ over periods of time becomes fixed and becomes increasingly difficult to remove.

All decontamination should be carried out using routine wet methods, the only difference is the reagents used for various materials. The routine procedure to be followed is the same for all equipment.

- Wash in detergent solution at raised temperature. This will remove all loose and grease-held contamination. It will be followed by swabbing and light scrubbing with the same solution.
- Decontaminated equipment should be washed in clean water and dried before monitoring.

- Further scrubbing and steeping technique may be used, where contamination remains after the above treatment. In the latter, the equipment is placed in solutions of suitable decontaminating reagents, preferably at raised temperatures, and is left there for suitable periods of time. Inclusion of complexing agents in the decontaminating solution is recommended to prevent redeposition of the contamination.
- Equipment is washed in clean water on removal from the decontamination solution and is then dried before being monitored.
- Further methods will depend upon the extent and nature of residual contamination when contamination remains after the above treatment. If the contamination is present in spots, a treatment known as *spotting* may be carried out using abrasive or strong acids on the small areas involved. Where acid is used, care should be taken to ensure that the surface of the equipment is not unduly etched.

  If the contamination is general, it may be possible to apply abrasive over the whole surface, but if this fails, seepage in acid solution will be necessary. Precautions should be taken to prevent the acids from damaging the surface of the equipment more than is necessary to remove the contamination. Special apparatus in the form of *fume hoods or gloves boxes* will be necessary for the acid treatment, because of noxious fumes.
- Equipment should be well washed and dried before monitoring.

Decontamination of Protective Clothing

Routine protective clothing should be cleaned regularly to avoid the build-up and fixation of contamination. For similar reasons, the clothing should not be left in storage for long periods before cleaning. Such storage results in the contamination being fixed and renders decontamination increasingly difficult. Another measure taken in such clothing to avoid build-up and fixation of contamination is to provide no pockets or belts and to minimize folds.

White Coats and Coveralls

In small establishments, it will not usually be necessary to segregate this clothing, before washing, according to the different contaminants and different levels of contamination. However, in larger establishments where a variety of radioactive material is used, it is often necessary to segregate the clothing to prevent cross contamination during the cleaning process.

Contaminated clothing should be handled as little as possible since it can give rise to airborne contamination. Process used in cleaning this type of clothing is not dissimilar to the processes adopted in conventional laundries. It is useful to remember that the more stringent washing solutions used necessitate the use of suitably resistant metals in the construction of washing machine.

The actual routine of washing will depend on experience, but as a guide it is usual to give clothing two full washes (of 10 minutes each) with a rinse (of 5 minutes) in clear water after each wash.

The reagents or soaps used will also depend upon experience, but a washing solution consisting of *unbuild detergents, sodium metasilicate, sodium acid phosphate, and citric acid* has given good results with this type of clothing. Clothing should be dried thoroughly before being monitored.

Rubber Gloves

It is essential that the personnel wearing these gloves, and particularly the heavy rubber gloves, should wash them on completion of their work. Bulk collection of contaminated gloves is most unsatisfactory, since there is no efficient way in which they may be washed in large numbers without transferring contamination to the inside.

Good-quality soap or detergents and scrubbing brushes should be provided at appropriate places where personnel may wash their gloves. Gloves should be well scrubbed and rinsed and then dried with paper towels or preferably with small pieces (say 2 × 1 ft) or towelling, which have proved economical and more satisfactory than paper towels. The small towels should be used once only and then placed in a suitable collecting bin.

Respirator and Dust Masks

The only satisfactory way in which these items may be cleaned is by individual swabbing with suitable detergents. Detergent used should be mild one and unlikely to cause skin complaints if it comes in contact with individual's face.

Small cloth or cotton swabs should be used all over and inside the face-pieces. These swabs should be changed frequently. Care should be taken to clean the outside first and then the inside using clean swabs. The face-pieces should be well swabbed with clean water, following the detergent treatment, and then dried.

Impressive Protective Clothing

On completion of an operation involving the use of this kind of clothing and where extra contamination is expected, it is essential that the operator, still wearing the suit should pass through some form of washing. This may consist of an installed shower or simply of a rinse with buckets of water. There is obviously a need to choose the correct position for this so as to prevent dispersal of contamination, and it should be followed by washing with detergent and soap solution, assisted by swabs and soft bristled brushes. Operations in these suits usually involve at least two individuals and it is a convenient practice for them to wash each other. Afterward, the suits should be rinsed in clean water and quickly dried.

When dry, the suit is removed and monitored. Any residual contaminating can be treated separately with mild abrasive pastes or similar material.

Suitable detergents should be used for washing these suits and it is also advantageous to use solutions containing weak *citric acid* and completing agents such as *ethylene-diamine-tetra-acetic acid (EDTA)*.

Footwear

Rubber-soled shoes may require decontamination from time to time. The soles should be scrubbed with detergent and complexing solutions, and for resistant contamination it may be necessary to remove the surface of the rubber by the application of *acetone or by mechanical buffing*. If mechanical buffing is used, it will be necessary to provide for local air extraction on the machine. The upper part of the shoes, if kept properly waxed, can be easily decontaminated.

Rubber boots should be cleaned after each operation. Scrubbing in detergent and complexing solutions should be followed using abrasive pastes necessary. Resistant contamination will necessitate the removal of the rubber surface by *acetone or mechanical buffing.* Precautions should be taken to prevent contaminated liquids from entering the boots.

MANAGEMENT OF RADIOACTIVE WASTE IN MEDICAL, INDUSTRIAL, AGRICULTURE, AND RESEARCH FACILITIES

Sealed and unsealed radionuclides, used in medicine, industry, agriculture, research, and other applications could result in generation of significant quantities of solid and liquid wastes and occasionally gaseous wastes. Much of the solid waste consists of contaminated items, such as paper, plastics, glassware, equipment, animal carcasses, excreta, and other biological waste. Some of the solid wastes may have considerable activity and small volumes as in the case of spent sealed sources.

Liquid radioactive wastes comprise aqueous and organic streams, such as patient's urine (primarily in thyroid cancer therapy) and effluents from decontamination processes. In many applications of radionuclides, the radioactive waste generated may comprise short-lived radionuclides, which may be managed by providing storage for decay.

Gaseous waste may be generated from the production and radiolabeling of chemical compounds and organisms, also during the production of radionuclides and from the treatment of solid and liquid waste.

However, in applications which involve long-lived radionuclides, an appropriate waste management program should be in place prior to the start of the work with radionuclides.

Principles and Philosophy of Radioactive Waste Management

Applications of these four principles as given below will ensure adequate safety in the management of radioactive waste.

Principle 1: Protection of human health and environment
Radioactive waste shall be managed in such a way as to provide an acceptable level of protection for human health and the environment.

Principle 2: Concern for future generations
Radioactive waste shall be managed in such a way that it will not impose undue burden on future generations and its predicted impact on the health of future generations, will not be greater than relevant levels of impact that are acceptable today.

Principle 3: Establishing legal framework
Radioactive waste shall be managed within an appropriate legal framework including clear allocation of responsibilities and provision for independent regulatory functions.

Principle 4: Waste minimization, management interdependency, and safety of facilities
Generation of radioactive waste shall be kept to the minimum practicable. Interdependency among all steps in radioactive waste generation and management shall be considered. The safety of facilities for radioactive waste management shall be assured during their lifetime.

DISPOSAL OF RADIOACTIVE WASTES

To achieve the above principle and philosophy of radioactive waste management, the methods adopted in practice includes (i) minimize the generation of radioactive waste, (ii) recycling and reuse the waste material, and (iii) minimize the exposure to operation staff and public. The basic approaches used in the management of radioactive wastes involve two stages, namely (i) collection and (ii) disposal. The waste must be identified and segregated within the area of work. Foot-operated collection bin, polythene bags, and polythene carboys (for liquid waste) are used for such collection. Each package is monitored and labeled for activity and radiation level and date, before deciding the nature of disposal. If two isotopes of different half-life are involved, separate waste collection bags and bins required, e.g., ^{99m}Tc and ^{131}I. In such case, isotope name, activity level, and date are labeled on the bag. General methods of radioactive waste disposal are as follows:

- Dilute and disperse
- Delay and decay
- Concentrate and contain
- Incineration
- Recycle and reuse

The delay and decay are suitable only for short half-life isotopes. For example, ^{131}I (HL-8 days) in small volumes may be retained till the activity levels come down to the desired values, suitable for release into the environment. Other methods are generally adopted in the management of all radioactive wastes.

General Methods of Disposal

Dilute and Disperse

Dilute and disperse refers to discharging low-level liquid radioactive effluent to the environment in a such a way that environmental conditions and processes ensure the concentrations of the radionuclides are reduced to such levels that the radiological impact of the related material is acceptable. Sometimes the principle of delay and decay is combined with dilute and disperse.

The principle of dilution and dispersion assumes that the environment has a finite capacity for dilution of radionuclides to an innocuous level. The application of this principle requires an understanding of the behavior of radioactive materials in the environment and of the ways in which the released radionuclides, particularly those that are critical, may lead later to the exposure of man. It is especially important to take into consideration environmental processes which may cause re-concentration of radionuclides.

Delay and Decay

Delay and decay refers to storing low-level liquid radioactive waste until the desired reduction in activity has occurred through radioactive decay, followed by discharging it into the sewage system without further dilution requirement.

It assumes that radionuclides lose their radioactivity through decay, and this fact may be utilized in the treatment not only of intermediate and high level solid, liquid, and gaseous wastes but in some cases also in that of low-level wastes. The aim is to ease problems in subsequent handling or to lessen risks of releases to the environment, taking advantage of the decay of some radionuclides—particularly those having short half-lives—with the passage of time. The principle is especially useful for those installations where a substantial reduction in the activity level of a waste stream can be achieved by delaying discharge of effluents for a few days.

Concentrate and Contain

Concentrate and contain principle refers to reduction of the volume and confinement of the radionuclide by means of a conditioning process to prevent dispersion in the environment. The principle of concentration and containment derives from the concept that majority of the radioactivity generated in nuclear programs must be kept in isolation from the human environment. Since some radionuclides take a long time to decay to innocuous level, some wastes must be contained for extended period.

Some radioactivity may have high activity level with long half-life period. Then delay and decay method is not suitable since it requires long-storage period. Therefore, radioactive waste is collected in designed and labeled containers and buried in exclusive burial sites, duly approved by the competent authority. Hospital may not come across such waste disposal.

Incineration

Incineration is used for insoluble waste like liquid scintillation system. It reduces the waste volume and reduces to small and concentrated volume so that it can be disposed further. Incineration will substantially reduce the volume of wastes, but the total radioactive content will not be reduced.

Incinerator releases part of the activity in the atmosphere and required to operate in controlled condition in segregated place. Depending upon the physical and chemical characteristics of the compound involved, the activity may be deposited in the gaseous effluents, inside surface of the incinerator and in the ash. The activity associated with the incinerated waste must be restricted to the public exposure limits. Ashes so collected are disposed as solid waste by burial. However, incineration and burial methods are rarely used due to environmental concern and public pressure.

This method is suitable in reducing the volume of the waste with little escape of activity to the environment. The incinerators are specially designed to remove the radioactivity from combustion gases using scrubbers and filters and to ensure that the radioactive ash is contained so that no airborne hazard is caused.

Disposal of Radioactive Solid Waste

Solid waste material is segregated into (i) compressible and combustible, and (ii) noncompressible and noncombustible waste. Waste material is concentrated and disposed by the following methods:

- Incineration
- Burial of solid waste in the ground
  - Unprotected material
  - Protected material
- Storage of protected material
- Sea dumping

Low-activity solid waste may be disposed as ordinary hospital waste if the activity does not exceed 50 kBq (1.35 μCi) or the overall package concentration will not exceed 5 MBq/m^3 (135 μCi/m^3). It may include vials, syringes, cotton swabs, tissue papers, etc. Occasional release up to 100 μCi in ordinary dustbin is allowed. Sealed sources >10 μCi should not be disposed, and they must be kept for decay. Higher activities can be buried or burnt and short-lived activity up to 1 mCi can be burnt.

Burial of Solid Waste

Any site chosen for such burial operations should be examined carefully about its geologic and hydrologic properties and an assessment should be made of the possible contamination of water supplies and of ecological systems that might lead to human exposures. The depth chosen for burial must be sufficient to prevent leakage of any harmful level of radioactivity into usable surface water or ground waters. The whole of the burial area and its immediate vicinity should be isolated suitably and fenced to prevent use of the area. A central record should be maintained of all burials to assure that the area is kept under continuing surveillance. Under such conditions some leaching of the radioactivity into the ground water can take place, and this may therefore be considered under the principle of dilute and disperse to a small extent.

Unprotected Material

The following method is suitable for low-level radioactive waste. The burial must be carefully controlled to avoid spread of contamination to surface ground waters. The choice of burial site is very important, and it should be suitably cordoned off. The solid type is also important since fixation on a good exchange material (e.g., montmorillonite) will reduce the movement of activity in the ground. In this method, one should ensure that the radioactivity is in the form of completely insoluble material. The size of the pits is 120 × 120 cm and depth of the pit should be such that there should be 120 cm of earth above. The amount in the pit should be restricted and the minimum distance between the pits should be 180 cm. Not >12 burial pits per year and after 7–8 half lives, the pits can be emptied into the municipal dump and reused. A record should be maintained about the location of each pit, the identity and quantity of each radionuclide buried in it.

Protected Material

Highly radioactive materials can also be buried in the soil if a material is treated in such a way that no leaching of the material can occur. In general, this involves packing the waste material in steel drums or concrete blocks. In the case of very high radioactive materials, a concrete tomb is constructed underground, and the material fed into the tomb via a chute from the surface. After the tomb is filled up the whole construction is filled with asphalt and sealed.

Municipal dumps can be used for protected burial because it is normally ensured that they carefully sited to prevent contamination of surface or other waters with conventional nonradioactive pollutants. The radioactive materials should be packed in steel bins and then must be buried beneath at least 1.5 meters of other rubbish. Up to 1 mCi can be buried in a municipal site in a form unattractive for salvage.

Storage of Protective Material

The purpose of protective storage is (i) to avoid dust hazard, (ii) to provide shielding, and (iii) to prevent accumulation in working areas. Normally short-lived isotopes are stored for decay. Long-lived radioisotopes are stored and disposed to centralized waste management facility (CWMF), IGCAR, Kalpakkam or BARC, Mumbai. There, the waste is disposed of in engineered structures such as reinforced concrete trenches and the tile holes depending upon the waste and the radioactivity. In the case of brachytherapy solid wastes, it is stored and then returned to the isotope supplier. The storage area should be in accessible to unauthorized persons. Usually, foot-operated dustbins with plastic bag are used in hospitals to store solid waste. Proper labeling of the container along with records is mandatory. The radiation level at 1 meter should not exceed 1.5 mR/h in such storages.

Sea Dumping

This method of disposal for solid active waste can be carried out after carefully choosing an area based on oceanographic studies. For low activity solid waste use is made of relatively shallow waters of approximately 100 fathoms (1 fathoms = 1.8 m). This method is practiced in the UK and in the US. Both packed and unpackaged wastes are dumped into water exceeding 1,000 fathoms in depth. Containers used for sea dumping should be designed, constructed, and filled in such a manner as to ensure the following:

- They cannot be easily damaged or broken and will reach the bottom without appreciable loss of contents.
- They are free from voids.
- They have density of 1.2 g/cc.
- They are provided with sufficient shielding for safe storage.
- They are of a size and shape to be handled quickly and conveniently.

Although no general legislative control exists for the dumping of material outside territorial water, it is highly desirable that careful records are maintained of the total activity content and weight of all consignments.

Discharge of Low-level Liquid Radioactive Effluents

Low-level radioactive waste must be managed as per the regulatory requirements. The principle involved is delay and decay, concentrate and contain and dilute and disperse. One must consider the (i) volume of the effluents generated, (ii) frequency of generation, (iii) activity or activity concentration in the effluents, and (iv) physical and chemical characteristics of the effluents for better waste management. While discharging low-level radioactive effluents the following points are considered:

- Population of the vicinity
- Extent of development of the sewage system of the country
- Number of establishments discharging in the same sewage system
- Discharge requirements of the institution
- Volume and activity levels of the proposed discharge
- Number of operational sewage treatment plants in that area
- Impact on the environment of the proposed discharge
- Acceptability of doses to the representative person
- Regulatory criteria

Discharge options of radioactive effluents include: (1) direct discharge to the sewage system, and (2) storage for decay and discharge to the sewage system. Clearance and exemption levels of the regulatory agency are strictly followed.

Direct Discharge to the Sewage System

Direct discharge is the preferred method since medical effluents activity is in the order of Bq to kBq per liter. Liquid waste of activity <μCi may be disposed in the sanitary sewerage system followed by water flushing.

TABLE 15.4 **Disposal limits for sanitary sewerage system.**

Radioisotope	*Maximum limit on total discharge per day (MBq)*	*Average monthly activity in discharge? (MBq/m³)*
Hydrogen-3 (Tritium)	92.5	3,700
Carbon-14	18.5	740
Sodium-24	3.7	222
Phosphorus-32	3.7	18.5
Sulphur-35	18.5	74
Calcium-45	3.7	10.1
Molybdenum-99 + Technetium-99m	3.7	185
Iodine-125	3.7	22.2
Iodine-131	3.7	22.2

Note: The gross quantity of radioactive material released into the sewerage system by any hospital should not exceed 37 GBq (1 Curie) in 1 year.

Courtesy: Khan S et al., 2010.

They are produced on daily basis and must be discharged on designated sinks. The tap should be turned ON before the discharge start for dilution. Water should flow from the tap even after discharge for further dilution. It is sufficiently flushed from the pipes and at the point of discharge. If the activity is low and within discharge limits, it can be discharged directly to the sewage system. If the activity is higher, the radiological impact on it be accessed before direct discharge of effluents to the sewage system. Any unacceptable impact may require regulatory consent and revision of procedures. Such disposal should not exceed the limits as given in the **Table 15.4**.

Storage for Decay and Discharge

Hospitals producing large volume, >0.5 m^3/year radioactive effluents with activity levels above the discharge limits can use store and discharge method. Medium activity waste and those isotopes with half-life less than a month can be stored. It follows the principle; delay and decay and use either (i) storage in containers within storage area or (ii) storage in decay tank. Such storage containers or tanks require labeling, record keeping, and secured storage. Urine collection containers of 5 L capacity with wide neck and provided with antimicrobial disinfection agent before use. Suitable volume containers should be chosen, and periodic diose rate measurements must be done.

The storage room is properly ventilated with an exhaust system passed through a duct line to roof top exit. Room shielding shall be 10 HVL to prevent radiation leakage. The waste is stored for 10 half-lives and monitored for residual activity. It makes the activity <0.1% of the original activity. Containers should be opened at the end of decay period. Transport of container with effluents is suitably shielded in a bin on a trolly. If the dose level is low, it is disposed as low-activity solid or liquid waste. Most of the hospital wastes arise from short low half-life radioisotopes. If the volume of effluents is high, storage with delay tanks is to be installed as discussed in the latter paragraphs.

Disposal of Radioactive Effluents into the Environment

The disposal of diluted waste can be done into the sea, river or into the ground. It will depend upon the proximity of the facilities producing or treating the wastes to the types of environments mentioned aforesaid. The principle involved is dilute and disperse.

Disposal of Radioactive Effluent into the Sea

Sea is a unique medium for disposal of low-activity waste because dilution factors are large and maximum permissible levels for discharge are higher than those for freshwater bodies, as drinking water tolerances are not involved. However, dilution may be partly offset by concentration of some radioactive species in marine life which may enter feed cycles ending in consumption by human beings.

Hence, any projected sea or river disposal scheme must be preceded by extensive trails to determine the dilution of foreign solution discharged at various points in the sea or river. By these the degree of horizontal and vertical mixing is obtained on discharge to the sea or river as well as the effects of winds and tides upon the dispersal of the material. Detailed biological experiments must also be done to determine the pattern of uptake of radioactivity by marine fauna and flora, especially those involved in food cycles.

For the disposal of liquid wastes into rivers the following factors should be considered: flow rate, nature of riverbed, turbidity, currents, etc. Consideration must be given to the types of water utilization such as drinking, industrial, and agricultural uses and appropriate correction factors should be applied to arrive at the permissible discharges. Dilution of low-level liquid wastes can be achieved by the following:

- Addition of uncontaminated liquid to reduce the concentrations prior to discharge
- Release of the liquid wastes at small rates over long periods of time
- Release of wastes into large bodies of water

Disposal of Radioactive Effluent into the Ground

The liquid waste injected into the ground will tend to percolate downward until it reaches the ground-water table, when it begins to travel forward in the direction of underground water flow; in doing so, the activity is diluted by the natural water flowing in the ground. In addition, if the permeability and porosity of the formation are such that underground water is appreciable in volume but not too rapid in rate, the combination of dilution and the decay afforded by an appreciable retention time may be such that the waste levels are below the dose equivalent limits, by the time the waste reaches the environment, by discharging to springs, streams, or the sea. The retention time may be extended by chemical reactions between the waste and the soil, and in very favorable circumstances very high retention times may be encouraged. The factors determining the applicability of ground disposal methods are two, namely (i) hydrological, and (ii) chemical. The desirable factors for hydrological factors for ground disposal can be summarized as follows:

- A deep-water table with good flow gradients
- Appreciable permeability to allow rates of flow sufficient to be useful
- Fairly high porous-thick formation to restrict rates of flow
- Wide spacing of water bodies such as lakes and streams so that long distances of underground flow are involved.

- Relatively low rainfall. Although the groundwater flow may then be slight, the porosity of unsaturated formation in an area of low rainfall may afford high-retention volumes.

In addition to the hydrological phase retention in the ground, there may be further retention of certain species due to chemical reactions with constituents of the soil or rock. These reactions are precipitation and ion exchange. The precipitation characteristics will depend upon the natural pH of the soil. Ion exchange properties of soil depend upon the type and amount of clay minerals present, and in soils rich in organic matter the humus content as well. In any case, ground disposal requires detailed study of hydrological and chemical characteristics of the soil where the disposal is contemplated.

Special Situation of Waste Management in Hospitals

Disposal of Sealed Sources

Sealed sources are used in hospitals in teletherapy, brachytherapy, blood irradiation, calibration, etc. These sources are small and have a few MBq activities except in teletherapy and blood irradiators. It requires replacement whenever it gets weaker, or the activity is low. Such sources are disposed safely to the manufacturer.

Disposal of Gaseous Waste

Radioactive sources like ^{131}I and ^{125}1 are volatile and release radioactive vapors, resulting airborne radiative waste. Containers of such sources shall be opened under fume hood connected to roof top exit via duct line. They should pass through charcoal and filters before the vapors get diluted and dispersed into the atmosphere. Use of radioactive gases in hospitals shall require efficient laminar air-flow system. Airborne radioactive concentration that would result in such disposal may be limited within the annual dose limits to occupational workers **(Table 15.5)**.

Radiopharmacy Laboratory Waste

Radiopharmacy laboratory attached to a nuclear medicine department generates number of wastes as stated earlier. Biological contamination is more series hazard and requires special consideration. Generally, waste is divided into controlled and uncontrolled waste and disposed. Controlled waste requires regulatory consent for disposal from the competent authority, e.g., ^{131}I (270 μCi), ^{99m}Tc (1.4 mCi).

TABLE 15.5 **Air borne radioactive concentration that would result annual dose limits to occupational workers.**

Radionuclide	*Air concentration borne (μCi/mL)*
^{18}F	3×10^{-5}
^{99m}Tc	6×10^{-5}
^{131}I	2×10^{-8}
^{14}C	1×10^{-6}
^{133}Xe	1×10^{-4}
Courtesy: Cherry SR et al., 2012.	

Technetium-99m Waste

Technetium-99m waste normally requires storage for only 48 hours in a plastic bag inside a shielded container. The container should be labeled with the radionuclide and date. Gallium-67, iodine-131, and other longer half-life materials should be placed in a separate labeled and dated plastic bag and stored safely. Sharp items, such as needles, should be separated and placed in a shielded plastic container for safety. When disposing of waste, attention should be paid to the following points:

- Normally once the surface dose rate in any individual bag of waste is below 5 mGy/h, it can be disposed of.
- Disposable gloves should be worn, and caution exercised when handling sharp items.
- Any labels and radiation symbols should be removed.
- Waste should be placed in a locally appropriate waste disposal container, for example, biological waste bag.
- Formulate practicable rules and discharge levels based on average water consumption and isotope concentration.
- Radiation hazard to sanitation workers and sewage personnel less than from accidental immersion of 0.1 mCi/L.
- Effective dose limits should not be exceeded.
- If the effluents are used for agricultural purposes the levels should be reduced by 10. Possible build-up of activity in irrigated land and crops to be considered.
- Total activity released should not exceeded 1 Ci/year.
- Long-lived isotopes other than ^{3}H and ^{14}C should not be released to sink.

Exhausted ^{99m}Tc Generators

A ^{99}Mo generator with activity of 345 mCi decays to 140 μCi after 31 days. It can be disposed under controlled conditions with proper authorization. Spent generators should be removed to a separate storeroom or bunker for the required decay period. Storage room should be provided with shielding, so that the exposure should not exceed the effective dose limits.

Management of Excreta and Urine in Therapeutic Iodine Patients

Patients are administered with high doses of iodine for therapeutic purposes and get under isolation in the ward. They stay in the ward until the radiation level from the patient comes to about 3 mR/h at 1 m from the patient. The excreta and urine of the patient is fleshed out through PVC pipes into the customized tanks through shortest route. Details of the tank are given in **Chapter 8: Planning a nuclear medicine facility (Fig. 8.10)**. The tank must be leak proof, corrosion free, has smooth surface inside and located in an area of minimal public activity. Either a single or double tanks are used, mostly the later version is preferred. In the case of single radionuclide, a number of tanks are connected in series. If different radionuclides are involved, different tanks are required:

- Tank for short half-life <100 days
- Tank for mixed beta/gamma with half-life >100 days
- Tank for alpha or alpha/beta/gamma emitters

Hospital with two patients' isolation ward requires about 6,000 L each at the rate of 100 L/day per patient over a period of month. After 1 month the tank is full, its value is closed, and the value of the second tank is opened. The first tank is kept

TABLE 15.6 Maximum radioactivity level of the corpse for disposal without any precautions.

Radioisotope	*Postmortem/embalming (MBq)*	*Burial (MBq)*	*Cremation (MBq)*
Iodine-131	10	400	400
Yttrium-90 colloid	200	2,000	70
Gold-198	400	400	100
Phosphorus-32	100	2,000	30
Strontium-89	50	2,000	20

Courtesy: AERB safety code, 2001.

closed for 1 month so that it holds the ^{131}I for 2 months that is enough for the decay of ^{131}I. Before releasing the effluents to the public drainage system, sample is taken from the tank and the activity is checked. It should be not >1.2 Ci per liter.

Management of Cadavers Containing Radioactive Material

Situation may arise that the patient administered with high dose of radioactivity may die in the hospital. Such patients may have high levels of radioactivity in the body. It is reported to the Radiological Safety Officer (RSO) of the institution immediately who should oversee the course of action along with the nuclear physician concerned. If high activity is nonconcentrated in an organ, then autopsy (removal of organ) is recommended. If a metastatic site has activity, efforts should be taken to remove the site. If the cadaver radioactivity is less the recommended limits, the dead body may be handed over to the relatives for final burial or crimination without precautions **(Table 15.6)**. If the activity levels are high, the body/corpse is retained in the hospital mortuary until the activity decays to safe limits.

Step-by-step Procedure

1. All reasonable efforts should be made to remove fluids or organs in which radionuclide is concentrated, provided the collective equivalent dose received in the procedure will be less than that in handling the cadaver as it is.
2. No special precautions are normally necessary for embalming, burial, or cremation of the corpse containing the quantities less than that specified.
3. The following precautions shall be observed in respect of dead bodies containing quantities more than that given in the above table.
   - Cremation: Prior authorization, and specific precautions to be observed during cremation, shall be obtained from RSO.
   - Burial: Relatives shall be prevented from coming into contact with the body and people must not stay near the coffin. The hospital staff and the persons involved in washing, preparing, and transporting the body to the burial ground shall be instructed by RSO on dose-reducing precautions. The body shall be handled with disposable gloves and kept on plastic sheets to control spread of contamination.
   - Embalming: Embalming is undesirable and, if unavoidable, shall be done by injection method. All contamination control measures shall be observed under the guidance of RSO.

4. Autopsy: Autopsy on contaminated cadavers shall be performed only in a special autopsy room provided with facilities such as a plastic-covered table, water-proof flooring, receptacles for organs, instrument cabinet and a washing stand for pathologist. A refrigerator for keeping the cadavers at temperatures below –10° shall be provided. The RSO shall supervise autopsy procedures and subsequent decontamination operations.

BIBLIOGRAPHY

1. Regulatory control of radioactive discharges to the environment and disposal of solid waste, AERB/NRF/SG/RW-10, 2021.
2. Selection of technical solution for the management radioactive waste, IAEA-TECDOC-1817, IAEA, 2017.
3. Management of discharge of low-level liquid radioactive waste generated in Medical, educational, research and industrial facilities IAEA-TECDOC-1714, IAEA, Vienna, 2013.
4. Cherry SR, Sorenson JA, Phelps ME. Physics in Nuclear Medicine, 4th edition, Elsevier, 2012.
5. Atomic energy regulatory board (AERB), safety code: CODE NO. AERB/RF-MED/SC-2 (Rev. 2), 2011.
6. International Atomic Energy Agency (IAEA) safety standards (SSR-5): Disposal of radioactive waste. IAEA, Vienna, 2011.
7. Khan S, Syed AT, Ahmad R, Rather TA, Ajaz M, Jan FA. Radioactive waste management in a hospital, International journal of health sciences. 2010;4(1):39-46.
8. Management of radioactive waste from the use of radionuclide in medicine IAEA-TECDOC-1183, IAEA, 2000. [online] Available from www.aerb@org.in [Last accessed December, 2022].
9. Atomic energy regulatory board (AERB), safety code: CODE NO. AERB/SC/MED-4 (Rev. 1), 2001.

CHAPTER 16

Transport of Radioactive Material

INTRODUCTION

Radioactive materials are used in nuclear reactors, medicine, and industry. There is a need to transport the radioactive material from the manufacturer to user and from the user to the disposal facility. International regulations are in place to transport such materials by road, air, and sea in a safe manner. International Atomic Energy Agency (IAEA) has given regulatory requirements for radioactive material transport duly approved by the United Nation (UN) in the form of UN numbers. In India, competent authority has given certain requirements in the safety code under Rule 16 of the Atomic Energy (Radiation Protection) Rules 2004.

REGULATORY ASPECTS OF TRANSPORT OF RADIOACTIVE MATERIAL

General Aspects

Transport includes any operation incidental to the whole course of carriage, such as loading, unloading, and storage in transit. Transport of radioactive material must adhere certain safety requirements to ensure the safety of persons, property, and the environment against radiological hazards. Hence, radioactive materials are transported in a variety of types of packages. To achieve radiation safety, several requirements are essential, which are as follows:

- Containment of the radioactive contents
- Control of external radiation levels
- Prevention of criticality, where applicable
- Prevention of damage caused by heat, where applicable

General provisions of radiation safety such as radiation protection, emergency response, noncompliance, special arrangement, and training should be followed during transport. Additionally, radionuclide values and UN numbers are required as given in the safety codes. These are given in the form of tables for: (1) basic radionuclide values for known radionuclides, (2) UN name and shipping numbers, and (3) basic radionuclide values for unknown radionuclides and mixtures. Radioactive materials should be properly packed prior to transport and should be accompanied by appropriate transport certificates. Prior to undertaking the transport of radioactive material, the consigner should approach the radiological safety division, Atomic Energy Regulatory Board (AERB) for permission and advice.

The AERB has issued certain guidelines in the form of codes AERB-NRF/TR/SC-1 (Rev. 1) and AERB/NRF-TS/SG-10 for transport of radioactive materials. The main objective of the above codes is that the doses to persons engaged in transport and other persons are as low as reasonably achievable, during such transport.

Classification and Terminologies

1. *Special form radioactive material*: It is either an indispersible solid radioactive material or a sealed capsule-containing radioactive material, conforming to the requirements specified and approved by the Competent Authority for special form radioactive material.
2. *Low dispersible radioactive material:* A solid radioactive material or a solid radioactive material in a sealed capsule (not in powder form) and which meets the requirements laid down by the competent authority in this regard.
3. *Low specific activity material*: Radioactive material that by its nature has a limited specific activity, or radioactive material for which limits of estimated average specific activity apply. External shielding materials, surrounding the low specific activity (LSA) material, should not be considered in determining the estimated average specific activity.
4. *Fissile material:* Fissile nuclides include Uranium-233, Uranium-235, Plutonium-238, Plutonium-239, Plutonium-241, or any combination of these nuclides. A material containing any of the fissile nuclides is called fissile material. The smallest external dimension of the fissile package shall not exceed 10 cm.
5. *Contamination:* The presence of a radioactive substance on a surface in quantities in excess of 0.4 $Bq.cm^{-2}$ for beta and gamma emitters and low toxicity alpha emitters, or 0.04 $Bq.cm^{-2}$ for all other alpha emitters.
6. *Surface-contaminated object (SCO)*: A solid object that is not itself radioactive, but it has radioactive material distributed on its surface.
7. *Criticality safety index (CSI)*: A number assigned to a package, overpack, or freight container-containing fissile material to provide control over the accumulation of such packages, overpacks, or freight containers-containing fissile material.
8. *Package*: The complete product of the packing operation, consisting of the packaging and its contents, prepared for transport.
9. *Packaging*: It refers to assembly of components necessary to enclose the radioactive contents completely. It may contain one or more receptacles and any other components necessary for the receptacles to perform containment and other safety functions. The packaging may be a box, drum, or similar receptacle, or a freight container, tank, or intermediate bulk container.

   Other components include absorbent materials, spacing structures, radiation shielding, service equipment for filling, emptying, venting, and pressure relief devices for cooling, absorbing mechanical shocks, providing handling and tie-down capability, thermal insulation, and service devices integral to the package.
10. *A_1 and A_2 package*: A_1 shall mean the activity value of special form of radioactive material whereas A_2 shall mean the activity value of radioactive material, other than special form radioactive material. The values of A1 and A2 of important clinical radionuclides are given in the **Table 16.1**.
11. *Transport index (TI)*: A number assigned to a package, overpack or freight container, or to unpackaged LSA-I or surface-contaminated object-I (SCO-I) that is used to provide control over radiation exposure.

TABLE 16.1 A_1 and A_2 values for clinical radionuclides (IAEA safety standards series, 2018).

Radionuclide	*A_1 (TBq)*	*A_2 (TBq)*	*Activity concentration limit for exempt material (Bq/g)*	*Activity limit for an exempt consignment (Bq)*
^{60}Co	0.4	0.4	10	1×10^5
^{137}Cs	2	0.6	10	1×10^4
^{131}I	3	0.7	1×10^2	1×10^6
^{192}Ir	1	0.6	10	1×10^4
^{32}P	0.5	0.5	1×10^3	1×10^5
^{226}Ra	0.2	3×10^{-3}	10	1×10^4
^{90}Sr	0.3	0.3	1×10^2	1×10^4
^{99m}Tc	10	4	1×10^2	1×10^7
^{125}I	20	3	1×10^3	1×10^6

12. *Unilateral approval*: An approval of a design that is issued by the competent authority of the country of origin of the design only.
13. *Multilateral approval*: Approval by the relevant competent authority of the country of origin of the design or shipment, as applicable, and where the consignment is to be transported through or into any other country, approval by the competent authority of that country.
14. *Consignee and consignor*: Consignee is any person, organization, or government that is entitled to take delivery of a consignment. Consignor is any person, organization, or government that prepares a consignment for transport, and is named as consignor in the transport documents.
15. *Competent authority*: Any official or authority appointed, approved, or recognized by the Government of India for the purpose of the rules promulgated under the Atomic Energy Act, 1962. Currently, the Chairman, AERB, is the competent authority.

TYPES OF PACKAGES

Radioactive packages are classified into eight types depending on total activity in a package, specific activity of the material, and whether the material is fissile or not. Sturdiness, shielding integrity of the packaging, and the quantity of radioactive material determine the type of the package. Various types of packages are:

- Excepted package
- Industrial package Type 1 (Type IP-1)
- Industrial package Type 2 (Type IP-2)
- Industrial package Type 3 (Type IP-3)
- Type A package
- Type B(U) package
- Type B(M) package
- Fissile package

Excepted Package

Excepted package means a packaging containing excepted quantities of radioactive material that is designed to meet the general requirements for all packaging and packages. These packages are permitted to contain small quantities of radioactive materials and are excepted from various specific packaging and labeling requirements. A package is said to be an expected package, if it meets one of the following conditions:

- Used for very small quantities of radionuclides, which would present a negligible hazard, if the package was destroyed
- No special protection other than containment for the radioactive contents
- Dose rate at any point on the external surface shall not exceed 5 μSv/h or exceed the activity **(Table 16.2)**.
- No external "radioactive" label. Vehicles carrying "excepted" packages do not require a placard.

Industrial Packages

- Used for physically large items of LSA material or SCOs; may be a drum or bulk tank.
- Intended only to prevent the loss of contents under normal transport conditions
- Should be labeled either "LSA" or "SCO".
- Include bulk consignments of low-level radioactive waste, or thorium or uranium compounds.

Type IP-1

It is designed to meet the general requirements plus the following: (1) smallest overall external dimension of the package shall not be <10 cm, and (2) meet the requirements of transportation by air.

TABLE 16.2 Activity limits for expected packages.

	Instrument or article		***Materials***
Physical state: Content	***Item limit***	***Package limit***	***Package limit***
Solids:			
Special form	10^{-2} A_1	A_1	10^{-3} A_1
Other forms	$10^{-2}$$A_2$	A_2	10^{-3} A_2
Liquids	10^{-2} A_2	10^{-1} A_2	10^{-4} A_2
Gases:			
Tritium	2×10^{-2} A_2	2×10^{-1} A_2	2×10^{-2} A_2
Special form	10^{-3} A_1	$10^{-2}$$A_1$	10^{-3} A_1
Other forms	10^{-3} A_2	10^{-2} A_2	10^{-3} A_2

Courtesy: AERB/NRF-TS/SC-1 (Rev.1), 2016.

Type IP-2

It is designed to meet the requirements of type IP-1 plus the following: (1) free drop test and (2) stacking test. It prevents loss or dispersal of radioactive material, and not >20% increase in maximum radiation level at any external surface of the package.

Type IP-3

It is designed to meet the requirements of type IP-1 and type A package except those containing liquids and gases.

Type A Packages

- Required to withstand normal conditions of transport without loss or dispersal of their contents or loss of adequate shielding integrity.
- Intended to provide adequate containment and shielding for limited quantities of radioactive materials, in a normal transport environment.
- Each package carries a "radioactive" label and a category designation ("I, II, or III, in red numerals") that is related to the dose rates at or close to the surface.

The total activity of radioactive material in type A package is limited. Type A packages must not contain activities greater than A_1 for special form radioactive material or A_2 for all other radioactive material. A_1 is the maximum activity of special form radioactive material permitted under provisions of the type A package. A_2 is the maximum activity of radioactive material, other than special forms of radioactive material permitted under provisions of the type A package.

In the case of mixtures of radionuclides whose intensity and activity are known, a special condition is followed as per the safety code. Special form of radioactive material refers to either an indispersible solid radioactive material or a sealed capsule containing radioactive material, conforming to the requirements specified and approved by the Competent Authority. The sealed capsule should be so constructed that it can be opened only by destroying the capsule.

Type B Packages

- Designed to withstand both normal and accidental conditions of transport.
- Usually cask shaped, intended to withstand severe accident conditions.
- Large transport flasks used by the nuclear power industry; those likely to be encountered in transport accidents are much smaller.
- Labeled as type B and category I, II, or III, and fireproof/waterproof designations.

Radioactive materials in quantities greater than those allowed in type A packages are shipped in type B packages. The design of the packages is subject to the approval of the competent authority. Type B packages must not contain: (1) activities greater than those authorized for the package design, (2) radionuclides different from those authorized for the packages design, or contents in a form, or a physical or chemical state different from those authorized for the package design, as specified in their certificates of approval.

Type B packages are divided into two basic categories namely: (1) Type B(U) and Type B(M), e.g., transport of teletherapy sources, gamma irradiators sources, and industrial radiography sources.

Type B(U) Package

Type B(U) packages meet the most stringent requirements; it is considered that safety is entirely built into these packages. The design of this package is subject to the approval by the competent authority of the country of origin. Design and shipment of type B(U) package are subject to multilateral approval (country of origin and the country through which it is transported).

Type B(M) Package

Type B(M) packages do not meet all the requirements applicable to type B(U) packages; however, they must incorporate alternative design features and operational controls must be instituted to achieve the same level of safety as for type B(U).

Type B(U) and Type B(M) packages, if transported in air, should not contain activities greater than:

- For low dispersible radioactive material—as authorized by the package design and specified in the certificate for approval certificate.
- For special form radioactive material—3,000 A_1 or 10^5 A_2, whichever is lower
- For all other radioactive materials—3,000 A_2

Type C Package

- Designed to transport large activities of radioactive material by air.
- They are designed to withstand severe accident conditions of transport.
- They are analogous to type B but designed to withstand more severe tests.

Fissile Packages

Package containing any of the fissile nuclides is called fissile material package. Critical safety in transport of fissile material is ensured by limiting the quantity and geometric configuration of the fissile material, package design features, and by controlling the number of packages to be carried on a single conveyance or to be stored together in transit. All packages containing fissile material must comply with the applicable activity limits specified in the safety code. The packages containing fissile materials, which may be LSA, SCO, Type A or Type B, are subjected to multilateral approval.

Packaging containing fissile material must not contain: (1) a mass of fissile material greater than that authorized for the package design, (2) any radionuclide or fissile material different those authorized for the package design, or (3) contents in a form or physical or chemical state, or in a spatial arrangement, different from those authorized for the package design, as specified in their certificates of approval.

Package Containing Uranium Hexafluoride

Uranium hexafluoride (UF_6) of >0.1 kg or more shall be packed for transport as per international organization for standardization document: ISO-7195 and the package design satisfies the following:

- Without leakage and unacceptable stress, be tested hydraulically at an internal pressure of at least 1.38 MPa. If the test pressure is <2.76 MPa, it requires multitravel approval. For retesting, nondestructive testing may be applied.
- Without loss or dispersal of UF_6 under the free drop test
- Without rupture of the containment under the thermal test
- Packages shall be provided with pressure relief devices
- Multitravel approval is required

Special Arrangement

Radioactive material shall be classified and transported under special arrangement when it is intended to be carried in accordance:

- Consignments for which conformity with the other provisions of the safety code is impracticable shall not be transported except under special arrangement.
- Provided the Competent Authority is satisfied that conformity with the other provisions of the safety code is impracticable and that the requisite standards of safety established by the provisions of this safety code have been demonstrated through means alternative to the other provisions, the Competent Authority may approve special arrangement transport operations for single or a planned series of multiple consignments.
- The overall level of safety in transport shall be at least equivalent to that which would be provided if all the applicable requirements had been met.
- For consignments of this type, multilateral approval shall be required.

GENERAL REQUIREMENTS FOR ALL PACKAGING AND PACKAGES

The package should satisfy the following general and specific requirements before they are used for actual transport:

- Packages are designed in terms of its mass, volume, and shape that—it could be easily and safely handled and transported. It is properly secured in or on the conveyance during the transport. [1]
- The design shall be such that any lifting attachments on the package will not fail when used in the intended manner and that if failure of the attachments should occur, the ability of the package to meet other requirements of the safety code would not be impaired. The design shall take account of appropriate safety factors to cover snatch lifting. [2]
- Attachments and any other features on the outer surface of the package that could be used to lift; it shall be designed either to support its mass in accordance with the requirements of point two or shall be removable or otherwise rendered incapable of being used during transport. [3]
- As far as practicable, the packaging shall be so designed and finished that the external surfaces are free from protruding features and can be easily decontaminated. [4]
- As far as practicable, the outer layer of the package shall be so designed as to prevent the collection and the retention of water. [5]
- Any features added to the package at the time of transport that are not part of the package shall not reduce its safety. [6]
- The package shall be capable of withstanding the effects of any acceleration, vibration, or vibration resonance that may arise under routine conditions of transport without any deterioration in the effectiveness of the closing devices on the various receptacles or in the integrity of the package. Nuts, bolts, and other securing devices shall be so designed as to prevent them from becoming loose or being released unintentionally, even after repeated use. [7]
- The materials of the packaging and any components or structures shall be physically and chemically compatible with each other and with the radioactive contents. Account shall be taken of their behavior under irradiation. [8]

- All valves through which the radioactive contents could escape shall be protected against unauthorized operation. [9]
- The design of the package shall consider ambient temperatures and pressures that are likely to be encountered in routine conditions of transport. [10]
- A package shall be so designed that it provides sufficient shielding to ensure that—under routine conditions of transport and with the maximum radioactive contents that the package is designed to contain, the dose rate at any point on the external surface of the package would not exceed the values specified in the IAEA safety standards. [11]
- For radioactive material having other dangerous properties, the package design shall consider those properties. [12]

Additional Requirements for Packages Transported by Air

- For packages to be transported by air, the temperature of the accessible surfaces shall not exceed 50°C at an ambient temperature of 38°C with no account taken for insolation. [13]
- Packages to be transported by air shall be so designed that if they were exposed to ambient temperatures ranging from –40° to +55°C, the integrity of containment would not be impaired. [14]
- Packages to be transported by air shall be capable of withstanding, without loss or dispersal of radioactive contents from the containment system, an internal pressure that produces a pressure differential of not less than maximum normal operating pressure plus 95 kPa. [15]

Additional Requirements for Type A Packages

- Type A packages should fulfill general requirements and additional requirements for air transport. [16]
- The smallest overall external dimension of the packaging must not be <10 cm. [17]
- The outside of the package must incorporate a seal that is not readily breakable, and serve as proof against tamper and ensure that the package not been opened. [18]
- Any tie-down facility on the package should withstand both normal and accidental conditions. The forces in those attachments shall not impair the ability of the package. [19]
- The design of the package must consider temperatures ranging from 40° to 75°C, for the components of the packaging. Attention is required for freezing temperatures in case of liquids and to the potential degradation of packing materials. [20]
- The design and manufacturing techniques must be in accordance with national and international standards. It is in accordance with the competent authority. [21]
- The containment system is securely closed by a positive fastening device. It cannot be opened unintentionally or by a pressure that may arise within the package. [22]
- Special form radioactive material may be considered as a component of the containment system. [23]
- If the containment system forms a separate unit of the package, it shall be capable of being securely closed by a positive fastening device that is independent of any other part of the packaging. [24]

- The design of any component of the containment system shall take into account, where applicable, the radiolytic decomposition of liquids, and other vulnerable materials and the generation of gas by chemical reaction and radiolysis. [25]
- The package containment system must retain its radioactive contents under a reduction of ambient pressure to 60 kPa. [26]
- All valves, other than pressure relief valves, shall be provided with an enclosure to retain any leakage from the valve. [27]
- A radiation shield that encloses a component of the package specified as a part of the containment system shall be so designed as to prevent the unintentional release of that component from the shield. Where the radiation shield and such component within it form a separate unit, the radiation shield shall be capable of being securely closed by a positive fastening device that is independent of any other packaging structure. [28]
- When the packages are subjected to specified tests, to demonstrate ability to withstand normal conditions of transport, it would prevent: (i) loss or dispersal of the radioactive material, or (ii) >20% increase in maximum radiation level on the external surface of the package. [29]
- The design of a package intended for liquid radioactive material shall make provision for ullage to accommodate variations in the temperature of the contents, dynamic effects, and filling dynamics. [30]
- Type A package with liquid radioactive material should have additional requirements:
    - Be provided with sufficient absorbent material to absorb twice the volume of the liquid contents. Such absorbent material must be suitably positioned to contact the liquid in the event of leakage
    - Be provided with a containment system composed of primary inner and secondary outer containment components designed to enclose the liquid contents completely and to ensure their retention within the secondary outer containment components, even if the primary inner components leak. [31]
- A package designed for gases shall prevent loss or dispersal of the radioactive contents if the package was subjected to the tests specified in the code. A Type A package designed for tritium gas or for noble gases shall be excepted from this requirement. [32]

Additional Requirements for Type B(U) Packages

- The package should meet all the general requirements and requirements for transportation by air, if required. [33]
- The heat generated within the package by the radioactive content shall not affect the package so that it would fail to meet the applicable requirements for containment and shielding if left unattended for a period of 1 week. [34]
- The temperature of the accessible surfaces of a package shall not exceed 50°C, unless the package is transported under exclusive use. [35]
- While transported in air, the maximum temperature of any surface readily accessible during transport of a package under exclusive use shall not exceed 85°C. [36]
- The ambient temperature shall be assumed to be 38°C. [37]
- The solar insolation condition shall be assumed to be as per the safety code. [38]
- Those packages subjected to thermal test, protection provided to withstand normal conditions of transport and mechanical tests. Ripping, cutting, skidding, abrading, or rough handling on the exterior of the package shall be avoided. [39]

- Package design—(i) should restrict the loss of radioactive content to not more than 10^{-6} A_2 per hour during the tests (water spray test, free drop test, stacking test, and penetration test) to demonstrate ability to withstand normal conditions of transport; (ii) in mechanical test, the shielding should ensure that the radiation level at 1 m from the surface of the package should not exceed 10 mSv/h. It should also restrict the accumulated loss of radioactive contents in a period of 1 week to not >10 A_2 for krypton-85 and not more than A_2 for all other radionuclides. [40]
- A package with activity >10^5 A_2, there would be no rupture of containment system during enhanced water immersion test. [41]
- Permitted activity release limits depend neither upon filters nor upon a mechanical cooling system. [42]
- Package should not include a pressure relief system from the containment system. [43]
- If package is at maximum normal operating pressure and subjected tests, the levels of strains in the containment system would not attain values that would adversely affect the package in such a way that it would fail to meet the applicable requirements. [44]
- A package shall not have a maximum normal operating pressure more than a gauge pressure of 700 kPa. [45]
- In package containing low dispersible radioactive material, any features added to the low dispersible radioactive material that are not part of it, or any internal components of the packaging, shall not adversely affect the performance of the low dispersible radioactive material. [46]
- A package shall be designed for an ambient temperature range of –40° to +38°C. [47]

Additional Requirements for Type B(M) Packages

- The package should meet all the general requirements and requirements for transportation by air, if required. Packages to be transported solely within a specified country or solely between specified countries are excluded, may be assumed with the approval of competent authority. [48]
- Intermittent venting of type B(M) packages may be permitted during transport, provided that the operational controls for venting are acceptable to the Competent Authority. [49]
- Subjected to tests for demonstrating ability to withstand accident conditions of transport. It includes mechanical test, thermal test, water immersion test, and enhanced water immersion test. [50]

Additional Requirements for Type C Packages

- The package should meet all the general requirements (1–12) + additional requirements for air (13–15) + additional requirements for Type A package (17–28, 30), + additional requirements for Type B(U) packages (34–38, 42–47). [51]
- A package shall be capable of meeting the assessment criteria prescribed for tests in Clauses 40 and 44 of the topic "Additional Requirements for Type B(U) Packages" after burial in an environment defined by a thermal conductivity of 0.33 W/mK and a temperature of 38°C in the steady state. Initial conditions for the assessment shall assume that any thermal insulation of the package remains intact, the package is at the maximum normal operating pressure and the ambient temperature is 38°C. [52]

- A package shall be so designed that if it was at the maximum normal operating pressure and subjected to: (i) water test, free drop test, stacking test and penetration test would restrict the loss of radioactive contents to not more than 10^{-6} A_2 per hour, (ii) specific test for type C package. It would retain sufficient shielding to ensure that the radiation level at 1 m from the surface of the package would not exceed 10 mSv/h with the maximum radioactive contents that the package is designed to contain. It would also restrict the accumulated loss of radioactive contents in a period of 1 week to not more than $10A_2$ for krypton-85 and not more than A_2 or all other radionuclides. [53]
- A package shall be so designed that there will be no rupture of the containment system following performance of the enhanced water immersion test. [54]

TESTS FOR PACKAGES

Tests are specific to special form radioactive material, low dispersible radioactive material, and packages. Special form radioactive material tests include impact test, percussion test, bending test, and heat test. Leaching test is required for low dispersible radioactive material. Test for packages is described in the following paragraphs.

Test for Demonstrating Ability to Withstand Normal Conditions of Transport

The type A package tests are: (1) water spray test, (2) free drop test, (3) stacking test, and (4) penetration test. These tests will demonstrate the ability of the package to withstand normal conditions of transport. After the specimen is subjected to tests, suitable assessment must be made to assure that the requirements of the packages are fulfilled in conformance with the performance and acceptance standards.

Target for Drop Test

The target for the drop test specified in respect of impact test for special form radioactive material, low dispersible radioactive material, free drop test for normal conditions of transport, additional free drop test for type A packages containing liquids and gases, mechanical test, and puncture-tearing test for type C packages shall be a flat, horizontal surface of such a character that any increase in its resistance to displacement or deformation upon impact by the specimen would not significantly increase damage to the specimen.

Water Spray Test

The specimen must be subjected to a water test that simulates exposure to rainfall of approximately 5 cm/h for at least 1 hour.

Free Drop Test

The specimen shall drop on to the target so as to suffer maximum damage in respect of the safety features to be tested—(1) the height of drop measured from the lowest point of the specimen to the upper surface of the target must be not less than distance specified in the code **(Table 16.3)**, (2) for rectangular fiberboard or wood packages not exceeding a mass of 50 kg, a separate specimen shall be subjected to a free drop onto each corner from a height of 0.3 m, and (3) for cylindrical fiberboard packages not exceeding a mass of 100 kg, a separate specimen shall be subjected to a free drop onto each of the quarters of each rim from a height of 0.3 m.

TABLE 16.3 **Distances for free drop test to test packages for normal conditions of transport.**

Package mass (kg)	*Free drop distance (m)*
Package mass < 5,000	1.2
Package mass 5,000–10,000	0.9
Package mass 10,000–15,000	0.6
Package mass >15,000	0.3

Courtesy: IAEA safety standards series, 2018.

Stacking Test

The specimen shall be subjected to a period of 24 hours to a compressive load equal to the greater of the following: (1) the equivalent of five times the maximum weight of the package, (2) the equivalent of 13 kPa multiplied by the vertically projected area of the package.

The load shall be applied uniformly to two opposite sides of the specimen, one of which shall be the base on which the package would typically rest.

Penetration Test

The specimen shall be placed on a rigid, flat, horizontal surface that will not move significantly while the test is being carried out: (1) a bar 3.2 cm in diameter with a hemispherical end and a mass of 6 kg, shall be dropped and directed to fall, with its longitudinal axis vertical, onto the center of the weakest part of the specimen, so that, if it penetrates sufficiently far, it will hit the containment system. The bar shall not be significantly deformed by the test performance and (2) the height of drop of the bar measured from its lower end to the intended point of impact on the upper surface of the specimen shall be 1 m.

Additional Tests for Liquid and Gases

A specimen, or separate specimens, shall be subjected to each of the following tests unless it can be demonstrated that one test is more severe for the specimen in question than the other, in which case one specimen shall be subjected to the more severe test:

- *Free drop test*: The specimen shall drop onto the target so as to suffer the maximum damage in respect of containment. The height of the drop measured from the lowest part of the specimen to the upper surface of the target shall be 9 m.
- *Penetration test*: The specimen shall be subjected to the test specified in penetration test, except that the height of the drop shall be increased to 1.7 m.

Tests for Demonstrating Ability to Withstand Accident Conditions of Transport

The tests for type B packages are: (1) mechanical test, (2) thermal test, (3) water immersion test, and (4) enhanced water immersion test. These tests will demonstrate the ability of the package to withstand accident conditions in transport. After the specimen is subjected to tests, suitable assessment must be made to assure that the requirements of the packages are fulfilled in conformance with the performance and acceptance standards.

Mechanical Test

This consists of three different drop tests, namely drop-I, drop-II, and drop-III. The order in which the specimen is subjected to the drops shall be such that, on completion of the mechanical test, the specimen shall have suffered such damage as will lead to maximum damage in the thermal test that follows:

- *For drop-I*: The specimen shall drop onto the target so as to suffer maximum damage, and the height of the drop measured from the lowest point of the specimen to the upper surface of the target shall be 9 m.
- *For drop-II*: The specimen shall drop onto a bar rigidly mounted perpendicularly on the target so as to suffer maximum damage. The height of the drop measured from the intended point of impact of the specimen to the upper surface of the bar shall be 1 m. The bar shall be of solid mild steel of circular section, 15.0 ± 0.5 cm in diameter and 20 cm long, unless a longer bar would cause greater damage, in which case, a bar of sufficient length to cause maximum damage shall be used. The upper end of the bar shall be flat and horizontal with its edge rounded off to a radius of not >6 mm.
- *For drop-III*: The specimen shall be subjected to a dynamic crush test by positioning the specimen on the target so as to suffer maximum damage by the drop of a 500 kg mass from 9 m onto the specimen. The mass shall consist of a solid mild steel plate 1 × 1 m and shall fall in a horizontal attitude. The lower face of the steel plate shall have its edges and corners rounded off to a radius of not >6 mm. The height of the drop shall be measured from the underside of the plate to the highest point of the specimen.

Thermal Test

The specimen shall be in thermal equilibrium under conditions of an ambient temperature of 38°C, subject to the solar insolation conditions specified, and subject to the design maximum rate of internal heat generation within the package from the radioactive contents **(Table 16.4)**.

Water Immersion Test

The specimen shall be immersed under a head of water of at least 15 m for a period of not less than 8 hours in the attitude that will lead to maximum damage. For demonstration purposes, an external gauge pressure of at least 150 kPa shall be considered to meet these conditions.

TABLE 16.4 **Insolation period versus form and location of surface.**

Form and location of surface	*Insolation for 12 h/day (W/m²)*
Flat surfaces transported horizontally—downward facing	0
Flat surfaces transported horizontally—upward facing	800
Surfaces transported vertically	200
Other downward facing (not horizontal) surfaces	200
All other surfaces	200

Courtesy: AERB/NRF-TS/SC-1 (Rev.1), 2016.

Enhanced Water Immersion Test

The specimen shall be immersed under a head of water of at least 200 m for a period of not less than 1 hour. For demonstration purposes, an external gauge pressure of at least 2 MPa shall be considered to meet these conditions. This test is required for Type B(U) and Type B(M) packages containing >10^5 A_2 and Type C packages.

Tests for Type C Packages

Puncture-tearing Test

The specimen shall be subjected to "for drop-I and for drop-II tests" as stated and follow the test sequence:

- The specimen, representing a package having a mass of <250 kg, shall be placed on a target and subjected to a probe having a mass of 250 kg falling from a height of 3 m above the intended impact point. For this test, the probe shall be a 20 cm diameter cylindrical bar with the striking end forming the frustum of a right circular cone with the following dimensions: 30 cm height and 2.5 cm diameter at the top with its edge rounded off to a radius of not >6 mm.
- For packages having a mass of 250 kg or more, the base of the probe shall be placed on a target and the specimen dropped onto the probe. The height of the drop, measured from the point of impact with the specimen to the upper surface of the probe, shall be 3 m. The probe for this test shall have the same properties and dimensions as specified above, except that the length and mass of the probe shall be such as to cause maximum damage to the specimen.

Enhanced Thermal Test

The conditions for this test shall be as specified in thermal test, except that the exposure to the thermal environment shall be for a period of 60 minutes.

Impact Test

The specimen shall be subjected to an impact on a target at a velocity of not <90 m/s, at such an orientation as to suffer maximum damage.

CONTROLS FOR TRANSPORT

Transport Index

The Transport index (TI) of a package is the number expressing the maximum radiation level in mSv/h at 1 m from the external surface of the package and multiplied by a factor. The values of TI are 0, 1–10, and >10.

Transport index for a package, overpack or freight container, or for unpackaged LSA-I or SCO-I shall be the number derived in accordance with the following: (1) the maximum radiation level in units of millisieverts per hour (mSv/h) at a distance of 1 m from the external surfaces of the package, overpack, freight container, or unpackaged LSA-I and SCO-I. The value determined shall be multiplied by 100 and the resulting number is the TI. For tanks, freight containers, and unpackaged LSA-I and SCO-I, the value determined in step (1) shall be multiplied by the appropriate factor from **Table 16.5**.

Categories of Package

There are three categories of packages namely: (1) category I—white, (2) category II—yellow, and (3) category III—yellow. Every package should contain the trefoil symbol as stated by the safety code **(Fig. 16.1)**.

Category I–White

The maximum radiation level at any point on external surface of the package should not be >0.005 mSv/h and the TI is zero. The category I: White label background color shall be white, the color of the trefoil and the printing must be black, and the color of the category bar must be red **(Fig. 16.2)**.

Category II–Yellow

The maximum radiation level at any point on external surface of the package should be >0.005 mSv/h, but not >0.5 mSv/h. The TI is >0, but not >1. In category II: Yellow label, the background color of the upper half of the label shall be yellow and the lower half white, the color of the trefoil and the printing shall be black, and the color of the category bar shall be red **(Fig. 16.3)**.

TABLE 16.5 **Multiplication factors for tanks, freight containers, and unpacked LSA-1 and SCO-1.**

Size of load	*Multiplication factor*
Size of load ≤1 m^2	1
1 m^2 < size of load ≤ 5 m^2	2
5 m^2 < size of load ≤ 20 m^2	3
20 m^2 < size of load	10

Courtesy: IAEA safety standards series, 2018.

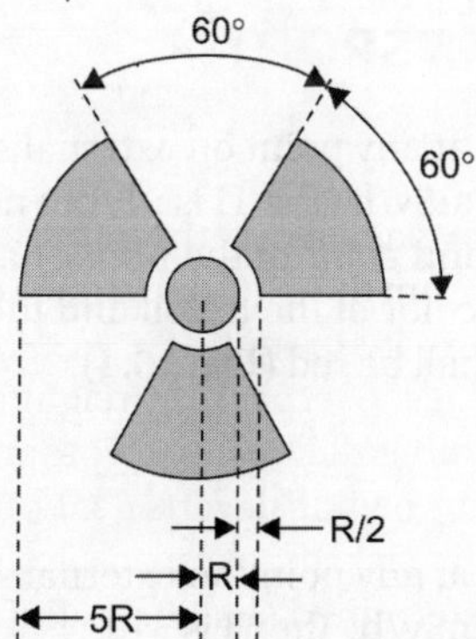

FIG. 16.1: The trefoil symbol with central circle of radius R and minimum R size shall be 4 mm. The inner circle of radius R, the inside radius of the blades is 1.5R and the outer radius of the blades is 5R. The blades are separated by 60° [AERB/NRF-TS/SC-1 (Rev.1), 2016].

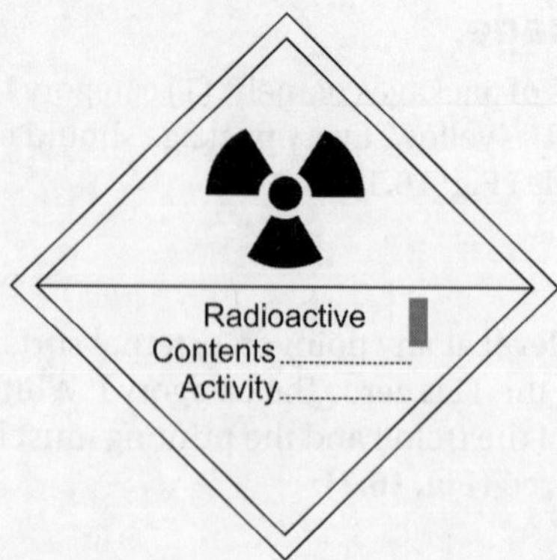

FIG. 16.2: Category-I WHITE label [AERB/NRF-TS/SC-1 (Rev.1), 2016].
(For color version, see Plate 2)

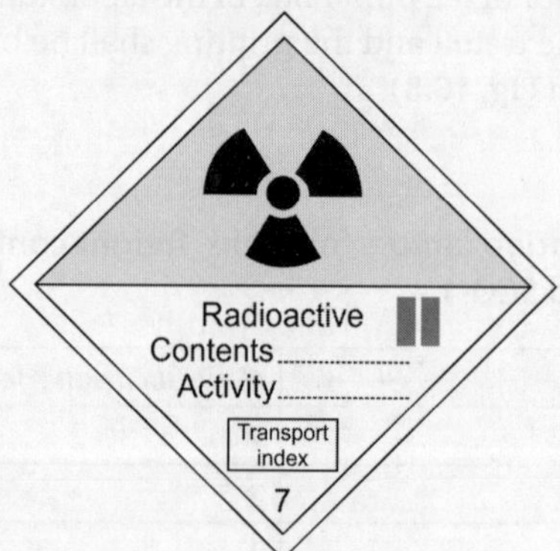

FIG. 16.3: Category-II YELLOW label [AERB/NRF-TS/SC-1 (Rev.1), 2016].
(For color version, see Plate 2)

Category III–Yellow

The maximum radiation level at any point on external surface of the package should not be >0.5 mSv/h, but not >2 mSv/h. The TI is >1, but not >10. In the case of category III: Yellow label, the background color of the upper half of the label shall be yellow and the lower half white, the color of the trefoil and the printing shall be black, and the color of the category bar shall be red **(Fig. 16.4)**.

*Category III–Yellow**

The maximum radiation level at any point on external surface of the package should not be >2 mSv/h, but not >10 mSv/h. The TI is >10.

---

*Shall also be transported under exclusive use except for freight containers.

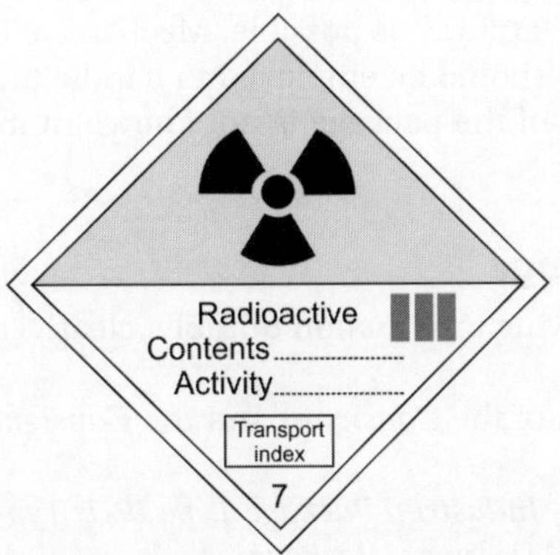

FIG. 16.4: Category-III YELLOW label [AERB/NRF-TS/SC-1 (Rev.1), 2016].
(For color version, see Plate 2)

PACKING, MARKING, LABELING, AND PLACARDING

Preparation of the Package for Transport

- Transport the source only in an approved transport container or use the original container in which the fresh source was received. Ensure that it is in good condition.
- Load the source in the container properly and carefully.
- Secure the source within the shielded container by means of appropriate locking mechanisms incorporated in the design of the shielded container.
- Close the lid of the container so that the source is not released during the transport.
- Load and immobilize (for example, fixing by bolts, with the help of spacers, etc.) the container in an outer sturdy container such as a wooden or metallic box. Ensure that the outer container deployed is in a sound condition and is provided with locking facility and strong lifting handles.
- *Lock and seal the outer container*: The seal should be tamper-proof, i.e., once a seal is disturbed/removed, it should not be possible to reuse. A recommended way of sealing is that the consignor may use weatherproof seals (e.g., laminated and self-adhesive type) with his/her signature. The key(s) of the lock(s) after putting in an envelope should be sealed with signature and handed over to the carrier to deliver the same along with the consignment (radioactive source) to the waste management agency.
- Using a working radiation monitor, measure the maximum radiation levels on the outer surface of the package and at a distance of 1 m from the surface and record them. The number obtained by measuring the maximum radiation level at 1 m expressed in mSv/h multiplied by 100 (or the number obtained by measuring the maximum radiation level at 1 m expressed in mrem/h) is called as the *Transport Index* of the package (TI).

Package Handling

Packages weighing <5 kg is not provided with handling facilities, and one can hold them with hands. Packages weighing not >30 kg is provided with manual handling facility. Two or more persons should be employed for handling the packages up to 100 kg. During manual handling, operations should be completed quickly, by keeping the packages as far away as possible. Mechanical handling devices (crane, chain pulley block, etc.,) should be employed to handle the packages, if the weight is >100 kg. If the weight of the package is not known, it must be handled only by mechanical means.

Marking of the Package

Write/inscribe the following information durably, clearly, and legibly on the outer surface of the package:

- Name and addresses of the *Consignor* and the *Consignee* with contact number details.
- Type of package (e.g., *Industrial Package Type IP-1, Type IP-2, Type IP-3, Type A Package, Type B(U)/(M), Type C Package*, etc.).
- *United Nations Number (UN Number)*, and the *Proper Shipping Name*. In case of *Excepted Packages*, proper shipping name is not required.
- Gross weight of the package if it exceeds 30 kg for domestic transport and 50 kg for international transport
- Competent authority identification mark along with its serial number if it is a type B(U)/type B(M)/type C package.
- In case of Type IP-2, Type IP-3, and Type A package, Vehicle Registration Code (VRI Code) of the country of origin and either the name of the manufacturer or other identification of the packaging specified by the Competent Authority of the country of origin.

Labeling

Each package, overpack, and freight containers shall be labeled with appropriate category. Any labels that do not relate to the contents shall be removed or covered.

Labels should be affixed on two opposite sides of the outside of the package overpacks. In the case of a tank or freight container, it should be on the outside of all four sides. The labels shall not cover the markings specified earlier. Both the limits should be satisfied for a package to belong to a specified category. If either of the limits is exceeded, the package would belong to the next higher but not more than category.

Labeling for Radioactive Contents

Each label should be completed with the information required, i.e., with the content, activity, and TI. Content is specified in the name of the radionuclide or mixture of radionuclide or LSA/SCO material. The maximum activity of the radioactive contents during transport expressed in units of becquerels (Bq) with the appropriate SI prefix symbol [system international (SI). For fissile material, the total mass of fissile nuclides in units of grams (g), or multiples thereof, may be used in place of activity. TI number is determined in accordance with the provisions and no TI entry is required for Category I: White. The criteria for determination of the category of the package are given in the **Table 16.6**.

Caution: If either the radiation level on the surface of the package is >2.0 mSv/h or TI is >10, the package should not be forwarded for transportation without prior permission of the competent authority.

In addition, each package, overpack, and freight container containing fissile material, other than fissile material excepted, shall bear labels conforming to the model in **Figure 16.5**. The labels conforming to the model where applicable shall

TABLE 16.6 Category of packages, overpacks, and freight containers (IAEA safety standards series, 2018).

Category	*Maximum radiation level at any point on external surface of the package (mSv/h)*	*Transport index*
I: White	Not >0.005	0
II: Yellow	>0.005 but not >0.5	>0 but not >1
III: Yellow	>0.5 but not >2.0	>1 but not >10
III: Yellow*	>2 but not >10	>10

*Shall also be transported under exclusive use except for freight containers

Both the limits should be satisfied for a package to belong to a specified category. If either of the limits is exceeded, the package would belong to the next higher category.

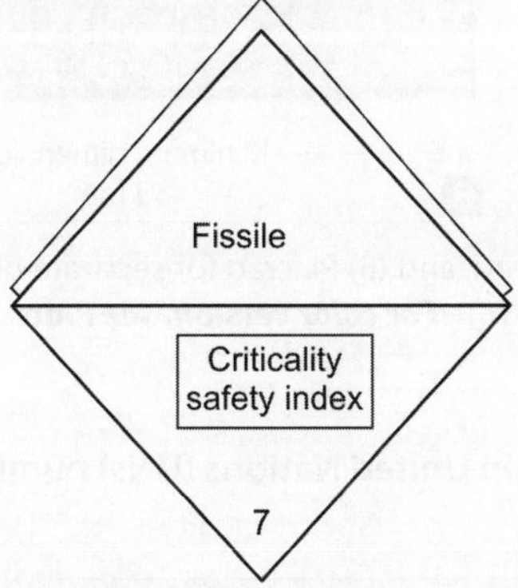

FIG. 16.5: Criticality Safety Index (CSI) label for fissile material [AERB/NRF-TS/SC-1 (Rev.1), 2016].

be affixed adjacent to the labels conforming to the applicable models. In this, the background color of the label shall be white, and the color of the printing shall be black. Each label is completed with CSI (Criticality Safety Index) number as stated in the certificate of approval of the containers. In the case of overpack or containers, it shall bear the sum of the CSIs of all packages contained therein.

Placarding

Large freight containers carrying packages other than excepted packages, and tanks must bear four placards as specified in the code. The placards shall be affixed in a vertical orientation to each sidewall and to each end wall of the large freight container or tank. Any placards that do not relate to the contents shall be removed. Instead of using both labels and placards, it is permitted, as an alternative, to use enlarged labels only, where appropriate with minimum size of 25 cm. The number 7 shall not be <25 mm. The background color of the upper half of the placard shall be yellow, and the lower half white. The color of the trefoil and printing shall be black. The use of the word "Radioactive" at the bottom half is optional.

Where the consignment in the freight container or tank is unpackaged LSA-I or SCO-I or where a consignment in a freight container is required to be shipped under exclusive use and is packaged radioactive material with a single UN number, the appropriate UN number for the consignment shall also be displayed, in black digits not <65 mm high. It can be displayed either in the lower half of the placard against the white background **(Fig. 16.6A)** or on the placard **(Fig. 16.6B)**. The later placard is used for separate display of UN number. The background color of the placard shall be orange, and the border and the UN number shall be black. The symbol ★★★★ denotes the space in which the appropriate UN number for radioactive material, as specified in the safety code is displayed **(Table 16.7)**.

- Transport regulations require placarding of vehicles and containers in most situations.

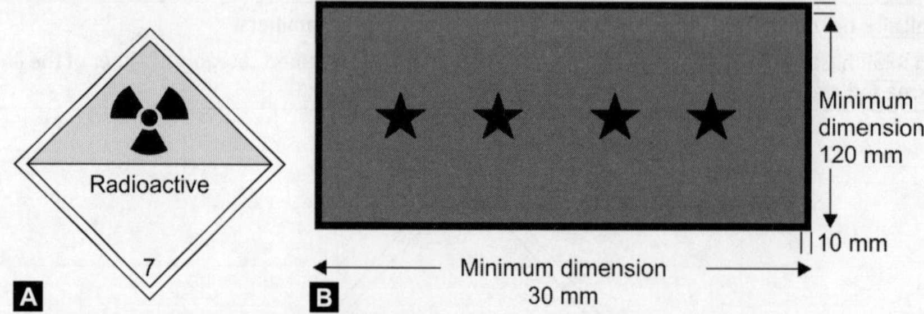

FIGS. 16.6A AND B: (A) Placard, and (B) Placrad for separate display of UN number [AERB/NRF-TS/SC-1 (Rev.1), 2016]. ***(For color version, see Plate 3)***

TABLE 16.7 **List of certain United Nations (UNs) number and proper shipping names.**

UN No	*Proper shipping name and description*
	Excepted package
UN 2908	Radioactive material excepted package: Empty packaging
UN 2909	Radioactive material excepted package: Articles manufactured from natural uranium or depleted uranium or natural thorium
UN 2910	Radioactive material excepted package: Limited quantity of material
UN 2911	Radioactive material, excepted package: Instruments or articles
	Low specific activity material
UN 2912	Radioactive material, low specific activity (LSA-I), nonfissile
UN 3321	Radioactive material, low specific activity (LSA-II), nonfissile
UN 3322	Radioactive material, low specific activity (LSA-III), nonfissile
	Surface contaminated objects
UN 2913	Radioactive material, surface-contaminated objects (SCO-I, SCO-II, or SCO-III), nonfissile
UN 3326	Radioactive material, surface-contaminated objects (SCO-I or SCO-II), fissile
	Type A package
UN 2915	Radioactive material type A package, nonspecial form, nonfissile
UN 3327	Radioactive material type A package, nonspecial form, fissile

Continued

Continued

UN No	***Proper shipping name and description***
Type B(U) package	
UN 2916	Radioactive material type B(U) package—nonfissile
UN 3328	Radioactive material type B(U) package—fissile
Type B(M) package	
UN 2917	Radioactive material type B(M) package—nonfissile
UN 3329	Radioactive material type B(M) package—fissile
Type C package	
UN 3323	Radioactive material, type C package—nonfissile
UN 3330	Radioactive material, type C package—fissile
Courtesy: AERB/NRF-TS/SC-1 (Rev.1), 2016.	

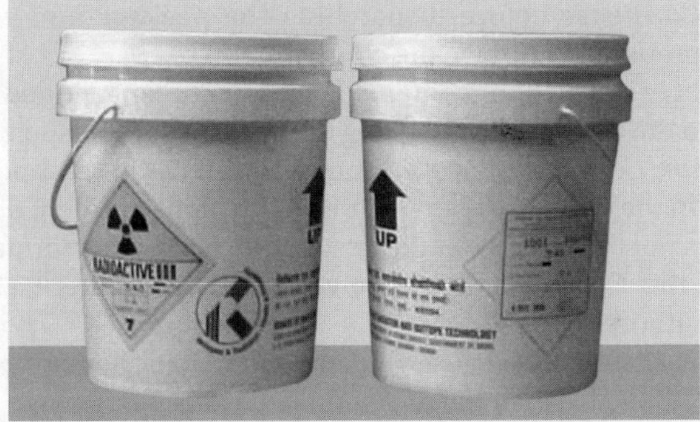

FIG. 16.7: Commercial transport packages with proper labeling.

- Freight containers or tanks should have placard with the United Nations Commodity Number describing the contents, which the police and fire services can interpret.
- Road vehicles should carry a warning placard on each side and the rear, and a fire-resistant notice in the driver's compartment. Packages transported by road require a consignor's certificate giving details of the material being carried; in most cases, the driver will carry a copy.
- Railway vehicles carrying radioactive materials together with parcels or other goods are not required to have placard. Certain professional users may carry radioactive materials in road vehicles without placarding and without consignor's certificates. These users are site radiographers and certain hospital staffs. However, appropriate packages must be used and correctly labeled, and a fire-resistant notice should be carried in the driver's compartment. Commercial transport packages are shown in **Figure 16.7**.

BOOKING, STORAGE, TRANSPORT, AND DELIVERY OF PACKAGE

General

- Do not transport the package as a personal luggage in a bus or in a shared taxi or in the passenger compartment of a train or in the passenger cabin of an aircraft.
- Always book the package as an item of cargo. Do not dispatch the package by post.
- Declare the package as a radioactive consignment in the transport documents. For road transport, in the lorry receipt (LR), the consignor shall declare the consignment by its proper shipping name.
- The transport documents include: (i) Consignor's declaration, (ii) TREM card (transport emergency card), (iii) Instructions to the carrier, (iv) Instructions about emergency measures in case of transport incidents.
- Send a key of the lock along with the transport documents to the *Consignee.*
- Do not dispatch the package without the prior permission of the *Competent authority.*
- Inform the *Consignee* before dispatching the package and ensure that the *Consignee* is prepared to receive the consignment.
- Furnish the set of instructions contained in the document entitled "*Instructions to the Carrier*" to the carrier while booking the package for transport.
- The *Consignor/Consignee/Carrier* should contact the competent authority immediately in the event of: (i) any untoward incident/accident during transport, (ii) nondelivery of the package at the destination within the normal period.
- Ensure that the *Consignee* has received the consignment and inform the Competent Authority accordingly.
- Fill in the checklist (copy enclosed) to ensure that all the requirements for safe transport of radioactive material are complied with.

Responsibilities of the Designer and the Consignor

It is the responsibility of the designer of radioactive material and designer of package, consignor, or their authorized representatives to apply for the necessary approval certificate from the competent authority.

Supplier shall ensure that if the period of validity of such certificate lapses, application for renewal should be submitted to the competent authority sufficiently in advance, so that domestic and international transport of radioactive material is undertaken with valid certificates only. The approval certificates, as applicable, issued by the competent authority conform to the international recommendations.

It is the responsibility of the consignor to ensure that: (1) the consignee of a radioactive consignment is duly authorized by the competent authority if the consignment is imported to India or by the relevant authority if the consignment is being exported from India, to receive the same; (2) multilateral approval is obtained, as necessary; (3) the carrier and cargo personnel are adequately instructed, through appropriate and effective means, about their responsibilities as to safe handling of package, accumulation of packages and segregation of packages from workers, public, undeveloped photographic films and other dangerous goods in conveyance and storage-in transit, emergency response actions during transport of storage-in transit and training of personnel and intimation of noncompliance as prescribed in this safety code; and (4) the consignor shall, prior to the dispatch of the shipment, inform the consignee and confirm that that the consignee is prepared to receive the consignment.

Transportation of radioisotope should follow transport regulation of International Air Transport Association (IATA), International Maritime Organization (IMO), and International Civil Aviation Organization (ICAO). The packages are categorized as expected, industrial, Type A, Type B, and Type C packages and labeled as per IAEA norms. These radioactive material transport labels are of th ree types and affixed on two opposite sides of the packages. The labels contain radioactive symbol, transport index, and hazards class number seven level of the radioactive isotope.

Transport and Storage-in Transit

- Packages, overpacks, and freight containers of radioactive materials and unpacked radioactive materials should be kept segregated during transport and storage-in transit: (i) from the members of public area, with dose criteria of 1 mSv/year, (ii) from workers from regularly occupied working areas, with a dose criteria 5 mSv/year, (iii) from undeveloped and photographic films so that these are not exposed to more than 0.1 mSv per consignment of such film, and (iv) from dangerous goods.
- Category II: Yellow or Category III: Yellow packages or overpacks shall not be carried in compartments occupied by passengers, except those exclusively reserved for couriers specially authorized to accompany such packages or overpacks.
- Consignments shall be securely stowed.
- The average surface heat flux does not exceed 15 W/m^2
- Loading of freight containers and accumulation of packages, overpacks, and freight containers shall be controlled: (i) total number of packages, overpacks, and freight containers abroad a single conveyance shall be limited so that the sum of the TI does not exceed the stated values, (ii) dose rate under routine conditions of transport shall not exceed 2 mSv/h at any point on the external surface of the vehicle or freight container, and 0.1 mSv/h at 2 m from the external surface of the vehicle or freight container, and (iii) sum of the CSI in a freight container and abroad a conveyance shall not exceed the stated values.

Consignor's Declaration

1. Consigner's transport document shall state the following:
   "I hereby declare that the contents of this consignment are fully and accurately described above by the proper shipping name and are classified, packaged, marked, and labeled/placard, and are in all respects in proper condition for transport in accordance with the applicable international and national governmental regulations."
2. If the intent of the declaration is already a condition of transport within a particular international convention, the consignor need not provide such a declaration for that part of the transport covered by the convention.
3. The declaration shall be signed and dated by the consignor. Facsimile signatures are acceptable where applicable laws and regulations recognize the legal validity of facsimile signatures.

4. If the dangerous goods documentation is presented to the carrier by means of electronic data processing (EDP) or electronic data interchange (EDI) transmission techniques, the signature(s) may be replaced by the name(s) (in capitals) of the person authorized to sign.
5. When radioactive material, other than when carried in tanks, is packed, or loaded into any freight container or vehicle that will be transported by sea, the consignor shall obtain from those responsible for packing the container or vehicle, a container/vehicle packing certificate specifying the container/vehicle identification number(s) and certifying that the operation has been carried out in accordance with the applicable conditions.
6. The information required in the transport documents and the container/vehicle packing certificate may be incorporated into a single document, if not, the documents shall be attached one to the other. If the information is incorporated into a single document, the document shall include a signed declaration such as: "It is declared that the packing of the goods into the container/vehicle has been carried out in accordance with the applicable provisions".

   This declaration shall be dated and the person signing it shall be identified on the document. Facsimile signatures are acceptable where applicable laws and regulations recognize the legal validity of facsimile signatures.
7. The declaration shall be made on the same transport document that contains the particulars of consignment **(Table 16.8)**.

TABLE 16.8 **Declaration of radioactive shipment.**

This is to certify that the package containing radioactive material as identified by the following details is safe for transport by: Rail☐ Road☐ Sea☐ Air☐.

Package Forwarded by (Consignor with Contact Number):			
Package Addressed to (Consignee with Contact Number)			
UN class of dangerous goods	7		
	Package 1	Package 2	Package 3
United Nations No			
Proper Shipping Name			
Subsidiary Risk, If Any			
Name of the Radioactive Material			
Quantity/Activity of Radioactive Material			
Package Details: • Dimensions of the package • Weight of the package • Type of package*			
Radiation Level on the Surface of the Package in mSv/h			

Continued

Continued

Transport Index of the Package			
Category of the Package	I-White/ II-Yellow/ III-Yellow	I-White/ II-Yellow/ III-Yellow	I-WHITE/ II-Yellow/ III-Yellow
*In case of type B package, Competent Authority identification number along with serial number should also be given. *Courtesy*: AERB: www.aerb.gov.in.			

I hereby declare that the contents of this consignment are fully and accurately described above by the proper shipping name and are classified, packed, marked, and labeled, and are in all respects in proper condition for transport according to the applicable regulations.

Date: Signature:

Name and Address:

Instructions to the Carrier

- The package should be transported by the most direct route.
- Intermediate offloading and reloading of the package should be avoided wherever possible.
- Package should be handled carefully. Suitable mechanical means should be deployed for handling packages weighing >30 kg.
- Persons should not be allowed to sit on the package or spend more time than the necessary time in the vicinity of the package.
- The package should not be transported along with other dangerous good such as explosives and inflammables.
- The package should not be transported/stored together with photosensitive films/plates.
- The package should be kept segregated from spaces occupied by passengers and public.
- If several packages containing radioactive material are to be transported, then the total number of packages loaded in a single vehicle should be so restricted that the sum of the transport indexes of the packages does not exceed 50, except in case of exclusive use. Further, the total number of packages stacked in a storage area should be so limited that, in a given stack, the above limit of 50 of the sum of transport indexes is not exceeded and such stacks containing radioactive consignments are separated by at least 6 m.
- If the shipment is under exclusive use, i.e., the entire conveyance is for the proposed transport of radioactive material then: (i) there should not be any intermediate loading and unloading operations of other goods, and (ii) nothing other than the intended radioactive material along with its accessories should be carried in this vehicle.
- At the destination, it should be ensured that the package is delivered to the consignee to whom it is indeed addressed.
- One copy of the TREM card should be carried in the vehicle carrying the radioactive cargo. If the package(s) get(s) involved in an accident or get(s) damaged during transport, the instructions specified in the TREM card should be implemented **(Table 16.9)**.

TABLE 16.9 **TREM card.**

Cargo	Radioactive material
Nature of hazard	Radioactive material, potential external and internal exposure
Protective device to be carried in the vehicle	One set each, for the driver and his assistant, of protective clothing (boots, gloves, overalls, caps). Six number of big polythene bags for collecting contaminated material
Emergency action	• Inspect the package visually. If it is intact, ensure onward journey in the same or another vehicle • In case of fire, fight from a distance • If the package appears to be damaged, cordon a distance of 3 m around the package • Obtain the names and addresses of persons who might have been exposed to radiation and convey the particulars to the Head, RSD, AERB and to the Head, RP and AD, BARC
Nature of hazard	Radioactive material, potential external and internal exposure
Protective device to be carried in the vehicle	One set each, for the driver and his assistant, of protective clothing (boots, gloves, overalls, caps). Six number of big polythene bags for collecting contaminated material
Emergency action	• Inspect the package visually. If it is intact, ensure onward journey in the same or another vehicle • In case of fire, fight from a distance • If the package appears to be damaged, cordon a distance of 3 m around the package • Obtain the names and addresses of persons who might have been exposed to radiation and convey the particulars to the Head, RSD, AERB and to the Head, RP and AD, BARC
First aid	Thoroughly wash the affected skin with plenty of water
Contact telephone numbers for advice and assistance	• Contact the consignor at the address given on the package • Emergency Control Room, Crisis Management Group, DAE, Mumbai, 400001 Telephone: 022-22023978; Telefax: 022-22021714; Fax-022-22830441 Mobile: +91-9969201364; E-mail: daeecr@dae.gov.in Alternate CMG: DAE Emergency Control Room (ECR) located at Anushakti Nagar (VSB) Telephone: 022-25991070; Telefax: 022-25515283; Fax: 022-25991080/022-25993080; Mobile: +91-9969201365; E-mail: vsbecr@npcil.co.in
Telegram	REGATOM, Chembur or HEAD, RP and AD, BARC, Chembur
Fax	022-25583230 (AERB), 022-255055151 (BARC)

(TREM card: transport emergency card; AERB: Atomic Energy Regulatory Board; BARC: Bhabha Atomic Research Center)

Courtesy: AERB/https://www.aerb.gov.in.

- If the package is not claimed by the consignee at the destination, it should not be auctioned or otherwise disposed of. The matter should be brought to the notice of the consignor and Head, RSD, AERB, Niyamak Bhavan, Anushaktinagar, Mumbai, 400094 and such measures as recommended in this regard by Head, RSD, AERB, Mumbai, should be duly implemented.

EMERGENCY MEASURES FOR TRANSPORT INCIDENTS INVOLVING RADIOACTIVE CARGO

About the Package

Packaging, which is permitted to be used for transport of radioactive materials, is generally designed to prescribe standards aimed at prevention of release of the contents and of excessive exposure of public to radiation. Commonly, there are two types of packages, namely, Type A and Type B(U)/(M).

Type A packages are designed to withstand minor mishaps, for example, falling of the package from the vehicle while loading/unloading, rain, falling of small objects on to the package, etc. If a Type A package is involved in a severe accident such as vehicle rolling over, then the package may be damaged through the loss of shielding or release of the contents. In such a situation, one follow instructions as given below under the heading *Emergency Action and First Aid.*

A Type B package is designed to withstand severe accidents. However, after severe accident, the package may be damaged, though the chances are remote. In such a situation, one follow instructions as given below under the heading *Emergency Action and First Aid.*

Nature of Hazard

The hazard associated with radioactive consignment is exposure to radiation. Such exposure may be external and/or internal in nature. If the radioactive content is an indispersible solid or capsule, the hazard is likely to be external. If the content is indispersible form, in the unlikely event of a severe accident, the potential for internal and sometimes, in addition, external exposure may exist.

Protective Devices to be Carried in the Vehicle

The driver of the vehicle and his assistant should each have some protective device if the vehicle carries a package containing dispersible radioactive material. The protective equipment should be carried in appropriate numbers and includes rubber shoes, latex gloves, coveralls, big empty polythene bags, big polythene sheets (3 × 3 m), cotton wool (for liquid radioactive material). If the vehicle does not carry any package containing dispersible radioactive material, the protective equipment would not be required from radiation safety standpoint.

Emergency Action and First Aid

If an accident occurs, do not be panic and rescue the injured. If life is at stake, save the life first. It is highly unlikely that in a transport accident involving the commonly deployed small type A and Type B(U)/(M) packages, any significant hazard to the rescuer will result from radiation. If any of the packages, which are damaged in the accident, but containing radioactive material in a dispersible form, one should hold a cloth towel or a handkerchief over his/her mouth and nose.

If there is fire, summon assistance from the local public and fire brigade. Fight fire from a distance. Follow these instructions: (1) fight fire as far upwind as possible, (2) keep out of smoke, fumes, and dust, (3) wear the coverall, gloves, and shoes and cover mouth and nose with handkerchief, (4) spend minimum time near the package, (5) keep bystanders upwind at least 5 m away, and (6) inspect the packages.

If the packages appear to be intact, ensure onward journey in the same vehicle. If the vehicle cannot be released for onward journey for a long time, then arrange for onward journey of the package in some other vehicle. If the package appears to be damaged, wrap it in a polythene bag, segregate the package, and cordon a distance 5 m around the package.

If the contents of the package appear to have spilled, then take the following measures: (1) assume that the area and the objects on which the spillage has occurred are contaminated, (2) wear the shoes, gloves, and coveralls, (3) collect the spillage, using cotton wool, in a polythene bag, (4) wrap the damaged package in polyethene bags, (5) cover the contaminated objects and contaminated area with polythene sheets, (6) do not eat, drink, or smoke within the cordon, (7) take measures to prevent a fire accident, (8) seek assistance from AERB/BARC as given below, and (9) do not allow the public within the cordon unless so advised by the radiological safety authorities from AERB/BARC, Mumbai.

All persons who were engaged in the emergency response measures should carefully and thoroughly wash the affected parts of the skin with plenty of water. Obtain the names and addresses of persons who may have been exposed to radiation and convey the particulars to the Head, RSD, AERB, Niyamak Bhavan, Anushaktinagar, Mumbai, 400094.

Assistance

Telephones for Advice and Assistance: Chairman, Crisis Management Group, DAE, Mumbai, 400001, Telephone (round the clock) 022-22023978, 22830441, 22862595; Fax: 022-22830441.

While seeking advice and assistance, furnish the following particulars: (1) the place where the accident occurred, (2) the date and time of occurrence of the incident, (3) whether the incident involved impact, fire, or both, (4) details of emergency action taken, (5) the condition of the packages, whether damage/spillage suspected, and (6) the name and addresses of persons who may have been exposed to radiation.

Act exactly in accordance with the instructions given by the above authorities. Onward journey of the packages which were damaged in the incident may be arranged only after obtaining clearance from the above authorities.

General

Every driver should ensure that he is completely familiar with the "Instructions in Writing......." and the procedures recommended in the TREM card. Prior to undertaking the journey, the driver should ensure that he carries the following items with him: the "Instructions in Writing..........", the "TREM card", the protective devices as specified under the heading *Protective Devices to be carried in the Vehicle* above. The assistant accompanying the driver should also be familiar with these instructions.

BIBLIOGRAPHY

1. Atomic Energy Regulatory Board. Security of radioactive material during transport: AERB/NRF-TS/SG-10, 2008. [online] Available from https://aerb.gov.in/images/PDF/CodesGuides/RadiationFacility/Transport/2.pdf. [Last accessed December, 2022]
2. Atomic Energy Regulatory Board. Safe transport of radioactive material, AERB safety code: AERB/NRF-TS/SC-1 (Rev.1), 2016. [online] Available from https://www.aerb.gov.in/images/PDF/CodesGuides/RadiationFacility/Transport/1.pdf. [Last accessed December, 2022]
3. International Atomic Energy Agency. Generic procedures for assessment and response during a radiological emergency, IAEA-TECDOC-1162, IAEA, Vienna 2000. [online] Available from https://www-pub.iaea.org/mtcd/publications/pdf/te_1162_prn.pdf. [Last accessed December, 2022]
4. International Atomic Energy Agency. Regulations for the safe transport of radioactive material-2018th edition, IAEA safety standards series ,No.SSR-6 (Rev.1) Vienna, 2018. [online] Available from https://www-pub.iaea.org/MTCD/Publications/PDF/PUB1798_web.pdf. [Last accessed December, 2022]
5. Atomic Energy Regulatory Board (AERB)website: https://www.aerb.gov.in

CHAPTER 17

Regulation for Medical Radiation Facilities

INTRODUCTION

Regulations are requirements that is applied to individuals, institutions and local organizations. It sets standards that will limit the hazards to the public and radiation workers. Radiation has both beneficial and harmful effects, regulation of medical radiation is very much essential. It not only protect the individuals but also the environment as whole. Hence, there is need to respect and follow current radiation regulations of an individual country. The radiation workers should understand the regulation and implement fully in their practices. This not only protects them from radiation hazards but also maintains the ethics and moral value of the profession.

NATIONAL LEGISLATION

Atomic Energy Act, 1962

The primary legislation to regulate the use of ionizing radiation, in India, is the Atomic Energy Act, 1962. The Act and the secondary legislation, viz., Radiation Protection Rules 1971 (RPR-1971) provide necessary regulatory infrastructure for effective implementation of radiation protection program (RPP). Atomic Energy (Radiation Protection) Rules, 2004, have replaced the RPR-1971 and provide the current regulation rules.

The Act empowers the Government of India to exercise control over production and the use of atomic energy. It offers special provisions to safety under Section 17 and powers to make rules under Section 30 of the Act. The Act envisages control over premises where radioactive substances are handled or radiation-generating equipment is operated. The Act emphasizes safety while working with radiation. It deals with control over possession, use, sale, and transport of radioactive materials and cognizance of offences.

Atomic Energy Regulatory Board

Atomic Energy Regulatory Board (AERB) was constituted on November 15, 1983, by the President of India by exercising the powers conferred by Section 27 of the Atomic Energy Act, 1962 (33 of 1962). It is an apex body that regulates the use of ionizing radiation in the country. The AERB is entrusted with the responsibility of developing and implementing appropriate regulatory measures aimed at ensuring radiation safety in applications involving ionizing radiations. The board is fully empowered to lay down standards and frame rules and regulations.

The Chairman, AERB, is the *competent authority*, recognized by the Government of India for enforcing provisions of radiation safety in the use of ionizing radiation. AERB has jurisdiction over all the units of the department of atomic energy and all radiation installations in the country. The mission of the board is to ensure that the use of ionizing radiation and nuclear energy does not cause undue risk to health and environment.

The board covers safety aspects of all areas of nuclear fuel cycle and use of radiation in medicine, agriculture, industry, and research and transport of radioactive materials. The board is assisted by Health, Safety, and Environment group of Bhabha Atomic Research Center (BARC), viz., Radiological Physics and Advisory Division (RPAD), advisory committees, and task groups.

The major objectives of AERB are to develop and publicize specific codes and guides, which will deal with radiation safety aspects of various applications of radiations. It will also issue authorization related to site, design, manufacture, construction, commissioning, operation, maintenance, and decommissioning and disposal of radioactive sources. The legislation and various rules related to radiation protection in medicine are given in the safety codes.

Safety Codes

- *Radiation safety in manufacture, supply, and use of medical diagnostic X-ray equipment*: AERB Safety Code No—AERB/RF-MED/SC-3 (Rev. 2), 2016
- *Safe transport of radioactive material*: AERB Safety Code No—AERB/NRF-TS/SC-1 (Rev. 1), 2016
- *Radiation therapy sources, equipment, and installations*: AERB Safety Code No—AERB/RF-MED/SC-1 (Rev. 1), 2011
- *Nuclear medicine facilities (NMFs)*: AERB Safety Code No—AERB/RF-MED/SC-2 (Rev. 2), 2011
- *Security of radioactive sources in radiation facilities*: AERB Safety Code No—AERB/RF-RS/SG-1, 2011
- *Security of radioactive material during transport*: AERB Safety Code No—AERB/NRF-TS/SG-10, 2008

Atomic Energy (Radiation Protection) Rules, 2004 (Published in the Gazette of India: September 11, 2004) Part-II: Section 3: Subsection (I) Government of India, Department of Atomic Energy, Mumbai, August 25th, 2004

G.S.R. 303

In exercise of the powers conferred by Section 30 read with Section 3 and clause (i) and subclauses (c) and (d) of clause (ii) of Subsection (1), Subsection (4) of Section 14, and Sections 16, 17, and other relevant Sections of the Atomic Energy Act (33 of 1962) and all other powers enabling it in this behalf, and in supersession of Radiation Protection Rules 1971 except as respects things done or omitted to be done before such supersessions, the Central Government hereby makes the following rules, namely:

Rule 1: Short Title, Extent, and Commencement

1. These rules may be called the Atomic Energy (Radiation Protection) Rules, 2004.
2. These rules shall apply to practices adopted and interventions applied with respect to radiation sources.
3. They extend to the whole of India.
4. They shall come into force from the date of their final publication in the official gazette.

Rule 2: Definitions

1. It defines various terms and terminology used in the atomic energy Act, 1962 and Atomic Energy (Radiation Protection) Rules, 2004 (Refer Act for details).

Rule 3: License

1. No person shall—without a license—(a) establish a radiation installation for siting, design, construction, commissioning, and operation; and (b) decommission a radiation installation.
2. No person shall handle any radioactive material or operate any radiation-generating equipment except in accordance with the terms and conditions of a license.
3. A *license* shall be issued for sources and practices associated with the operation of (i) nuclear fuel cycle facilities, (ii) land-based high-intensity gamma irradiators other than gamma, irradiation chambers, (iii) particle accelerators used for research and industrial applications, (iv) neutron generators, (v) facilities engaged in the commercial production of radioactive material or radiation-generating equipment, (vi) telegamma and accelerators used in radiotherapy, (vii) computed tomography (CT) unit, (viii) interventional radiological X-ray unit, (ix) industrial radiography, and (x) such other source or practice as may be notified by the competent authority, from time to time.

   Provided that for sources and practices associated with the operation of (i) brachytherapy, (ii) deep X-ray units, superficial and contact therapy X-ray units, (iii) gamma irradiation chambers, (iv) nuclear medicine facilities, (v) facilities engaged in the commercial production of nucleonic gauges and consumer products containing radioactive material, and (vi) such other source or practice as may be notified by the competent authority, from time to time, an *authorization* shall be necessary.

   Provided further that for sources and practices associated with the operation of (i) medical diagnostic X-ray equipment including therapy simulator, (ii) analytical X-ray equipment used for research, (iii) nucleonic gauges, (iv) RIA laboratories, (v) radioactive sources in tracer studies, (vi) biomedical research using radioactive material, and (vii) such other source or practice as may be notified by the competent authority, from time to time, a *registration* shall be necessary.

   Provided, also that for (i) approval for siting, design, construction, commissioning, and decommissioning of a radiation installation, (ii) approval for sealed sources, radiation-generating equipment, and equipment-containing radioactive sources, for the purposes of manufacture and supply, (iii) approval for package design for transport of radioactive material, (iv) approval for shipment approval for radioactive consignments, and (v) such other source or practice as may be notified by the competent authority, from time to time, *consent* shall be necessary.

4. The license shall not be transferable without the prior approval of the competent authority.

Rule 4: Fees for License

The competent authority may prescribe by notification in the Official Gazette, appropriate fees payable for issuance of license specified in these rules.

Rule 5: Exemption

The use and disposal of a substance and materials, which spontaneously emit radiation not exceeding the level of radiation prescribed by notification issued under clause (i) of Subsection (1) of Section 2 of the Act and the use of radiation-generating equipment, devices, or appliances emitting radiation not exceeding the limit determined by the Central Government under clause (g) of Section 3 of the Act, are exempted from the purview of Rule 3.

Rule 6: Exclusion

Exposures resulting from naturally occurring radionuclides present in the human body, cosmic radiation at the earth surface, unmodified concentrations of radionuclides in raw materials, and from other sources and practices, which may be prescribed as not amenable for control, are excluded from these rules.

Rule 7: Conditions Precedent to the Issuance of a License

1. An application for license shall be made by the competent authority and by an employer or a person duly authorized by him.
2. No license to handle radioactive material, or to operate radiation-generating equipment, shall be issued to a person unless, in the opinion of the competent authority:
    a. The application for such license is for purposes envisaged by the Act.
    b. Documentation relevant to the license and complete in all respects is submitted to the competent authority.
    c. In respect of approval for siting, design, construction, commissioning, and decommissioning of a radiation installation, the proposed equipment, facilities, and handling procedures afford adequate protection during normal or intended operations.
    d. The applicant has demonstrated compliance with the provisions of the relevant safety codes and safety standards specified by the competent authority
    e. In respect of license for operation of a radiation installation:
        i. All the requirements relating to safety specified by the competent authority in the relevant safety codes and safety standards have been satisfied in the construction of the radiation installation
        ii. Workers have appropriate training and instructions in radiation safety, in addition to the appropriate qualification and training required for performing their intended tasks,

iii. A Radiological Safety Officer (RSO) is designated in accordance with Rule 19

iv. Appropriate radiation monitors and dosimetry devices are available with the applicant for purposes of radiation surveillance

f. The equipment, facilities, and handling procedures afford adequate protection during normal operations, minimize occurrence of potential exposures, and enable appropriate remedial actions to be taken in the event of an accident.

3. No type approval of sealed sources, radiation-generating equipment, and equipment containing a radioactive source for the purpose of manufacture and supply or package design approval for transport of radioactive material or shipment approval for radioactive consignment or any other approval as notified under third provision to Rule 3, by the competent authority, may be issued unless, in the opinion of the competent authority, the applicant has demonstrated compliance with the relevant safety codes and safety standards specified by him.

Rule 8: Issuance of License

The license shall be issued within a period of 180 days from the date of receipt of the application subject to the condition that all the requirements for issuance of the license have been duly fulfilled.

Rule 9: Period of Validity of License

Every license issued under Rule 3 shall, unless otherwise specified, be valid for a period of 5 years from the date of issue of such license.

Rule 10: Suspension, Modification, or Withdrawal of a License

The competent authority may—(i) if in its opinion, the licensee has contravened any of the provisions of these rules, or (ii) considers it to be necessary in public interest pertaining to radiation safety; after giving a show-cause notice to the licensee and giving him an opportunity to make a representation within a period of 30 days from the date of receipt of the notice by him against the action proposed to be taken and on consideration of his representation; (a) suspend the operation of the license for a specified period of time, or (b) revoke or modify the terms and conditions of the license.

Rule 11: Modification of Radiation Installation or Change in Working Condition

No modification to an existing radiation installation or no change in working conditions, therein, affecting safety shall be done without the prior approval of the competent authority.

Rule 12: Restrictions on Use of Sources

1. The licensee shall not handle any source:
   a. Other than those specified in the license
   b. For any purpose other than those specified in the license
   c. In any location except as specified in the license.
2. The licensee shall ensure that individuals other than those who may be specified in the license do not handle the source.

Rule 13: Restriction on Certain Practices

1. Practices such as deliberate addition of radioactive substances in foodstuffs, beverages, toys, personal ornaments, and cosmetics or any other commodity or product intended for ingestion, inhalation, or percutaneous intake by, or application to, a human being and sale, import or export of such products shall not be permitted.
2. Activation of the aforesaid products shall not be permitted.

Rule 14: Radiation Symbol or Warning Sign

1. The radiation symbol or warning sign shall be conspicuously and prominently displayed at all times: (a) on externally visible surfaces of radiation equipment, and containers for storage of radioactive materials, packages for radioactive materials, and vehicles carrying such packages, (b) at the entrance to the room housing the radiation-generating equipment, and (c) at the entrance of controlled area and supervised area.
2. The radiation symbol shall not be used for any purpose other than those mentioned in these rules.
3. The specification of the radiation symbol or warning sign shall be as prescribed by the competent authority, by order for that purpose.

Rule 15: Dose Limits and Other Regulatory Constraints

The licensee shall ensure compliance with the dose limits and other regulatory constraints specified by the competent authority by order under these rules.

Rule 16: Safety Standards and Safety Codes

The competent authority may issue safety codes and safety standards, from time to time, prescribing the requirements for radiation installation, sealed sources, radiation-generating equipment and equipment containing radioactive sources, and transport of radioactive material and the licensee shall ensure compliance with the same.

Rule 17: Prohibition of Employment of Persons below Certain Age

1. No person under the age of 18 years shall be employed as a worker.
2. No person under the age of 16 years shall be taken as trainee or employed as an apprentice for radiation work.

Rule 18: Classified Worker

The employer shall designate as classified workers, those of his employees, who are likely to receive an effective dose in excess of three-tenths of the average annual dose limits notified by the competent authority and shall forthwith inform those employees that they have been so designated.

Rule 19: Radiological Safety Officer

Every employer shall designate, with the written approval of the competent authority, a person having appropriate qualifications as RSO.

Rule 20: Responsibilities of the Employer

1. Every employer shall: (a) ensure that provisions of these rules are implemented by the licensee, RSO, and other worker (s), (b) provide facilities and equipment to the licensee, RSO, and other worker(s) to carry out their functions effectively in conformity with the regulatory constraints, (c) prior to employment of a worker, procure from his former employer, where applicable, the dose records and health surveillance reports, (d) upon termination of service of worker provide to his new employer on request his dose records and health surveillance reports, (e) furnish to each worker dose records and health surveillance reports of the worker in his employment annually, as and when requested by the worker and at the termination of his service, (f) inform the competent authority if the licensee or the RSO or any worker leaves the employment, and (g) arrange for health surveillance of workers as specified under Rule 25.
2. The employer shall be the custodian of radiation sources in his possession and shall ensure physical security of the sources at all times.
3. The employer shall inform the competent authority, within 24 hours of any accident involving a source or loss of source of which he is the custodian.

Rule 21: Responsibilities of the Licensee

1. The responsibility for implementing the terms and conditions of the license shall rest with the licensee.
2. The licensee shall comply with the surveillance procedures, safety codes, and safety standards specified by the competent authority.
3. Every licensee shall establish written procedures and plans for controlling, monitoring, and assessment of exposure for ensuring adequate protection of workers, members of the public and the environment and patients, wherever applicable.
4. The licensee shall comply with the provision of rules for safe disposal of radioactive waste issued under the Act.
5. Without prejudice to the generality of the above, the licensee shall (a) not allow workers, other than those specified in subclause (ii) of clause (e) of subrule (2) of Rule 7 and already dealt with under Rule 17, (b) maintain records of workers as specified under Rule 24, (c) arrange for preventive and remedial maintenance of radiation protection equipment, and monitoring instruments, (d) in consultation with the RSO, investigate any case of exposure in excess of regulatory constraints received by individual workers and maintain records of such investigations, (e) inform competent authority promptly of the occurrence, investigation, and follow-up actions in cases of exposure in excess of regulatory constraints, including steps to prevent recurrence of such incidents, (f) carry out physical verification of radioactive material periodically and maintain inventory, (g) inform appropriate law enforcement agency in the locality of any loss of source, (h) inform the employer and the competent authority of any loss of source, (i) investigate and inform the competent authority of any accident involving source and maintain record of investigations, (j) verify the performance of radiation monitoring systems, safety interlocks, protective devices, and any other safety systems in the radiation installation, (k) in consultation with RSO, prepare emergency plans, as specified in Rule 33, for

responding to accident to mitigate their consequences and ensure emergency preparedness measures, (l) conduct or arrange for quality assurance (QA) tests of structures, systems, components, and sources and related equipment, (m) advise the employer about the modifications in working condition of a pregnant worker, (n) inform the competent authority if the RSO or a worker leaves the employment, and (o) inform the competent authority when he leaves the employment.

6. The licensee shall ensure that the workers are familiarized with contents of the relevant surveillance procedures, safety standards, safety codes, safety aides, and safety manuals issued by the competent authority and emergency response plans.

Rule 22: Responsibilities of the Radiological Safety Officer

1. The RSO shall be responsible for advising and assisting the employer and licensee on safety aspects aimed at ensuring that the provisions of these rules are complied with.
2. The RSO shall: (a) carry out routine measurements and analysis on radiation and radioactivity levels in the controlled area, supervised area of the radiation installation, and maintain records of the results thereof, (b) investigate any situation that could lead to potential exposures, (c) advise the employer regarding: (i) the necessary steps aimed at ensuring that the regulatory constraints and the terms and conditions of the license are adhered to; (ii) the safe storage and movement of radioactive material within the radiation installation; (iii) initiation of suitable remedial measures in respect of any situation that could lead to potential exposures; and (iv) routine measurements and analysis on radiation and radioactivity levels in the off-site environment of the radiation installation and maintenance of the results thereof, (d) ensure that—(i) reports on all hazardous situations along with details of any immediate remedial actions taken are made available to the employer and licensee for reporting to the competent authority and a copy endorsed to the competent authority; (ii) QA tests of structures, systems, components, and sources, as applicable, are conducted; and (iii) monitoring instruments are calibrated periodically, (e) assist the employer in—(i) instructing the workers on hazards of radiation and on suitable safety measures and work practices aimed at optimizing exposures to radiation sources, (ii) the safe disposal of radioactive wastes, and (iii) developing suitable emergency response plans to deal with accidents and maintaining emergency preparedness, (f) advise the licensee on—(i) the modifications in working condition of a pregnant worker and (ii) the safety and security of radioactive sources, (g) furnish to the licensee and the competent authority the periodic reports on safety status of the radiation installation, and (h) inform the competent authority when he leaves the employment.

Rule 23: Responsibilities of Worker

1. Every worker shall observe the safety requirements and follow safety procedures and instructions and shall refrain from any willful act that could be detrimental to self, co-workers, the radiation installation, and public.

2. The worker shall: (a) provide to the employer information about his previous occupations including radiation work, if any, (b) make proper use of such protective equipment, radiation monitors and personnel monitoring devices as provided, and (c) inform the licensee and the RSO, of any accident or potentially hazardous situation that may come to his notice.
3. A female worker shall, on becoming aware that she is pregnant, notify the employer, licensee, and RSO in order that her working conditions may be modified, if necessary.

Rule 24: Records of Workers

1. Every licensee shall maintain complete and up-to-date records of: (a) personnel monitoring under clause (b) of subrule (2) of Rule 27, in the format as specified by order by the competent authority, and (b) the health surveillance specified in Rule 25.
2. Such records shall be preserved during the working life of each worker, and afterwards until the worker attains or would have attained the age of 75 years, or not less than 30 years after the termination of the work involving occupational exposure whichever is later.
3. A worker shall have access to his personnel monitoring and the health surveillance records.

Rule 25: Health Surveillance of Workers

1. Every employer shall provide the services of a physician with appropriate qualifications to undertake occupational health surveillance of classified workers.
2. Every worker, initially on employment and classified worker, thereafter at least once in 3 years as long as the individual is employed, shall be subjected to the following: (a) general medical examination as specified by order by the competent authority and (b) health surveillance to decide on the fitness of each worker for the intended task.
3. The health surveillance shall include: (a) special tests or medical examinations as specified by order by the competent authority, for workers who have received dose in excess of regulatory constraints and (b) counseling of pregnant workers.

Rule 26: Medical Exposures

The licensee carrying out diagnostic or therapeutic work using radiation-generating equipment, sealed or unsealed sources, shall for optimizing the medical exposure ensure that: (a) performance of the equipment is verified periodically by appropriate QA tests, (b) records are maintained for a period specified by the competent authority of—(i) radiation doses received by therapy patients, (ii) activity administered to patients for diagnostic and therapeutic purposes, and (iii) other relevant parameters, (c) the exposure of humans for biomedical research is carried out only on healthy volunteers with their prior consent in writing. The methodology, the number of volunteers, and the radiation dose they are subjected to shall be reviewed by the ethical review committee constituted by the employer, and (d) any accidental medical exposure is investigated, and a written report is submitted to the competent authority.

Rule 27: Radiation Surveillance Requirements

1. The competent authority may by order specify appropriate radiation surveillance requirements and procedures and the employer and the licensee shall comply with them.
2. Without prejudice to the generality of the foregoing provisions, such radiation surveillance requirements and procedures may provide that: (a) the siting, design, construction, commissioning, operation, servicing, and maintenance and decommissioning of facilities involving the use of radiation, and disposal of radioactive material shall be done in accordance with the specifications laid down by the competent authority in the relevant safety codes and safety standards, (b) the workers shall be subjected to personnel monitoring and health surveillance and appropriate records shall be maintained, (c) transport of radioactive material in public domain shall be in accordance with the procedures laid down by the competent authority and in accordance with the other regulations pertaining to transport by different modes, and (d) appropriate QA requirements in the above.

Rule 28: Directives in the Cases of Exposures in Excess of Regulatory Constraints

1. When, in the opinion of the competent authority, any worker has exceeded the dose constraints, the competent authority may, without prejudice to other course of action available, issue appropriate directives for controlling further exposure and the employer shall comply with the directives.
2. If a worker discontinues radiation work under the directives of the competent authority issued under this rule, the employer shall assign alternative work not involving exposure to radiation, until the competent authority is satisfied about the fitness of the worker to resume radiation work.
3. The employer shall comply with restrictions, if any, that the competent authority may impose in this regard.

Rule 29: Power to Appoint or Recognize Persons or Agencies

The competent authority may, from time to time, appoint or recognize persons or agencies having the qualifications and expertise, prescribed in the relevant safety code, for the purpose of performing any of the functions entrusted to them by the authority and for ensuring compliance with radiological surveillance.

Rule 30: Inspection of Premises, Radiation Installations, and Conveyances

1. Any person duly authorized under Subsection (4) of Section 17 of the Act may, for the purposes of enforcement of these rules, inspect any premises, or radiation installation, or conveyance.
2. The date and time of inspection may or may not be informed to the employer or the licensee prior to the inspection.
3. The employer and the licensee shall extend all assistance to enable the inspection to be carried out effectively and unhindered.
4. The findings of the inspection shall be forwarded to the licensee for necessary corrective actions.

5. Inspection may be carried out at all licensing stages, namely, siting, construction, commissioning, operation, and decommissioning.
6. The person authorized to conduct inspection may: (a) inspect, from safety point of view, to ensure that the licensee has fulfilled the radiological safety requirements for carrying out the practices at the radiation installation as per the stipulations laid down in the license. This shall include: (i) checking, whether the safety-related structures, systems, components, and devices are of approved quality based on the relevant safety codes and safety standards specified by the competent authority and that they are functioning as per the design intent, checking that respective operating personnel are competent to operate the facility, (ii) that the facilities are operating as per the approved technical specification; and (iii) conducting all such examinations including verification of relevant records as may be considered necessary, (b) make such tests and measurements as may be necessary for the purpose of assessing radiation safety, (c) investigate unusual incidents or accidents, if any, that had occurred at the radiation installation and arrive at the reasons for the same and recommend corrective measures, (d) review and verify whether the corrective actions have been implemented, and (e) inspect radioactive consignments in any conveyance carrying radioactive material and inspect any package containing radioactive material.

Rule 31: Power to Investigate, Seal, or Seize Radiation Installation or Radioactive Material and to Give Direction to the Employer

1. Any person duly authorized under Section 17 of the Act, may, after inspection, carry out investigation for the purposes of determining contravention of any of the provisions of these rules.
2. The investigation may be carried out against a complaint or on suspicion or after an unusual incident or accident.
3. The person authorized to investigate may—(a) seal any radiation installation or any conveyance carrying radioactive materials or seize any radioactive material or contaminated equipment, and (b) indicate in writing to the employer any recommendation aimed at ensuring adequate protection and the licensee shall comply with the same.

Rule 32: Directives in Case of Accidents

1. In the event of an accident involving the source or release of radioactive material, the competent authority may—(a) intervene and issue such directions as deemed fit and proper under the circumstances in the interest of radiation safety and the employer shall act as per the directions of the competent authority and shall make every effort to mitigate the consequences of the accident, or (b) the competent authority may assign experts to give advice or render assistance in mitigating the consequences of the accident and the expenses incurred, if any, shall be reimbursed by the employer.
2. In the interest of safety of the radiation installation, workers, public, and the environment, the competent authority may issue such directions as it may deem fit for ensuring safety including the immediate shutting down of the radiation installation and the employer shall comply with the directions.

Rule 33: Emergency Preparedness

1. The licensee shall prepare emergency response plans as specified by the competent authority in the relevant safety codes and maintain emergency preparedness.
2. The licensee shall submit the response plans for plant emergencies and site emergencies to the competent authority for approval.
3. The licensee shall submit the response plans for off-site emergencies prepared by the appropriate authorities to the competent authority for review.
4. In respect of radiation installations governed by clause (a) of subrule (3) of Rule 3 and clause (b) of subrule (3) of Rule 3, emergency response plans shall be submitted to the competent authority prior to the commissioning of the installations.
5. Any modification to the emergency plan shall require prior approval of or review by the competent authority.

Rule 34: Decommissioning of Radiation Installation

1. When a radiation installation or radiation-generating equipment ceases to be in use, the employer shall ensure its decommissioning.
2. No employer shall decommission a radiation installation without the prior approval of the competent authority.
3. The decommissioning plan shall take due cognizance of disposal of radioactive wastes, recycling of materials, and reuse of equipment and premises.
4. The licensee shall comply with such directive as may be issued by the competent authority to ensure adequate protection of the persons in and around the decommissioned installation.

Rule 35: Offences and Penalties

Any person who contravenes the provisions of these rules or any of the terms and conditions of license issued hereunder shall be punishable as provided for under the Act.

RESPONSIBILITIES OF EMPLOYER, LICENSEE, RADIOLOGICAL SAFETY OFFICER, AND RADIOISOTOPE SUPPLIER

Registration of Institute in e-LORA

e-LORA stands for e-licensing of radiation application. It is a web-based ICT (Information and Communication Technology) application establishing direct communication channel between AERB and its stakeholders for exchange of information and communication transaction for delivering its regulatory services as well as for achieving higher efficiency, reliability, and transparency in dealings. The e-LORA system is designed to automate the comprehensive business processes of radiological application regulations targeted to large number of facilities using ionizing radiation as well as radiation workers for safe service.

To access the AERB e-LORA system, employer needs to register his/her institute for obtaining login credentials and get user ID and password. The details can be referred by visiting AERB website *www.aerb.gov.in*.

Employer

As the owner of the facility using a radioactive source, the employer has the primary responsibility for ensuring and maintaining the safety and the security of the sources. He should prepare appropriate security plan for the facility, which needs to be submitted to the competent authority for review. The employer is primarily responsible for ensuring that the security plan at the facility is implemented in letter and spirit. The employer is responsible for:

- Ensuring that all personnel and their contract workers who use or have access to the sources are reliable
- Reporting to the competent authority of a source in the facility, provide the origin, and/or identity of which cannot be established
- Promoting a security culture and establishing a management system commensurate with the security need to ensure that problems affecting security are promptly identified and corrected, clear lines of authority are defined for security-related decision-making, and sensitive information is identified and protected on a "need to know" basis
- Promptly responding to any request from the local law-enforcing authorities in the recovery of any lost or stolen source.

Licensee

As the individual who is responsible for preparing a security plan and submitting to the competent authority and obtaining the license in his/her name, the licensee has a major responsibility in ensuring the security of the radioactive sources at the facility. The licensee's responsibility commences from the moment the authorized radioactive material is received in the radiation facility. The licensee should ensure that the following actions are carried out:

- Assess the security threats, evaluate the security requirements, design the security provisions, and prepare a security plan for the facility in consultation with the security personnel.
- Implement the security plan along with its administrative and technical measures to ensure the safety and security of the radioactive sources at the facility.
- Bring to the notice of the employer any additional actions specified by the competent authority for implementation.
- Establish a specific security clearance procedure for those persons in the radiation facility who would be involved in the use of the source, as also those personnel who would be deputed to collect the source from the supplier or carrier on behalf of the facility.
- Procure radioactive material only from an authorized supplier.
- Maintain a complete inventory of all sources in the facility.
- Ensure that the storage of a source not in use, its transfer to any other person/agency is done in accordance with procedures and requirements prescribed by the competent authority.
- Promptly respond to any request from the local law-enforcing authorities in the recovery of any lost or stolen source.
- Submission of reports to the competent authority at prescribed intervals in the prescribed format, on the status relating to the safety and security of sources handled in the facility. This should include any unusual events that have a bearing on the security of the sources and would include among others, loss of control, unauthorized access, unauthorized use, malicious acts threatening the

authorized activities, failures of equipment containing sources which may have security implications and discovery of any unaccounted source.
- Any attempt to actual breach of security including attempted thefts and actual thefts, and even misplacement or loss of radioactive material or loss/theft of sensitive information is reported to the law-enforcing authorities and the competent authority within 24 hours of the event.

Radiological Safety Officer

While the RSO's primary responsibility is to implement radiological safety requirements at the facility, he/she should be fully aware of the fact that any breach of security has safety implications. Consequently, regarding ensuring security of radioactive sources, the RSO should:

- Ensure that persons entering the area/zone where a radioactive source is used/or in use have been permitted by the Concerned Authority
- Implement when required, the procedure for mitigating the consequences of a breach of security
- Inform and train all the personnel working with radiation in the facility and other personnel as well about the safety and security of sources
- Secure the records appropriately and update the routine source inventory. This should also include source use history.
- Bring to the notice of the licensee, the employer and the security personnel of the facility, any situation which could be a potential threat to the security of source(s) in the facility.

Responsibilities of Radioisotope Supplier

The source supplier should register their institute in e-LORA as supplier of radioisotope. He should possess a license from the competent authority (Chairman, AERB) to supply radioactive material as required in the Atomic Energy (Radiation Protection) Rules, 2004, and should further ensure that the radioactive material is being supplied only to the person authorized to receive and handle the source. While obtaining authorization as supplier, following details are to be furnished:

- Letter from the principles declaring the applicant as authorized supplier of their products used for nuclear medicine (NM)/radiotherapy, e.g., Mo-Tc generator and other radioisotopes in India/Abroad
- Certificate, from the country of origin, regarding the approval of transport package for the generator and other radioisotopes
- Details of the generator or sealed source including the shielding provided
- Range(s) of activity to be imported and whether the activity mentioned on the package corresponds to activity on date of dispatch or as on date of delivery to the customer.
- Provisions made to export the spent generators/sealed sources to the original supplier after their useful life.

Supply of radiopharmaceutical/radioisotopes to authorized radiation facilities shall be done only on intimation received by the supplier from the competent authority and shall be within the authorized quantity.

In the case of radiotherapy, the isotope supplier or vendor shall: (i) make available along with the radiation therapy equipment, manuals for installation, operation and maintenance, and detailed procedures for equipment-specific QA tests; (ii) provide the user with a representative set of (a) central axis depth dose data and isodose curves in case of beam therapy, and (b) source specification and encapsulation information in case of brachytherapy; (iii) provide the necessary gadgets and accessories for the normal operation of the radiation therapy equipment and for handling emergency situations; (iv) ensure that the equipment is serviced and maintained by service engineer certified by the competent authority; and (v) ensure the availability of essential spare parts of the radiation therapy equipment for its useful life.

REGULATORY REQUIREMENTS SPECIFIC TO DIAGNOSTIC RADIOLOGY

General Requirements

The employer and licensee of the organization as defined in Atomic Energy (Radiation Protection) Rules, 2004, shall fulfill the responsibilities prescribed in this safety code [AERB/RF-MED/SC-3 (Rev. 2)].

Procurement of X-ray Equipment

The employer shall procure no objection certificate (NOC) validated/type approved X-ray equipment from authorized suppliers and after obtaining procurement permission from the competent authority.

Operation of X-ray Equipment

No diagnostic X-ray equipment shall be operated for patient diagnosis unless license for operation is obtained from the competent authority.

Prerequisites for Obtaining License for Operation of X-ray Equipment

X-ray room layout and shielding requirement: The room housing X-ray equipment shall have an appropriate area to facilitate easy movement of staff and proper patient positioning. Appropriate structural shielding shall be provided for walls, doors, ceiling, and floor of the room housing the X-ray equipment so that radiation exposures received by workers and the members of the public are kept to the minimum and shall not exceed the respective limits for annual effective doses as per directives issued by the competent authority. Appropriate overlap of shielding materials shall be provided at the joints or discontinuities.

The control console of CT equipment shall be installed in a separate room located outside but adjoining to CT room and provided with appropriate shielding, direct viewing, and oral communication facilities between the operator and the patient. The gantry and couch shall be placed such that it enables the operator to have the complete view of the patient from the control room viewing window.

Interventional radiology equipment room shall have an adjoining control room with appropriate facilities for shielding, direct viewing, and oral communication.

In case of room housing radiography equipment, chest stand shall be located in the X-ray room such that no significant stray radiation reaches at control console/entrance door/areas of full-time occupancy such that the dose limits to radiation worker and members of public are not exceeded.

Mobile X-ray equipment, when used as fixed X-ray equipment, shall comply with all the requirements of those of fixed X-ray installation. Movement of mobile X-ray equipment shall be restricted within the institution for which it is registered.

A permanent radiation warning symbol and instructions for pregnant/likely to be pregnant women shall be pasted on the entrance door of the X-ray installation, illustrating that the equipment emits X-radiation.

Vehicle-mounted X-ray Equipment

X-ray equipment installed in a mobile van or vehicle shall be provided with an appropriate shielding enclosure to ensure adequate built-in protection for persons likely to be present in and around the vehicle. Shielding shall be provided around the equipment from all the sides up to height of 2 m from external ground surface. Radiation warning symbol shall be displayed on all sides of the vehicle.

Staffing Requirements

X-ray installations shall have a radiologist/related medical practitioner/X-ray technologist with adequate knowledge of radiation protection to operate the X-ray equipment. The employees involved in these activities are considered as radiation workers and shall comply with the duties and responsibilities as prescribed in this safety code. The minimum qualification and training shall be as prescribed by the competent authority. All installations having X-ray equipment with fluoroscopy facility, CT, and all establishments performing special procedures shall have the services of a qualified radiologist or related medical practitioner, with adequate knowledge of radiation protection for interpretation and reporting.

Radiological Safety Officer

X-ray department shall have an RSO approved by the competent authority. The RSO may either be the employer himself/herself or an employee to whom the employer shall delegate the responsibility of ensuring compliance with appropriate radiation safety/regulatory requirements applicable to his X-ray installation. The minimum qualification and training shall be as prescribed by the competent authority.

Radiation Protection Devices

Appropriate radiation protection devices such as barrier, apron, goggles, and thyroid shields shall be used during operation of X-ray equipment. These devices shall be verified periodically for their shielding adequacy.

Personnel Monitoring Service

Personnel monitoring services shall be provided to all the radiation workers.

Quality Assurance Requirements

The end user shall ensure that periodic QA of the equipment is carried out by agencies authorized by the regulatory body.

Servicing

The end user shall ensure that servicing of the X-ray equipment is carried out by agencies authorized by the regulatory body.

Periodic Safety Reports

The user shall submit periodic safety reports in the format and frequency specified by the regulatory body.

Renewal of License

The license accorded by the competent authority shall be renewed before its expiry.

Decommissioning of X-ray Equipment

Decommissioning of the X-ray equipment shall be carried out by authorized agencies with prior intimation to the competent authority.

REGULATORY REQUIREMENTS SPECIFIC TO NUCLEAR MEDICINE

License

The licensee can obtain a license, authorization, registration, and consent by applying through e-LORA system from the competent authority. The licensee shall be a fulltime employee of the institution. The licensee shall ensure compliance with the mandatory requirements specified in the Atomic Energy (Radiation Protection) Rules, 2004, in addition to the specific requirements given in the safety code [AERB/RF-SC/MED-2 (Rev.2)].

Approval of Layout Plan of Nuclear Medicine Facility

Room layout drawings and site layout drawing are prepared in consultation with RSO, Architect, and the supplier of the nuclear medicine equipment (SPECT, SPECT-CT, PET-CT, PET-MRI, etc.) unit. It should be submitted to AERB "Site and Layout Approval". The drawings will be reviewed by AERB, and approval is issued from radiation safety standpoint on satisfactory compliance with all the relevant requirements.

Radiation Safety Officer

The employer shall designate with the approval of the competent authority a person having qualifications prescribed by the safety code to function as an RSO. RSO shall be a full-time employee of the institution.

Nuclear medicine facilities shall have RSO-II as per qualifications specified in the code. Facilities with radioisotope-producing accelerators such as medical cyclotron shall have RSO-III as per qualifications specified by the safety code.

Appointment of Staff for the Nuclear Medicine Facility

Appoint adequate staff as per the qualification and experience stipulated in AERB Safety Code. It may be noted that only "Radiation Professional" (RP) registered nuclear medicine (NM) staff can be declared for your institute in e-LORA. These RPs are the radiation workers whose qualifications comply with the code requirement. Obtain RP registration ID and date of birth of appointed staff for declaring them in your institute's e-LORA account.

Procurement of Personnel Monitors Badges

Procure Personnel Monitoring Badges (i.e., TLD badges) from the agency accredited by AERB for all the radiation workers. Pocket dosimeters for the radiation workers may also be procured, which are meant for measuring radiation dose received by the radiation worker during his work.

Measuring and Monitoring Instruments

Procure appropriate measuring instruments for measurement of activity to be administered to the patients (dose calibrator/isotope calibrator), appropriate radiation monitoring instruments (survey meter, contamination monitor, gamma zone monitor, etc.), and QA tools. The requisite instruments should be declared in e-LORA system and their calibration details must be updated as and when instruments are being calibrated.

Other Associated Handling Accessories

The other associated handling accessories such as localized shields in the form of lead bricks, L-bench, tongs, syringe carriers/shields, and tongs should be made available.

Equipment and Source Procurement Permission

Obtain permission from AERB for procurement of equipment (such as PET-CT, SPECT-CT) and radioactive sources to be used for QA/radiological survey.

Equipment Receipt Intimation

Provide intimation of receipt of the equipment through e-LORA within 15 days of its receipt.

Quality Assurance Tests and Radiological Survey Report

After installing the NM equipment, QA should be undertaken, and its report should be submitted through e-LORA. Radiation survey is required to be carried out and its report is required to be submitted to AERB through e-LORA.

Precommissioning Inspection

The nuclear medicine facility (NMF) shall not be commissioned until the competent authority approves the facility. Any change or modification to an already approved facility shall be carried out only with the prior approval of the competent authority.

When the NMF is constructed as per the approved plan and ready for commissioning, a precommissioning inspection of the facility may be arranged. Any modifications/suggestions made at the time of precommissioning inspection by this division shall be complied with.

License for Operation

License in the form of authorization from competent authority is required to procure radioactive material. The licensee shall be responsible for the safety and security of the radioactive material, its proper use, and the safe disposal of waste.

After completion of all related QA tests, submit application for obtaining license for operation. A report on the action taken on the recommendations during the precommissioning inspection shall also be submitted along with the application for license.

The licensee shall not lend, gift, transfer, sell, or receive any radioactive material other than those specified in the authorization without the prior approval of the competent authority.

Permission for Procurement of Sources for Clinical Use

On receipt of the license for operation, permission for procurement of source for clinical use should be submitted. While submitting the application for procurement of source, appropriate installation (PET-CT/SPECT/LDT/HDT/NIT/β therapy, etc.) should be chosen depending on the intended use of the source.

Source Procurement Intimation

The NMF shall place its source requirement to a specific source supplier through e-LORA and the supplier shall in turn acknowledge the request and supply the quantity which shall be within the AERB authorized limit.

Annual Report on Status of Radiation Safety for NMF

It is mandatory for all NMFs to submit safety status report by the end of calendar year but not later than January 31st of the next year. Nonsubmission of annual safety status report is considered as noncompliance.

Periodic Quality Assurance

Periodic QA should be undertaken as per the National Electrical Manufacturers Association (NEMA) protocol for all the NM equipment and the report for same should be uploaded on e-LORA during the renewal of license for all imaging equipment.

Disposal and Transport of Disused Radioactive Sources

Any disused/decayed sealed source shall be returned to its original manufacturer/supplier by obtaining the requisite permission through e-LORA portal. Disposal of all radioactive waste arising from the use of unsealed radioisotopes should be managed as per the requirements of the Atomic Energy (Safe Disposal of Radioactive Wastes) Rules, 1987.

Radioactive material shall not be disposed of without prior approval of the competent authority. The licensee shall obtain authorization, as per Rule 4 of the Atomic Energy (Safe Disposal of Radioactive Waste) Rules, G.S.R. 125, 1987, from the competent authority.

Transport of radioactive material in public domain shall be in accordance with provisions of AERB safety code on "Safe Transport of Radioactive Material', AERB/NRF-TS/SC-1 (Rev.1), 2016, currently in force. The licensee shall not take radioactive material out of the approved premises.

Inspection

Any person duly authorized by the competent authority shall inspect the NM facility, the radioactive sources available in-house, the radioisotope inventory, logbooks, records of area monitoring, and contamination monitoring, instruments, and devices used for the above and/or QA program, records of unusual occurrences during handling of the sources and transport of radioactive materials, records of radioactive waste generated and disposed of, and emergency response plans.

Decommissioning of NMF

The NMF shall be decommissioned only after prior approval of the competent authority and after removing all radioactive and contaminated materials from the facility. Prior approval of the competent authority is necessary for reuse of the facility.

A prior consent for decommissioning of NMF shall be obtained from AERB. On receipt of the permission from AERB, decommissioning shall be undertaken under the guidance of RSO, and its report shall be submitted through e-LORA while submission of the intimation on decommissioning.

REGULATORY REQUIREMENTS SPECIFIC TO RADIATION THERAPY

License

Radiation therapy sources and equipment shall be handled only in accordance with the terms and conditions of the license issued by the competent authority. License shall be in the form of a license, authorization, registration, or consent:

- *License*: License shall be issued for sources and practices associated with the operation of—(i) telegamma unit and accelerator used in radiotherapy, (ii) CT unit for simulation purpose, (iii) such other source or practice as may be notified by the competent authority, from time to time.
- *Authorization*: License shall be an authorization for sources and practices associated with the operation of—(i) brachytherapy, (ii) deep X-ray units, superficial and contact therapy X-ray units, and (iii) such other source or practice as may be notified by the competent authority, from time to time.
- *Registration*: License shall be a registration for sources and practices associated with the operation of—(i) therapy simulator and (ii) such other source or practice as may be notified by the competent authority, from time to time.
- *Consent*: License shall be a consent for—(i) approval for siting, design, construction, commissioning, and decommissioning of a radiation installation, (ii) approval for sealed sources, radiation-generating equipment and equipment containing radioactive sources, for the purposes of manufacture and supply, (iii) approval for package design for transport of radioactive material, (iv) approval for shipment of radioactive consignments, and (v) such other source or practice as may be notified by the competent authority, from time to time. Compliance with the specifications of the code is a prerequisite for the issuance of the said license by the competent authority.

Design Certification

Every radiation therapy source and equipment shall meet the design safety specifications stipulated in the Code. The manufacturer/vendor shall obtain design certification from the competent authority prior to marketing, manufacturing the therapy source and equipment.

Type Approval/No Objection Certificate

Indigenously Made Radiation Therapy Equipment/Radioactive Source

Prior to marketing the radiation therapy equipment/radioactive source, the local manufacturer shall obtain an NOC or a type approval certificate from the competent authority for supply of radiation therapy equipment or radioactive source, respectively. Type approval certificate shall be issued only if the equipment/radioactive source satisfies the safety specifications prescribed in the applicable standard. The local manufacturer shall demonstrate type approval testing and performance verification of the equipment/radioactive source to representatives of competent authority for type approval. Based on the satisfactory demonstration of type approval testing and performance verification, type approval certificate for such equipment/radioactive source shall be issued by the competent authority. Only type-approved equipment shall be used in the country.

Approval of Building Design and Layout of the Proposed Rooms for Housing Radiation Therapy Equipment/ Radioactive Source

The drawings of building design and the layout of the proposed rooms for housing radiation therapy equipment/radioactive source shall be submitted as stipulated by the competent authority. Room housing radiation therapy equipment/radioactive source shall not be constructed unless the competent authority approves the building and the layout drawing of the proposed room housing radiation therapy equipment/ radioactive source from radiation safety standpoint. Any change in the approved building and the layout design shall be carried out only with the prior approval of the competent authority.

Selection of Radiotherapy Equipment

Verify from the supplier that the radiotherapy equipment (which is either radiation-generating equipment such as medical accelerator/simulator or houses sealed radioactive material such as telecobalt/gamma knife/brachytherapy unit) is either type approved or NOC is issued by AERB to the local supplier. For this, copy of type approval certificate or NOC issued by AERB may be demanded from the local supplier. It may be noted that—license to operate equipment procured based on NOC will not be issued by AERB till local supplier demonstrates its compliance with AERB requirements and user fulfills all the regulatory requirements.

Radiotherapy Staffs

Appoint adequate number qualified staff such as Radiation Oncologist(s), Medical Physicist(s), and Radiation Therapy Technologists as per the qualification and experience stipulated in AERB Safety Code AERB/RF-SC/MED-1 (Rev.1). In case of appointment of Medical Physicists, it is to be ensured that at least one of them is eligible to work as RSO.

Nomination and Approval of Radiological Safety Officer

The employer shall designate a qualified person from his employment to function as RSO in a radiotherapy installation with the approval of competent authority. The nomination in the prescribed application shall be submitted to the competent authority application through e-LORA. It is essential to obtain RSO approval for obtaining procurement permission for any radiotherapy equipment in new radiotherapy facility.

Measuring and Monitoring Instruments

Procure appropriate measuring instruments for measurement of output and other dosimetric parameters (thimble ionization chamber, parallel plate ionization chamber, well type ionization chamber, electrometer, dosimetric phantom, radiation field analyzer, etc.). Also, procure appropriate monitoring instruments for area monitoring (survey meters, contamination monitors, gamma zone monitors etc.), security systems, and QA instruments.

Detail on requisite instruments for each type of radiotherapy installation is provided in "user manual for radiotherapy", available in "help" menu of e-LORA. It may be noted that gamma zone monitor for telecobalt unit and remote after loading brachytherapy unit should be of autoreset type, whereas that for manual brachytherapy must have manual-reset button. The requisite instruments must be declared in e-LORA system and its calibration details must be updated as and when instruments are being calibrated.

Other Associated Equipment and Accessories

The associated equipment for radiotherapy includes simulator/CT-simulator for simulating the patient prior to radiation therapy. The layout plan of simulator installation also requires site and layout approval from AERB as mentioned above and need authorization prior to its procurement. The other associated equipment/ accessories include treatment planning system (TPS), last man out switch (LMOS), beam modifiers, and patient immobilization devices such as molds and QA test tools.

Authorization for Procurement of Equipment/Radioactive Source

Prior authorization shall be obtained from the competent authority for procurement of radiation therapy equipment or/and radioactive source.

Equipment/Source Receipt Intimation

Provide intimation of receipt of the equipment/source within 15 days of its receipt. Install the teletherapy/brachytherapy unit as per the approved plan and carryout the mechanical and electrical tests thoroughly prior to source loading or switching on the radiation beam in case of radiation-generating equipment (e.g., medical accelerator, simulator).

Security of Sources

The employer/licensee shall make adequate provisions for the security of sources during all stages of handling, as required by the competent authority.

Loading of the Source (Obtain Source Supervision Authorization)

In case of telecobalt source, the source shall be loaded (as well as unloaded) by the certified service engineer under supervision of the medical physicist/RSO, who has been authorized by AERB for supervising the source transfer operation. Source supervision authorization is also required to obtain for first source loading in remote afterloading brachytherapy unit.

Commissioning

Room housing radiation therapy equipment/radioactive source shall be commissioned only with prior approval and as per the terms and conditions specified by the competent authority.

Survey Report

After obtaining commissioning approval, a radiation survey is required to be carried out and survey report is required to be submitted to AERB. Only after approval to survey report, radiation-related QA tests should be carried out thoroughly.

License for Operation

After completion of all mechanical, electrical, and radiation-related QA tests, submit application for license. Patient treatment can be started only after obtaining license for operation. The license shall be renewed before expiry of license.

Radiation Therapy Technologist

The employer/licensee shall employ only qualified radiation therapy technologist in a radiotherapy installation as prescribed in the code.

Certification of Radiation Therapy Service Engineer

The employer/licensee shall employ vendors who have qualified service engineers as prescribed in the code. Each such vendor shall obtain a certificate for their service engineers in the prescribed format from the competent authority.

Annual Report on Status of Radiation Safety in Radiotherapy Department

It is mandatory for all radiotherapy facilities to submit safety status report by the end of calendar year but not later than January 31st of the next year. Nonsubmission of annual safety status report is considered as noncompliance.

Quality Assurance/Dose Reports

Perform periodic QA test of the teletherapy/brachytherapy unit and the report of the same must be kept in the institute records. The personnel monitoring dose reports must also be maintained by the institute. These reports are to be produced while inspection of radiotherapy department of an institution by AERB personnel.

Notifications/Directives

The employer/licensee shall ensure that persons handling radiation therapy equipment/radioactive source shall abide by the provisions of this Code and their further elaboration in the various notifications/directives, issued by the competent authority from time to time. The employer/licensee shall also ensure that other measures of radiation safety stipulated by the competent authority are promptly implemented.

Inspection

The radiation therapy installation, equipment, and radioactive source shall be made available for inspection to the representative of the competent authority to verify the compliance with the regulatory requirements including the provisions of this code.

Transport of Radioactive Source

The employer/licensee shall not lend, gift, transfer, sell, or dispose of radioactive source without the prior approval of the competent authority.

Radioactive source shall not be transported in public domain without prior approval of the competent authority. The requirements that shall be complied with for transport of radioactive materials are given in the AERB safety code for "Transport of Radioactive Materials" (AERB/SC/TR-l, 1986).

Change of Premise/Location

Radiation therapy equipment/radioactive source shall be used only in the approved premise/location and the same shall not be taken out of the approved premise/location for any purpose without the prior approval of the competent authority.

Disposal and Transport of Disused Radioactive Source

After end of useful life of radioactive source used in radiotherapy, the source should be disposed safely with the disposal agency. A consent must be obtained from AERB for disposal and transport of disused radioactive source to disposal agency. It may be noted that any radiotherapy source not in used for >1 year is deemed to be called as disused source and institute has to take immediate action for disposal of such disused source.

Decommissioning and Disposal

When the radiation therapy unit or radioactive sources are no longer to be used, the employer/licensee shall:

- Submit a proposal to competent authority to undertake decommissioning of radiation therapy installation/equipment or disposal of radioactive sources to obtain approval
- Remove the radioactive sources, contaminated materials, if any, and depleted uranium, if present, and return them to the supplier/disposal agency for safe disposal
- Upon completion of decommissioning and disposal, submit to the competent authority a detailed report on: (a) decommissioning operations, (b) safe disposal of the radioactive material, and (c) personnel doses received during these operations.

Penalties

Any employer/licensee, who contravenes the provisions of the Atomic Energy Act, 1962, and/or Atomic Energy (Radiation Protection) Rules, 2004, or as elaborated in this Code, or any other terms or conditions of a license issued to him by the competent authority, is punishable under Sections 24, 25, and 26 of the Atomic Energy Act, 1962. The punishment may include imprisonment, or fine, or both.

PHYSICAL PROTECTION OF SOURCES, SAFETY, AND SECURITY OF SOURCES DURING STORAGE, TRANSPORT, AND DISPOSAL

Physical Protection Systems

Physical protection system (PPS) refers to the entire range of systems and equipment, which physically protect the radioactive source or the facility using a radioactive source. The design of these systems is governed by physical protection principles and physical protection can be effectively implemented through human actions supported by equipment. An effective PPS makes a judicious combination of human surveillance and physical protection equipment. Its design and evaluation involve concepts of design basis threat (DBT) and vulnerability assessment (VA).

Physical protection design for a given source consists of three steps, namely—(i) assessment security check, (ii) establishment of performance objectives for the PPS commensurate with the security risk, and (iii) identification of a combination of security measures that meet the performance objectives. The security risk is associated with all the security levels and can be estimated by carrying out threat assessment and vulnerability analysis. Physical protection is achieved by human actions with supported equipment. Such equipment includes turnstile gates, which will regulate the entry and exit of individuals enabling direct surveillance, entrance doors operated by electronic recognition of security cards, provision of intrusion alarms, video cameras, etc. An effective PPS makes a judicious combination of human surveillance and physical protection equipment.

AERB/RF-RS/SG-1 (Appendix-V) gives details on PPS, which covers these aspects and could be used as a guide to develop an effective security plan.

Source Storage and Inventory Control

Radioactive sources both sealed and open isotopes are stored in a source storage which is specially designed. The integrity of sources and shielding must withstand all envisaged accident conditions. The storage room must be well ventilated under lock and key when not in use. The room should be designated as source storage room and marked as such at the entrance. The source capacity must be clearly indicated outside the safe along with radiation symbol. The design of the safe must be duly approved by the competent authority.

Brachytherapy-sealed sources may require source storage safe in the room. The safe is designed in such a way that it should provide adequate protection to the operating personnel, prevent unauthorized access to the sources, and prevent damage to the sources in case of an accident and fire, flood, or mechanical impact. Arrangement of sources inside the storage safe must permit easy handling with minimum exposure to personnel. Inventories of sources and dummy must be maintained and verified once in 3 months. Stock of the brachytherapy sources must be notified to the competent authority annually.

Records of sources such as date of procurement/sale/transfer/loss/disposal/damage, type and specifications, and details of the acceptance tests carried out shall be maintained. A chart indicating the location, type, and activity of the various sources in storage shall be displayed in the vicinity of the storage safe. Records of sources with comparatively short half-lives, such as ^{125}I and ^{192}Ir, shall be updated in the chart at suitable intervals. Only persons duly authorized by the licensee shall release and receive back the sources.

A logbook must be maintained for the movement of sources FROM and TO the storage room:

- Type, number, and activity of sources required
- Name and signature of the person receiving the sources with time and date
- Name, hospital number and address of the patient, site of treatment, and locations of use in the hospital
- Proposed time and date of termination of treatment
- Date and time of actual return of the sources to storage and signatures of persons returning and receiving the sources

Sources, which are leaky and damaged, shall not be used. Sources contaminated, but not leaky, must be used before proper contamination. If there is missing source, RSO must initiate suitable action to locate and recover the source. Movement of personnel, patients, all hospital waste, and use of toilet and washbasins must be stopped in the suspected areas to prevent escape route. All occupied areas in and around the hospital shall be monitored to confirm radiation-free conditions. The competent authority is informed about the loss of source, if any.

Security of Radioactive Sources during their Transport and Disposal

A radioactive source could be in storage at the facility or in use there. It could also be in transport either from the supplier of the source to the facility or from one location to another for operational reasons, or the source is being sent to a disposal facility. As mentioned earlier, transport of a radioactive source needs special consideration from the view of safety and security. The guidance for this purpose is available separately in the AERB Safety Guide No. AERB/NRF-TS/SG-10 [7] and these should be used by the licensee whenever the source is in transport.

SECURITY PROVISIONS

Administrative Measures

Administrative measures are the use of policies, procedures, and practices which direct personnel to securely and safely manage the sources. Administrative measures are used to support or supplement technical measures. Among others, administrative measures would include:

- Access control procedures [e.g., personal identification number (PIN) or biometric features to activate a door control reader or a badge system which may also activate an electronic reader]

- Intrusion alarms at access points (e.g., with radiation detectors)
- Key control procedures
- Video cameras or personal surveillance supported by adequate area lighting systems (even if surveillance measures involve the use of intrusion detectors instead of human observation, they are still considered as administrative measures since they do not provide a physical barrier)
- Records related to management of sources
- Inventories
- Reliability and trustworthiness of personnel
- Preparation of emergency plans to respond to the loss of control of higher risk radioactive sources and carrying out exercises (the envisaged scenarios including a suspected or threatened malicious act, or a public demonstration which has the potential to threaten the security of sources or an intrusion into the security area by unauthorized persons with violent and malicious intent)
- Information security (protecting the confidentiality of information, the unauthorized disclosure of which could compromise the security measures, e.g., information relating to the specific location and inventory of sources, the relevant security plan and detailed security arrangements, security systems such as intruder alarms, weaknesses in the security arrangements, means of response to a breach of security planned dates, routes and mode of transport/shipment or transfer of sources)
- Quality assurance measures
- Establishment and maintenance of a safety culture and a security culture. The extent to which the above measures would need to be implemented would depend upon the security level applicable to the practice.

Technical Measures

Technical measures pose a physical barrier to the radioactive source, device, or facility to prevent inadvertent or unauthorized access, to deter, or to prevent removal of a radioactive source. The design of technical measures and the level of QA should be appropriate to the threat and the potential consequences of the defined malevolent act. Technical measures generally comprise hardware or security devices and would include among others:

- Fences
- Walls, rooms/vaults
- Cages
- Transport packaging
- Locks and interlocks for doors with alarm systems
- Intrusion-resistant source-holding devices

The extent to which these measures would need to be implemented would depend upon the security level applicable to the practice.

The description of security measures includes access control, cages, CCTV surveillance, communication, fences and gates, intrusion detection systems (IDS), key control procedures, locks, hinge, and interlock for doors, locked, shielded containers, maintaining and testing of security technology, pass system, QA, security and area lighting, special security doors and door sets, standby power, and walls. Detailed discussion is given in AERB/RF-RS/SG-1 (Appendix-IV) under, security of radiation sources in radiation facilities.

Security Threat

Security means measures to prevent unauthorized access or damage and loss, theft, or unauthorized transfer of radioactive sources. Security measures are designed for specific sources as design basis threat assessment method. It should be commensurate with threat and the level of risk acceptance. Security measures are based on generic assessment performed at the government or organization level or could be specific in nature. Threat assessment provides the means of adjusting security provisions in accordance with the results of that analysis and more specifically for addressing the potential consequences associated with loss of control over each specific source.

Security threats are dynamic in nature and could vary with space and time, hence, continuous review is required. If it indicates deterioration of security, the licensee should prepare a revised security plan, upgrade the security level, and implement required measures. If it is a short-term issue, the licensee could revert to the original security plan. In both cases, the competent authority is informed accordingly.

Graded Approach in Security Provision

Graded approach will ensure that the level of security measures in place is commensurate with the potential consequence associated with the possible breach of security with respect to that source. Based on the security threat associated with radioactive sources, four security levels: A, B, C, and D have been defined **(Table 17.1)**. These levels provide a systematic way of categorizing the graded performance objectives required to cover the range of security measures that might be needed, depending on the assessed risk.

- *Security level A*: Prevent unauthorized removal of a source by timely detection and response action. Measures should be established to deter and detect unauthorized access and acquisition of the source in a timely manner. These measures should be such as to delay acquisition until a response is possible.

TABLE 17.1 Security levels based on categorization of sources.

Security level	*Source category*	*Examples of practices*
A	*1*	Radioisotope thermoelectric generators (RTGs), irradiators, teletherapy, and fixed multibeam teletherapy (gamma knife)
B	*2*	Industrial radiography, high-/medium-dose rate brachytherapy
C	*3*	Fixed industrial gauges incorporate high activity sources (e.g., level, dredger, and conveyor) and well-logging gauges
D	*4*	Low-dose rate brachytherapy (except those given against Category 5), industrial gauges that do not incorporate high-activity sources [e.g., thickness/fill-level gauges, portable gauges (e.g., moisture/density)], bone densitometers, static eliminators, diagnostic isotope generators
	5	Low-dose rate brachytherapy eye plaques and permanent implant sources [positron emission tomography (PET) check sources, X-ray fluorescence (XRF) devices, electron capture devices, Mossbauer spectrometry sources], radiopharmaceuticals, and other unsealed sources

Courtesy: AERB safety code No. AERB/RF-RS/SG-1, 2011.

- *Security level B*: Minimize the likelihood of unauthorized removal of a source by immediate detection without having to interrupt the act. Measures should be established to deter and detect unauthorized access and acquisition of the source in a timely manner.
- *Security level C*: Reduce the likelihood of unauthorized removal of a source. Measures should be established to deter unauthorized access and verify the presence of the source at set intervals.
- *Security level D*: Measures should be established to ensure safe use of the source and adequately protect it as an asset, verifying its presence at set intervals.

Radiation Protection Program

Radiation protection program is generally implemented in handling ionizing radiation gauging devices (IRGDs) in industrial radiography, especially in well-logging sources. In each facility handling an IRGD, an RPP including standard operating procedures commensurate with the work involving the IRGD should be prepared and implemented. The RPP should be formulated addressing all the safety-related procedures to be implemented in the facility on a day-to-day basis. The elements of the RPP are included in Annexure-III, AERB/RF-IGD/SG-1.

Radiation protection program should be integrated with other documented safety procedures and work practices that exist within the organization. Any modifications in the integrated safety procedures and work practices should not negatively impact the RPP. The RPP should be reviewed and updated at appropriate intervals. It should reflect the changes in the equipment, operators, or work practices which have a bearing on safety.

REGULATORY REQUIREMENTS FOR IMPORT/EXPORT, PROCUREMENT, USE, HANDLING, TRANSPORT AND DISPOSAL OF RADIOISOTOPES

Vendor shall obtain an NOC from the competent authority, for import of one such equipment for obtaining type approval, prior to marketing. NOC for such equipment/radioactive source shall be issued only if the equipment/radioactive source satisfies the safety specifications of the prescribed standards applicable for the equipment/radioactive source. Upon import and installation of the equipment in the country, the vendor shall demonstrate type, approval testing and performance verification of the equipment to representatives of competent authority for type approval. Based on the satisfactory demonstration of type approval testing and performance verification, type approval certificate for such equipment shall be issued by the competent authority. Only type approved equipment shall be used in the country.

International Shipments

For air transport, the shipment should be carried in accordance with applicable security provisions. For maritime transport, shipments should be carried out in accordance with the applicable security level provisions of the international ship and port facility security (ISPS) code of the International Maritime Dangerous Goods Code as required with the International Convention of the Safety of Life at Sea (SOLAS 74 amended). These provisions should be supplemented by the guidance in this document. Before undertaking an international shipment, the originating country should make adequate provisions to ensure that the security requirements of the receiving country or any country through which the material will transit will be met.

BIBLIOGRAPHY

1. Atomic Energy Regulatory Board. (2008). Security of radioactive material during transport: AERB Safety code No. AERB/NRF-TS/SG-10, 2008. [online] Available from https://aerb.gov.in/images/PDF/CodesGuides/RadiationFacility/Transport/2.pdf. [Last accessed December, 2022]
2. Atomic Energy Regulatory Board. (2011). Nuclear medicine facilities: AERB Safety code No: AERB/RF-MED/SC-2 (Rev. 2) [online] Available from https://www.aerb.gov.in/images/PDF/CodesGuides/RadiationFacility/MedicalApplicationsInvolvingRadiation/3.pdf. [Last accessed December, 2022]
3. Atomic Energy Regulatory Board. (2011). Radiation therapy sources, equipment, and installations: AERB safety code No. AERB/RF-MED/SC-1 (Rev. 1). [online] Available from https://www.aerb.gov.in/images/PDF/CodesGuides/RadiationFacility/MedicalApplicationsInvolvingRadiation/4.pdf. [Last accessed December, 2022]
4. Atomic Energy Regulatory Board. (2011). Security of radioactive sources in radiation facilities: AERB Safety code No. AERB/RF-RS/SG-1. [online] Available from https://aerb.gov.in/images/PDF/CodesGuides/RadiationFacility/RadioactiveSources/1.pdf. [Last accessed December, 2022]
5. Atomic Energy Regulatory Board. (2016). Radiation safety in manufacture, supply, and use of medical diagnostic X-ray equipment: AERB safety code No. AERB/RF-MED/SC-3(Rev.2) [online] Available from https://www.aerb.gov.in/images/PDF/RF-MED-SC-3.pdf. [Last accessed December, 2022]
6. Atomic Energy Regulatory Board. (2016). Safe transport of radioactive material: AERB safety code No. AERB/NRF-TS/SC-1 (Rev.1) [online] Available from https://www.aerb.gov.in/images/PDF/CodesGuides/RadiationFacility/Transport/1.pdf. [Last accessed December, 2022]
7. Atomic Energy Regulatory Board. Nucleonic gauges and well logging applications; AERB/RF-IGD/SG-1, 2015. Mumbai: AERB; 2015.
8. Government of India, Department of Atomic Energy. (2004). Atomic energy (Radiation protection) Rules, 2004: Published in the Gazette of India: September 11, 2004. [online] Available from https://www.barc.gov.in/about/07.pdf. [Last accessed December, 2022]
9. International Atomic Energy Agency. (2003). Manual for reactor produced isotopes, IAEA TET-DOC-1340, IAEA, Vienaa. [online] Available from https://www-pub.iaea.org/MTCD/publications/PDF/te_1340_web.pdf. [Last accessed December, 2022]

CHAPTER 18

Radiation Emergencies and Medical Management

INTRODUCTION

Radiation emergencies may arise whenever radiation accident occurs and cause radiation injuries to the individuals. Hence, there is a need of guidelines to healthcare professional to carry out correct diagnostic procedures, assessment and medical management of an individual/people, affected with such injuries. Guidelines should also offer multidisciplinary approach to medical preparedness and response to medical emergencies.

RADIATION ACCIDENTS

A radiation accident is an unusual occurrence resulting from the loss of control over a radiation source which could directly or indirectly involve hazards to life, health, and property. It could occur at any stage of an operation involving radiation sources. For example, a beam of X-ray could be inadvertently turned towards a wall to which it should not normally be directed. As a result, persons in the adjoining room who may be nonradiation workers could be exposed to relatively high levels of radiation. Radiation accidents would be in one of the following headings:

- Accidental external exposure to excessive amounts of radiation, e.g., a person remains inadvertently close to a strong source or accidentally exposed to beam of radiation.
- Accidental spill or explosion in a working place resulting in surface and air contamination of the surroundings and contamination of personnel. In such cases, the intake of radioactive substances into the body could be by inhalation through open wounds or absorption through skin.
- Dispersal of radioactive material to the environment because of an explosion, fire, mechanical shock, or other incident occurring in a public place, e.g., transport of radioactive substances.

On-site Radiation Accidents

High levels of exposure to radiation occur because of a person inadvertently entering a high-radiation field, for example, a person walking towards an X-ray beam, when the machine is ON. In such places, where there is potential for accident, appropriate control measures should be taken well in advance to ensure that the chances of any person being accidentally exposed to high levels of radiation are minimized.

Such measures include—(i) provision of interlocks which could ensure that no person can enter the radiation area when the exposure is in progress, (ii) provision of visual or aural indication to identify high radiation level areas, (iii) provision of adequate radiation alarms which can be either located at strategic points or carried by individuals whenever they are near high radiation level areas, and (iv) the absorption of detailed administrative procedures such as provision of suitable cordoned-off areas and prohibition of entry into such areas during radiation operations.

A second category of accidental radiation exposure, which could arise in a radiation work area, could result from one of the following contingencies:

- The inability to get a remotely controlled source back into its shielded container because of mechanical or pneumatic failure
- Accidental breakage of a sealed source or the container of an open source, resulting in high contamination of both surface and air in the vicinity
- Breakdown of crucial ventilation systems in areas where open sources are being handled
- Accidents which could involve fire or explosion, and which could result in the breakdown of the integrity of shielding or dispersal of radionuclides in the environment of the laboratory, e.g., criticality accident in nuclear reactor

Off-site Accidents

This type of accident may occur in areas to which public have access and may result from one of the following contingencies:

- Unplanned release of airborne activity to the environment of a radiation facility owing to unusual conditions such as fire, explosion, breakdown of the ventilation system, or breakdown of the filter system
- Accident to consignments of radionuclides when such consignments are in a carrier such as a truck, train, or aircraft, or when such consignments are held in storage during transit

Classification of Radiation Accidents

Accidents involving radiation sources and radioactive minerals can be classified as—(i) external radiation and (ii) radioactive contamination. External radiation can result in whole body exposure, partial body exposure, or localized skin exposure. Radioactive contamination may be external or internal. External contamination can occur because of spillage of radioactive material on skin or hands that in contact with loose radioactive material. It can cause irradiation of the skin and underlying tissues as well as provide a potential for the material to enter the body subsequently. The possibility is high, if the integrity of the skin is lost due to wounds, abrasions, or chemicals.

Internal contamination occurs most often because of inhalation of radioactive materials in finely divided form. As mentioned above, it may also occur when contamination present on the skin penetrates the outer layer and enters systemic circulation. Internal contamination can also occur because of eating with contaminated hands or consuming contaminated water which is quite uncommon.

In the case of external irradiation, first aid is not required, unless it is accompanied by traumatic injury. In radioactive contamination, there is no immediate risk to life. To minimize the long-term sequelae, it is necessary to block or minimize systemic uptake and hasten the biological elimination of the contaminant. First aid, if administered to the person within a short period at the accident place, is sufficient.

International Atomic Energy Agency Classification of Accidents

International Atomic Energy Agency (IAEA) has classified the causes of accidents based on the techniques such as—(1) external beam therapy, (2) low-dose rate brachytherapy, (3) high-dose rate brachytherapy, and (4) unsealed sources. External beam therapy includes—(i) events related to equipment affecting many patients and (ii) events involving many patients. Origin of accidents arises from radiation measurement system, treatment machine, simulators, and treatment planning system (TPS), prescription, and execution of treatment. Low-dose rate brachytherapy includes—(i) events related to equipment affecting many patients and (ii) events involving single patients.

Causes of accidents include verification of activity, batch uniformity, and identification of markers, storage, and inventory, performance of leakage test, applicator, etc. High-dose rate brachytherapy includes events related to equipment affecting many patients. Accidents rise from training of personnel and malfunction of equipment. In the case of unsealed sources, the causes are planning and dispensing, administration, and safety and contamination.

Radiation Injury

Radiation injury is a damage caused by ionizing radiation exposure. Large dose of ionizing radiation can cause acute illness by reducing the production of blood cells and damaging the digestive track. At very high doses, skin, heart, and blood vessels, and brain will be affected. Radiation injury caused by very large dose is referred as tissue reaction. Severity of tissue reaction depends on dose, dose rate, part of body exposed, sensitivity of tissue, and presence of genetic abnormalities that impact normal DNA repair, presence of age, and general state of health, etc.

Radiation Emergency

An emergency is a nonroutine situation that necessitates prompt action, primarily to mitigate a hard or adverse consequence for human health and environmental safety. Radiation emergency is an emergency in which there is, or perceived to be, a hazard due to—(1) the energy resulting from a nuclear chain reaction or from the decay of products of a chain reaction and (2) radiation exposure. The hazard includes sealed and unsealed radioactive source which may lead to uncontrolled release of ionizing radiation or radioactive material into the environment or to the individuals. Sources in medicine and industry include ^{60}Co, ^{137}Cs, or ^{192}Ir and unsealed sources of nuclear medicine. Hazards due to X-ray units and linear accelerators/particle accelerators are in lesser degree. The employer is the custodian of the radiation source. It is his responsibility to handle radiation emergency, mitigating the consequences, and making preventive measures to avoid any recurrence of such situation in future.

Radiation Accidents and Emergency in Diagnostic Radiology

In India, two incidents were reported with X-ray fluoroscopy, during cardiac catheterization and pacemaker insertion and two patients received very high doses to the skin of their back.

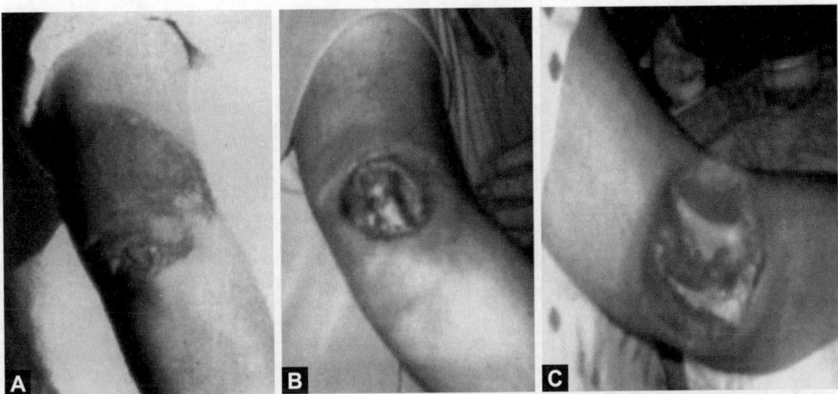

FIGS. 18.1A TO C: 49-year-old woman with 8-year history of refractory supraventricular tachycardia; Photographs show: (A) sharply demarcated erythema above right elbow at 3 weeks after radiofrequency cardiac catheter ablation; (B) tissue necrosis 5 months after procedure; and (C) deep ulceration with exposure of the humerus at 6.5 months. ***(For color version, see Plate 3)***

Courtesy: AJR:177, July 2001.

Interventional radiology using fluoroscopy equipment for image guidance may pose greater risk of X-ray-induced injuries. The reason for higher risk includes—(i) more extended periods of time, (ii) multiple uses of radiography, and (iii) relatively high-radiation exposure for both patients and personnel. About 3.6 billion procedures are carried out per year globally, and >70 injuries have been reported.

Fluoroscopy exposure may lead to deterministic effects that include erythema, skin ulcer, temporary epilation, and dermal fibrosis. However, these effects vary with fluoroscopy time, dose rate, fractionation of dose, mode of operation, patient age, and site of exposure. Skin injuries have been reported in patients who undergone prolonged fluoroscopy-guided interventional procedures such as percutaneous transluminal coronary angioplasty (PTCA), radiofrequency cardiac catheter ablation, and vascular embolization. The cumulative skin doses in some patients may exceed 10 Gy, which is sufficient to cause radiation-induced skin injury **(Figs. 18.1 to 18.4)**. These injuries may appear only after a threshold period of several months.

The risk of deterministic and stochastic effects of radiation exposure varies for different areas of the skin. The age of the patient undergoing long fluoroscopic time of imaging is also an important factor. PTCA and percutaneous transluminal angioplasty (PTA) are used in patient population over 40 years of age. Lesser numbers of adults and children are also treated using interventional procedures. It is essential to differentiate between interventional procedures in adults, in young adults, and in children. If areas of the skin are exposed to levels of absorbed doses that approach the skin tolerance, the patient should be informed in advance about the possible effects of treatment. All relevant parameters should be documented for all interventional procedures.

RADIATION EMERGENCIES IN RADIOISOTOPE LABORATORY

Radiation emergencies in radioisotope laboratory would normally involve only spillage of radioactive liquids. The procedures for handling spills and emergency preparedness are much important.

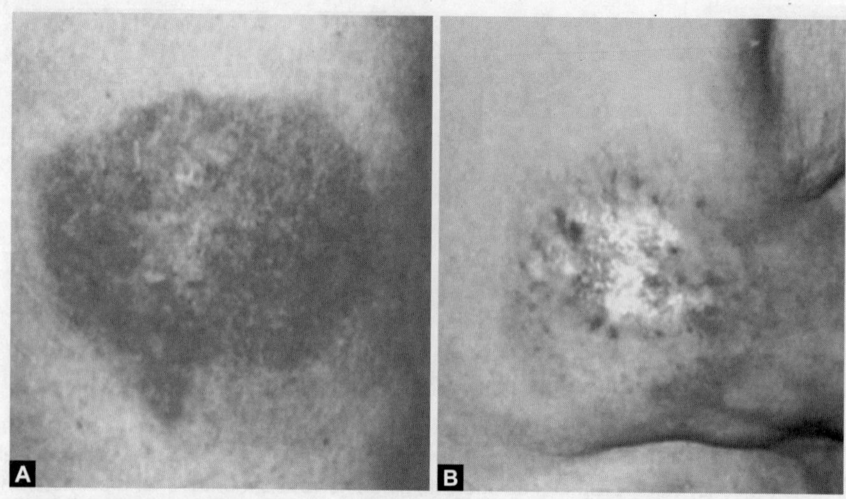

FIGS. 18.2A AND B: (A) 56-year-old man with obstructing lesion of right coronary artery. Photograph of right posterolateral chest wall at 10 weeks after percutaneous transluminal coronary angioplasty shows 12 × 6.5 cm hyperpigmented plaque with hyperkeratosis below right axilla; (B) A 75-year-old woman with 90% stenosis of right coronary artery. Photograph of right lateral chest obtained 10 months after percutaneous transluminal coronary angioplasty shows area of hyper- and hypopigmentation, skin atrophy, and telangiectasia (poikiloderma). ***(For color version, see Plate 4)***

Courtesy: AJR:177, July 2001.

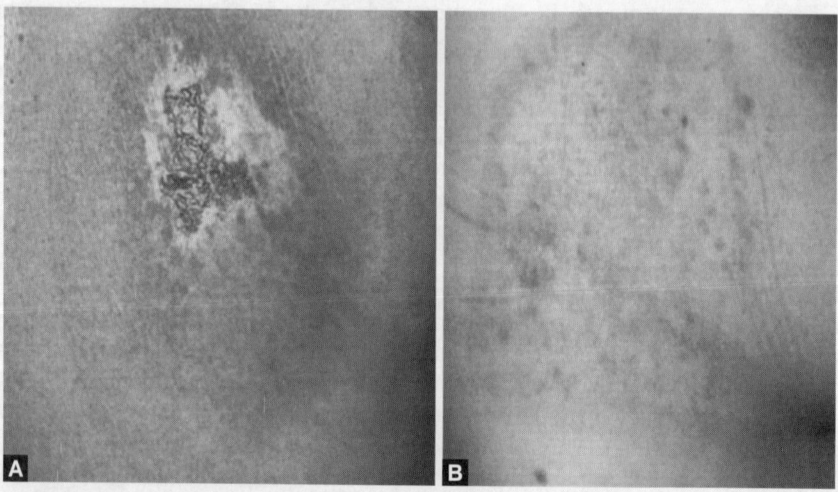

FIGS. 18.3A AND B: (A) Skin necrosis (erythema and hyperpigmentation), 3 years after angioplasty examination; (B) A17-year-old girl with history of cardiac arrhythmia underwent two cardiac ablation procedures in 13 months. Photograph taken 2 years after last intervention shows atrophic indurated plaque with skin telangiectasia at right lateral chest wall involving posterolateral aspect of breast. Induration resulted in limited movement of right arm. Risk of breast cancer is increased. ***(For color version, see Plate 4)***

Courtesy: AJR:177, July 2001.

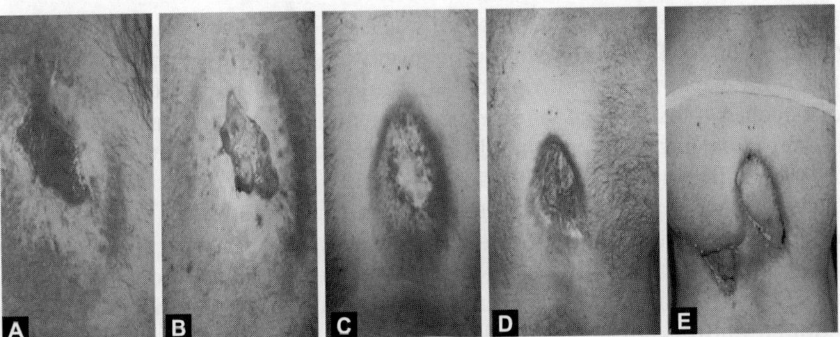

FIGS. 18.4A TO E: A 49-year-old man with history of liver cirrhosis and intractable upper gastrointestinal bleeding who underwent two transjugular intrahepatic portosystemic shunt (TIPS) placements and one attempted TIPS placement within a week. Photographs show progression of ulceration. (A) Secondary ulceration with surrounding rings of depigmentation and hyperpigmentation 6 months later; (B) Small blisters developed at 7.5 months after procedure. Wound is very painful; (C) Wound has progressed in size and depth at 10 months; (D) Nonhealing ulcer with exposure of deep tissues, including spinous process of vertebra, at 22 months; (E) At 23 months, musculocutaneous skin grafting was performed. Disfigurement is permanent. ***(For color version, see Plate 5)***

Courtesy: AJR:177, July 2001.

Procedures for Handling Spills

Accidental spills of radioactive materials are quite common in nuclear medicine departments, but they are not life-threatening hazards. Hence, spills should be treated as events completely without hazard, and the staff should be aware of the procedures to be followed. Steps involved in the radioactive spill are—(i) to inform, (ii) to contain, and (iii) to decontaminate. Individuals in the immediate work area should be informed that the spill has occurred so that they can avoid contamination if possible. Individuals outside the immediate area should be warned so that they do not enter it. The Radiation Safety Officer (RSO) should be informed so that he/she may begin supervising further action as soon as possible.

The laboratory personnel should attempt to control the spill to prevent further spread of contamination, without risking themselves. A flask that has been tipped over should be uprighted. Absorbent pads should be thrown over a liquid spill. Doors should be closed to prevent the escape of airborne radioactivity. The spill area should be closed off to prevent entry, especially by persons who might not be aware of the spill. Personnel monitoring for contamination should be started as soon as possible, so that contamination and uncontaminated persons can be segregated. To prevent further spread of radioactivity, contaminated individuals should not be allowed to leave the area until they are decontaminated. The uncontaminated individuals should not be allowed to enter the spill area. Contamination monitoring should be done using a sensitive radiation-monitoring instrument appropriate for the type of radioactivity involved. It is advisable that each laboratory has on hand a thin window Geiger Müller (GM) counter survey meter cum contamination monitor for handling such situations.

Personnel decontamination procedures should be the first step followed by decontamination of work areas, etc. Personnel involved in decontamination procedures should wear protective clothing to avoid becoming contaminated themselves in the process. Contaminated skin should be flushed thoroughly with water. Special attention should be given to open wounds and contamination around the eyes, nose, and mouth. Contaminated clothing should be removed and placed in plastic bags for storage. After major localized areas of personnel contamination have been attended to, a shower bath may be required to remove more widely distributed contamination.

Decontamination of laboratory and work areas should not be attempted except under the supervision of RSO. If the work surfaces and floors are constructed from a nonabsorbent material, soap and water are generally used for decontamination. Contaminated areas should be cleaned "from outside in" to minimize the spread of contamination. Porous or cracked surfaces may create difficult problems. If complete decontamination is not possible, it may be necessary to cover and shield the affected surfaces or perhaps even to remove and replace them.

It is very difficult to make rules to manage variety of radiation accidents. However, spillage of radioactivity is the most likely accident in radioisotope laboratory, for which following procedures are recommended in dealing with such emergencies:

- Tongs or forceps should be used to remove the contamination by absorbent material. The absorbent material and other wastes collected during decontamination should be kept in a polythene bag as radioactive waste. It should be disposed, as per Atomic Energy Regulatory Board (AERB) safety guidelines.
- After as much contamination as possible has been removed, the surface should be washed with damp-not wet-paper towels held by forceps, always working towards the center of contaminated area, rather than away from it.
- A contamination monitor should be used to monitor the area as well as personnel during the procedure of decontamination. It should be operated by someone who is not involved in the clean up so that the instrument does not become contaminated when the decontamination procedure is over. Contaminated gloves, shoe covers, etc. should be kept in a polythene bag for decay or ultimate disposal as radioactive waste. The forceps/tongs should be kept separately covered in polythene bag for decay of radioactivity in it.
- In case of a large release of radioactive powder or aerosol in a room, such a room must be immediately isolated from its surroundings by shutting off mechanical ventilation and by closing windows and doors. A room with heavy air contamination can be decontaminated from within by drawing air of the room through an appropriate filler.
- Maintain complete records of the accident giving details of the radioisotope, activity involved, etc. and follow-up procedures.

For effective management of any kind of radiation emergency, the RSO should educate and familiarize all radiation workers with steps to be taken to meet the emergency. Use of radionuclides in research applications will not give significant exposure to public, provided certain basic precautions are taken. These precautions mainly involve good accuracy for the radionuclides, good work practice, and a well-controlled program for the disposal of radioactive waste.

Emergency Preparedness

- Charts detailing various steps to be taken by the radiation workers in case of emergency should be conspicuously displayed in the laboratory.
- All radiation monitoring and measuring instruments should be routinely checked and kept in working condition. Handling equipment such as tongs, forceps, etc. must be kept in ready access.

- Ventilation system of the radioisotope laboratory should be routinely checked and maintained properly.
- Ready availability of a decontamination kit containing all the items of decontamination should be ensured to deal with an accidental spill effectively.
- A proper inventory of radioisotopes received, used, and disposed should be maintained.

Nuclear Medicine Case Studies

Case Study 1

The IAEA report 17 (2000) has reported seven accidents in the case of unsealed sources. A therapeutic dose of 370 MBq was prescribed to a wrong patient because two patients had the same name. Among the two patients, one for iodine administration and other for treatment of a lung disease with identical name were there. The physician familiar with the patient was not available and another physician was assigned to administer the dose. The lung disease patient was administered with ^{131}I of 370 MBq activity.

Case Study 2

In another event, a patient came for a diagnostic bone scan was administered with 333 MBq of ^{131}I, instead of 740 MBq of ^{99m}Tc for bone scan study.

Case Study 3

In another event, a 60-year-old woman was referred to the nuclear medicine for thyroid ablation. The physician prescribed 6475 MBq of ^{131}I by oral administration. The technician without reading the labels picked up two vials containing 6475 MBq and 5180 MBq of ^{131}I and administered both the activity to the patient.

Case Study 4

In another event, a patient was prescribed 370 MBq for a thyroid treatment. A capsule containing 370 MBq was ordered. The supplier sent a capsule containing 444 MBq. Though the technician calibrated the dose but misread the activity of 444 as 370 MBq. The patient was administered with 444 MBq, which resulted in an overdosage of 20%.

Case Study 5

Another event includes administration of 180 MBq of ^{131}I for a whole-body scan to a feeding mother. The scan indicated an unusual high breast uptake of ^{131}I, which resulted in a 300-Gy thyroid dose and 0.17-Gy whole body dose to the infant. Both the physician and technologists have failed to confirm that the patient was not breastfeeding.

Case Study 6

In another event, a therapy dose of 7400 MBq was administered to an 87-year-old patient. After 34 hours, the patient experienced cardiac failure and 16 staff members attempted to resuscitate the patient to insert pacemaker, etc. Blood and urine contaminated with radioactivity were spilled, but the personnel clothing was not checked for activity. A dose of 0.3 Gy was reported in one of the nursing staffs.

Case Study 7

In another event, a patient was to be administered with 259 MBq of ^{131}I. There were two capsules of 130 MBq each in the vial, which were labeled correctly. When the vial is inverted only, one capsule fell out and the same was administered. That is patient was given 130 MBq instead of 259 MBq activity, 50% of the prescribed dose.

RADIATION ACCIDENTS AND EMERGENCIES IN RADIATION THERAPY

A situation in a beam therapy facility can be considered as an emergency, if it could result in higher actual or potential radiation doses than those in normal situations to personnel, patients, or public. In 2000, the IAEA published its report no. 17 "Lessons Learned from Accidental Exposures in Radiotherapy", it described 92 accidents resulting in an incorrect dose to the patient. Out of 92, 32 of these accidents were related to the use of sealed sources (brachytherapy).

In the case of telegamma units, two potentially hazardous situations may arise: (1) the source does not, or only partially, go back to OFF position; in other words, it continues to be in the "ON" position even after the termination of the set treatment, and (2) the source falls off from the source head.

The type of situations where the telegamma source continues to be in the "ON" position, vary with the source "ON-OFF" mechanism in the unit. It includes failure of—(i) pneumatic system, (ii) shutter to close, and (iii) drum to rotate, to bring the source back to "OFF" position at the end of the set treatment time. Emergency continues until the source is completely shielded by mechanical or manual or other means. In certain systems, emergency may be caused by leakage of mercury which functions as a shield, thus leaving the source in the "ON" position even after the set treatment time is over.

In medical accelerators, normally such type of emergency does not occur. However, recently, a few cases of computer software mix-up, resulting in the wrong selection of electron mode, have been reported. The following paragraph discusses several instant of such emergency situations in teletherapy units which have occurred in this country and abroad. In India, six incidents have been reported in radiotherapy applications. They were associated with teletherapy units, due to which 24 persons received low-radiation doses, and one person received a high dose on hand, requiring amputation.

Emergency Situations in Radiation Therapy: Case Studies

Leakage of Mercury (Shutter)

In September 1980, the film badges worn by the radiation therapist, the physicist, and the technologist of a hospital recorded high doses. On investigation, it was noted that this was caused by an emergency of an Eldorado A Unit 2. Here, the source is stationary and shielded in "OFF" position by mercury between the source and the collimator. When the source is made "ON", the mercury is pumped out and stored in a reservoir and held there against gravity. Small mass of mercury started leaking from this reservoir when the source was "ON". The leakage of mercury was noted, and they arranged to collect the leaking mercury and put it back into the unit as immediate remedial measure. However, some quantity of mercury was lost in this process and, hence, the efficiency of mercury as the shield was gradually reduced. This process continued until December 23, 1980, when the treatment by the unit had to be discontinued for want of spare parts. Later, the hospital staff developed a special filter, which, when incorporated into the unit, completely prevented the leakage of mercury. Several overexposures to personnel were reported during this period. Based on chromosome aberration test reports, the individual equivalent dose, ranging from 20 to 50 rem, was estimated to have been caused by this emergency.

Failure of Shutter Movement

Case study 1: In July 1984, a case of malfunctioning of the mobile shutter of a *Theratron-B* unit was reported. The shutter mechanism was working only when the unit was pointed downward. The mobile shutters were encountering the obstructions on its path and as a result, the shutter used to remain partially open during the "off" position. The source was unloaded, and the shutter was removed and examined. It was observed that the mobile shutter had lost its integrity and that a tiny particle removed from it got embedded in the housing and caused the obstruction. The shutter was thoroughly cleaned, polished, and lubricated, and the unit recommissioned. During this emergency, the doses to personnel involved in the repair work were negligible.

Case study 2: The shutter mechanism of a *Gammatron* unit, serviced during the source replacement on December 13, 1984, failed to function and remained open at the end of set treatment time on January 23, 1985. The service engineers reported that the shutter developed extraordinary friction. Treatment was stopped until April 16, 1985, when the source was unloaded, and shutter repaired. The individual doses received by personnel during the repair were <10 mrem.

Case study 3: In another emergency, on November 23, 1985, the shutter of a *Gammatron* unit remained in open position and could not be closed, even manually. The service engineers reported that the source had to be unloaded prior to shutter repair. It was ascertained that the shutter mechanism had developed extraordinary friction due to damage in the ball-bearing movement system. For want of spare parts, to be imported, the unit could not be used for treatment for about 16 months. The source was unloaded on April 14, 1987, and the unit was repaired. The personnel dose during the repair was <10 mrem.

Case study 4: In another case of *Gammatron* unit, the shutter failed to close at the end of the set treatment time in October 1986. The patient was immediately removed, and defect was rectified by the hospital engineer.

Pneumatic System Failure

Two cases of source "stuck" in the "ON" position for *Gammarex-R* unit have been reported. In both cases, the source drawer did not return to the parking position at the end of the set treatment time, and the sources were pushed back to "OFF" position manually with the T-rod. Personnel exposures were well within permissible levels. In one case, subsequently the source was unloaded, the drawer and its passage area thoroughly cleaned, and the source reloaded.

Improper Functioning of Timer

A typical case of improper functioning of the timer of *Picker* unit has been reported. The timer was observed to reset the time automatically at the end of the set treatment time. This resulted in the source to be in the "ON" position continuously until the timer was manually interrupted. Even though such an incident has not been reported in India, a formal intimation regarding this malfunction was sent to all users of Picker unit. It was confirmed that the timers in the Picker units in India were functioning properly.

Software Mix-up in Accelerator

Two incidents of massive overdoses of patients took place in a hospital in USA from *Therac-25 accelerator* on March 21 and April 11, 1986, with "Malfunction-54" occurring in both the cases. A third case with the same accelerator, which occurred on April 25, 1985, was reported later. Another similar incident from a different hospital using the same model of accelerator occurred on January 17, 1987, though the reported malfunction was of a different nature. The first two patients died, and the third patient was seriously maimed.

The "Malfunction-54" occurred when the technician inadvertently selected photon beam mode for a patient who was to be treated with electron beam of lower energy. The operator realizing the mistake promptly corrected for the mode using the edit-key facility. The computer displayed the electron beam mode and the "beam ON" command was given to start the treatment. The treatment was abruptly terminated after 1 second with the patient writhing in pain calling for help from inside treatment room. The physicist later simulated the malfunction and measured the dose in water phantom as 25,000 rads in 1 second. Atomic Energy of Canada Limited (AECL) subsequently informed all Therac-25 users to suspend the use of this accelerator. A plan for correcting the errant software was submitted by AECL to Food and Drugs Administration, USA.

In the fourth incidence, though the photon beam mode was selected, the heavy metal target did not come into position into the path of the electron beam, instead a light field mirror came in position to intercept the electron beam. Corrective action plan was amended accordingly.

San Jose, Costa Rica Accident

A radiotherapy overexposure occurred at the *San Juan de Dios Hospital* in San Jose, Costa Rica in August and September 1996. About 115 patients, who were treated for neoplasm by radiotherapy, were affected. Out of the 115 patients, 42 died and 73 were alive. The radiation exposure was a major factor for death in three patients and partial in four patients. The event occurred on August 22, 1996, when a Cobalt-60 source was replaced. After the source loading, the new source was calibrated, and an error was made in calculating the dose rate. The miscalculation had resulted in administration of higher doses to the patients than prescribed.

Panama Accident

A radiation accident occurred in the *National Institute of Oncology, Panama*, in May 2001, in which 28 patients undergoing radiotherapy in cobalt unit were affected. The IAEA team visited the place on May 22, 2001, and reported that out of 28, eight patients had died. The death of five is due to radiation overexposure, one death is related to cancer, and, in remaining two deaths, no conclusion was made.

The cause for the accident is due to wrong data entry into the TPS computer. The spatial coordinates of the shielding block have to be fed into the TPS in way that-one shield at time. From August 2000, the coordinates of all the shielding blocks were entered as a single block, which resulted in incorrect dose and treatment times. Lack of written procedures and manual check, when the data input procedure was changed, resulted in radiation overexposure to the above patients.

Ottawa Hospital Cancer Center Accident

A relocation of an orthovoltage treatment unit from one campus to the other in the *Ottawa Hospital Cancer Center* in the Fall of 2004 was followed by an error at the time of recommissioning. The error was reflected as incorrect output tables for all four beam qualities and for all field sizes other than $10 \times 10\ cm^2$. A total of 1,019 treatments were delivered to 620 patients using the incorrect orthovoltage output tables during November 2004 to November 2007. Patients were underdosed to a maximum of 17%. No overexposure was reported, and the cause was due to the omission of a backscatter conversion factor for all the fields other than $10 \times 10\ cm^2$ (*www.iaea.org*).

Overexposure during Source Exchange

Two radiation workers, while working on a source exchange of a decayed cobalt-60 source in a hospital in the state of *São Paulo, Brazil* on July 21, 2008, received significant overexposure. The workers transferred the source drawer from the unit head to the transfer flask with the help of tool. When the tool was pulled out, the source drawer momentarily came out of the transfer flask before the worker pushed back. They received a whole-body equivalent dose of 135 mSv and 0.7 mSv, respectively. Later, on August 15, 2008, it was found that one of the fingers of the individual was blistering. The extremity dose was estimated as 25 Sv.

Different types and degrees of emergency as discussed above can potentially occur in beam therapy facilities. The facility and the RSO must be prepared to meet such kinds of emergencies at any time. Line of action to be followed may vary with the type of emergency and the personnel must be clearly aware of the same.

Radiation Emergencies: Fall of Source Drawer

During source replacement or source head repair of telegamma therapy units with source "ON–OFF" mechanism, serious accidents can take place unless proper care is taken. Two such serious accidents have taken place in India in two different institutions. In each case, sources loaded in parallelepiped shape source drawer fell from the source head during repairing of shutter mechanism. In one case, it was Cobalt-60 source of 6000 RHM and in the other it was Cesium-137 source of 2050 Ci.

First Incident

The first incident took place when two undertrained staff members of the institution tried to repair the shutter mechanism of a *Gammatron-3* teletherapy unit. They removed the gearbox mounted at the back side of the drum shutter to look for any foreign particles obstructing the movement. Later, they removed the front plate as well as the arresting strip of the drawer. The head was tilted through +30° in the forward direction and the unit was rotated to bring it to a convenient position. The source drawer, which was lying freely in the cavity, slipped down from the head. Realizing the seriousness of the situation, they came out and locked the room

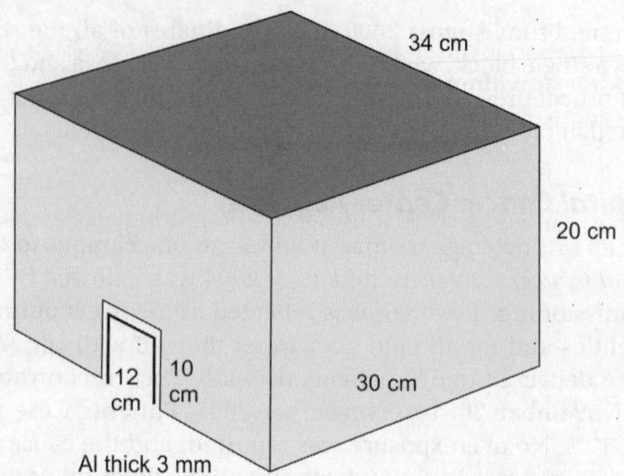

FIG. 18.5: Aluminium tray designed to cover the source drawer.

Courtesy: AERB/BARC,2014.

immediately. They received whole body equivalent dose of 29.50 mSv (2950 mrem) and 12.40 mSv (1240 mrem).

Source retrieval operation: The retrieval operation was planned based on information collected during a preliminary visit to assess the situation. The details available from the layout of the installation were also useful in planning the management of the accident. Temporary extra shielding was planned for secondary walls to be provided by piling up sandbags up to 1 meter height. An aluminum tray with a groove-like depression at the bottom to sit on the source drawer was designed and fabricated (**Fig. 18.5**). It was planned to cover the source drawer with the above tray and to fill it up with lead shots through a polystyrene pipe by personnel positioned behind the maze wall.

Area monitoring of the entrance to the treatment area and other areas of interest was carried out using a Teleflex cable of 12-m length connected to the detector, keeping the meter of the monitoring instrument outside the room. The radiation levels at various points measured before and after providing temporary shielding are given in **Table 18.1**. The various locations in which radiations were measured are given in **Figure 18.6**. Since there was no lead glass viewing window and since the CCTV was focused to the couch, a mirror mounted on a wheel trolley was employed at the entrance of the treatment room to locate the source drawer. With the help of this mirror, it was observed that the major length of the source drawer was hidden by the base drum of the couch, which was locked to the ground. Further, a raised wooden platform made of interlocked portions was provided in the room for the convenience of patients, as it lowered the height of the couch. The source drawer was lying on this platform. As such, positioning the aluminum tray to cover the source drawer and to fill it up with lead shorts were not viable to persons positioned behind the temporary shielding erected at the entrance position.

A rehearsal of the operation with a dummy drawer was conducted in the adjacent teletherapy room. It was concluded that aluminum tray can be placed over the source drawer by one person entering the room with a remote handling tong of 2.0 m length and that the equivalent dose for this operation will be about 15 mSv (1500 mrem). However, this job could have been carried out with an equivalent dose of 12.5 mSv (1250 mrem) to the operator.

TABLE 18.1 **Radiation levels in and around the telecobalt facility before and after providing temporary shielding at the entrance and maze region [the source drawer with ^{60}Co source of 222 TBq (6,000 Ci) was lying on the wooden platform inside the treatment room. The source was facing the ceiling. The locations where radiation levels were measured are numbered and marked in Fig. 18.6]. (AERB/BARC, 2014)**

Radiation levels in and around the telecobalt facility					
		Before providing temporary shielding		***After providing temporary shielding***	
Location number	***Location description***	***Air kerma rate (mGy/h)***	***Exposure rate (mGy/h)***	***Air kerma rate (mGy/h)***	***Exposure rate (mR/h)***
1.	Behind the maze wall	1.74	200	0.35	40
2.		0.87	100	0.87	100
3.		0.44	50	0.44	50
4.		0.87	100	0.87	100
5.		1.74	200	1.74	200
6.		6.97	800	1.31	150
7.	Entrance to Treatment room	43.50	5×10^3	5.22	600
8.		522.00	60×10^3	522.00	60×10^3
9.		104.40	12×10^3	43.50	5×10^3
10.	Door maze reg.	0.17	20	0.04	4
11.	Control panel	0.02	2	8.70×10^3	1

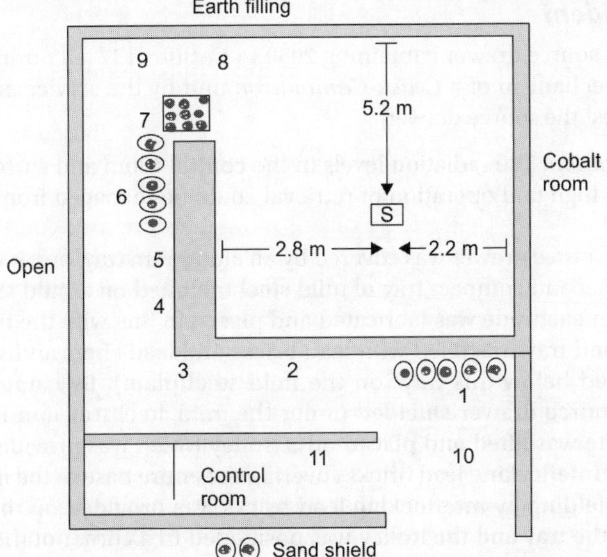

FIG. 18.6: Layout of the teletherapy facility, where radiation levels are measured.

Courtesy: AERB/BARC, 2014.

In the wall common to control room and treatment room, a tapered hole was drilled at the height of 2.5 m from the floor for the passage of polystyrene pipe, to facilitate filling up of the aluminum tray with lead shots. In order to reduce the radiation level at the drilling position, radiation source had to be shielded, temporarily. Lead shots (about 40 kg) packed in cloth bags were used for this purpose. This was carried out for a collective equivalent dose of 0.025 man-Sievert (2.5 man-rem). The exposure rate at the drilling position was then reduced to 5 mR/h from 200 mR/h.

Polystyrene pipes of 5 cm in diameter and 6 meter in length were extended to the aluminum tray through the hole drilled on the wall at control room. About 350 kg of lead shorts of diameter 1–2 mm were poured into the aluminum tray through this pipe. This brought down the radiation level inside the treatment room to a workable level. All unwanted materials and a major portion of the wooden platform inside the room were quickly removed.

The source drawer was lying at the middle of the platform. To transfer the drawer into a transport flask, the drawer had to be brought to the edge of the platform. Another aluminum tray of slightly larger size and smaller groove for source drawer to exactly fit in (to reduce streaming) was fabricated and positioned in line with the aluminum tray with lead shots in it, which was covering the source drawer. The source drawer was then transferred to the groove of the second tray. After emptying the first tray, it was used in line with the second tray for shifting the source drawer further close to the edge of the platform to enable it to be loaded into the transportation flask. Before loading source drawer into the transportation flask, shielded source drawer had to be lifted through 20 cm to bring the source drawer in line with the cavity loading the fallen source drawer into transportation flask, the teletherapy unit was repaired, and subsequently the source loading was carried out. The equivalent doses received by personnel involved in the retrieval operation are given in **Table 18.1**. The total collective equivalent dose was about 0.07 man-Sievert (7.0 man-rem).

Second Incident

In this case, a source drawer containing 2050 Ci Cesium-137 fell during repairing of the shutter mechanism of a *Ceasa-Gammatron* unit by the service engineers, who missed to arrest the source drawer.

Retrieval operation: The radiation levels in the control room and surrounding areas were not very high and operation of retrieval could be managed from the entrance door.

The fallen source drawer was covered by an aluminum tray, and it was filled with lead shots. A second compact tray of mild steel mounted on a mild steel plate with three hooks on each side was fabricated and placed in line with the first aluminum tray. The second tray was filled with lead bricks and lead shots and source drawer was transferred below this tray (on the mild steel plate). By using chain pulley system, the source drawer shielded under the mild steel tray and resting on the mild steel plate was lifted and placed on a trolley which was provided with 10-cm thick layers of interlocking lead bricks covering the entire base of the mild steel tray. Additional shielding by interlocking lead bricks was provided on three sides and on the top of the tray and the trolley was positioned in a corner of the room. Later, the source drawer was loaded into the teletherapy head after the repair of the unit. The total collective equivalent dose in the operation was about 0.02 man-Sievert (2 man-rem).

TABLE 18.2 Type and number of accidents reported in brachytherapy treatments (IAEA, 2000).

Accident caused by	*Number of cases*
Dose calculation error	6
Error in quantities and units	2
Incorrect source strength	7
Equipment failure	4
Others	13
Total	32
(IAEA: International Atomic Energy Agency)	

From the above incidents, we can conclude that unless proper care is taken during servicing or source loading, serious accidents involving high exposure to personnel and long down time of machine can take place. In addition, skillful planning of management of accident is necessary for keeping radiation dose to the minimum to personnel involved in the operation.

Radiation Accidents: Brachytherapy

The IAEA report no. 17 presents 32 accidents related to brachytherapy. The type and number of accidents are summarized in **Table 18.2**. Errors in the specification of the source activity, dose calculation, or the quantities and units resulted in doses that were up to 170% of the prescribed dose. Some accidents were related to human mistakes, for example the use of an incorrect source due to fading of the color coding. This is listed under "other" in the table, which also includes accidents caused by badly implanted sources, removal of the sources by the patient or otherwise dislodged sources. The most severe accident was due to equipment failure, where a lethal dose was delivered to a patient.

High-dose rate (HDR) brachytherapy units have higher potential for damage to patients because of misadministration. In one HDR event, the patient was prescribed a dose of 35 Gy to lung. There was a kink in the catheter which positioned the source 26 cm away from the target site. The error was not discovered until the treatment was over. Because of this error, hypopharynx received 35 Gy and the target received only 1 Gy.

The other events include using an HDR prescription for the wrong patient, and malfunction of the HDR equipment, etc. Overall, the treatment delivery errors can be summarized as follows:

- Positioning of the active source train outside the treatment volume
- Mispositioning of dose prescription points
- Failure to detect a source that separated from its cable and remained in the implanted catheter for 91 hours

International Atomic Energy Agency reported that the misadministration is due to malfunctioning equipment, such as catheters do not allow full movement of sources. It also mentioned the inadequacy of personnel training which caused the misadministration. The above demonstrates the need for a well-designed program of quality assurance in any brachytherapy department. Its goal should be the consistency of the administration of each individual treatment, the realization of the clinical intent of the radiation oncologist, and the safe execution of the treatment with respect to patient and staffs.

MEDICAL MANAGEMENT OF RADIATION EMERGENCY

The objective of medical management is to—(i) save lives and perform required emergency medical procedures, (ii) treat treatment injuries and injuries resulting from emergency situations, and (iii) perform required public heath actions including providing advice and counseling and long-term medical follow-up. Medical management is required for (1) external exposure, and (2) contamination with radionuclides, or both.

External Exposure

Exposure is an act or condition of being subjected to irradiation. In external exposure, no radioactive material is transferred, and the source is outside the body. It poses no radiological hazard to any one or an individual and can be local, partial, or whole-body exposure. Medical consequences depend on the dose received by different tissues and organs and the volume of body irradiated. Variables such as source activity, energy of the radiation, duration of exposure, and dose rate will provide information for dose assessment and treatment guidance. After an external exposure, two conditions may emerge, namely (1) acute radiation syndrome (ARS) and (2) local radiation injury.

Acute Radiation Syndrome

Acute radiation syndrome (ARS) is an acute illness caused by exposure to high dose of radiation at one time or over a short period. It is a deterministic effect to the whole body or partial volume of the body, above a threshold dose of about 1 Gy. It induces set of clinical and biological manifestations in the organs and tissues. ARS is divided into—(i) hematopoietic syndrome, (ii) gastrointestinal syndrome, and (iii) neurovascular or cerebrovascular syndrome. ARS progresses in three stages, which are as follows:

1. *Stage 1*: Early symptoms such as nausea, loss of appetite, vomiting, tiredness, and diarrhea
2. *Stage 2*: Symptom-free period
3. *Stage 3*: Various pattern of symptoms based on the radiation dose received

The symptoms and its rate of progression depend upon the radiation dose. Higher the dose, earlier will be the symptoms which progress more rapidly. The severity and time course of the early symptoms are consistent from person to person. It is possible to estimate the radiation dose based on the timing, nature, and severity of early symptoms. For detailed discussion on ARS, refer Chapter 2, Radiation Biology.

Local Radiation Injury

In localized radiation injury (LRI), radiation exposure is restricted to limited area of the body. Most commonly, skin, hands, feet, legs, and face are irradiated but any other part of the body may also be involved. Extensive involvement of skin which may jeopardize life is referred as *cutaneous radiation syndrome (CRS)*, which is different from LRI. LRI caused by gamma radiation is a matter of concern in accidental overexposures in terms of frequency and deeper skin injury. Shallow skin injuries caused by extensive exposure by external beta radiation are referred as *beta burns*. Beta radiation injuries are nonhomogeneous pattern and mostly protected by clothes. In this, the radiation dose is a function of time taken to the removal of beta source from the cloth or skin. Observed data reveals that radiation workers, public, and patients are the targets for LRI from the following:

- Radiotherapy and interventional radiology accidents
- Industrial radiography sources accidents
- Accidents with irradiators
- Accidents at nuclear power plants
- Criminal or terrorist acts involving radioactive material

Symptoms of Local Radiation Injury

Radiation therapy used to treat cancer is the common source of LRI. Its symptoms depend on quantity of dose, dose rate, and the area of the body. Nausea, vomiting, and loss of appetite may occur after irradiation in brain or abdomen. Skin changes are hair loss, redness, peeling, sores and thinning of skin, and dilated blood vessels. Irradiation in mouth and jaw results in dry mouth, number of dental caries, and damage of jawbone. Radiation to lungs can cause lung inflammation (pneumonitis), severe scarring of lung tissue (fibrosis). It may cause disabling shortness of breath and later death. The heart and its protective sac become inflamed and cause pain and shortens of death. High doses of radiation to the spinal cord can cause catastrophic damage, leading to paralysis, incontinence, and loss of sensation. Abdomen irradiation can cause chronic ulcers, scarring, and narrowing or perforation of the intestine. It involves symptoms of abdominal pain, vomiting, vomiting blood, and dark, tarry stools.

Severe injuries may appear occasionally in kidney after high dose of radiation therapy, and kidney function may decline after 6 months resulting anemia and high blood pressure. Irradiation to muscles may cause muscle wasting (atrophy) and calcium deposits in the irradiated muscle. Radiotherapy may cause cancer rarely >10 years after irradiation.

Skin Injuries Following Exposure

Localized radiation injury is a deterministic effect, and its severity follows dose-dependent pattern. It is a dynamic process, develops over time in an unpredictable way. Skin is the first organ to be exposed following irradiation. The earliest response to skin irradiation is primary erythema that appears in few hours after high acute exposure due to capillary dilation. It may be unnoticed in an individual due to dark skin and its severity is dose indicator.

Acute radiation induces oxidative stress resulting in a cascade of inflammatory responses, reduction and impairment of functional stem cells, endothelial cell changes, and epidermal cell death through apoptosis and necrosis. High-dose radiation can interfere with normal maturation, reproduction, and reproduction of germinative epidermal cell populations. At much higher dose, the mitotic activity of the germinal cells of the sebaceous glands, hair follicles, basal cell layer, and intimal cells of the microvasculature may be compromised. Primary erythema is followed by secondary erythema dry desquamation, moist desquamation, blistering, ulceration, and necrosis **(Table 18.3)**.

TABLE 18.3 Local radiation injuries and threshold radiation dose (IAEA, safety report series no. 101, Medical management of radiation injuries, 2020).

Radiation effects	*Threshold dose of X- and γ-rays (Gy)*	*Time of onset (days)*
Second phase erythema	3	14–21
Temporary epilation	3	14–18
Definitive epilation	7	25–30
Dry desquamation (dry epithelitis)	10	20–28
Moist desquamation (exudative epithelitis)	15	15–25
Necrosis	25	>21

(IAEA: International Atomic Energy Agency)

Phase-1 erythema: Primary erythema is followed by secondary erythema and dry desquamation in about 1–5 weeks due to release of proteolytic enzymes from the damaged epithelial cells. It follows dose-dependent time relation and moves next manifestation stage if dose is high. At high doses, late erythema may occur between 6 and 18 months postirradiation and follow vasculitis crises. Phlogistic and painful edema with paresthesia on the erythema area may appear at high doses.

Phase-2 epilation: Epilation or hair loss occurs if there is sufficient reduction in the replicative capacity of germinal cells or the matrix of the hair follicles. A dose of 2 Gy may cause follicular dysplasia. Temporary epilation may occur after doses of about 3 Gy, with an onset at about 2–4 weeks, after irradiation. Hair regrows after 2 months and gets completed within 6–12 months. For doses of >7 Gy, epilation is permanent. Hair follicle reaction to radiation indicates retrospective dose indicator. Biopsy is not advisable since it induces formation of ulcer in that zone due to fragile condition by radiation.

Phase-3 desquamation: The manifestation phase includes dry desquamation, moist desquamation, blistering, ulceration, and necrosis for doses >25 Gy. Pain, because of deep ulceration and necrosis is a matter of concern and treatment is difficult. Severity of pain is an indicator for future recurrence over time which is a prognostic indicator of the evaluation of LRI.

Transepidermal Burn

This is like second-degree thermal burns with a latent period of 1–2 weeks. Radiation burns are sometimes deceptive on superficial appearance as damage to important organs in subcutaneous tissue nerve endings, hair follicles, sweat glands, and endothelium of blood vessels may not be obvious. Among these, the injury to the endothelium of blood vessels is the most serious. It produces endarteritis obliterans, leading to necrosis of overlying tissues, which continues to progress for several months. The severity of burns depends on the dose and dose-rate and at doses of 30 Gy (300 rad) or above, blistering, and skin loss may take place. In such cases, besides subcutaneous tissues, other internal structures are affected and may give rise to radiation necrosis of bone, muscle, and other internal organs. Initial symptoms are erythema, pain, swelling, itching, or tingling and epilation.

Full-thickness Radiation Burn

This is like third-degree burns and a serious version of transepidermal injury. The injury extends up to the dermis and produces prompt and severe pain. If damage to circulation is present, the healing will take long time and surgical intervention may be required. Pain is an important feature of the exposure of skin, particularly in the extremities, to high doses of radiation. This pain is maximum with the appearance of vascular lesions. The pain is experienced during the first few days, lasting several hours, and it may last for long periods.

Long-term Effects

Long-term sequelae include changes in pigmentation, atrophy of epidermis, sweat glands, sebaceous glands and hair follicles, fibrosis of derma, and increased susceptibility to trauma and chronic ulceration. Sweet and sebaceous glands may undergo functional and structural changes after radiation. Telangiectasia, angioma formation, nail and nail bed changes, dermal erythematous reactions, atrophy, induration, fibrosis, and nonmelanoma skin cancer are the possible late effects. Radiation can cause hyperpigmentation through the activation of melanogenesis. At high doses, hyperpigmentation and depigmentation may appear due to death of large number of melanocytes.

Muscular damages were observed after high dose of radiation to human skeletal muscle. Severe reduction of fiber diameter and area, degree of fibrosis is abundant in the irradiated area, and loss of cytoplasm in the myofibers was noticed. In the irradiated tissue, microvascular circulation is disturbed, and numbers of micro-vessels are reduced. Irradiated bone biopsy may reveal greater volume of trabecular bone volume indicating morphological changes in a time and dose-dependent pattern. Medical management bone tissue necrosis includes surgery and may lead to even amputation.

Radio-osteonecrosis has been observed month–years after high dose of radiation. Radiation skin burns are sometimes considered as insect bites, skin allergies, thermal or chemical burns, and pemphigus foliaceus. Nonradiation exposure burns provide shrinking evidence for diagnosis of lower respiratory infection (LRI).

Diagnosis of Radiation Injury

Radiation injury can be diagnosed by history, symptoms, severity of symptoms, and time of onset of symptoms after radiation exposure, and lymphocyte counts.

History

A detailed history of accident with name, age, and sex of the person, the nature of radiation and energy, possibility of whole-body exposure or contamination, etc. should be collected. Personal thermoluminescent dosimeter (TLD) badges will provide some idea about the exposure. Sometimes, the patient may not be aware of irradiation and dose. Complete examination of the skin repeatedly from the first day is required to see—is there any prodromal erythema? The time at which transient erythema occurred, along with other symptoms, will enable the physician to come to a rough conclusion regarding the dose and the ultimate prognosis, with the development of fixed erythema.

Investigations

Radiation exposure is suspected if there are symptoms of illness or skin redness or sores in patients after radiation accident. No specific test is available; however, some tests can be used to detect infection such as low blood counts or organ malfunction.

Lymphocytes can be measured to determine the severity of radiation exposure. Lower lymphocyte count after 48 hours of radiation will indicate worsened situation. Radioactive contamination can be detected by GM counter survey, swipe test from nose, throat, and any wounds. Early symptoms of ARS are nausea, vomiting, and tremors due to anxiety. Procedures useful for medical evaluations of LRI are:

- Serial high quality and standardized color photography
- Ultrasonography
- Computed tomography (CT)/Magnetic resonance imaging (MRI)
- Thermography
- Early physical dose reconstruction
- Complete blood count (CBC)
- Blood lymphocyte culture and chromosomal analysis
- Sperm count
- Culture and antibiotic sensitivity test
- Estimation of radionuclides in urine and stools
- Noninvasive vascular studies
- Radioisotope scintigraphy
- Slit-lamp examination of eyes
- Physical dosimetry

Samples should be taken immediately for some tests in the above list. Concurrently, photographs should be taken, and dosimeters sent for evaluation of dose. Scintigraphy may be done before slit examination in view of blood contamination with ^{99m}Tc. Even after the area of burn becomes apparent, the underlying damage cannot be observed with accuracy clinically. Thermography and scintigraphy offer a means of detecting areas affected significantly by localized irradiation and the functional status of the organ. This information is helpful in planning any surgical intervention without waiting for the clinical symptoms to unfold fully. If there is leukopenia in the 1st week, it is suggestive of whole-body exposure. There is danger of infection which should be treated vigorously. Surgical intervention should be kept to the minimum during this phase of bone marrow depression which usually lasts about 4–8 weeks.

Prevention of Radiation Injury

After nuclear power plant accident or high-level environmental contamination of release of radioactive material, people should adhere the advice of public health officials through TV and radio. Advice includes evacuation of the contaminated areas to the shelters. It depends upon the time elapsed after the incident, availability of shelters. Concrete or metal structures preferably in basement (below grade) are advisable. Alternatively, halfway between top and bottom of the tall building may be occupied.

Nuclear detonation near the ground produces a fireball into the atmosphere and pulls up thousands of tons of dirt and debris, which create iconic mushroom-shaped cloud. The cloud stabilizes in the upper atmosphere and the radioactive material released in the explosion mix-up with dirt and small debris. This may return to earth (fallout), gets deposited on the surface, and gives dangerous radiation. Fallout may extend up to 10–20 miles away from the nuclear accident site. Those who are in the shelter may not be affected by the fallout. However, people should move to the shelter after 10–15 minutes of detonation to avoid such radioactive fallout. Change of clothes and warm water showering are recommended if contaminated with radioactive material.

Prognosis of Radiation Injury

The outcome of radiation injury depends on dose, dose rate, and part of the body exposed. Whether they receive medical care or not is also an important factor. It is stated that half of the people who receive >3 Gy or all the people who receive >8 Gy whole body exposure may die if medical treatment is not provided. Those who receive <2 Gy will recover within 1 month, though long-term cancer induction is not ruled out. In the case of medical care, half of the people who received whole body dose of 6 Gy may survive. Some people have survived even after 10 Gy whole body radiation exposure.

Cerebrovascular syndrome is fatal within hours to few days, whereas gastrointestinal syndrome fatal is within 3–10 days. People with hematopoietic syndrome, if medically treated, may survive depending upon the dose and state of health. Those who do not survive may die within 4–8 weeks after exposure.

Clinical and Radiological Triage

Triage refers to sorting of patients into priority groups as per need and availability of resources as first step. It is based on severity of medical conditions using conventional triage systems and not on radioactive exposure or contamination.

Second step is to identify the individuals as exposed or contaminated. Severity of radiation injury depends on radiation dose, dose rate, radiosensitivity of affected tissues and organs, and area and extent of the body exposed.

In radiation accidents, radiation exposure may combine with trauma, thermal, chemical, or other exposures, which make the prognosis poorer. Hospitalization depends on presence of early clinical signs, and it is necessary based on patient condition, medical diagnosis, and estimated dose. Alternatively, the skin lesion appearance of the patient is monitored, and laboratory reports are analyzed in the first 48 hours.

Treatment of radiation injury:

- Treatment of life-threatening injuries first
- Decontamination of wounds, skin, and hair
- Treatment of internal contamination
- Specific measures for some radionuclides
- Treatment of compromised immune system
- Supportive care

Serious physical injuries should be treated first since they are life-threatening. Contamination should be removed to prevent radioactive material. Contaminated wounds are treated before the skin, by flushing with saltwater solution and wiping them with surgical sponge. Later, wounds are covered to prevent recontamination to other sites. Contaminated skin should be gently scrupled with large amount of warm water and soap, given attention to skin folded and nails. If hair cannot be decontaminated with soap and water, clipping it off with scissors is preferred. This is continued until GM counter reads either zero or acceptable levels of contamination. As per AERB, decontamination level on skin due to spillage shall not exceed 3.7 Bq/cm^2.

In the case of internal contamination, intake of few chemicals can reduce the absorption or removal of radioactive material. *Potassium iodide (KI)* tablet can be administered but only useful for radioactive iodine release. People with other radioactive contamination, iodine sensitivity, and other thyroid conditions should avoid KI. Other drugs can also be used as intravenously or orally as follows:

- *Zinc or calcium diethylenetriamine pentaacetate (DTPA)*—for plutonium, yttrium, californium, and americium
- *Calcium or aluminum phosphate solution*—for strontium
- *Prussian blue*—for cesium, rubidium, and thallium

Potassium iodide is effective up to 90%, whereas other drugs are useful up to 25–75%. Nausea and vomiting are reduced by drugs and dehydration is treated with intravenous fluids. Gastrointestinal or hematopoietic syndrome patients are isolated to minimize their contact with infectious microorganisms. Blood transfusions and injection of growth factor stimulate blood cell production. This will decrease bleeding and anemia and fight against infection. If bone marrow is damaged, hematopoietic stem cell transplantation is preferred.

Persons with gastrointestinal syndrome require *antiemetics, intravenous fluids, and sedatives*. Antibiotics are given by mouth to kill bacteria in the intestine. Antibiotics and antifungal and antiviral drugs are given intravenously, if necessary. Cerebrovascular syndrome is treated for relieving pain, anxiety, and breathing difficulty and control seizures. Radiation-induced sores can cause pain which can be treated by analgesics, may need surgical intervention at later date. Surviving people are monitored for thyroid and cataract disorder.

Treatment of LRS and ARS is beyond the scope of the book and one can refer safety series no. 101, IAEA for further details. Generally, it requires hospitalization with plastic and reconstructive surgery. Management of pain relief is obtained with *conventional analgesics, nonsteroidal anti-inflammatory drugs, central action analgesics, and sedatives*.

Treatment of radiation-induced skin burns:

- *Mild erythema*: Mild erythema may become dry and start itching in 3–4 weeks. A bland lotion or steroid ointment should be applied locally. No tight clothing should be worn on the affected part.
- *Transepidermal burn*: Pain should be relieved by analgesics, and drug such as phenylbutazone, which causes bone marrow depression, should be used. Sterile-protective dressings should be used. Systemic antibiotics should be given for prevention of infection. Usually, the burns will heal without skin grafting in the absence of infection.
- *Full-thickness radiation burn*: The burns may progress from initial blistering to skin loss and deep tissue necrosis, giving rise to severe pain, tissue loss, and infections. This will require surgical intervention, the timing of which will be difficult to decide due to slow progression of burn. Bone marrow depression may further complicate the condition. In case there is leukopenia at 1 week, surgical treatment should be at minimum until hematopoietic recovery takes place (usually in about 8 weeks). In case the involved area is more than a few square cm (2–3 cm^2), skin grafting will be required. Larger areas involving necrosis and gangrene of distal portions of fingers or extremities will require amputation. In beta-ray burns, early excision and skin grafting may spare the patient from pain and discomfort. Lastly, follow-up of such cases is important because healed radiation burns may result in weak atrophic skin that is subject to chronic and recurrent ulceration. The time for amputation and reconstructive surgery depends on the following determinants:
    - Intractable pain
    - Size and location of injury
    - Degree of control over infection

- Degree to which vascular damage can be estimated
- Value of the part

Contamination with Radionuclides

Contamination with radionuclides may be external or internal or involving both. Radiation material is deposited on the skin surface, wounds, or internally via inhalation or ingestion.

External Contamination

External contamination occurs when radioactive material from an unsealed or broken source is deposited on the skin or clothing. It can be assessed by direct monitoring of the skin and clothing. These patients have potential for spreading the contamination; hence, special precautions are required. Whenever external contamination is suspected or present, life-saving action is required and the risk is less, if universal biosafety precautions are used.

Management of external contamination: Priority of patient management depends on radiological condition of the patient. Once medical condition of the patient is stabilized, if external contamination is suspected, the internal contamination must be ruled out. Radiation survey at the site should be performed. The clothing of the patient should be removed and kept in a sealed plastic bags along with sheets and blankets. This will remove 90% of external contamination and reduce risk of exposure for healthcare personnel. Clothes can be used to identify the contaminant radionuclides. Radiological survey of the patient can be done to find the presence and levels of contamination on the body surface. The personnel items such as watch, buttons, and mobile phones shall be collected, labeled, and stored.

Workers are considered as contaminated and should be decontaminated before the intake of skin. Otherwise, physician may consider the contaminated wounds as internal contamination. Treatment is based on half-life, solubility, radiotoxicity, and the amount of radioactive material. It is beneficial to prevent or minimize the uptake of radioactive material into the organs or tissues. Decontamination is done by gently irrigating of the wound with saline solution or water and may be repeated. Embedded material or detritus containing radioactive material are removed with forceps for analysis. Healthcare staffs should change their gloves often. Priority of decontamination is wounds, orifices, skin area. Body orifices include mouth, nose, eyes, and ears. Warm water is used to decontaminate intact skin. Mild soap or surgical scrub soap can be used additionally.

Internal Contamination

If radioactive material is taken into the body through different pathways, it is referred as internal contamination. It is checked by taking biological sample from the person or by direct measurement. Patients present only internal contamination may not cause direct hazard to other people. If the contamination is higher involving gamma emitters, it causes external exposure to other personnel, but the overall effect is minimal. Various pathways of internal contamination are:

- Intake of radioactive particle or gases
- Ingestion of radioactive material
- Absorption of radioactive material through wounds
- Absorption of radioactive material through intake skin
- Ingestion of radioactive material in the body

Radioactive material undergoes series of physiological process. It is retained or released from the organs or tissues that depend on physical and chemical forms, the intake of pathway and physiological conditions. Main priority is to stabilize and provide medical support to the patient. Secondary priority includes dose estimation, decontamination procedures, and decorporation.

Use of unsealed radioactive sources can cause risk of internal contamination. If universal safety standards are used, the radiological risk is lower. It will not cause immediate clinical manifestations. Internal contamination with radionuclides has four phases, namely (1) intake, (2) uptake, (3) deposition, and (4) decorporation.

Health consequences: Health risks from internal contamination are influenced by the following: (i) amount of radionuclide material that enters the body, (ii) chemical form of radioactive material, (iii) kind of emission and half-life, (iv) radiosensitivity of the organ or tissue, (v) patient's age, (vi) individual's physiological factors, and (vii) contamination pathway. Internal contamination with radionuclides is a stochastic late effect of cancer development. Risk coefficient for cancer development with different radionuclides has been reported.

Diagnosis and assessment: Internal contamination occurs when unprotected personnel ingest, inhale, or have wounds contaminated with radioactive material. Person without respiratory protection and also externally contaminated should be evaluated for internal contamination. Internal contamination is more if significant contamination is found on the face, in/around nostrils, or mouth or in/around the open wounds.

Internal doses are assessed by—(i) assessing certain biokinetic model for the radioactive substance in different organs and tissues and (ii) doses are committed doses. Internal dose assessment is done by bioassay, whole body counting, and gamma camera measurement. Urine and feces bioassays are most common methods for assessing intake. Generally, 24-h urine sample is collected, labeled, and recorded for sampling. After assessing the activity concentration in the urine, the activity entered in the body is calculated.

The assessment provides information on the nature of radionuclide, quantity of radioactive matter in the body, and estimation of effective dose. It also helps the required short- or long-term treatment. Treatment of internal contamination details is available in safety series no. 101, IAEA.

Case study: In *Goiania, Brazil* accident, four patients died out of ARS and autopsies showed that the bodies had both internal and external contamination with ^{137}Cs source. In a 6-year-old girl patient, the dose close to the skin was 2.5 mSv/h with massive internal contamination. During autopsies, the personnel were rotated in every 10 minutes and the gloves were changed often. All radiation protection and conventional biosafety measures were adopted. Personnel monitoring and dose rate were measured. Autopsy room was well prepared so that nobody had received significant radiation dose or contamination.

Emergency Communication and Mental Health

Communication is one of the important elements of emergency management. It addresses—(i) emergency communication during radiation emergencies and (ii) mental health aspects of radiation emergencies. Communicating the public will help the public to understand the risk, supporting the implementation of protective measures and remove negative psychological effects. Effective risk information should include—(i) dialogue exchange between the affected and controllers and (ii) delivering actual information about the risk. Immediate short-term and long-term actions may be provided.

Short-term actions include counseling, establishing link with family, providing psychological first-aid, recreational activities, and providing training in preparedness. Long-term action includes medical and mental health follow-up and assistance to population. Communication, risk perception, and impact of mental health of radiation emergencies are related factors. Social assistance is required for the affected population for those evacuated or relocated, which will prevent additional stress and restore self-confidence. Responsible organization should offer constant flow of information, and updates about situation. People in distress should understand the information and physician explanations must be simple and clear.

Psychological factors is an integral part of radiation emergency training, preparedness, and response. It is often underestimated or even ignored. Fear may be an important driver of human actions during emergency situations. Emotional reaction impacts how people feel and perceive risk. A clear and direct message will reduce the stress level and limit the risk perception in the population.

Long-term psychological stress will result in physiological changes, psychosomatic and mental health problems, and cognitive effects. Psychosocial support related to affected population should be addressed. Religious, cultural, and other social aspects will be addressed while performing survey, decontamination. Responders may be under stress, periodic heath examinations, group discussion about the problem, or distress they face should be addressed. Real risk of emergency responders is regularly provided.

Records

Records need to be maintained about patient care, dosimetry, and follow-up including medicolegal, which is useful for future actions. Information of (i) identification and notification of emergency, (ii) related circumstances, and (iii) individuals involved should be collected. From RSO point of view, exposure rate and surface contamination, type of accident, sources, nature of radioactivity, and dosimetry that affects the subjects and contamination of environment, details are collected.

LESSONS LEARNED FROM ACCIDENTAL EXPOSURES IN RADIATION THERAPY

Safety series no. 17, IAEA (2000), has listed the various accident exposures took place in radiotherapy and reviewed the accidents under the following headings as 92 events:

- Radiation measurement system (1–5)
- *External beam therapy*: Machine commissioning and calibration (6–20)
- *External beam therapy*: Treatment planning, patient setup, and treatment (21–46)
- Decommissioning of a ^{137}Cs machine (47 and 48)
- Mechanical and electrical malfunction (49–52)
- *Brachytherapy*: Low-dose rate sources and applicators (53–81)
- *Brachytherapy*: High-dose rate brachytherapy (82–84)
- Unsealed sources (85–92)

Lessons Learned from Accidents

Basic safety standard of IAEA has grouped the lessons learned from various radiation exposures in radiotherapy as follows: (i) resources—personnel and equipment, (ii) human factors, (iii) training, (iv) communication, (v) equipment, (vi) human-machine problems, (vii) improper decommissioning of equipment and unsafe storage of radioactive sources, (viii) documentation, (ix) integration of safety and quality assurance, (x) safety assessment, and (xi) regulatory control.

Radiotherapy department should have sufficient staffs proportional to the number of patients. Shortage of staffs leads to increase in errors. Assessment of staff and training needs to be undertaken as the workload increases. Radiotherapy is performed by many personnel who work together and potential for mistake is large if enough care not taken. The lack of alertness or awareness on human performance is much important. Oncologist, physicist, and other paramedical staff require formal training and should attend professional meeting and refresher courses. New equipment installation requires training from the manufacturer. Nurses and ancillary personnel should be trained in radiation safety. They should recognize emergencies and trained to handle both usual and unusual events.

Communication between staff member is essential. Mistakes may arise due to lack of adequate communication, incorrect information, or poor understanding of correct information. Equipment failure accounts only small percentage of accidents. However, equipment malfunction may affect patients. Personnel need to understand the functionality of every equipment including alarms, signals, and displays that indicate a malfunction.

Unauthorized handling, dismantling, or abandonment of teletherapy isotope units leads to large-scale series consequences, including fatality and environmental contamination. Measures for prevention and mitigation of consequences need to be taken. Documents are important for high quality and safe radiotherapy and foster communication among staff and communication of public overtime. Instructions misinterpreted, displays and interlocks, and signal relating to unusual events have been reported. Maintenance mistakes are related to lack of training and continuing education.

Systemic assessment of both equipment and treatment procedures, followed by application of *defense in depth* measures, should be the main approach. Defense in depth is defined as "the application of more than one single protective measure for a given safety objective such that, the objective is achieved even if one of the protective measures fails" (BSS). All health professionals need to demonstrate *culture of safety*, independent checks, internal and external, are the methods of avoiding errors or detecting them early. Check up the data, measurements, or repeat calculations by a second person are essential. Safety culture refers combining personnel attitude and habits of thoughts and organizational policies and priority. Objective of safety culture is that: "all duties important to safety should be carried out correctly, with due thought and full knowledge, sound judgment, and a proper sense of accountability".

Safety assessment requires systemic approach to identify events that lead to potential exposure and to estimate probability and magnitude of such exposures. Safety assessment can be deterministic and probabilistic methods. Deterministic methods are the first line of safety that includes equipment design or operating procedures with relevant training of personnel and formulation of contingency plans. Probabilistic method is used to identify weakness in safety measures that may be overlooked often. It calculates the expected frequency of events leading to potential exposures and calculates the expected detriment. It also gives relative importance of individual events with quantification.

Regulatory control must ensure assessment of safety, reduction of unwarranted or unjustified radiation exposure. It requires incorporation of safety measures in the management system and the development of safety culture. Regulatory framework involves authorization, inspection, and enforcement. Radiotherapy is under license, and it involves all aspects of acquisition, use, storage, and disposal of radiation sources including decommissioning. Plans for prevention of mistakes and emergency preparedness are to be assessed before issuing the license.

BIBLIOGRAPHY

1. Atomic Energy Regulatory Board. (2014). Radiation safety certification programme for regularization of radiation therapy technologists: AERB and RPAD, BARC, Mumbai, 2014. [online] Available from https://www.aerb.gov.in/storage/images/PDF/09-January-2014.pdf. [Last accessed December, 2022]
2. Bushberg JT, Anthony SJ, Leidholdt EM, Boone JM. The essential physics of medical imaging, 3rd edition. Philadelphia: Wolters Kluwer/Lippincott Williams & Wilkins; 2012.
3. International Atomic Energy Agency. (2000). Safety report series no. 17: Lessons learned from accidental exposures in radiotherapy, IAEA, Vienna, 2000. [online] Available from https://www-pub.iaea.org/MTCD/publications/PDF/Pub1084_web.pdf. [Last accessed December, 2022]
4. International Atomic Energy Agency. (2020). Medical management of radiation injuries, IAEA, Safety report series no. 101, 2020. [online] Available from https://www-pub.iaea.org/MTCD/Publications/PDF/PUB1891_web.pdf. [Last accessed December, 2022]

CHAPTER 19

Emergency Response Plans and Preparedness

INTRODUCTION

Radiation emergency are nonroutine situations. It may result from misuse of radioactive sources during industrial, medical or research applications, accidental exposure to uncontrolled radiation sources, accidents during transport of radioactive materials. It also be combined with conventional emergencies, natural disasters, military conflicts etc. It involves variety of accidents, injuries, and intentional incidents. It requires a prompt action to mitigate a radiation hazard or its adverse effects for human life, health, property, or the environment. Suitable radiation emergency action plans are needed to be initiated. The objective of such emergency action plan should be to mitigate the consequences and manage any emergency situation. This requires planning, preparedness with suitable accessories, and personnel's training and responsibilities.

Radiotherapy uses sealed radioactive sources whereas, in nuclear medicine unsealed radionuclides are used. Hence, the nature and magnitude of accidents and injuries and causes are different in the above areas. Hence, the emergency response plans and preparedness are different in the above departments.

NORMAL AND POTENTIAL EXPOSURES

Radiation exposures both in medicine and industry may result in normal and potential exposures. Normal exposure refers to exposures with predictable magnitude or with some degree of uncertainty. It is controlled by restriction of dose delivery. In the case of patients, only required dose to achieve the required diagnostic and therapeutic intent is to be delivered.

Potential exposure refers to the exposure that is unexpected but feasible and no certainty that exposure will occur. Potential exposure becomes actual exposure, if the unexpected situation occurs, e.g., equipment failure, design problem, and operating error. Potential exposures are controlled by optimizing the design of installation, equipment, and operating procedures. The objective is to restrict the probability of occurrence of events that could lead to unplanned exposures and restrict the magnitude of exposures that could result if such events were to occur.

Normal and potential exposures consist of: (1) occupational exposure; (2) medical exposure; and (3) public exposure. Occupational exposure refers to exposure of workers incurred in the course of their work. Medical exposures refer to exposures incurred: (i) by patients as part of their own medical/dental or treatment; (ii) by persons other than occupationally exposed, knowingly, or voluntarily helping in the support and comport of patients; and (iii) volunteers in a program of biomedical research involving their exposure. Public exposure is defined as the exposure incurred by the members of public from radiation sources, excluding any occupational or medical and background radiation. It includes exposures to authorized sources and practices and from intervention situations.

Modes of Exposure to Radiation and Radioactive Sources

Modes of exposure to radiation and radioactive sources are divided into: (1) external exposure to an individual from a source in very close proximity; (2) external exposure from an unshielded source involving several individuals; and (3) exposure following rupture of source casing. Medical response planning depends on various factors, namely (i) number of individual involved; (ii) possible radiological and other health consequences; and (iii) presence of contamination or combination of radiation exposure with thermal or chemical exposure or trauma. Radiation injury in an exposed individual depends on the characteristics of nuclear or radiological facility and the type of radioactive sources and their activity **(Table 19.1)**.

TABLE 19.1 **Potential exposure modes in radiation emergency.**

Group	*Facility/Source*	*Potential external exposure*	*Potential contamination (internal/external)*	*Both external exposure and contamination*
1	• Critical assembly	Yes	Yes	Yes
	• Reactor	Yes	Yes	Yes
	• Fuel element manufacture	Yes	Yes	Yes
	• Radiopharmaceutical manufacture	Yes	Yes	Yes
	• Fuel processing plants	Yes	Yes	Yes
2	*Radiation devices*:			
	• Particle accelerator	Yes	No*	No*
	• X-ray generator	Yes	No	No
3	• Sealed source (industrial radiography)	Yes	No	No
	• Unsealed source (airborne, volatile liquid, or powder)	Yes	Yes	Yes
4	• Nuclear medicine department	Yes	Yes	Yes
	• In vitro assay laboratory	Yes	Yes	Yes
5	Source transport	Yes	Yes**	Yes**
6	Radioactive waste	Yes	Yes	Yes

*Neutron capture results to induced radioactivity and produces Na-24 and K-40 in the human body.

**No significant contamination has been reported.

(IAEA: International Atomic Energy Agency)

Courtesy: Safety Series 101, IAEA, 2020.

ACCIDENTS SITUATIONS INVOLVING RADIOISOTOPES

Sealed radioactive sources (SRSs) are used in medicine, research, agriculture, and industry. It is sealed in a capsule or closely bounded and in a solid form. Encapsulation is done in a strong metal housing by stainless steel. They were not manufactured with current standards and have increased risk of mishap. There are about millions of such sources of varying activity from kilo Bq to peta Bq. SRSs, which are not in use and no further use if foreseen, are referred as spent sources, whereas source, which is taken out of service temporarily or indefinitely, is called disused source. Such sources represent special risks and cause accidents. Disused source causes accident due to leaking, or damaged source, obsolete equipment, alternative technology, changes in priorities, lost, stolen, and unknown sources, and source transition.

About 417 radiation accidents have occurred between 1944 and 2000 including 3,000 overexposures and 127 fatalities. These accidents are related to sealed radiation sources such as ^{192}Ir, ^{60}Co, and ^{137}Cs or X-ray sources used in industry. About 52% accidents are due to ^{192}Ir, whereas ^{60}Co accounts for 23%, and the remaining is due to ^{137}Cs, radium, uranium, transuranic elements, and other isotopes. About 630 thefts of radioactive material were reported between 1993 and 2021, out of which 310 occurred during transport. In 57% cases, the stolen radioactive material were not recovered [International Atomic Energy Agency (IAEA)]. In another study, 634 radiation overexposures involving 2,390 peoples have been reported between 1980 and 2013. In this, 64% of overexposures are due to radiotherapy and fluoroscopy (Karen Coeytaux, 2015).

Medical interventions have increased the cases of overexposures in individuals. Sealed sources accidents used in radiotherapy and industry are common. *Any unintended radiological event, including operator errors, equipment failure, or other mishap or consequences which are not negligible from the point of view of radiation protection or safety are referred as accident.* Over 20 years, about two accidents/year have been reported due to spent sources, exposing large number of people. Radiation accidents by SRS may consist of:

- Radiation injuries due to involving SRS to individuals
- Contamination material or the environment due to breaching of the encapsulation and dispersion of the radioactive content of SRS
- Internal and external contamination of individuals
- Economic losses due to medical treatment, accident-related radiation surveillance, decontamination, dismantling, waste management and disposal, and cost due to loss of production capability, monetary compensation to cover exposed individual, so that expenses and the loss of use of source itself
- Each accident is associated with a specific probability, which is a function of the characteristics of the source, environment factors, and the actions of the persons involved.

International basic safety standard (BSS) specifies requirements of security of sources: (i) sources should be kept secure to prevent theft or damage as per national regulation; (ii) not transferred unless the receiver possess valid authorization; and (iii) periodic inventory of movable sources at suitable intervals. Noncompliance of the above requirements may cause major accidents which are difficult to predict. Probability of accident may increase by the following factors **(Fig. 19.1)**:

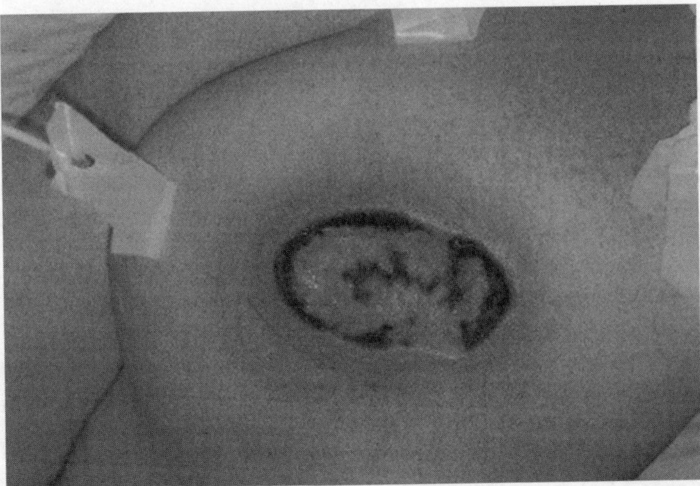

FIG. 19.1: Iridium source kept in the back pocket caused radiation burn in the buttock of a worker. ***(For color version, see Plate 5)***

Courtesy: IAEA-TECDOC-1205, IAEA, 2001.

- Inefficient regulatory control
- Lack of management commitment to safety and security of the disused sources
- Lack of funds to implement safety requirements related to storage, decommissioning, conditioning, and disposal of disused and spent sources
- Poor safety culture with deviation from written management procedures and relevant radiation protection guidelines
- Improper maintenance or handling of equipment leading to failure and malfunction
- Lack of proper planning of scheduled work
- Poor management of sources and recordkeeping

Nuclear medicine involves number of facility and devices which contain unsealed sources of low activity and short half-lives. Accidents of such radioisotopes, during transportation, waste management, and military application are much rare with low potential. The causes of radiation accidents in such sources are:

- Lack of information on physical appearance and hazards of radiation sources
- Lack of knowledge in radiation protection and regulations
- Violation of radiation protection and safety procedures
- Human error
- Inappropriate training
- Unauthorized repair of γ- and X-ray sources
- Misuse and misadministration of radioisotopes
- Unregulated disposal of radiation sources and waste

EMERGENCY PLANNING AND PREPAREDNESS

Categorization of Facilities for Emergency

Emergency situation in radiological facility may be widely classified as: (1) emergency alert; (2) plant emergency; (3) on-site emergency; and (4) off-site emergency.

Based on hazard potential and safety requirements, nuclear and radiological facilities are categorized as five categories:

- *Category I*: Nuclear power plants <100 megawatt of thermal output (MWth) and freshly discharged spent fuel pool storage.
- *Category II*: Spent fuel pool storage and reactors <100 MWth
- *Category III*: Industrial irradiation facilities, sealed source manufacturing, hospital, radiopharmaceutical manufacturing, teletherapy, high- and medium-dose rate, brachytherapy, and fuel fabrication
- *Category IV*: Dangerous sources, transport of radioactive or fissile material, severe overexposure, and mobile radiography source
- *Category V*: Accidents in category I and II resulting into contamination at distant place

The licensee should identify the event and prepare emergency operating plans to mitigate the events. He should also declare emergency alert in the facility and report the competent authority within 24 hours.

In the case of plant emergency, emergency preparedness and response plan suitable for hazard assessment should be in place before commissioning. It should be tested periodically, reviewed, and modified based on the experience. Plant emergency should address multiple sites if any and should be intimated immediately to the regulatory body. Operation should be suspended during plant emergency and may be restarted only after getting consent from the regulatory body.

Site emergency preparedness and response plan should be in place prior to commissioning. Licensee should intimate the site emergency to the regulatory authority with details including plant parameters and workers exposure levels. It should be tested periodically and reviewed based on experience. If it is a multi unit facility, all the facility should be shut down. The role of site emergency response team should be defined and tested periodically. Licensee should implement remedial measures to mitigate emergency. Operation may be restarted only after getting consent from the regulatory body.

An approved off-site emergency preparedness and response plan should be in place prior to commissioning. It should involve all responsible persons and agencies. It should be tested periodically and reviewed based on experience. It should be in line with national disaster management plan and get approved by the state and district administration.

Elements of Emergency Planning and Preparedness

Emergency planning preparedness has the following components namely: (i) identification of potential accident situation; (ii) evaluation of identified accident situations; (iii) preparation of emergency response plan; and (iv) training and exercises. Emergency response capability method must be integrated in terms of user, local and national. The step-by-step emergency plans are:

- Information flowchart
- Allocated tasks and responsibilities of authorities and organization involved
- Identification of emergency response team (team manager, radiological and industrial safety manager, instrumentation specialist, public relations, media contact, and persons trained in relevant technical and medical disciplines)
- Measurements to be made and equipment to be used to identify, locate, and recover the source (remote handling tongs, measuring instruments, and shielding containers)

- Radiation protection measures (radiation warning signs, ropes, overalls, shoe covers, gloves, and respirators)
- Decontamination (equipment, chemical, and procedures)
- Postaccident assessment and monitoring
- Temporary storage arrangement
- Transport to an authorized storage facility
- Final handling, possible conditioning, and storage of the involved sources and any contaminated material (postaccident management)
- Coordination of public information activity

Emergency Procedures in General

The first step in dealing with radiation accident is to identify, segregate, and treat all persons who are exposed to radiation, both external and internal. Immediate steps should be taken to assess the extent of exposure by sending the personnel monitoring thermoluminescent dosimeter (TLD) badges used by the exposed persons for dose evaluation. Biological monitoring and body burden measurements must also be conducted immediately.

If the radiation fields are higher, special radiation measuring devices will be required. These instruments must be capable of measuring much higher dose and dose rate, which are not common. Sometimes, they are telescopically coupled to the meters, so that the detector would be in proximity with high-radiation field and the person reading the meter is away from the radiation field. Such instruments should be periodically calibrated and kept in good working conditions. Air and surface contamination samples should be analyzed urgently to take further action. The instruments required to carry out this work should also be made available. The following guidelines may be adopted during emergency:

- Evacuate the immediate area, by ensuring that the radiation field and the extent of contamination are kept minimum
- Identify and isolate all persons, who might have exposed or contaminated. Arrange immediate evaluation of their TLD badges and collect samples from body fluids such as blood, urine, etc., for analysis.
- In the case of personnel contamination, carry out decontamination.
- Regulate entry to the area of accident, so that further exposures and contamination may be prevented.
- Notify promptly to the appropriate authorities through media such as fax, mobile, and telephone, and seek suitable advice. Arrange for immediate availability of experts, who are trained to deal with emergencies.
- Contain contamination within the accident site. In case of radioactive liquid spillage, clean up the contamination immediately. Routine protective measures such as wearing gloves and segregating the mop as radioactive waste should be adopted. If there is relatively large release of radioactive powder or aerosol in the room, that room must be immediately isolated from its surroundings by shutting off mechanical ventilation and by closing windows and doors. Entry into the room except the experts should be forbidden. A room with heavy air contamination will be decontaminated from within by drawing the air of the room through an appropriate filter.
- Priority should be given to human safety and the personnel dose should be restricted within limits (ICRP has recommended 100 mSv dose limits for planned special exposures). The staffs are instructed in basic emergency procedures

including the persons to be contacted in case of an accident. The same may be displayed at suitable locations in the radiation installation. Mock-up operations for dealing with complicated situations associated with high-radiation fields and contamination areas should always be part of a radiation emergency procedure.
- Maintain complete records of the accident and follow-up procedures. This simple instruction is often not followed, resulting in enormous complications in investigating such incidents and in the adoption of subsequent remedial measures.
- If the accident is in the public area, the area should be cordoned off and appropriate authorities will be contacted for further action.

Communication

Communication is essential part of emergency response preparedness. Early messages and actions of an emergency response will form the foundation. It will strengthen the actions to bring emergency under control and the aim of communication is:

- To provide public information
- To manage public response
- To establish responsible organization for information
- To prevent rumors and conflicting information
- To maintain credibility of authorities
- To allow the operating personnel to concentrate on their work
- To reduce psychological impact

Leaflets with general information are prepared and circulated. It should cover general terms and units used, emergency arrangements, and putting risks in perspective. Information of the use of radiation and emergency plans should be given to the media in the first few hours.

The target audience is important whether it is a small-scale or large-scale accidents.

Small-scale accidents are restricted to site and few workers and their family members, whereas large-scale accidents involve public. Communication is necessary throughout the emergency and sometime later. Communication must prevent reoccurrence of such incidents. In large-scale accidents, leaflets and documents shall be targeted to public. It should brief circumstances and consequences of the accident.

The media must have deadlines to meet for newspapers, radio, and television. Hotlines for people to telephone, meetings with interested groups and access to internet, and placing material on dedicated website are essential. Communication with public and media is through an authorized spokesperson by the organization. In large-scale accidents, the government and the organization must be involved. The information to the public and media should be coherent, consistent but not with conflicting information. The manner of communication in interviews and public meeting is crucial to enhance people confidence.

Procedures for Notification

All radiation emergencies shall be notified. After receiving the notification, response initiator should provide initial advice. If there is no radiation hazard, no further action is required but details are recorded. If it involves radiation hazard, emergency manager is alerted who will access the hazard as low, medium, and high. If it is low hazard type, radiological accessor is only activated, and he will be sent to the scene to reaccess the radiation hazard and perform recovery actions as required.

Response initiator is the first official of the country who will be informed about the emergency, and he has authority to initiate response plan. Emergency manager is an appointed official in-charge of overall emergency operations.

If it is medium and high hazard category, activate first responder, radiological accessor, and nominate on-scene controller. The first responder's duty is to perform actions to mitigate the accident and implements protective and initial recovery actions. It is from the local response organization. Senior official of the organization will assume the role of on-site controller and manage all response actions at the scene of an accident. Emergency manager shall determine whether the emergency is serious and has public interest or not. Radiological accessor shall access the hazards and recommend protective actions and recovery and clean-up operations. Overall, all should generate information required to provide media and the public.

First responder is a person or team to arrive at the scene of an accident and has role to play in accident response. The team includes police, fire service, emergency medical responder, and facility responder. One of the site controllers is a senior member of the first responder team. Radiological accessor is a senior member of the radiological assessment team sent to the scene of an accident.

Emergency Response Actions

If an accident with a radioactive source has occurred, emergency response actions may be taken to:

- Determine the actual disposition of the radioactive source
- Prevent access to the area
- Identify strategies, procedures, and tools to regain control of the source
- Rehearse adopted procedures for source recovery and containment
- Regain control of the radioactive source to restore the normal situation
- Arrange for medical assistance, if necessary
- Notify all relevant parties and organizations including IAEA emergency response unit
- Implement appropriate radiation protection measures to reduce risk to the health of the public and members of the emergency response team
- Identification of waste management procedure to be carried out to remediate any postaccident conditions that pose a danger to staff or the public (management of the sources as spent, collection of any secondary waste, decontamination of affected area, and conditioning of the resulted waste)

EMERGENCY RESPONSE ACCESSORIES

Radiation Survey Instruments

- High range survey instruments, preferably with an extendible probe
- Low-range survey instrument
- Contamination monitor
- Check source for low-range survey instruments

Personnel Monitoring Devices

- Self-reading dosimeters for each team member
- Permanent dosimeters for each team member
- First aid kit

Communication Equipment

Portable radio communications

Supplies

- Appropriate shielding (sufficient to significantly attenuate the radiation, for example, at least two bags of lead shot, i.e., 5 kg each for ^{192}Ir and 10 kg each for ^{60}Co or lead bricks or slabs)
- Tongs at least 1 m long suitable for safely handling the source assembly
- A shielded container
- Appropriate hand tools
- Radiation warning labels and signs
- Plastic for preventing contamination of instruments and isolation of contaminated objects
- Logbook

Supporting Documentation

- Equipment operation manuals
- Response coordination procedures
- Procedures for conducting monitoring
- Procedures for personal radiation protection

Personnel Protective Equipment

In radiation emergency, workers should be protected by using either one or combination of methods, namely (i) engineering controls; (ii) administrative methods; and (iii) personnel protection equipment. Engineering control uses barrier against radiation which is inherently safe and protects workers from external and internal exposure. Administrative control involves warning notice and a tag on the drainpipe to prevent unauthorized entry. Selection of personnel protective equipment (PPE) depends on the nature of exposure, performance data for PPE, and acceptable limits of radiation.

Personnel protective equipment refers to clothing or special equipment that is issued to individual workers to provide protection against actual or potential exposures to ionizing radiation. Every worker involved in emergency operation should wear PPE. It will protect from the risk of external and internal exposure, and it is reasonably practicable to provide complete protection. Adequacy of personnel protection depends on correct selection of PPE, fitting, and maintenance. One should be aware of its capability and limitations.

Personnel protective equipment is designed to cover large areas of the body or individual organs such as eye against external radiation. However, it can also be used against radioactive internal contamination. Different types of PPE are used in radiation emergency, which include protective clothing and respiratory protective equipment (RPE). Later type is intended to prevent inhalation of radioactive substance which will irradiate lungs.

Aprons, Gloves, and Sleeves

Apron: Flexible aprons of 0.33 mm of lead can be used as apron to protect the upper torso. Double-sided apron protects both front and backside of the worker's body. It attenuates 90% of low-energy scattered radiations. However, it is ineffective in penetrating radiations of >100 keV energy, especially in nuclear medicine and radiotherapy. Wearing apron for prolonged period gives tiring and slows down the work; hence, thin aprons are manufactured. Damaged aprons are removed from use and discarded.

Gloves and sleeves: Shielding gloves and sleeves containing up to 0.33 mm Pb are used against ionizing radiations. It provides local shielding and reduces dexterity. They are ineffective compared to aprons except in beta and low-energy X-rays. Since sleeves are flexible, these are useful to cover extremities and keep fingers free. Double thickness provides better protection against external exposure. If it is worn inappropriately, it will result in significant hand and body doses.

Apron and gloves should be stored in flat position or in rounded hangers to avoid cracks. It should be periodically tested radiographically/fluoroscopically to ascertain its integrity as annual basis. Minor contamination of the outer cover can be removed by water and mild detergent.

Laboratory Coat

Laboratory coat made up of cotton or synthetic fibers are used in laboratory and hospitals to avoid minor radioactive contamination. The fabric selection should address flammability and short jackets and smoke does not protect the lower body; hence, full-length coat is required. Full-length coat should be fastened to avoid spills or splashes of radioactive contamination which will contaminate inner garments. It is fastened along one shoulder and the side of the body with Velcro instead of buttons to ensure. If the contamination is high, a plastic disposable bib apron may be worn over the lab coat.

Lab coats should be monitored after the work and before laundering. Color coding in the pocket or collar can help to identify the process. Heavily contaminated coats need decontamination by decay before sending to laundry. Seams should be checked before reuse to avoid irradiation of underneath body surface by contamination.

Industrial Suits

Industrial suit is a single piece, covers overall or slicker suits, and protects against radioactive contamination in industry. There are three types of industrial suits: (1) unventilated and permeable; (2) unventilated and impermeable; and (3) ventilated and impermeable. These are available with or without head cover or hood to suit different RPE. Elasticated hoods and arm and leg cuffs cover the body surface with comfort. Permeable suits are common, suitable for long duration wear, and comfortable. Woven garments retain contamination and minimize resuspension. Impermeable suits made up of rubber or plastic coated or nonwoven fabrics are suitable for severe contaminations.

These suits provide resistance to chemicals, flames, and heat but vary in comfort and cost. It tends to cause and retain perspiration. Suits are generally ventilated by sleeves, seams, values, filters, or small-concealed holes. Encapsulated, impermeable, and pressurized suits offer highest level of protection. Suits are decontaminated before removal or be sprayed with a fixative if possible. It will avoid transferring or resuspending contamination during removal. Especially, seams should be checked for their decontamination. Damage, if any, needs repairs as per vendors' instructions.

Gloves for Radioactive Contamination

Gloves are made up of polythene and synthetic materials such as fabrics and elastomers, leather, mineral fiber, glass fiber, or mixture of materials. These are available in different sizes or stitched to fit or disposable type or separate item or fixed and detachable part of a suit. Gloves should extend above the elbows or small hand pads and mitis just cover the fingers and thumbs. Advantage of glove is that it mechanically locks onto the suit.

Lightweight polyvinyl chloride (PVC) or thin natural rubber latex (NRL) surgeon's glove may be suitable for laboratory use. It provides maximum sensitivity and flexibility and required grip. Heavyweight PVC gloves suit harsh material environment. They act not only as barrier but also protect harmful agents such as solvent, chemicals, physical hazard, and severe climate. Some users of NRL may get allergy, skin, and eye irritations including asthmatic conditions and systemic shock due to contact with gloves of glove powder. It can be avoided by changing the powder or cream or gloves of different version. Elasticated sleeves pulled down over the gloves or tape around the cuffs prevents exposure to the wrist. Gloves that are damaged should be disposed, but it is not possible if the glove is integral part of the suits. Those gloves that are not disposable require decontamination in special facility.

Footwear

Footwear includes overshoes, booties, and shoes and boots. Overshoes are used in areas of minor spills or drips contaminating the floor. It is disposable, single size, and have foot-shaped plastic bags with elasticated openings. It is available as: (i) hard soles and booties; (ii) fabric overshoes with legging supported at the knee by elastic or drawstrings; (iii) outsized plastic shoes; (iv) rigger boots; (v) steel toecaps and color coded; and (vi) rubber safety boots. The elasticated trouser cuffs may be pulled down over the bootleg to offer full protection. Fabric overshoes are decontaminated by decay or soaking or laundering before use. Deodorizing and hard brushing or grinding may be required to remove contamination in boots and shoes.

Respiratory Protective Equipment

There are two categories of RPE, namely: (1) respirator with filter purifies air by filtering particulate matter (dust, or low concentrations of gas or vapor); and (2) breathing equipment provides purified air or oxygen from an independent source. The former respirator includes filtering face piece respirator, half mask respirator, full mask respirator, and powered respirator fitted with a fan and filter.

The later breathing equipment type includes fresh air hose equipment, constant flow compressed air equipment, and breathing apparatus with full facemasks and full suits supplied either from compressed airlines or from compressed air cylinders.

National regulation defines assigned protection factor (APF) for RPE/PPE and some RPE, and the inward leakage (IL) is being tested. The IL is the ratio of the concentration of the dust particles inside the RPE to the concentration of dust particle in the test chamber. It is expressed in percentage as 100:IL for normal RPE.

The effectiveness of a respirator to minimize IL depends on integrity of face seal and filtration capability of filter medium.

Emergency Protective Clothing

Provision of the protective clothing is usually indicated in areas where the operations concerned will expose the personnel involved to a high risk of contamination and of breathing contaminated air. Before wearing emergency protective clothing, one must have a full change, which implies removal of all personnel clothing and the wearing of simple clothing supplied by the laboratory. A typical change would be drill trousers underwear, shirt, socks, and shoes.

Fully impervious clothing: This consists of garments so designed that they cover the individual completely, except for the head and neck and hand and feet with a layer of impervious material. As breathing apparatus to be worn at the same time, hoods of similar material are used. Finally, complete exclusion from contamination is obtained by wearing rubber gauntlet gloves pulled well over the cuffs of the protective suit and rubber boots with bottom of the impervious suit trousers brought over them.

Pressurized clothing: This suit is made of impervious material which completely encloses an individual. Such a suit effectively isolates the individual inside, from any contamination on the surfaces or in the air. Compressed air supplied to the suit enables normal breathing during operations.

The compressed airline delivers its air immediately in front of the face, as this arrangement provides plenty of air for breathing and, at the same time, helps to reduce the misting of the transparent headpiece. Complete protection of hands and wrists is afforded by wearing rubber gloves, which are securely taped to the suit to prevent the ingress of any contamination. Rubber boots are usually worn with the suit.

Assistance is always necessary to dress an individual in any impervious clothing. Such assistance is essential when impervious clothing is being removed. If the individual concerned undresses, it is likely that he will become contaminated from the active material present on that suit.

Breathing apparatus: When compressed air supply is not available for use in the pressurized suits described above, breathing sets may be used. These comprise a well-fitted face piece in which suitable goggles are inserted and the face piece is attached to a cylinder. Regulating valves attached to the cylinder enable the wearer to control his air supply. This breathing set may be used in conjunction with fully protective impervious clothing and so desired, the individual concerned can enter a contaminated atmosphere under emergency or maintenance conditions.

RADIATION EMERGENCY IN NUCLEAR MEDICINE AND PREPAREDNESS

A large number of unsealed radionuclides are used in nuclear medicine. Accident may happen due to error, carelessness, and absence/failure of safety/equipment. Emergency may arise due the following:

- Spillage of radiopharmaceuticals
- Misadministration of radiopharmaceuticals to patient
- Loss of sources in the department or in transit

Such accident may cause personnel exposure, internal/external, or both. Hence, emergency response plans should be in place to prevent such accident. Two important mishaps often occur without the control of staff members:

1. Vomiting of radiopharmaceutical by the patient
2. Death of a patient with administered radiopharmaceuticals in the body

Factors Leading to Spillage

While working with radiopharmaceuticals, spillage can take place due to tilt of vial containing radiopharmaceutical, leakage from the syringe, or splash of liquid. Sometime, vomiting of administered radiopharmaceutical by the patient resulting spread of radioactivity.

Prevention of Spillage

- Performing wet and dummy trials prior to handling the radiopharmaceutical
- Keeping vial containing the radiopharmaceutical in an appropriate outer container with heavy base to avoid tilting of the vial
- Performing all wet operations in a tray lined with polythene and absorbent paper so that the spilled radioactivity is contained, and spread of contamination is restricted
- Transporting the radiopharmaceuticals within the lab in appropriate shielded transport containers
- Preparation of doses in a careful manner by a skilled person
- Adopting standard code of practice in the preparation of dosages/ radiopharmaceuticals
- Ensuring stable condition of patient to avoid vomiting

Handling Procedures of Spillage

- Confine the spill immediately, by dropping paper towels or other absorbent material onto it.
- Evacuate the immediate area so that persons will not walk over the spill and spread the contamination.
- If the spilled material has splashed onto a person or clothing, immediate steps should be taken to remove the clothes and collect the same in a polythene bag and to be kept in the radioactive waste storage room. It should be ensured that the person with contaminated clothes does not leave the area before removing the protective clothing.
- Hands and other contaminated areas of the body should be washed thoroughly with soap and water. Care should be taken not to aerate or inflame the skin surface.
- Possible care must be taken to prevent intake of radioactive material. If intake of radioactive material has taken place, immediate action should be taken to prevent or minimize the deposition in organs or tissues. If necessary, steps should be taken to bring out the ingested radioactive material under the expert medical guidance.
- The internal deposition of radioactive material should be estimated by carrying out bioassay, whole body counting or both.
- Contaminated area should be decontaminated by expert team using appropriate methods by wearing surgical gloves, shoe covers, and a surgical facemask, if available.

- The waste collected during decontamination should be treated as radioactive waste and disposed as per Atomic Energy Regulatory Board (AERB) safety guidelines.

Misadministration of Radiopharmaceuticals

Type of Misadministration

- Administration of radiopharmaceutical to a wrong patient
- Administration of wrong activity
- Administration of wrong radiopharmaceuticals
- Administration through wrong route
- Administration of radiopharmaceutical in pregnant female patient without confirming pregnancy

Consequences of Misadministration

It is reported that about 80% of accidents are due to administration of wrong radiopharmaceuticals, 10% by administration to wrong patient, and about 2% by administration of wrong activity:

- Nonjustified exposure
- Increased radiation risk
- Delayed diagnosis
- Increase in cost
- Increase in workload
- Reduction in confidence

Causes of Misadministration

- Communication problems or gaps
- Busy environment or distraction
- Bypassing local rules or code of practice
- No training in emergency situations
- Absence of clearly defined responsibilities
- Absence of efficient quality assurance program

Prevention of Misadministration

- Using transparent vial and syringe shields
- Tagging and segregating the vials and syringes
- Write activity, source, patient on vial or syringe containing dosages
- Check labels of vial or syringes before administration
- Measuring the activity in radiopharmaceutical
- Identifying name, number, and case of the patient
- Ensuring that the female patient is not pregnant

General Methods of Prevention of Accidents

Accident of spillage and misadministration can be avoided by: (i) preparing safety code of practice; (ii) educating the staffs; (iii) inculcating safety culture in the department; and (iv) identifying emergency situations and assessing the causes and probability of occurring accidents in critical and normal situations. Accident should be attended immediately with countermeasures suitable for the type of situation. The same is informed to all the staff members, head of the institution, and AERB. The following points should be followed to prevent or manage such accidents:

- There should be adequate number of trained staff available in the department to carry out the emergency plan
- The personnel/staff should be instructed to exercise care in respective areas to avoid situations that may lead to an accident
- All radiation monitoring, measuring instruments and safety devices should be routinely checked and kept in working condition. Handling equipment, e.g., tongs forceps, etc., should be kept in ready access
- A proper inventory of radioisotopes received, used, in stock, and disposed off should be maintained.

Emergency Response Team

To handle emergency, every institution must have emergency response committee as given below with experts and is assigned specific jobs. The members of the committee are familiar with their jobs and offer full coordination. It should have periodic discussion and the same is recorded:

- Authorized nuclear medicine physician
- Physicist
- Laboratory assistant
- Radiation safety officer (RSO)
- Administrative personnel
- Electronic instrumentation expert
- Emergency director

Death of a Patient Administered with Radiopharmaceuticals

If a patient dies with radiopharmaceuticals in the body, the body can be handed over to the relatives, if the level of acidity is within the permissible levels for cremation, burial, postmortem, or embalming, as per AERB norms. If the activity is higher than the limits, the body should be kept in morgue to decay of activity and handed over to the relatives when the activity falls below the limit. In case of emergency release of the body, the organ with accumulated activity should be removed before the release. It is ensured that the radiation levels in the body are within the prescribed limits. The removed organ with activity is disposed of as per disposal rules.

EMERGENCY PREPAREDNESS IN RADIOTHERAPY: ACTIONS RELATED TO TELECOBALT SOURCE

In radiotherapy, sealed radioactive sources (SRS) are used. Despite preventive measures, accidents or unusual events may occur. The safety assessment will identify accident scenarios and situations, and countermeasures for mitigation to be designed. Some of the actions in the emergency response plan need to be taken immediately, without hesitation or mistakes. To achieve this, personnel need to be trained and simulation drills are carried out. A clear and concise list of actions and responsible officers is posted in relevant places. There is a written documentation of rules for action and training, including simulating exercises, for the emergency response plan, which needs to be periodically reviewed.

TABLE 19.2 Generic criteria to minimize acute deterministic and stochastic effects.

Generic criteria	*To minimize severe deterministic effects*	*To minimize risk of stochastic effects*
Whole body (bone marrow)	1 mSV	
Skin	10 Sv to 100 cm^2	
Internal exposure from acute intake (delivered in 30 days)		
Thyroid	2 mSV	
Lung	30 mSv	
Thyroid dose		50 mSv in the first 7 days
Whole body dose		100 mSv in the first 7 days
Food, milk and drinking water, vehicles, equipment		
Whole body		10 mSv per annum
Fetus effective dose		10 mSv for full period

Courtesy: AERB/NRF/SG/EP-5 (Rev. 1), 2014.

Line of Command of Actions

The RSO must establish the line of command of actions to be taken, in the case of any emergency. This will include the type of immediate action to be taken and persons to be contacted. The addresses and telephone numbers, if any, of these persons must be conspicuously displayed.

Source not Returning to "OFF" Position

Removal of the Patient

If the source does not return to "OFF" position after the set treatment time is over, the technician must remove the patient without himself getting directly exposed to the primary beam. This would also imply that an audio-type gamma zone monitor is available, calibrated, and working, which will indicate that the source is "ON" or "OFF". To facilitate such action, the RSO must routinely advise the workers regarding the route to be taken by them inside the treatment room for various directions of primary beam. It must be clearly demonstrated to the staff that the dose equivalent to the worker for such a procedure will be only of the order of mSv **(Table 19.2)**. They must also be told to be in the treatment room only for the minimum time required and, in any case, not to expose any part of their body including hands to the primary beam. After patient is removed, the technician must lock the room, inform the RSO immediately, and wait for further instruction.

Restoring the Source to "OFF" Position

The RSO must try to return the source to the "OFF" position as specified for the unit concerned and with appropriate care. This may involve procedure such as pushing the source drawer to the parking position with a T-rod, pressing a popped-up button on the source head, rotating a wheel in the gantry, or by switching off electric power as specifically directed in the instruction manual supplied by the manufacturer.

If this procedure does not result in returning the source to the "OFF" position, the RSO must leave the treatment room. The room must be closed immediately, and the service engineers of the company concerned may be called for appropriate assistance. Administrative actions will include vacating or shielding adjacent rooms and areas and cordoning off the facility as required.

Requirement of Equipment and Accessories

The following materials and equipment must be available in the hospital and be kept outside the telegamma room. It must be possible to procure items such as sandbags, lead shots, etc., at very short notice in case of emergency.

- *Survey meter*: Properly calibrated and maintained survey meter of appropriate range must be available. A wide range survey meter with long cable facility is desirable.
- *T-rod*: T-rod or other such equipment meant for the unit.
- *Manual*: Operation/service manual of the unit, which will give details regarding type of source drawer, etc., must be kept at easy accesses. In one of the major incidents, the instruction manual was located only at after prolonged search.
- *Binoculars*: Binoculars could be of help to verify whether the source is in the "ON" or "OFF" position, as also its location, if it has fallen down.
- *Lead shots*: About 300–400 kg of small-sized lead shots of about 1–2 mm diameter will be needed to shield the source in case it falls off from the unit.
- *Lead wool*: Several kilograms of lead wool preferably packed in bags will be needed to be thrown over the source from a safe distance, so that the source can be initially shielded, before its actual retrieval. This will enable personnel to approach closer to the source for the retrieval work.
- *Lead bricks*: Several lead bricks of standard size, regular and interlocking type, will be useful to shield the source further once the lead shots and lead wool are thrown to cover the source.
- *Sandbags*: Generally, a telegamma particularly telecobalt room is designed such that two walls will act as primary walls and the remaining two as secondary walls. However, if the source falls on the floor, all walls become primary walls. Hence, additional shielding may be needed for the secondary walls, and, in some cases, depending on the location in the room where the source has fallen, for primary wall too. Number of sandbags may need to be arranged on these walls, so that the exposure rates outside are within permissible levels.
- *Long-handled tongs*: Long-handled tongs on which the radiation probes could be fixed will be needed to monitor the radiation levels at various locations in the telegamma room. This will help in deciding the course of action to be followed.
- *Long pipe and funnel*: A long pipe is needed so that the lead shots can be dropped through a funnel connected to one end kept near the door or maze in such a way that radiation is avoided by the worker to the extent possible. The pipe must be in an inclined position, in such a way that the other end is over the source.
- *Transport container*: The transport container (source flask) must be available locally with the servicing firm, so that remedial action can be initiated immediately in the case of the source fall. It must also be stressed that in case of major repairs of the head, drawer, or shutter, the source, if needed, must be unloaded prior to such work.
- *Personnel monitoring dosimeters*: All personnel in the telegamma room including casual workers must wear personnel monitoring dosimeters.

Reports

The RSO must send a report of the emergency to the Head, Radiological Safety Division, AERB, Mumbai. The report should give details of the incident including the causes, remedial action, dose received, and steps taken to avoid such emergencies in future.

Prevention of Emergency

Generally, emergencies arise in the case of old and poorly maintained units. It must be stressed that proper work discipline, as well as regular servicing, maintenance, and quality assurance tests of the teletherapy unit and associated equipment will help to prevent potential emergencies. It must be pointed out that most of the major incidents involving telegamma units have occurred during source transfer or repair work. It must be ensured that any servicing of the source head must be done only by experienced engineers and in the presence of the RSO. In many cases, emergencies arise because of temptations to compromise on or bypass of—simple requirements of radiation safety. These should never be resorted to. Typical example includes arrestor not provided to prevent movement of source drawer and transport container not immobilized during source transfer operation. Periodic drills must be arranged by the RSO to simulate emergency situations. This will also help to avoid tendency for complacency among the staff.

MANAGEMENT OF RADIATION EMERGENCY: RESPONSIBILITY OF RSO, LICENSEE, EMPLOYER, AND RADIOISOTOPE SUPPLIER

The purpose of the radiation emergency action plan shall be to mitigate the consequences and manage any emergency situation. The intervention, if any, shall aim at limiting external exposure. In the event of an accident, every possible care shall be taken to prevent radiation injury, e.g., by direct contact with unsealed sources. In case of release of contamination, the affected area shall be isolated, and its use is permitted only after proper contamination. The internal contamination of affected personnel shall be assessed to initiate remedial measures as appropriate. All monitoring instruments such as radiation survey meter and contamination monitor are made available with good working condition. If internal contamination facility is not available, assistance from the nearby institution should be sought. Safety measures recommended by the competent authority shall be implemented expeditiously to restore normal conditions. This includes: (i) radiation emergency action plan; and (ii) reporting radiation emergency.

Licensee

Licensee, in consultation with Radiological Safety Officer, shall prepare emergency response plan and ensure emergency preparedness measures. The emergency response plans shall mitigate any consequences of emergencies and address the following events:

- Radioactive source rack stuck in an unshielded position
- Radioactive contamination (detection of leaking radioactive sources, contamination of source storage water pool)

- Fire, explosion, or gas leakages inside the accelerator equipment area, radiation cell or product storage area
- Loss of source shielding
- Malfunctioning or deliberate defeat of the safety interlock systems and access control systems
- Accidental radiation exposure of individual(s) more than dose limits
- Breach of security, natural occurrences such as earthquake, flood, and tornadoes.

Foreseeable Emergencies

Licensee shall prepare emergency action plans, consisting of a set of procedures to be implemented for all foreseeable emergencies, including the following:

- Radioactive source failing to return to the safe shielding position
- Damage to, or dislodge/loss/theft of, radioactive source at the installation during use, storage, transport, loss of source shielding or natural calamities such as fire, flood, or earthquake; death of a patient with radioactive source in situ
- Teletherapy emergencies such as selection of wrong treatment mode, selection of wrong beam modifiers, and wrong dose delivery; spillage of radioactivity
- Misadministration of radiopharmaceutical
- Radiation levels more than the baseline/normal values recorded during the installation
- Fire accident, explosion, or natural disaster such as earthquake
- Malevolent actions by the antisocial elements leading to damage of radioactive source
- Death of patient, with sources in situ

Emergency response plans shall be specific to each situation and should include the following:

- Identification of reasonably foreseeable accidents and other incidents or occurrence
- Communication procedures
- Availability of emergency tools and training
- Availability of first-aid equipment, its list, and location
- Specify the authorities to be contacted during emergency
- Outline of postemergency recovery procedures

All the workers are familiar with emergency action plan. In situ sources in dead bodies should be removed first, accounted, and monitored by RSO, before handing over the dead body to claimants.

Emergency Response Measures

- The response measures shall be concise, unambiguous, easily practicable, and aimed at restoring normal operation keeping exposures to individuals as low as reasonably achievable (ALARA).
- In case of injury to any individual, medical attention shall be provided as priority.
- In case of external emergency, area shall be cordon off and decontaminated.
- Response to an emergency shall consist of initial actions to be implemented immediately and follow-up actions subsequently.

Emergency Preparedness

- Contact numbers of emergency response persons including licensee/employer, RSO, fire services, ambulance, medical center, manufacturer, and the competent authority shall be displayed at control panel and other relevant locations.
- Periodic review of emergency plans shall be carried out to enhance the effectiveness of the plans.
- The employer shall report every unusual event to the competent authority immediately and certainly within 24 hours of its occurrence. The details shall include: (i) date and time of occurrence; (ii) status of radiation protection factor (RPF) at the time of incident; (iii) source activity at the time of incident; (iv) brief description of the event; (v) action implemented; and (vi) probable cause of incident.
- The immediate notification shall be followed by a detailed report after carrying out investigations.
- The manufacturer/supplier shall provide assistance to handle any emergency situations involving radiation source.
- The licensee shall conduct an emergency exercise at least once in a year and report of the exercise shall be prepared immediately upon completion of exercise and made available to the competent authority, when required.

Radiation Emergency Action Plan

The aim of radiation emergency action plan is to mitigate the consequences and manage any emergency situations. Any intervention, if any, shall limit the external exposure and intake of radioactive materials and spread of contamination. The initiation and termination of intervention shall be to maximize the averted dose. In case of spillage of radioactivity, the residual fixed contamination (beta/gamma) after decontamination shall not exceed the levels specified by the competent authority. The licensee shall prepare action plans, as per Rule 33 of Atomic Energy (Radiation Protection) Rules, 2004 in coordination with the RSO. It should envisage various emergency sceneries/situations that may be encountered and action plans for responding to emergencies to mitigate their consequences. The emergency plan shall be specific to each situation and shall include as appropriate:

- Identification of reasonably foreseeable accidents and other incidents or occurrences and their predicted consequences
- Communication procedures, including an emergency call-out list, recommended actions for specified situations, a list of persons identified for implementing the specified action plan, and specification of situations requiring evacuation together with procedures for implementation
- A statement regarding immediate life-saving actions, statutory responsibilities, and the names of persons identified for implementing actions to discharge them
- Availability of emergency equipment, including a list of the equipment available and their locations
- Availability of first aid equipment, including a list of equipment available, their locations, and the names of persons trained to use them
- An outline of the postemergency recovery procedures designed to restore normal operating conditions.

Display of Emergency Procedures

Emergency procedures to be followed should be posted conspicuously at appropriate locations. It should be concise, unambiguous, easily followed, practicable, and simple to restore normal situation by keeping exposures to individuals at ALARA. It should include responsible personnel to be contacted in case of emergency. In addition, contact details of local police, fire brigade, source supplier, and AERB should also be displayed.

In the case of radiotherapy, emergency procedures to be followed in the event of failure of beam control mechanism, source movement mechanism, dislodgement, and damage or loss of the source shall be established and posted conspicuously near the control panel in the case of teletherapy and remote afterloading brachytherapy equipment, and near the source storage and other appropriate locations in the case of manual brachytherapy system.

Identification and Training of Emergency Handling Personnel

The emergency action plan shall: (i) identify personnel for handling radiation emergencies and make them familiar with the responsibilities and functions, line of authority, and most direct and alternate lines of communication; (ii) provide for initial training and drills, and periodic retraining and drills, in their respective tasks to ensure effectiveness of the plans; (iii) provide for training needed to recognize abnormal exposures, as well as formal procedures, and for prompt communication to the RSO; (iv) provide for appropriate tools, radiation monitoring instruments, and personnel monitoring devices to be kept and maintained in working condition; and (v) specify the authorities to be contacted at the initial phase, during progress, and at termination of an emergency.

The licensee shall ensure that all workers are familiar with the emergency action plan. Their radiation exposure during emergency handling should not exceed the regulatory limits. Generic criteria to minimize acute deterministic and stochastic effects are shown in **Table 19.2**.

Release of Dead Bodies

Any dead body containing sources in situ shall not be handed over to the claimants until all the sources have been removed and accounted for, and the body duly monitored by the RSO to confirm removal of all the sources.

Legal and Regulatory Requirements

Rule 20 of Atomic Energy (Radiation Protection) Rules, 2004 stipulates that the employer is the custodian of radiation sources in his possession and shall always ensure physical security of the sources.

The worker shall inform the licensee and RSO of any accident or potentially hazardous situation that may come to his notice. The licensee shall prepare emergency response plans and submit to the competent authority for approval. Licensee should arrange to carry out prompt investigation on equipment failure, accident, mishap, miscalculation, or unusual occurrences causing different dose to the patient. Investigation should also include treatment of wrong patient or tissue or source or dose or dose fractionation.

It is the duty of the RSO to investigate and initiate prompt and suitable remedial measures in respect of any situation including emergencies that could lead to radiation hazards. He should develop suitable emergency response plans to deal with accidents and maintaining emergency preparedness. RSO should also make a report, giving details of the incident, including the causes, remedial action, dose received, and steps taken to avoid such emergencies in future to the competent authority.

The employer shall inform the competent authority within 24 hours of any accident involving a source or loss of source of which he is a custodian. In the case of theft of radioactive source, if not traced within 24 hours, a complaint shall be lodged to the nearest police station.

Reporting Radiation Emergency

- RSO shall: (i) report to the licensee immediately about any emergency situation, initiate necessary remedial actions, and endorse a copy of the report to the competent authority; and (ii) carry out prompt investigation on causes of the emergency, evolve means to prevent recurrence, and submit a detailed report to the competent authority.
- Licensee shall: (i) report to the employer immediately and to the competent authority regarding the incident within 24 hours of its occurrence; (ii) submit to the competent authority a detailed report on the emergency/unusual occurrences, which have hazardous consequence or potential to cause hazardous consequences; and (iii) arrange to carry out prompt investigation on any emergency situation, including—(a) any equipment failure, accident, mishap, miscalculation, or other unusual occurrence with the potential for causing a patient dose significantly different from that intended; and (b) any therapeutic treatment delivered to either the wrong patient, or the wrong tissue, or using wrong source, or with a dose or dose fractionation differing substantially from the value prescribed by the radiation oncologist, or that may lead to undue acute secondary effects. The report shall contain the following:
    - Date and time of occurrence
    - Brief description of the unusual incident
    - Radionuclide, its activity, and radiopharmaceutical composition
    - Action taken
    - Probable causes of the incident
    - Personnel radiation exposure, if any
    - Lessons learned to prevent such reoccurrence in future
    - Improvement in the emergency plans and preparedness, if any
- The employer shall: (i) report to the competent authority regarding the incident within 24 hours of its occurrence; and (ii) lodge a written complaint with the police in case of loss or theft of the radioactive sources, if they are not traced within 24 hours.

Nuclear and Radiological Emergency Monitoring Cell

It is the responsibility of the district, state, and national authorities to implement off-site emergency preparedness and response plan. However, to strengthen the monitoring the progress of the response action and review the response action, AERB has established the Nuclear and Radiological Emergency Monitoring Cell (NREMC).

It consists of experts who demonstrate exercise in activating the cell on short notice to analytically assess an emergency situation, and the action performed by various agencies to handle the emergency. The NREMC has infrastructure of communication facilities, documents, and protocols to obtain the information from concerned agencies. Standard operating procedures (SOPs) will be activated during the off-site emergency exercises.

BIBLIOGRAPHY

1. Atomic Energy Regulatory Board. (2011). Radiotherapy sources, equipment, and installations. AERB safety code: AERB/RF-MED/SC-1 (Rev. 1). [online] Available from https://www.aerb.gov.in/images/PDF/CodesGuides/RadiationFacility/MedicalApplicationsInvolvingRadiation/4.pdf. [Last accessed December, 2022]
2. Atomic Energy Regulatory Board. (2014). Criteria for planning, preparedness and response for nuclear and radiological emergency: AERB/NRF/SG/EP-5 (Rev. 1). [online] Available from https://aerb.gov.in/images/PDF/Criteria-for-Planning-Preparedness-and-Response-for-Nuclear-or-Radiological-Emergency.pdf. [Last accessed December, 2022]
3. International Atomic Energy Agency. (2000). Generic procedures for assessment and response during a radiological emergency, IAEA-TECDOC-1162, IAEA, Vienna. [online] Available from https://www-pub.iaea.org/mtcd/publications/pdf/te_1162_prn.pdf. [Last accessed December 2022]
4. International Atomic Energy Agency. (2004). Practical radiation technical manual—Personnel protective equipment, IAEA, Vienna. [online] Available from https://www-pub.iaea.org/MTCD/Publications/PDF/PRTM-5_web.pdf. [Last accessed December, 2022]
5. International Atomic Energy Agency. (2020). Medical management of radiation injuries, IAEA, Safety report series No. 101. [online] Available from https://www-pub.iaea.org/MTCD/Publications/PDF/PUB1891_web.pdf. [Last accessed December, 2022]

Index

Page numbers followed by *b* refer to box, *f* refer to figure, and *t* refer to table.

D

E

I

M

N

Q

R

T